Springer Series on
Health Care and Society

Steven Jonas, M.D., *Series Editor*

Volume 1

Quality Control of Ambulatory Care:
A Task for Health Departments
Steven Jonas

Volume 2

Community Medicine in the United Kingdom:
Medical Education and an Emerging Specialty within the Reorganized National Health Service
William S. Jordan, Jr.

Volume 3

Social Medicine:
The Advance of Organized Health Services in America
Milton I. Roemer

Forthcoming:

Change in State Psychiatric Hospitals:
Thirteen Case Studies
Paul D. Greenberg

Milton I. Roemer has been Professor in the School of Public Health at the University of California, Los Angeles, since 1962. He taught previously at the Cornell University Institute of Hospital Administration (1957–61) and at Yale Medical School (1949–51). Dr. Roemer earned the M.D. degree in 1940 and holds also master's degrees in sociology and in public health.

Dr. Roemer has served at all levels of health administration—as a County Health Officer in West Virginia, a state and provincial health official in New Jersey and Saskatchewan, Canada, a commissioned officer of the U.S. Public Health Service in Washington, and a section Chief of the World Health Organization headquarters in Geneva, Switzerland. He is a Diplomate of the American Board of Preventive Medicine (1949); he was an elected councillor of the American Public Health Association for nearly a decade and Chairman of its Medical Care Section in 1956–57. In 1972 he was elected President of the California Academy of Preventive Medicine and in 1974 was elected to the Institute of Medicine of the National Academy of Sciences.

As a consultant to international agencies, Dr. Roemer has studied health care organization in 46 countries on all the continents. He is the author of 16 books and over 250 articles on the social aspects of medicine. In 1977, he was the recipient of the American Public Health Association International Award for Excellence in Promoting and Protecting the Health of People.

Social Medicine

The Advance of Organized Health Services in America

Milton I. Roemer

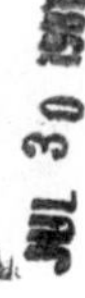

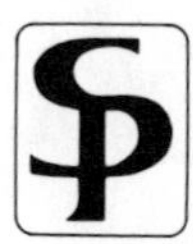

Springer Publishing Company / New York

Springer Publishing Company, Inc.
200 Park Avenue South
New York, N.Y. 10003

78 79 80 81 82/10 9 8 7 6 5 4 3 2 1

Library of Congress Cataloging in Publication Data

Roemer, Milton Irwin, 1916-
Social medicine.

(Springer series on health care and society ; v. 3)
Includes bibliographical references.
1. Social medicine—United States—Addresses, essays, lectures. 2. Medical care—United States—Addresses, essays, lectures. I. Title. II. Series.
[DNLM: 1. Health services—Organization and administration—United States. 2. Social medicine—United States. WA31 R715s]
RA418.3.U6R63 362.1'0973 78–17621
ISBN 0–8261–2600–6
ISBN 0–8261–2601–4 pbk.

Printed in the United States of America

Contents

Introduction

Observers of the current American health care scene are sometimes frustrated and angry at the slow progress in solving our problems. Speaking of "dynamics without change," they would give the impression that obvious difficulties persist and no improvements are or have been made in achieving a more equitable distribution of health services in relation to human needs.

Yet there have, in fact, been enormous improvements in many aspects of American health services over the last several decades. These have come about as a result of social pressures to organize and rationalize both the financing and delivery of health care. Nearly always, there is resistance to change, and idealistic goals are seldom fully reached, but countless changes have occurred toward modifying health care patterns to meet needs more effectively.

This volume offers 38 papers which document these trends of social medicine in America. Thirty-two of the papers have been published in diverse English-language journals; one was published in Yugoslavia; four were "processed" reports; and one has not been previously published. Aside from convenience for the interested reader, the assemblage of all 38 papers in one place may convey a message not otherwise very clear. All the papers were written or presented in the 1960s and 1970s, but most refer to trends from earlier periods as well. I hope that by presenting the views of one observer, they may offer a cohesive interpretation of developments in social medicine in America.

The papers are presented in eight parts. Part One offers several broad panoramas of trends toward organization in health care, from differing perspectives. Part Two examines special programs developed to compensate for the health handicaps of poverty, and various difficulties in the way that the American health care system impinges on the poor. In Part Three, health insurance—the principal strategy for easing the economic burden of medical costs on the general population—is probed in several of its aspects. Part Four analyzes the mounting organization of ambulatory health services which have historically been most individualistic. The growing importance of hospitals, their increased structuring, and their impacts on the total health care system are explored in Part Five. In Part Six, methods of evaluating organized health programs are analyzed, along with the expanding regulation that social pressures generate. With the increasing organization, greater attention to systematic health planning is inevitable, and various features of this planning are explored in Part Seven. Based on these trends of the past, Part Eight concludes with some forecasts and recommendations on the American health care system of the future.

Not every facet of social medicine is examined, but the principal components of this large field are discussed. In a collection of this sort, moreover, some major developments—such as the expanding impact of government or the heightened structuring of hospitals—are inevitably discussed in more than one place. It is hoped that such repetition is warranted by the different contexts in which the topic appears.

Most of these papers offer general interpretations of events made at professional meetings, but several report the results of empirical research projects. In aggregate, the content reflects the thoughts of one American public health worker about the changes taking place in the social institution of medicine, that is, in "social medicine." My interpretation is clearly one of an expanding organization of health services along several dimensions. While the basic social or political motives may vary, the general effect of the organization has been to better meet the health needs of people through more effective application of medical knowledge and technology.

The processes analyzed in these chapters are obviously still going on. This is not to deny the persistence of many serious problems in health care or even that some difficulties are growing worse. The exposure of problems, however, tends to generate social pressures for their correction. There is still a long way to go before many deficiencies in the American health care system are eliminated and the potentialities of social medicine are fully realized. But I believe trends of the last several decades give reason for optimism.

Social Medicine
The Advance of Organized Health Services in America

Part One

General Organizing Trends

For reasons springing from developments in all of society, not only in the health sciences, the provision of health care has become increasingly complex and organized. The organization has applied both to the economic support of health services and to the manner of their delivery. The trend is seen in all countries, although at different paces and in various forms.

Chapter 1 examines the variety of social forces that influence and shape the organization of health services. Chapter 2 probes the nature of some of the more significant organizational innovations in the United States. The traditional public health movement, oriented initially to the community prevention of disease, has slowly changed its character as pressures have mounted for equivalent organization of the treatment services, and these changes are explored in Chapter 3. In Chapter 4, we review the broad scope of governmental roles in the management of health programs, from the perspective of the American family.

1

Social Determinants of Changing Health Service Patterns

The social institution of health services, like all other social institutions, is a product of forces in the world around it. A comprehensive analysis of these forces would entail an encyclopedic accounting of all the economic, political, technological, cultural, demographic, and related factors that describe the dynamics of a society at each time and place.

In this paper, the highlights of the principal such forces shaping health care are reviewed, as seen in the environment of the United States of the early 1960s. Since then, it is quite clear that the trends of all the major movements identified have moved along in the same direction; one can say that the pressures of the late 1970s are essentially "more of the same."

IN ALL HISTORICAL periods, the patterns of medical service have depended on the existent technology and the structure of society. The current period is no exception, and the many changing patterns of health service organization in current-day America can easily be traced to larger developments in science, on the one hand, and society, on the other.

These changing patterns are found in all the major spheres of health service: in hospitals, in ambulatory medical care, and in the public health services. They are found in the professions of medicine, dentistry, nursing, pharmacy, all the related disciplines. They are found in the sphere of private action no less than in government. They characterize the organizational aspects of curative as well as preventive health service.

Rather than cataloguing the new and changing patterns in each of these sectors, the dependence of medicine on the world around it may perhaps be better demonstrated by starting from the other side and examining the forces at play which are inducing the changes. What, then, are some of these social forces and their consequences?

Technological Developments

First and most obvious are the enormous technological developments in medicine itself, with innovations emerging at a geometric rate over the last century. The knowledge to be encompassed has grown rapidly beyond the competence of even

Chapter 1 originally appeared as "Changing Patterns of Health Service: Their Dependence on a Changing World" in *The Annals of the American Academy of Political and Social Science,* 346:44–56, March, 1963, and is reprinted by permission of that journal.

the most exceptional human minds, so that the only answer was specialization. It has occurred along several dimensions: the organs of the body—ophthalmology, cardiology, or dermatology; the techniques used—surgery, internal medicine, radiology; age groups served—pediatrics or geriatrics; even the physician's social role—public health, teaching, industrial medicine. Some twenty "specialty boards" have been established to certify qualifications in those fields—a form of superlicensure under nongovernmental auspices. Specialization has occurred not only within the ancient medical art, that itself evolved from the priesthood, but it has led to the fragmentation of healing into a score of other separate occupations: pharmacy,an early offshoot of the Middle Ages; nursing, a much later offshoot of the nineteenth century; dentistry; laboratory technology; physiotherapy; dietetics; medical social work, a newcomer to the health scene. And within each of these paramedical or auxiliary health professions are many further subspecialties to cope with the needs of an ever-expanding science.[1]

If the enormity of knowledge has caused the fractionation of medicine, the needs of people, sick or well, do not fall neatly into such cognitive departments. The countervailing movements, therefore, have been great. Not so great, perhaps, as the human need, for no better example of Ogburn's cultural lag could be cited than the slowness of medicine to adapt its social organization to its technical inventions. But the complexities of specialization have, nevertheless, produced in all American cities an elaborate network of formal and informal relationships among the various practitioners. These are reflected in codes of ethics and etiquette governing the process of referral of patients from one doctor to another, prohibiting the "splitting of fees," and opposing the "stealing" of a patient by a consultant. They are seen in "medical arts buildings" where a galaxy of private practitioners is brought close together physically, if not professionally. They are seen in increasingly elaborate schemes of departmental organization in hospitals, with accumulating committees on credentials, records, medical audits, hospital utilization, drugs, and other functions. Specialization has also produced a pattern of medical teams for the care of ambulatory cases—group practice clinics assembling numerous specialists, technicians, and aides for the treatment of the patient who, more often than not, requires a multiplicity of skills to serve his total health needs.

The development of group medical practice in America has not been a sweeping revolution, for the resistances against it have been great. Private medical practice is not only a professional skill but also a proprietary business, and it has resisted competitive schemes of marketing the wares in much the same way as early artisans resisted factories by throwing wooden shoes—sabotage—into the machinery. The modes of resistance to group practice have been a saga in the dynamics of social change. Groups have grown most rapidly in regions of the United States where private solo practice was weakest rather than where medical technology was most advanced; thus, group practice is much stronger in the newer West than in the older East. Nevertheless, grown it has, and today some 6 to 8 percent of clinically practicing physicians—depending on how the pattern is defined—are so engaged. While still only an eddy in the larger stream of clinical medicine, the proportions of group medical practice are slowly swelling.[2]

Other consequences of specialization are seen within the bounds of the predominant pattern of solo office practice. The office secretary has become a staple, and record systems are mechanized in an endless variety of ways. The telephone answering service has become a necessity in urban practice, where the doctor's office is no longer attached to his home. There are clinical laboratories to do diagnostic tests and collection agencies to handle the nasty financial side of private practice. In a significant minority of communities, doctor's offices are being established within or next to hospitals, so that these elaborate resources are more accessible for the care of the ambulatory patient.[3]

Urbanization

Specialization in the larger society has produced the city, and, in the world of medicine, the city has had further effects on the patterns of health service. Medical specialization could hardly have developed without concentrations of population; thus, urbanization, along with the accretion of knowledge, is doubtless a parent of the medical specialties. In the nineteenth century, it was the epidemics and squalor of urban living that gave rise to the whole public health movement. In the large city today, moreover, we see other developments which change the face of modern medicine.

Most impressive is the medical center, the great constellation of basic and applied health sciences devoted to teaching and research as well as clinical service. The impact of the medical center is very wide. It sets the standard of technical performance in all the specialties. Along with the medical school, it produces doctors, as well as nurses, technicians, and other personnel. It provides the locale of clinical research for improved diagnosis and therapy of disease. It serves as the court of last resort in the management of difficult cases. It may, if its leadership is not parochial, offer postgraduate training to physicians in smaller hospitals situated around it.

Indeed, the impressive development of medicine in the big city has made conspicuous the disparity with the level of service in rural areas. It is these recognized inequalities that are responsible for another important pattern in modern health service: the concept of regionalization. Although applied largely to hospitals and the planning of their construction, their location, size, and functions, the regionalization idea has meaning for all of health service. It involves the use of transportation and referral of both patients and technical resources in defined geographic areas so as to assure the same technical level of service to all sick persons, wherever they may live. In a few selected regions, where special grants have supported demonstration plans, this two-way flow has been developed to a high point. But, in all states of the nation, the concept has been embodied at least in the master planning for hospital construction under the federal subsidy (Hill-Burton) program.[4]

Urbanization has brought in its wake many other social movements—increased literacy, communication, and democratic participation of people in public life—the effects of which on health service will be noted below.

The Cost Problem

The enormous expansion of medical technology has also had an economic dimension, leading to continual changes in the patterns of health service. As early as the fifteenth century, medieval guilds appreciated the problem of catastrophic illness, and the pooling of money in mutual-benefit funds to help a guild brother in distress was seen as a solution. As medical-care costs rose higher and the industrial worker came to be more dependent on his job for his total income, the cost problem became more serious. Insurance to buffer the costs of medical care evolved as the answer in Europe throughout the nineteenth century, spreading to America in the twentieth. The leadership in Europe was taken initially by the trade unions, later by the government. In America, on the other hand, the strongest and most successful leadership came from providers of health service—hospitals and doctors—and from the commercial insurance industry.[5]

The Blue Cross and Blue Shield plans for insurance in hospitalized illness and the indemnity plans for hospital, surgical, and medical expenses of private insurance companies have come to enroll some 70 percent of the United States population. Although these programs basically have been systems of pooled payment for medical expenses in serious illness, they have inevitably had some influence on the patterns of rendering service. They have certainly led to an increased utilization of medical care. They have supported a great enrichment of the equipment and personnel for all health service. They have led to standardization of the cost accounting of institutions and the fees of private medical practice. They have changed the social character of hospitals, with marked reductions in their "charity" wards and increases in their provisions for private patients. They have provided financial support for the growth of the medical specialties. As in Europe, however, it may be said that these insurance plans have fortified the pattern of private solo medical practice by providing it economic underpinning. Likewise for general hospitals under nongovernmental auspices.

More far-reaching in their conceptual influence on patterns of medical care, though much smaller in coverage, have been the health service insurance plans organized by various consumer groups. Under the sponsorship of cooperatives, labor unions, or sometimes broadly representative community groups, these programs have engaged or contracted with teams of doctors in group practice clinics. This pattern has, indeed, altered the framework of private solo medical practice. It has meant reduction in "free choice of doctor" by the patient but surveillance over the quality of medical care through the internal discipline of a group practice clinic.[6] Examining group practice clinics as a whole, however, the greatest proportion are found to be independent of any prepayment organization.

The cost problem has had other major impacts on health service organization through the role of government. A vast network of medical services for certain population groups—indigent, veterans, children; for particular diseases—mental illness, tuberculosis, venereal disease; and for special services—hospitalization, laboratory tests, dental care—have evolved under the wing of local, state, and federal governments in the United States. Of course, each of these programs has been stimulated by a constellation of social needs—hazards of contagion, pity for the poor, fear of the insane, political obligations to veterans, and so on—but, in all of them, the problem of cost is an essential component. Combined with the other needs, it has been the high cost of the appropriate medical care that has induced governmental action. Each of these programs involves a different pattern of technical organization, the general effect of which is to place medical services in a more organized framework for reasons of maximum economy and efficiency in the use of public funds.[7]

Another response to the cost problem has been expressed by voluntary support for a great variety of health agencies tackling specific diseases, for the provision of visiting nurse services, for construction of hospitals, for advancing research and professional education. The base of philanthropy has widened in recent decades from the huge grants of a handful of millionaires to the small contributions of large numbers of people. The concept, however, remains that of giving money to aid one's fellowmen who, because of the costs, cannot always help themselves. Although some of this voluntary action has been undertaken in the frank effort to forestall action by government, the net effect, nevertheless, has been to widen the sector of social, as distinguished from individualistic, patterns of health care.[8]

With these many social measures for spreading medical-care costs over the population, the utilization of services has greatly increased. The current National Health Survey discloses about five physician contacts per person per year outside the hospital in the United States; studies in the 1928–1931 period—although based on smaller samples—found only about half this rate. The rise in rate of hospital admissions has been even greater. Increased utilization applies also to drugs, dental services, laboratory and X-ray procedures, and so on. This elevated volume of medical care, in turn, has raised suspicions of abuse, on the supposition that the elimination of cash barriers leads to frivolous and unnecessary demands. Objective study has usually implicated the doctor, more than the patient, in such abuse, for it is his decision that controls expensive diagnostic and therapeutic procedures, all hospital admissions, and most other services as well, except initial office visits. In any event, the utilization problem has induced a chain of controls over the practice of medicine, particularly in hospitals, which make further inroads on the unbridled freedom of the American doctor.[9]

All these social measures, springing from the problem of medical costs, have been associated with resistance and controversy in that they tend to change the old ways of medical practice. Little by little, physicians have gone along with collective systems of financing, but only after initial opposition. Voluntary insurance, launched by hospitals or private groups of citizens, engendered as much hostility twenty-five years ago as proposals on governmental insurance for hospital care of the aged today. Even the most limited public health programs of local government, like well-baby clinics or poliomyelitis immunizations, have led to battles with the local medical society. There are many explanations for this resistance to change by private physicians—fear of reduction in income, objection to loss of professional freedom, the doctor's social-class background, and so on—and doubtless all play a part.[10]

Changing Disease Burdens

Another constellation of forces shaping the patterns of modern health service must be sought in the changing nature of the diseases presenting medicine its challenge. Just as the epidemic diseases in an earlier period gave rise to the organization of public health services, the major health problems of today in the United States are provoking other forms of social organization. Within the sphere of public health itself, attention is shifting—perhaps at too slow a rate—from the communicable to the chronic noninfectious diseases. Cancer stimulates the effort at early detection, and mass-screening procedures are promoted. The obesity problem changes the main themes of nutritional education, and the consumption of fats and cholesterol has become a national issue. With lung cancer now exceeding the annual toll of tuberculosis in the United States, the inhalation of tobacco smoke has become another national health issue.

The higher proportion of aged in the population, with associated chronic illness, creates a whole chain of special problems. The general hospital, proud of its evolution over the last century into a center for the alert scientific management of acute illness, is now finding itself with more and more long-stay cases. Of all patient-days of care in so-called short-term general hospitals, 25 percent are now referable to those patients who remain for over a month. To cope with the problem, hospitals have taken various steps. A small but important number of them have organized home-care programs by which the services of the hospital are extended to patients—usually chronically ill—in their own homes. This is believed to provide more appropriate care for the patient while releasing the hospital bed for another case. Hospitals have also put greater emphasis on rehabilitation services to hasten recovery of long-term patients. Some have developed special pavilions for long-stay cases, where a more homelike atmosphere can be offered. "Progressive patient care" is a new hospital slogan, referring to the classification of patients according to their needs for active nursing care rather than their clinical diagnosis. Social-service departments now find their raison d'être more in the field of geriatrics than in the means testing for indigency of an earlier period. All these features of today's general hospital spring essentially from the changing nature of disease and the altered age composition of the population.[11]

A galaxy of other institutions has also entered the medical scene. Nursing homes, long a background feature of the institutional landscape, have now mushroomed to provide nearly as many beds in the nation as do general hospitals. They are predominantly small, proprietary places operated for profit by retired nurses or small businessmen, and the quality of their services is generally poor. Voluntary religious or nonsectarian agencies have been relatively slow to respond to the need for these long-term facilities; where they have, however, the scope of services tends to be more nearly adequate. Governmental institutions, mostly city- and county-owned, have also been expanded; the old county almshouse has frequently been revitalized with a better nursing service and a rehabilitation program. Homes for the aged under various auspices have had to face the survival of their residents into the eighties and nineties; thus, they inevitably become chronic-disease institutions with many bedridden patients. The problem of financing institutional care for aged persons, through social-security benefits or other means, has become a national legislative issue.[12]

The inexorable growth of the chronic-disease problem has led to an avid search for preventive approaches. Epidemiological research has turned from the classical problem of infectious disease to the riddles of cancer and heart disorders. Aspects of our way of life, our diets, our patterns of work and play, our habits, even our sexual practices are being probed to find positive correlations with particular types of cancer and heart disease. In the absence of effective clues to prevention—except for the smoking-lung cancer connection—the main emphasis is placed on early diagnosis through simple tests. A battery of such tests, which can be done without involving the expensive time of a physician, has made a new slogan of "multiphasic screening."[13]

Mental illness has doubtless occurred in all societies, but, more than any other type, its extent is based on the accepted definitions of the time and place. Without examining the complex question of whether or not there has been a real increase in mental illness in modern America, there can be no question about the increased attention to its care. Mental hospitals—quite unlike those in any other country of Europe or elsewhere—have come to have as many beds as all general hospitals. Psychiatric sections have been established in hundreds of general hospitals. Mental health clinics have been organized in almost all cities. Psychiatric concepts have entered into the everyday practice of medicine, as well as into the operations of school health services, public health clinics, and industrial medicine. Psychoanalysis, as a philosophy, has influenced not only child-rearing and everyday interpersonal relations but also the world of art, literature, and drama.[14]

Labor and Industry

The industrial revolution, of course, had enormous effects on the technology of medicine itself, through the developmnent of optical instruments, X-ray, biochemical analyses, drug manufacturing, and hosts of other techniques. Patterns of medical care also have been influenced in many ways by the vast growth of industry.

It was the enlarging epidemic of industrial accidents that led, in the United States, as it had in Europe, to the first widespread form of social insurance in the state workmen's compensation programs. All the state laws incorporate some provision for medical care to the injured worker. Ordinarily, the compensation laws simply require that the employer carry insurance with a private company, and the necessary medical services are provided by private physicians who are paid on a fee basis. These programs have furnished rank-and-file physicians with their longest experience in prepaid medical care, and, under them, a great volume of service has been provided—about $500,000,000 worth annually in recent years. The problems in this program today spring from the tie-up of cash awards to persistent disability, so that effective rehabilitation may be discouraged. And the roots of change lie in the maturation of the rehabilitation movement, which is slowly being felt in the compensation field.[15]

Partly because of the pressure of compensation laws—which penalized, through higher premium charges, those employers with higher accident rates—and partly from recognition of the value of good health for effective manpower, American industries have developed special health services for workers. Large factories have done more than small ones, and the range of services is usually quite limited, but a great deal of emergency medical care and preventive service is given under these auspices. Some firms have provided comprehensive health care programs for the workers and their families, especially in isolated localities. The railroads, mines, and lumber companies that opened up the West in the nineteenth century financed general medical care through periodic wage deductions. Aside from the old Marine Hospital Service started by the federal government in 1798, these industrial programs constituted the earliest form of health insurance in the nation.

When the hospital insurance movement, under the Blue Cross emblem, began to grow in the 1930s, industrial groups provided a natural base for large collective enrollments. This was even truer for commercially sponsored health insurance, for various forms of group insurance for death and disability were already commonplace in industry. Indeed, it is likely that the whole health insurance movement, with its vast impacts on hospital and medical care in the United States, would never have flowered without the great facilitation of enrollment and premium collection through industrial organization. The so-called voluntary character of this insurance has been successful largely insofar as coverage was provided to millions of workers as an automatic feature of their employment.

Moreover, the transfer of all or part of these enrollment costs to management, as "fringe benefits," has become a routine object of collective bargaining by unions—which has further extended the health insurance idea.[16]

Though it is quite recent, one of the most significant impacts of industry on health service in America has come from maturation of the interests of labor unions in improved care for their members. Aside from collective bargaining for fringe benefits, by way of coverage under commercial or Blue Cross-Blue Shield plans, hundreds of unions have used payroll contributions to establish special health-and-welfare funds. These are used to provide various benefits directly. One of the most impressive of such funds is that of the United Mine Workers of America—a program that has rendered extensive specialty services to coal miners and their families, that has built a network of ten general hospitals, and has stimulated the organization of many community group practice clinics. Scores of unions have used welfare-fund money for building "labor health centers" where the worker may get various scopes of ambulatory medical care. Through "their own" doctors, union members feel a greater sense of confidence in the medical care received, especially in compensation cases involving disputes with management or insurance companies. The rising voice of organized labor in the health field, moreover, is being felt in the selection of union members for the boards of directors of hospitals and voluntary health agencies.

Transportation and Communication

Though it is part of our general technological development, the enormous strides in transportation and communication of the current century have had an impact on patterns of health service that warrants special comment. Because of the greater ease of transportation for the vast majority of people, the whole character of medical practice has changed. Almost every American family has access to an automobile or good public transportation, so that the usual response to a symptom is to go to the doctor's office or clinic, rather than calling the doctor to the home. The physician encourages this, of course, because he can usually do a better examination in the office setting and he thereby also saves time, enabling him to see more patients per day—the social cost of the patient's travel time might be worth studying. For many medical specialties—for example, ophthalmology or radiology—home calls by the doctor are virtually unknown; even for general practitioners or internists, the ratio of office to home calls is now about ten to one. Only in pediatric practice does the home call remain a significant service. The telephone has further reduced the need for home calls by permitting the patient to communicate with his doctor day or night.

This major shifting of the site of medical care away from the home has, despite its technical advantages, engendered problems as well. Perfunctory telephone medicine has been the subject of many jibes, in back of which lies serious criticism. The heavy demand on the doctor's time in his office, on the other hand, often means long waiting periods for the patient, in spite of an appointment schedule. Moreover, when the doctor sees his patient only on the office examining table, his insight is bound to be more limited than it would be from a view of the patient's family setting in a particular home and neighborhood. Despite these limitations, however, the increasing concentration of medical service in more efficient technical settings, made possible by modern transportation and communication, has doubtless contributed significantly to the improved quality and quantity of medical care received by the average American.

The whole problem of rural medical care, with its serious deficiencies of personnel and facilities, has been greatly mitigated by improved roads and transportation. In the last thirty years, the maldistribution of doctors between urban and rural areas has actually not diminished—despite corrective efforts, such as rural medical fellowships and construction of rural hospitals. In some states, like Missouri, the rural shortage has grown worse. Nevertheless, the provision of medical service to rural people has greatly improved, simply through easier physical access to doctors and hospitals.[17]

The concept of regionalization in hospital planning depends, of course, on transportation. In fact, the ease of transportation has even nullified some of the theoretical expectations of the regional hospital concept. Thus, rural people, who might be expected to go to a distant urban medical center only for major and difficult conditions, often bypass the local rural hospital even for common ailments. The concept of community, district, and base hospitals, with three levels of complexity of service, is seldom applied in practice simply because easy transportation permits all sorts of variations in the theoretical scheme.

Another effect of modern communications relates to health education. More through popular media like newspapers, magazines, radio, and television than through formal public health programs, the population has become remarkably sophisticated about medical subjects. Much of the mystery of the doctor's skills has been removed, and patients increasingly demand an understandable explanation of their illness and how it is being treated. The illegible Latin prescription of a many-splendored drug mixture is replaced by orders for penicillin or phenobarbital or insulin, the action of which is quite well understood by most patients. Not that the art of medicine has been totally replaced by scientific technology, but the times call for another kind of art that does not depend on naiveté or ignorance in the patient.

Democracy and Humanism

Still another social force shaping modern health service in the United States is a corollary of our urban and industrialized society but must be examined because its impacts are so great. This is the whole constellation of pressures, policies, and practices embodied in the concepts of democracy and humanism. The idea is more and more widely accepted that all people have a right to proper health service which a mature society must somehow provide them. The individual patient is to be respected and treated with dignity. Decisions on health policy in a community, moreover, should be subject to the influence—if not the complete determination—of the recipient as well as the professional provider of service.

These principles of humanism and democracy are reflected in the great extension of governmental authority over standards of health service, as measures for protection of the public. Food and drug control legislation is designed to shield people from the possible evil effects of commercialization. Although tragedies, such as the recent thalidomide scandal, show the gaps in such laws, the movement has clearly been toward tighter controls. The extension of governmental medical services for the indigent is a mark not only of political good sense but also of humanism. A thousand and one voluntary charities may serve to meet psychological needs for their sponsors while, at the same time, they express humanitarianism in the larger community.

In clinical medicine, great and growing emphasis has been put on the importance of "treating the patient as a person." A large literature has been produced in the last thirty years on the obligation of the physician to understand the social and psychological background of the patient. The whole field of medical social work represents this humanism in patient care. Medical schools have introduced the concept of comprehensive medicine, which means simply taking account of patient's total life situation.[18] Hospitals have been subjected to criticism in popular magazines for not showing sufficient sensitivity to the personal needs of patients—and this at a time when the average general hospital provides almost 2.5 nurses, technicians, and other personnel per patient each twenty-four hours. The point is that the public conscience has come to expect hospitals to give tender, loving care to every patient every day.[19]

The democratic ideal has certainly not yet been achieved everywhere in American medicine. The structure of wards, semiprivate rooms, and private rooms in hospitals is an obvious reflection of class lines. The service of the doctor in his private office tends to differ from that given in a public clinic not only in the time spent per case but in the interpersonal attitudes. Nevertheless, the right of the patient to be heard, to express grievances and have them redressed, is becoming widely recognized. The rash of malpractice suits in recent years is one expression of the laymen's loss of inhibitions. In general hospitals, it is common practice to ask patients for written reports of any dissatisfactions. In health insurance plans, there are usually established procedures for making complaints. The basic structure of boards of directors of hospitals and health agencies, indeed, brings the public will formally into the management of medical affairs. And, in governmental programs where an executive has the final authority, advisory boards, representing various professional and civic groups, have become a conventional way of incorporating public participation in policy formulation.

The Overall Effect

There can be no doubt that the overall effect of all these social processes is to make American health service more and more socially organized. Yet the organization occurs in segments. Particular needs are met with particular programs. Actions are taken by government at all levels and by hundreds of voluntary agencies. Special efforts are applied to a certain population group, a certain disease, or for the provision of a certain type of technical service. The focus may be preventive or therapeutic or it may be both. The organization may involve direct provision of some health service by a structured social entity, or it may involve the imposition of certain formal standards and economic arrangements over the provision of services by individual medical practitioners. Social organization may also apply to the world of medical research or professional education.[20]

The resulting structure is organized, but it is a polyglot picture. It reflects the historic origin of each program more than a rational approach to the meeting of current needs. A vast new need has emerged, therefore, for the coordination of health services. In government, this has long been appreciated with the periodic appointment of "reorganization" commissions federally and in most of the states. At the local community level, councils of social agencies and health committees have tackled the problem. In 1962, a new National Commission on Community Health Services was established to analyze the problem on a nationwide scale.[21]

The difficulty at the local level is that there are various constellations of power with quite different concepts of an ideal pattern of health service coordination. The private physician, and his medical society, sees the doctor as the natural leader of health affairs. The various institutions and agencies, in his view, should serve principally to support the private practice of medicine and the private relationship between doctor and patient. Anything that invades that relationship he tends to see as destructive. Questions of public policy should be determined predominantly by the doctors as a group through their medical society.

The professional public health worker sees the situation differently. To him, the application of mass measures for prevention of disease are most important, and local government is the logical focus of power. Individual medical and allied practitioners are regarded as the manpower necessary to cope with disease in individuals but not to determine or control social policy. The health department should be the logical authority over matters affecting the public health and should coordinate the multiple agencies concerned.

Still another view is held by hospital leaders. Here is an institution, the modern general hospital, where the most skilled medical personnel do their work and where the most seriously ill patients are treated. Here is the center of diagnosis and therapy, the place where doctors rub shoulders with each other, where technical issues are decided, where nurses and other health professionals are trained, where research is conducted. Whether the patient is indigent or wealthy, whether his disease is infectious or degenerative, the hospital has a place in his care. Is this not the logical center for coordination of all health services in a community?

Each of these three groups—medical society, public health agency, general hospital—makes claim to be the logical center around which all health services in a community should be structured. There is no question about the critical position held by the practicing doctor, who holds the power of life and death not only over individuals but over health programs as well. Yet the nature of his work surely does not endow the private practitioner with a spirit of social responsibility. The public health agency has built-in social responsibility, but, with its focus on mass measures of disease prevention, it has, in fact, been quite isolated in America from the day-to-day problems of personal medical care. The hospital is surely close to the problems of medical care in its most crucial forms, but it is usually nongovernmental and, moreover, one of many such institutions in a city or county. Which hospital among the several would take leadership in an area?

The answer to the obvious and pressing need for coordination of health services in American communities has not yet been found. Health councils, hospital councils, councils of social agencies, councils for patient care, all are efforts to tackle the problem, though seldom are any of these comprehensive in scope. We are a relatively rich nation and, despite the waste of in-coordination, our health status and health services show steady improvement. The pinch seems to be felt most sharply, at this point, in the problems of chronic illness. This burden is increasing, as people live on with heightened susceptibility to physical and mental disorders and reduced financial resources to cope with them. That a more orderly pattern of health service organization will be achieved in America can be safely predicted, but its precise social and political form remains to be seen.

References

1. Richard H. Shryock, *The Development of Modern Medicine* (Philadelphia: University of Pennsylvania Press, 1936).
2. E. P. Jordan, *The Physician and Group Practice* (Chicago: Yearbook Publishers, 1958).
3. C. Rufus Rorem, *Physician's Private Offices at Hospitals* (Philadelphia: Hospital Council of Philadelphia, 1952).
4. Leonard S. Rosenfeld and Henry B. Makover, *The Rochester Regional Hospital Council* (Cambridge: Harvard University Press, 1956).
5. Herman M. Somers and Anne R. Somers, *Doctors, Patients, and Health Insurance* (Washington: Brookings Institution, 1961).
6. American Medical Association, *Report of the Commission on Medical Care Plans* (Chicago: American Medical Association, 1958).
7. Bernhard J. Stern, *Medical Services by Government* (New York: Commonwealth Fund, 1946).
8. Selskar M. Gunn and Philip S. Platt, *Voluntary Health Agencies: An Interpretive Study* (New York: Ronald Press, 1945).

9. Benjamin J. Darsky, Nathan Sinai, and Solomon J. Axelrod, *Comprehensive Medical Services Under Voluntary Health Insurance* (Cambridge: Harvard University Press, 1958).
10. Michael M. Davis, *Medical Care for Tomorrow* (New York: Harper and Brothers, 1955).
11. Commission on Chronic Illness, *Care of the Long-Term Patient* (Cambridge: Harvard University Press, 1956).
12. U. S., Social Security Administration, *The Health Care of the Aged* (Washington, D.C.: Government Printing Office, 1962).
13. American Public Health Association, *Chronic Disease and Rehabilitation: A Program Guide for State and Local Health Agencies* (New York: American Public Health Association, 1960).
14. Joint Commission on Mental Illness and Health, *Action for Mental Health* (New York: Basic Books, 1961).
15. Herman M. Somers and Anne R. Somers, *Workmen's Compensation: Prevention, Insurance, and Rehabilitation of Occupational Disability* (New York: John Wiley and Sons, 1954).
16. Joseph W. Garbarino, *Health Plans and Collective Bargaining* (Berkeley and Los Angeles: University of California Press, 1960).
17. Frederick D. Mott and Milton I. Roemer, *Rural Health and Medical Care* (New York: McGraw-Hill, 1948).
18. Peter V. Lee, "Medical Schools and the Changing Times" in *Medical Education and Medical Care,* Part 2 of *Journal of Medical Education,* December 1961.
19. Leo W. Simmons and Harold G. Wolff, *Social Science in Medicine* (New York: Russell Sage Foundation, 1954).
20. Milton I. Roemer and Ethel A. Wilson, *Organized Health Services in a County of the United States* (Washington, D.C.: Government Printing Office, 1952).
21. Berwyn Mattison and T. L. Richman, *Community Health Services: The Case of the Missing Mileposts* (New York: Public Affairs Committee, 1962).

2

New Organized Patterns for Providing Health Services

Many facets of the health services have responded to the social pressures toward increased organization in the American setting. Even in individual medical practice–the keystone of American medicine–various forms of systematization of health care delivery have been occurring. More striking has been the expansion of other forms of organized ambulatory services, as well as the internal structuring of hospitals, relations among hospitals in various forms of area-wide systems, and a generally widening role in the health services of state and national governments.

This text analyzes the five paths along which health care delivery has become more organized, and also some associated issues about what is happening to mainstream medicine and the personal freedom of doctor and patient. While published in 1966, the same trends and issues continue today. The following chapter was presented during a conference on "New Directions in Public Policy for Health Care," held in New York on April 21 and 22, 1966.

THE ECONOMIC AND legislative foundations of a steadily increasing demand for health service have been reviewed elsewhere. Even if medical technology had been standing still, the very volume of this mounting demand would compel us to find more efficient ways of meeting it through a given supply of personnel and facilities. But the vast growth of scientific potential has compounded the problem; the galaxy of specialized skills and instrumentation requires organization if they are to be delivered at all. On top of this, the enlargement of democratic humanism has put further stresses on our health service system; expectations of more and more sensitive patient care have created—paradoxically to some—still further requirements for social organization of services.

These four sets of pressures—economic, legislative, scientific, and humanistic—have induced responses in the social institution of medicine in scores of ways. They can be classified, I think, in terms of five levels of medicosocial structure: 1. individual medical practice, 2. organized ambulatory service, 3. hospital organization, 4. interhospital systems, and 5. state and national governments. There is a stream of increasing social responsibility for health services along these five levels of increasingly collective actions. Within each level, furthermore, there is evidence of systematization of health functions to higher degrees.

Chapter 2 originally appeared as "New Patterns of Organization for Providing Health Services" in *The Bulletin of the New York Academy of Medicine*, 42:1226–1238, December, 1966, and is reprinted by permission of that journal.

Individual Medical Practice

Despite the basic trends just outlined, at this point in history the prevailing pattern of personal health service in the United States is still the individual doctor in a private office. This is by no means true on a world scale, and the rate of change in the United States is rapid, but the independent private medical or dental practitioner is still the commonest model in the country. Yet, within this basic model, the evolutionary ferment is clear.

The general physician who practices in true isolation has become a rare bird. In the great majority of offices are medical aides, some of whom are registered nurses. The specialist may have a laboratory or X-ray technician or a physical therapist. Equipment may be elaborate and record systems well developed. The office assistant may take the patient's history through a standardized form, like the *Cornell Medical Index*. It is commonplace for several clinical rooms to be in use, so that one patient is being examined while another is disrobing. The telephone is, of course, a powerful channel to the patient at home. These and many other measures are forms of organization of the individual physician, whether in general or specialty practice.

The proportion of individual practitioners who share office suites is continually rising. A recent national survey by *Medical Tribune and Medical News* reported that 46 percent of doctors have shared office quarters, with higher proportions among the young, among specialists, and in the Western states. In the larger cities, office sharing is getting to be the general rule. Although patients and incomes are quite separate, waiting rooms, clerical files, laboratory or X-ray apparatus may be fully shared. Usually these shared facilities serve two or three specialists in the same field; sometimes in complementary specialties. If one doctor is away, his suite partner may cover for him. At a more elaborate level is the "medical arts building," where a score or more of independent doctors are served by a private laboratory, and perhaps an optometrist or a physical therapist, in the same building. A pharmacy on the ground floor is an obvious convenience for patients. One study of such buildings in Washington, D.C., moreover, found 68 percent of doctors in them to be in "associated practice," ranging from office sharing to full partnership.

Aside from these physical forms of coordination of solo practitioners, there are functional relationships through a variety of influences. Attachment of the large majority of practicing physicians to one or more hospitals brings them into frequent contact with others. Channels of specialty referral develop through these connections. The medical society or academy serves a similar purpose. Postgraduate educational programs sponsored by voluntary health agencies or medical schools, as well as hospitals and medical societies, are further antidotes to isolation.

Thousands of individual practitioners spend some hours each week at part-time salaried posts in various organized programs. *Medical Economics,* the magazine, estimates that 65 percent of practicing doctors have some such appointments in public health clinics, industrial medicine departments, Veterans Administration facilities, schools of medicine, voluntary hospitals, insurance companies, and the like. Another study of that magazine reports that about half of the 64-hour working week of the average practitioner is spent in activities other than direct patient care in his office. It is interesting to observe in the biographical notes of the *Directory of Medical Specialists* the multitude of connections with organized programs that each diplomate proudly claims. The education of the physician, of course, is almost entirely carried out through such social frameworks. When the private doctor, furthermore, serves a patient with an industrial injury, a crippled child, a home-town veteran, or even a Blue Shield plan beneficiary—even though he holds forth in a single office—he articulates with an organized system of health service.

Organized Ambulatory Service

The impact of organization on the performance and behavior of the doctor is greater at the next level in our typology. When groups of three or more physicians form a team for coordinated services to the individual patient, the rationalization of medical and surgical specialties can be much greater. There are all degrees of group practice, and much depends on the range of physicians of different specialties involved, as well as the system of income sharing. A medical group can make fuller use of auxiliary personnel and expensive equipment. When group practice embodies a full sharing of earnings, the dysfunctional incentive to "hold onto" patients is replaced by uninhibited referral, but the opposite evil of excessive and expensive work-ups may result. When it is combined, however, with prepayment by a population, the economic incentive favors both economy and quality of care—as shown in several comparative studies.

The movement to coordinated medical teams for ambulatory patient care takes various forms throughout the world. In the underdeveloped countries it is the standard pattern in larger cities. The Chilean National Health Service provides ambulatory service through health centers staffed by a range of specialists and paramedical personnel. The polyclinics of Germany or the Soviet Union have long embodied this concept, as do similar facilities in Israel, Yugoslavia, or Japan. In Great Britain or Scandinavia, the multispecialty clinics are nearly always attached to hospitals, as in the outpatient departments in this country, but their services are, of course, not confined to the poor.

The growth of private group medical practice has probably been more rapid in the United States in recent years than is generally recognized. The count of organized groups by the U.S. Public Health Service in 1949—using the definition of three or more physicians with some form of shared income—found only 368 such entities. In 1959 the count was 1,546 such practices. But in 1965, when a national inventory of virtually all physicians was made by the American Medical Association, Chicago, Ill., it was revealed recently that 5,450 group practices were identified with about 26,000 physicians. This is about 15 percent of all doctors in community practice. In the Western states, where traditions are younger, the growth of group practice is very prominent.

Programs serving special populations have developed teams of physicians for ambulatory care outside of private practice. The Veterans Administration operates free-standing multispecialty clinics in most large cities. Industrial medical care programs, since the pioneering of the Endicott-Johnson Shoe Corporation, Binghamton, N.Y., do likewise, especially in large enterprises such as public utilities or railroads. The ordinary public health clinic for children or mothers, for tuberculosis, venereal disease, or cancer detection is not to be overlooked in an accounting of organized ambulatory services. And recently, the antipoverty program has broken precedent with establishment of comprehensive medical care centers in numerous blighted urban or rural sections.

The well-organized group practice clinic is able to introduce services difficult in a one-man office. Multiple screening procedures for early disease detection, handled mainly by paramedical personnel, are quite feasible. A visiting nurse, social worker, psychologist, or rehabilitation therapist can be readily employed. Health education can be offered. The family physician, of course, can be backed up by appropriate specialists not only at critical stages of illness (common enough in solo practice) but all along the way. These more comprehensive services can be offered at lower costs because of economies of scale, although these savings are often translated into higher medical incomes rather than lower patient fees. The reality of the savings has been well demonstrated in the economic achievements of organizations such as the Kaiser-Permanente medical care plan.

Some of the larger ambulatory care clinics have sprouted branch clinics in metropolitan areas. The pioneer prepaid Ross-Loos Medical Group in Los Angeles, Calif., now has 12 satellite units. Branches are also being established by purely fee-for-service medical groups. In such clinic networks the scarcer specialists serve patients from any branch unit. Group practice is probably the most feasible way to adjust for the steady decline in general practitioners, while still meeting the psychosocial needs of patients. The recently proposed federal legislation for encouraging construction of group clinics through mortgage insurance and low-interest loans will, if enacted, doubtless accelerate the whole trend.

Hospital Organization

General hospitals served as a setting for systematic organization of medical care centuries before community medical practice. From the beginning, hospitals have brought together many types of medical workers and equipment. Since about 1900 the rate of hospital organization has accelerated everywhere.

The European hospital has always been essentially a public place, staffed mainly by physicians attached to the organization. We take this for granted in mental hospitals, but in other countries it has been the prevailing pattern for general hospitals as well. In the United States, the trend within general hospitals has been in the same direction, although the form taken is different. Departments and committees, appointment procedures and by-laws, clinical conferences and medical audits—all these measures of group discipline heighten the social controls in medical staffs. An increasing proportion of physicians working in hospitals are being appointed through some form of contract, under which their rewards come from the hospital organization rather than the private patient. These include not only radiologists and pathologists (about whom we hear so much controversy), but directors of medical education, researchers, out-patient department directors, and full-time members or chiefs of clinical departments.

Our own research in this field suggests that hospitals with a higher proportion of contractual physicians, even when correction is made for hospital size, are more likely to be providing the full gamut of services expected of an ideal institution. These hospitals are more likely to be offering education to interns and residents, to be doing research, to be engaged in preventive medicine (e.g., routine chest X-rays), to be operating strong out-patient departments or coordinated home-care programs, to be admitting psychiatric cases, to be furnishing newer modalities such as intensive care or rehabilitation services.

The spectacular growth of hospital "emergency-room" services in recent years is an important straw in the wind of medicine in the United States. Relatively few of the patients coming to these units are genuine emergencies; they are mainly sick people who want attention and feel that the hospital—rather than a private medical office—is the place to get it swiftly and competently. Hundreds of hospitals with no previous organized out-patient clinics have had to set up special medical staff patterns to cope with the demand. In spite of the extension of the "free choice" pattern in welfare medical programs, the American Hospital Association, Chicago, Ill., reports total (i.e., both emergency and formal clinic) out-patient visits to have reached an all-time high in 1965. The rate of approximately 8,000,000 visits per month indicates that such services now constitute about 14 percent of all doctor-patient contacts.

Here and there a full group practice clinic is attached to a hospital, and some of the largest (such as the Ochsner Foundation Hospital in New Orleans, La.) operate their own hospitals. Private doctors' offices in a medical arts building near the hospital or even in an attached wing are becoming more frequent. Large prepaid group practice plans, such as Kaiser-Permanente and those in Seattle, Ore., and Detroit, Mich., also provide comprehensive care through their own hospitals. Medical schools and their teaching hospitals have been slow to affiliate with health insurance plans, but the need for a balanced population to teach medical students properly is arousing increasing interest in such affiliations.

A major force for enriching the structure of medical staffs in hospitals has been the Joint Commission on Accreditation of Hospitals, Chicago, Ill. The requirements of the Council on Medical Education and Hospitals of the American Medical Association, for approval of internship and residency programs, has been another positive extramural influence. The quality of medical staff leadership itself, of course, can be decisive, and physicians seem to be increasingly sensitive to the responsibilities of such leadership. Medical performance is also influenced by a board of directors, especially if it is oriented by an imaginative administrator. Indeed, the whole temper of modern hospitals has been vitalized by the professionalization of the discipline of hospital administration.

The new Medicare law is confined largely to the aged and the indigent, but it has other specific implications for hospital organization. Aside from general certification—which should lead to an upgrading of customary state hospital licensure standards—the special requirement for a "utilization review" process will doubtless enhance medical staff self-discipline. The relatively generous support for "home health services" under the new law should stimulate the expansion of organized home-care programs based in hospitals and other agencies. While the focus of these programs has been largely on the care of chronic illness, their long-run significance may be greater by way of extending hospital influence over day-to-day community medicine in all fields.

It has become trite to say that the hospital is increasingly becoming the health center of the community, but the full significance of the statement is not always realized. It is not only the hospital's functions in patient care, professional education, and research that shape its central role. It is its capacity for *organizing* a symphony of skills around patients—both in bed and on foot—that gives it force in the total span of health service. This includes the ambulatory services generally and the preventive services. Such scope is seen more clearly in Chile, Brazil, the Soviet Union, India, or even Ethiopia, where the public health services and the ambulatory care services for a district are often headquartered at the general hospital. In the United States, such curative-preventive unification is seen only in 40 or 50 counties where local health departments and local governmental hospitals are under the same physical and administrative roof. But the movement in this direction is more than meets the eye, as the "public utility" character of hospitals, on the one hand, and the necessity of public health agency involvement in medical care, on the other, become more widely recognized.

Interhospital Systems

More recent and more spotty than the increased organization within hospitals—but perhaps more important in the long run—has been the movement for enhanced relationships between hospitals. Within cities or larger geographic regions, these relationships have taken many forms.

It was the National Hospital Survey and Construction Act (Hill-Burton) in

1946 that launched on a nationwide scale the concept of planned hospital networks in geographic regions. As a device for allotting federal subsidies for needed construction, each new hospital as well as each approved existing hospital had to have its theoretical place in a system of "community," "intermediate," and "base" facilities. In such systems patients would be referred from the periphery inward and consultant services from the center outward. Every state drew its "master plan," and the maps enabled state hospital agencies (usually in state health departments) to make reasonable decisions on subsidized construction, even though day-to-day hospital operations rarely corresponded to the image of the maps.

In spite of the disparity between theory and reality in the Hill-Burton regional plans, the isolation and sovereignty of individual hospitals have been reduced in many ways. State hospital associations have brought administrators and trustees together to discuss common problems. Radiologists, pathologists, and physiatrists based at a large hospital often render part-time services in smaller hospitals nearby. Schools of nursing enrich their training programs by affiliations between hospitals and exchanges of students. Recruitment and training of personnel, bulk purchasing of certain supplies, negotiations with third-party payers (Blue Cross or governmental agencies), and other administrative functions are often carried out jointly by the hospitals in a region. Postgraduate education of medical staffs has been greatly facilitated. The most impressive demonstrations of such regional interhospital cooperation have been in foundation-supported programs radiating from Boston, Mass., and from Rochester, N.Y.

Within metropolitan areas, the tempo of interhospital councils has been higher than in larger geographic regions. Most of the nation's great cities have set up councils whose primary objective has been to exercise direct or indirect control over new hospital construction (independent of the Hill-Burton program), but usually bringing about other administrative liaisons as well. These metropolitan hospital councils are composed in a variety of patterns, representing different blends of large industrial donors, hospital administrators, medical leaders, Blue Cross executives, and so on. In the last few years, federal grants for "area-wide planning" have given a further boost to these local efforts. Their long-run significance doubtless extends beyond the capital cost problem, which has usually stimulated them, toward genuine coordination of hospital services.

The advantages of large-scale operation have led to outright merger of several groups of hospitals in cities such as Newark, N.J., Wilmington, Del., and St. Louis, Mo. The administrative marriages of several pairs of voluntary and municipal hospitals here in New York City are well known to this audience. Within particular religious sponsorships—Catholic, Jewish, Lutheran, and so on—various forms of integration, ranging from simple cooperation to full merger, have been growing for years. The goal of these relationships is often to develop first-class centers embodying the ultimate in scientific technology, with or without medical school affiliation. The university medical centers, in the meantime, have also expanded, bringing under their wing specialized hospitals for children, for mental disorder, for chronic disease, for orthopedic conditions, as well as the older general hospital at the hub. They are offering an increasing range of postgraduate instruction to physicians practicing in the surrounding area. Professor Thomas McKeown of England has spoken of the "balanced hospital community" in which patients are flexibly transferred to the type of facility that meets their needs rather than kept in the one they happen to enter initially. This is basically the goal of any regionalized hospital system, but it is more readily attainable within a multidivisional medical center.

These varied expressions of interhospital cooperation have one thing in common: they embody an increasing organization of skilled and scarce medical resources to meet needs with optimal quality and economy. Whether the goal is achieved or not, there is no doubt that some form of organization, as distinguished from sovereign individualism, is the path toward it.

The new Medicare law has two provisions specifically designed to promote further such interfacility relationships. The mandatory "transfer agreements" between extended care facilities and general hospitals, as a condition for participation, have been discussed in other places. The second provision is the assignment of a specific task of "coordination" to the state health agencies. This may be expected to encourage better relationships in the full continuum of health service, from organized home care through the intermediate levels to the complex medical center.

A more direct legal push to the interhospital coordination movement is given by the 1965 federal amendments on "heart disease, cancer, and stroke." The focus of attention in this law on the three leading causes of death in the nation is obviously only a means to the end of promoting "regional cooperative arrangements" between medical centers and peripheral hospitals for research, training, and "related demonstrations of patient care." I believe we may look upon this law as the 1966 approach, on a functional level, to the regionalization idea launched, on a structural level, by the Hill-Burton Act 20 years ago.

State and National Governments

Interwoven among the four levels of medical-social organization we have briefly discussed is a widening role for state and national governments. Within individual medical practice, the basic licensure laws exert their influence, as do the food and drug control laws, the malpractice statutes, and enactments such as the 1965 medical disciplinary measures in California. At the level of organized ambulatory service, government has been relatively timid, but we are now seeing more interest on the part of Congress in bills to promote the extension of group medical practice. Senator H. A. Williams, Jr.'s, new "Preventicare" bill on organized multiple screening centers is another augury. As in internal hospital organization, the impact of government has been extensive through the hospital licensure laws, the Hill-Burton Act, and the quality standards demanded of many programs for defined beneficiaries such as crippled children or compensably injured workers. At the level of interhospital networks, the influences of government have just been mentioned.

Beyond these four levels, national and state governments are influencing the ultimate patterns of health service in other far-reaching ways. The whole underpinning of economic support for health care—through general revenues or social insurance—means more than dollars. If due only to elevated utilization of service, the medical and hospital resources of the country are daily influenced by publicly financed health programs. Beyond the quantitative pressure is the impact of qualitative standards imposed on providers of service under these programs. Public agencies are, in effect, becoming a mentor to the patient in his choice of doctor or hospital; "free choice" is being replaced by guided choice where technical sophistication is required for intelligent decision.

Government is also influencing patterns of care indirectly through its strong support of medical research. Advanced technology leads to changed social adjustments in spite of the usual cultural lag. Research on patterns of health service organization itself is also financed by government, and its impact may be seen directly in the fashioning of new programs; Medicare is one such product of years of data gathering and analysis. Government support of professional education, of course, has further influences on the quality of medical care.

The whole public health movement, in local, state, and national governments, also affects patterns of personal health service. Environmental prevention, of course, changes the spectrum of disease, reducing the infections and contributing to the higher burden of chronic metabolic disorders. Mass case-finding programs detect cases that are referred to personal physicians. Health education induces people to live hygienically and to seek attention for suspicious symptoms. School health examinations direct many handicapped children to the doctor's office.

Several governmental programs, of course, operate as separate and parallel systems of health services. The Veterans Administration, the Indian and merchant marine health service, the state mental and tuberculosis programs, the municipal or county hospitals for the poor—these entities maintain their own personnel and facilities. While these programs are often contrasted with the so-called mainstream of United States medicine, one must not underestimate their importance; they affect millions of people according to highly structured patterns of medicine. Whether the quality of care is conceded to be high, as in the Veterans Administration system, or low, as in most state mental hospitals, these programs are part and parcel of health services in the United States. They preempt a substantial sector of health needs into frameworks organized at both the ambulatory and hospital levels.

Beyond these various specific roles of government, there is a further overall role of which we may expect to see more in the future. "Planning" is no longer a dirty word in our political vocabulary, and it is being undertaken increasingly by local, state, and national governments. It has been done for years in such fields as transportation, public power systems, city zoning, education, agriculture. It has been done informally by the more imaginative public health officials on problems of environmental sanitation, child health services, chronic disease control, accident prevention, or home nursing. Now we are coming to a time when the overall planning of health services will probably be a designated task of government at all levels; a bill introduced in the U.S. Senate a few months ago provides for earmarked grants to the states for such purposes. In some form or other, overall governmental health planning is bound to arrive eventually.

Some Issues

Several questions arise from this review of the five levels at which new patterns of health service organization are evolving in our society. I should like to close these remarks with consideration of just two of them.

One concerns the issue, alluded to briefly, of segregated medical care systems versus the "mainstream of medicine" approach. Segregated programs have often meant poor quality care, epitomized perhaps in the crowded public clinic for the poor. It is easy to see why clinic attendance has implied second-class citizenship and why many organized programs have favored the use of public moneys to channelize patients to private medical offices. Such offices, however, are far from guarantees of good medical care; welfare clients with "free choice of doctor" may be badly served, as any physician in welfare medical administration knows. On the other hand, a public clinic may give first-class service if it is adequately staffed and supervised, as it often is at good teaching hospitals.

The dilemma, it seems to me, is not insoluble. Segregation and mainstream patterns alike are poor if they lack resources and standards. Both can be good with adequate resources and standards. The segregated system, however, runs the constant political danger of weak economic support—hence meager resources. There are also undemocratic overtones. The task, then, is to move toward a single mainstream of personal health service for all persons in the United States, but to upgrade its quality continuously. This can be done only by ample economic support, sound technical organization, and carefully supervised standards. Such influences will change the character of the mainstream while widening its encompassment.

The second issue concerns personal freedom of patient and doctor, which is so often alleged to be reduced by all the organization of health services we have reviewed. The burden of proof, it seems to me, is on those who repeat this cliché. It is hardly reasonable to express pride in the medical and health records of the United States and, in the same breath, to regret the social organization of the past and to oppose the social trends of the future. The scientific achievements of

United States medicine are not matters divorced from social organization: they have been largely products of such organization. The reduced mortality and increased longevity are of similar derivation. The professional effectiveness of United States doctors, both in the quantity and quality of their output—not to mention their personal affluence—is not independent of health insurance and public health and hospitals, but is largely attributable to them.

Where, then, is the loss of personal freedom from social organization? Is the child immunized in a public clinic less free because he is spared from diphtheria or poliomyelitis? Is the veteran served by a surgeon in a government hospital less free because the Veterans Administration requires that the doctor be board-certified to do the operation? In today's complicated world, one must conclude that organization is not merely consistent with personal freedom; it is a requirement for the attainment of that freedom. Others may argue the issue in other spheres of life, but in the health services the evidence is overwhelming. Social organization has moved us forward toward greater personal freedom. There are still many gaps and problems, but they will be resolved in the future as they have been in the past, by further organization of our resources in men, things, and knowledge.

3

Organized Medical Care in the Public Health Movement

A key indication of the dominance of private sector interests in America has been the pressure to confine governmental public health activities to the sphere of prevention; all treatment of the sick would be considered the province of private medical practice. In spite of the general effectiveness of these pressures, public health agencies have come to encompass more treatment services in their jurisdiction. More important, numerous organized medical care programs have developed in government even though under auspices other than Health Departments.

The irregularities of this evolution have been reflected in the history of the professional body of public health workers, the American Public Health Association. On its one hundredth anniversary in 1972, I was invited to examine the role of the Association over the past century with respect to organized medical care.

AS A FORCE influencing the organization of medical care in the United States, the American Public Health Association has reflected the larger social environment around it. The professional health workers who make up its ranks have inevitably brought with them into the Association the attitudes, restraints, or enthusiasms shaped by their job experiences. These attitudes have, in turn, formulated APHA positions and actions—at times crusading, at other times in conservative compliance with dominant social pressures.

The story of APHA influence on medical care in America, therefore, is not entirely a saga of courageous and forward movement. It is a story with ups and downs, in relation to the social and political climate of the day. It is a story also that reflects internal conflicts within the Association—contention between the voices of conservatism and those advocating change. Perhaps because medical care, more than most other components of health service, involves issues between private and governmental power, the course of events surrounding it within APHA has been a sensitive barometer to larger social and political forces.

Chapter 3 originally appeared as "The American Public Health Association as a Force for Change in Medical Care" in *Medical Care,* 11:338–351, July–August, 1973, and is reprinted by permission of that journal.

Early Decades

For the first 40 years after its founding in 1872, the American Public Health Association was dedicated exclusively to the prevention of disease. At the time, of course, this was a controversial task, for there was plenty of opposition to the social actions necessary for achievement of a sanitary environment and for control of the communicable diseases. The year 1872, as George Rosen has pointed out, was also a time when the Marine Hospital Service was reorganized and steps were taken to establish a federal public health authority—a subject discussed at this first Association meeting.[19]

It was not until 1910 that any stream of interest appeared in the APHA relating to the general health needs of people, especially the poor, aside from the organized prevention of disease. This was the same type of ideological current which a generation later gave rise to the robust movement that we now think of as "medical care." By 1910, America was rapidly growing in population and economic vitality, largely because of massive immigration from Europe. The cities became marked by working class slums, peopled by central Europeans, Italians, Irish, Germans, and others in search of a new life; there were those who fled from the famines in Ireland and the abortive 1905 revolution in Russia.

It was in this atmosphere that the field of social work arose. In several large cities, settlement houses were founded, and, in Boston around 1905, Richard Cabot pioneered the idea of medical social work—giving aid to poor patients seen at hospital clinics. Special interest groups had begun to take form in the APHA in 1899, with the initiation of the Laboratory Section, followed by the Vital Statistics Section and the Health Officers Section in 1908. Then, in 1910, a Sociological Section was founded in the APHA, evidently to give a voice to social workers and others who were concerned with the "social and economic aspects of (health) problems."[20] It is relevant that the first Workmen's Compensation Law for injured workers had been passed in New York State in that year, and the idea of social insurance for coping with the burden of sickness was beginning to diffuse to America from Europe. Indeed, in 1916, the Conference of State and Territorial Health Authorities, meeting in Washington, passed a resolution calling for state health insurance funds to cover all workers, and urging "close cooperation of the health insurance system with state, municipal, and local health departments and boards."[15] It does not appear that this viewpoint, however, was expressed within the APHA, where *municipal* public health officers were evidently the dominant group.

The Sociological Section, however, did not have a very robust life in the APHA. The dominant theme of the day was bacteriological control, and calls for social reform were not warmly received. The general pall of post-World War I conservatism ("back to normalcy") was reflected around 1919–20 in a violent rejection of "alien ideas" by the new leadership of the American Medical Association.[11] The effect of this professional climate was undoubtedly to constrain the scope of what local health officers considered proper for public health, both inside the APHA and on their jobs. Compounding these constraints was the rising influence of Freudian psychiatry, which turned the attention of social workers from social reform to individual casework. In 1920, the Committee on Municipal Public Health Practice was organized in the APHA, with a focus exclusively on sanitation and quarantine at the local city level (maternal and child health services, for example, were not considered). In this environment, it is no surprise that, by 1922, the APHA Sociological Section died a quiet death.

A few years later, nevertheless, the need for a broader view of public health, both functionally and geographically, became recognized. In 1921, the Sheppard-Towner Act was passed, providing federal grants to the states for establishing infant health clinics. Recognizing the boundaries of public health to be wider than the individual city, the Committee on Municipal Public Health Practice changed its name in 1925 to the Committee on Administrative Practice (CAP).[23] Indeed, a subcommittee of CAP which had worked since 1921 with the American Hospital Association on questions of handling communicable disease cases in hospitals was reorganized, in 1926, as a Subcommittee on Organized Care of the Sick, chaired by Michael M. Davis. This subcommittee's concern also became widened to consider more general questions like the community's need for hospital beds.[24]

In 1926, C.E.A. Winslow was President of the APHA, and the concept of the public health role had by then broadened a great deal in the minds of its enlightened leaders. The main thrust of Winslow's presidential address was actually to call on public health officers to concern themselves with the organization of medical care. He said:

> Future progress in the reduction of mortality and in the promotion of health and efficiency depends chiefly on the application of medical science to the early diagnosis and preventive treatment of disease. . . . In the last analysis, it will be the duty of the health officer of the future to see that the people under his charge, in city or country, in palace or tenement, have the opportunity of receiving such service and on terms which make it economically and psychologically easy of attainment.[26]

Depression Years and World War II

The tone of Winslow's address, however, suggested that he was making a plea to a skeptical audience, and subsequent events show that he really did not succeed. A few years later, in 1928, Winslow became Vice-Chairman of the Committee on the Costs of Medical Care. Despite the fact that the CCMC had issued 27 volumes by 1932, there is nothing in the APHA annals of those years to suggest that the public health movement became involved in the ideological battles that the CCMC helped to launch. By 1932, the nation was deep into the Great Depression, Roosevelt was elected, breadlines were long, and welfare rolls were heavy. In 1929, hospitalization insurance had been started (later called Blue Cross), and, in 1934, the Federal Emergency Relief Administration put the first federal monies into medical care of the poor, through grants to local welfare departments. In 1935, the first National Health Survey was launched with the aid of the WPA, revealing an enormous volume of sickness and unmet medical care needs among lower income groups. In that year also, the Social Security Act was passed, with Titles V and VI to strengthen state and local public health, MCH, and crippled children's services.

The fact that the APHA appeared to play very little if any part in these important medical care events of the 1930s is not hard to explain. The Association was clearly dominated in those years by local Health Officers. With no strong tradition of public health professionalism yet developed, most of these men were part-time or retired private medical practitioners. With some remarkable exceptions, their usual allegiance was to their fellow-doctors, not to the people. We have noted the conservative, even commercialized, ideology that came to characterize the private medical profession after 1920. As a result, the significant organizational developments in medical care occurring throughout the 1920s and most of the 1930s took place outside the world of public health. Medical care for the poor, health insurance, hospital regionalization, group medical practice plans—all these movements evolved under the auspices of other agencies. Even academic training for hospital administration, inaugurated in 1934, had to be located in a School of Business because the then-existent Schools of Public Health had no interest in such a field.

As the Depression wore on, however, and the New Deal matured, larger events began to have an influence in the APHA's attitude toward medical care. The first National Health Conference was held by a federal interdepartmental committee in Washington in 1938, and the *Journal* of the Association published a favorable editorial on this Conference's recommendations for great extension of health insurance plans. In 1939, the Committee on Administrative Practice began to reorganize its Subcommittee on Organized Care of the Sick, which had previously been rather weak, to give it greater strength. When Senator Wagner introduced the first National Health Bill, in 1939, calling for federal promotion of general health insurance plans in the states, APHA President Abel Wolman, a distinguished sanitary engineer, testified on behalf of the Association in favor of it. Dr. Haven Emerson, however, speaking as an individual testified against it; at the time, Emerson was a leading member of the CAP and he was manifestly, if not officially, a spokesman for the main body of local Health Officers in the APHA.

Thus, by the late 1930s and early 1940s, a schism was taking shape within the APHA between those who favored keeping public health out of the contentious arena of medical care and those who favored broadening public health's scope to include medical care. The former were evidently the large number of local Health Officers in the Association, and the latter were a minority of public health physicians and others mainly in the federal government and the universities. The anti-medical care forces tended to favor not only confinement of public health to the sphere of disease prevention, but also a general minimization of public as against private enterprise and of federal as against local authority.

Post-War Period

World War II had started in 1939 and, by 1943, discussion was beginning on post-war planning to help achieve the social benefits for which the war was supposed to have been fought. As part of the war effort, the Emergency Maternity and Infant Care (EMIC) program had been enacted, assigning to state health departments responsibility for administering obstetrical and pediatric services to the dependents of military men—a straight medical care task. Within APHA, a new sense of concern for medical care was expressed by still another reorganization of the CAP Subcommittee on Organized Care of the Sick, to widen its scope. Dr. Reginald Atwater, Executive Secretary, in an obvious attempt to reconcile the conflicting factions in the Association—as brought out in Viseltear's valuable study of primary sources[25]—proposed that the reconstituted unit be called a CAP "Subcommittee on Post-War Health Department Participation in Medical Services." The views of a dynamic federal public health worker, Dr. Joseph W. Mountin, prevailed, however, and the new unit was called simply the Subcommittee on Medical Care, with Mountin as its first Chairman. This was in 1943, and most important, the Subcommittee soon got financial support to maintain a full-time technical staff.

In my opinion this action in 1943 was the important turning point in APHA's hundred-year history, launching its involvement in a significant way in the American movement for improved organization of medical care. From this time forward to the present, APHA has functioned as a force for change in medical care in the United States. The influence has not always been powerful, nor unified, but it clearly has been in the direction of increasing the social organization of medical services, strengthening public as against private responsibility, achieving greater equity between rich and poor, and elevating the standards of care for all.

The first major achievement of the Subcommittee on Medical Care was the formulation of a now classic policy statement on "Medical Care in a National Health Program," which was adopted by the Association in 1944.[4] There was strong opposition to this statement by Emerson, Wilson Smillie, and other spokesmen for the traditional Health Officers, but it was adopted by a solid majority of the Governing Council. Perhaps this defeat for the "old guard" was a harbinger of future developments in the American medical care movement, which—as in the 1930s and 1940s—have continued to take place, as we shall see, mainly outside the bailiwick of local health departments.

The post-war years set in motion many important currents relevant to medical care. Stimulated by the several proposals for national health insurance (through the Wagner-Murray-Dingell bills in several versions), the voluntary health insurance movement gained great momentum. One title of the original W-M-D Bill, for federal subsidy of local hospital construction, was enacted as the Hill-Burton Act in 1946, and its administration was, indeed, assigned to state health departments. Public assistance medical care programs expanded, as did the federal program for veterans. Low income farm families and migrant agricultural workers became the beneficiaries of special medical care programs. With thousands of young doctors returning from military service to build a new professional life, group medical practice increased. All these currents generated an increasing body of health workers concerned about the problems of medical care organization and administration.

The APHA Subcommittee on Medical Care made important contributions to technical knowledge through a series of policy statements on various facets of the field. The first was in 1947 on "Planning for the Chronically Ill"—a set of recommendations formulated jointly with the American Hospital Association, the American Medical Association, and the American Public Welfare Association.[5] Further policy statements, some done jointly with other national organizations, were issued over the next 5 years on "Coordination of Hospitals and Health Departments" (1948), "The Quality of Medical Care in a National Health Program" (1949), and "Tax-supported Medical Care for the Needy" (1952). The Subcommittee also gave technical advice on medical care problems in selected communities, did research (e.g., "Medical Care Activities in Local Health Departments," 1949), issued several annotated bibliographies, and stimulated the establishment of other influential bodies, like the national Commission on Chronic Illness (1949).

Technical contributions, however, were not enough to respond to the mounting demands for discussions of medical care issues by the growing number of health workers in this field. Some outlet for these demands was provided by other organizations, such as the Physicians Forum or the Cooperative Health Association of America (both started around 1940) or even to some extent the American Hospital Association as well as various consumer organizations of workers or farmers. But in the APHA itself, the appropriate forum for discussion of medical care issues was the Health Officers Section, and the leaders of this prestigious unit were not very friendly to the idea of discussing medical care issues at their annual sessions. As one of the young Turks eager to discuss the struggles surrounding rural medical care in those days, I remember vividly these repeated rejections from the Health Officers group. Even the *Journal* of the APHA, under the fine editorship of Dr. Winslow, did not seem to have sufficient space for medical care articles, and in 1947 some of us attempted to launch a new "Journal of Social Medicine"—this verv attempt, in fact, leading to a broader policy in the APHA *Journal*.

The Medical Care Section

In this atmosphere, it was inevitable that steps would be taken to organize a Section on Medical Care in the APHA, where a hospitable forum could be provided for discussion of this whole dynamic field. Such had been the history of growth of other special fields within the Association, from the founding of the Laboratory Section in 1899, to the Dental Health Section in 1943. For those of us interested in the idea, it was not an easy battle, because we faced not only the opposition of the Health Officers, but even of many of our friends who feared that this would be a disruptive move in the Association. Eventually, however, the idea attracted adherents, most important of whom were Dr. Martha Eliot, as President-Elect of the Association in 1947, and Dr. Joseph Mountin as Chairman of the CAP Subcommittee on Medical Care. Perhaps it was some of the strain between the Subcommittee and its parent CAP, dominated by traditional Health Officers, that led Dr. Mountin to throw the resources of his Subcommittee staff (especially Dr. Milton Terris) in back of an organized effort to create a Medical Care Section. The details of these events have been well recounted by Viseltear.[25] In any event, a Medical Care Section was established by vote of the Governing Council in 1948.

Immediately, the new Section grew rapidly in membership, not so much by drawing persons from other sections (although many came from the "Unaffiliated" group), as by bringing new blood into the Association. Never had a new section in APHA expanded so rapidly. Within a few years it passed the 1,000 mark, in 1965 it outstripped the enrollment of the Health Officers Section, and, by 1966, with 2,163 members, it had grown to be the largest section in the entire Association. The vitality and also the scholarly quality of papers presented at the annual meetings exceeded the expectations of the Section's most earnest promoters. These sessions, it is fair to say, became the high points of many of the annual APHA conventions, attracting listeners from throughout this large multidisciplinary association.

This popularity and growth of the APHA Medical Care Section contributed to American health developments not only by providing an opportunity for exchange of technical ideas in a complex field. More important perhaps, it clarified to many skeptics that discussion of problems in the organization of medical care could be held in a spirit of scientific objectivity—as constructively or more so than discussion in other sectors of the public health field. Before 1948, in spite of the scholarly quality of the CCMC reports and much other research, there had been a common tendency in public health circles, not to mention clinical medicine, to regard medical care as a matter only for political haggling. These views were soon dissipated by an impressive output of scientific papers, analyzing America's medical care problems. Some sessions at annual APHA meetings were devoted to selected topics, like prepaid group practice or medical care of the poor, while others were open to contributed papers about any subject on which scientific work could be reported.

Not that the founding of an APHA Medical Care Section suddenly removed the field from political controversy. Far from it; the early 1950s were a conservative era in American life, with the rise of McCarthyism, the Cold War and the hot one in Korea, a placid Presidency from 1952 to 1960, and more. One small but significant reflection of the times was my own experience as a Consultant to the Subcommittee on Medical Care, with respect to a policy statement on "Federal-State-Local Relationship in a National Health Program." I was engaged to draft this statement in 1948, working jointly with representatives of the Health Officers Section. The document, which attempted to outline how state and local health departments would function under federal standards in administration of a nationwide health insurance program, went through no less than seven drafts. By the time the seventh draft was finally approved by the Subcommittee in 1952, the general political atmosphere had changed so much that the statement no longer seemed appropriate; it was quietly filed away and never presented for CAP or Governing Council approval. In 1957, as outgoing Chairman of the Medical Care Section, after commenting on a past decade of achievements I felt compelled to say:

> I would not want to give the impression that all is now milk and honey in the relationships between medical care organization and the rest of the public health movement. There are still many public health workers, within government and in voluntary agencies, who look upon medical care as dangerous territory.[17]

The Apprehensive 1950s

In spite of this continuing apprehension about medical care in the overall public health movement, the 1950s yielded further maturation of the field. The Medical Care Section in APHA gave it legitimacy and respectability, so that workers and scholars on medical care problems did not have to fear epithets about "plotting to bring about socialized medicine." As an offshoot of the Section, the Committee on Medical Care Teaching (only later affiliating with the Association of Teachers of Preventive Medicine) brought out in these years the first standard textbook in the field: *Readings in Medical Care,* 1958.[12] Additional policy statements were issued, mainly on medical care of the needy and on relationships between public health and social welfare agencies. Numerous resolutions on medical care were passed which, if they did not visibly influence public policy, helped to educate many public health workers.

Most important, perhaps, was the influence of the new influx of Medical Care Section members in stimulating the established leadership of the Association to reexamine the goals of the entire field. The theme of the 1955 Convention was "Where Are We Going in Public Health?" and the next year, after a soul-searching conference at Arden House, New York, the whole Association was reorganized. Among other things, the Committee on Administrative Practice, which had restrained the efforts of its Subcommittee on Medical Care, was eliminated. Under a new Technical Development Board, several Program Area Committees were established in 1957, including one on Medical Care.

The Program Area Committee on Medical Care did not actually produce so many policy statements as its more constrained predecessor, perhaps because it was no longer a group fighting an uphill battle. A policy statement adapted by the Association, in 1959, on the "Public Health Role in Medical Care" was really much more modest than the clarion call of 1944, and simply said that "whether or not a health department will be given responsibility for the administration of such (medical care) programs should be left to the discretion of each state or local government."[7] Likewise a statement adopted, in 1963, on "The Organization of Medical Care and the Health of the Nation" called mainly for better coordination of personal health services at the local level.[9] It did not demand national health insurance but only that "prepayment and other types of medical care financing must be expanded."

The Energetic 1960s

With the election of President Kennedy in 1960, the dignity with which the APHA had helped to endow the medical care movement exerted a visible influence on the federal health establishment. For the first time, in 1962, a Medical Care Administration Branch was established at a fairly high level in the U.S. Public Health Service, evolving by 1965 into a Medical Care Division. The close relationship between this federal office and the APHA is reflected by the publication between 1964 and 1967 of the three-volume book, *Medical Care in Transition,* based entirely on articles published over the years in the *American Journal of Public Health* (most of them emanating from presentations before the Medical Care Section).[22] These volumes, like the earlier *Readings,* helped to establish the scholarly quality of the medical care field, to facilitate training of administrative personnel, and ultimately to influence public policy.

The crucial medical care event of the 1960s in America was undoubtedly the enactment of Titles XVIII and XIX in the Social Security Act—Medicare and Medicaid. The rising costs of medical care, the aging of the population, and the inadequate coverage of the aged by voluntary health insurance were the main forces in back of this 1965 legislation. For better or for worse, however, one cannot attribute either the enactment or the content of this legislation to the APHA. With the strong voice that medical care specialists had attained in the Association by the mid-1960s, the APHA testified favorably before Congress on the proposed bill, but the public health movement as a whole did not really promote its enactment. In the face of bitter opposition from the American Medical Association, state and local health officers remained essentially silent. Whatever the basic causes, once again history passed the public health agencies by, and the administration of Medicare was assigned to the Social Security Administration and a network of fiscal intermediaries drawn from the world of private health insurance. Medicaid remained almost everywhere in welfare departments. Except for their now established role in hospital licensure under the Hill-Burton program, the state Health Departments might not have been given their modest duties to certify institutional providers under the Medicare program.

Other important medical care developments of the 1960s were the rise in 1964 of "neighborhood health centers" (as part of the rediscovery of poverty in America and the launching of a "war" against it), the Regional Medical Program for Heart Disease, Cancer, and Stroke (RMP) in 1965, and the Comprehensive Health Planning (CHP) legislation in 1966. Time does not permit discussion of these programs—all three involving an extension of governmental responsibility for medical care—and the relationship of the APHA to them, but it may simply be noted that each of them has been entrusted mainly to agencies other than the Health Department. One is reminded of the evolution of the British National Health Service two decades earlier, when the significant responsibilities were assigned to the established hospitals (through Regional Hospital Boards), to the previously existent insurance committees (through Executive Councils), and to academic centers (through Teaching Hospitals), while the scope of local public health authorities was somewhat reduced. Correspondingly, the OEO "neighborhood health centers," and even later offshoots sponsored by the Department of HEW, were operated by various new community bodies; the RMP activities went mainly to medical schools; and the CHP program—while often under State Health Departments at the state level—was assigned at the all-important local or "area-wide" level to local hospital councils or their offshoots.

This bypassing of the traditional public health agencies created further administrative fragmentation in the already superpluralistic American health service system, but it fortunately did not weaken the APHA. In fact, personnel from the new medical care programs simply joined the APHA, swelling the ranks of the

Medical Care Section. In a study by Anzel and Roemer of the membership of the Medical Care Section in 1967, 82 percent of members were found to come from agencies other than health departments at all levels (local, state, national, or international).[18] The distribution of 1,480 members who responded to our questionnaire was as follows:

Type of Agency or Program	*Percentage of Members*
Public health agencies (all levels)	17.8
Other government agencies	6.9
Health insurance programs (all types)	13.1
Voluntary health associations	7.0
Health planning agencies (all levels)	6.8
Hospitals and clinics	27.4
Academic institutions	20.3
Agency unspecified	0.3
All types of agency	100.0

This influx of health workers into the APHA from many sources outside the local and state Health Departments doubtless added to the overall vitality of the Association. Formal recognition of this input, in a sense, was given by election to the Presidency of the Association, in 1966, of Dr. Milton Terris, a man proposed formally by the Medical Care Section in recognition of his key role in the founding and early development of the Section.

The resolutions passed at Annual APHA Conventions were no longer confined to topics within the traditional bailiwick of Health Departments, but were addressed to problems like:

- Home care of the sick (1952)
- Diagnostic and treatment centers in rural areas (1959)
- Use of drugs in public medical care programs (1960)
- High quality health services for the aged (1961)
- The Civil Rights Act in relation to medical care (1966)
- Neighborhood health centers (1969)
- The consumer and comprehensive health care (1970)

The influence of resolutions by professional associations on public policy determination is anybody's guess, but they surely play some part in defining the political atmosphere of the health field. The color of APHA resolutions since about 1960, when the voice of medical care advocates in the Association began to be fairly strong, has clearly been on the liberal side of the sociopolitical spectrum. In this sense, respectability and legitimacy are given to viewpoints which, in an earlier period, were regarded as dangerous or deviant.

The Program Area Committee on Medical Care meanwhile continued its technical outputs. A policy statement on "The Local Health Department—Services and Responsibilities" issued in 1963 and listing "medical care" as the first among numerous functions—a far cry from "the basic six" of 1943—reflected the influence of this Committee.[8] Likewise one sees the influence of the Committee in the Policy Statement on "The State Public Health Agency" issued by the Association in 1965.[10] In 1965, the Program Area Committee produced *A Guide to Medical Care Administration: Concepts and Principles,* which did much to establish technical standards,[16] equivalent at least in intent to such APHA staples as *The Control of Communicable Disease in Man* or *Standard Methods for the Examination of Dairy Products.* In 1969, a second volume of this *Guide* was produced, devoted to "Medical Care Appraisal—Quality and Utilization," a contribution which has done much to eliminate the mystique from the task of evaluating the quality of medical care.[14]

Professional journals add to the vitality and continuity of any technical field. In 1940, Michael Davis had founded the first national journal of *Medical Care,* but it lasted only 4 years. Then in 1963, British colleagues took up the challenge and produced another such journal, which also lasted only a few years. Then in 1967, the APHA Medical Care Section undertook sponsorship of the current journal, *Medical Care,* which seems to be enjoying robust health and to be exerting a positive educational influence. Another distinct contribution of APHA to the medical care movement has been a series of "Faculty Institutes on Medical Care" held each summer since 1969, at which teachers from medical schools and other educational institutions have learned about this field—better preparing them for enlightening their students.

The "Health Crisis" and Recent Events

When Comprehensive Health Planning legislation was enacted in 1966, the APHA Technical Development Board brought together the Program Area Committee on Medical Care and its sister Committee on Public Health Administration to issue "Guidelines for Organizing State and Areawide Community Health Planning."[2] The CHP field, whose personnel were originally welcomed mainly into the Medical Care Section, eventually gained sufficient identity to form a new Section on Community Health Planning in 1969. With the new wave of interest in a nationwide health insurance program, emerging in 1969—as an aftermath of Medicare, precipitous rising costs, and White House recognition of a national "health crisis"—the APHA issued still another official policy statement on "A Medical Program for the Nation."[6] Like its antecedents, this statement has helped to align public health workers with the forces for social change in the structure of American health services. The ideological development was carried still further, with "A National Program for Personal Health Services" passed by the APHA Governing Council in 1970.[1]

Once again in 1969, the APHA felt it was time to reexamine itself in relation to the needs of the country's health services, and there can be no doubt that the widely heralded "crisis" in health care played a large part in this decision. Following another planning conference (more spirited perhaps than the Arden House session of 1956), the Association was again reorganized with a new Constitution in 1970. Under the new Constitution, it is significant to note, there is no longer a technical committee on "medical care" nor on "public health administration," but rather a single Council on Personal Health Services. Thus, it took nearly 30 years from the establishment of the Subcommittee on Medical Care under the Committee on Administrative Practice—dominated by local public health officers—for the two fields of "public health" (read: "preventive service") and "medical care" to become firmly unified in the technical structure of the APHA.

We are too close to the origins of the Council on Personal Health Services (on which I am pleased to be serving as one of the initial members) to have perspective on its contributions. A policy statement of the Council, on "Health Maintenance Organizations" issued in 1971, may perhaps influence the formulation of federal legislation currently pending in this field.[3] Other current issues, like "peer review," "consumer participation," "proprietary facilities," and so on are on the agenda of the Council, and are generating technical reports passed along to the APHA Action Board, also established under the new Constitution.

Another relevant APHA development to be noted is the founding in 1971 of a New Professional Health Workers Section. The constituency of this section is mainly from the ranks of allied health workers in neighborhood health centers and other programs generated in response to medical care needs. Its influence is not yet clear, but one can assume that it will be exerted on the side of democratization of the control of health services of every type.

Conclusions

What, then, has been the impact of the American Public Health Association as a force for change in the medical care realities of the United States? To answer this question, one must first realize that, as this paper has attempted to show, the APHA has not always been of one voice on the social issues involved in medical care. From as far back at least as 1910, there have been forces within APHA pressing for conservation of the status quo and other forces pressing for social change with respect to medical care. Inevitably, these forces have reflected the larger environment in which the members of the Association have lived and worked. They have also reflected the dominant political climate of the period. The play of these forces is as evident today as in the past, although the relative strengths of the contending sides are different.

In general, so far as medical care organization is concerned, the pressure for conservatism has emanated from members of the Association who have identified themselves principally with the private medical profession. For many reasons documented elsewhere, the private physicians of America, particularly through their medical societies, have resisted the social organization of health services in general, and the enlargement of public responsibilities in particular.[13] Public health officials and their staffs who looked mainly to other local physicians for moral support, in a kind of medical fraternity spirit, usually have ended up opposing or counselling extreme caution in the modification of our system of medical care.

On the other hand, members of the Association who, for a variety of reasons, identified mainly with groups other than the private doctors of the nation, have constituted the forces for changing the system. The reasons have come from the types of professional position they hold, the agencies they work for, the constituencies of their programs, and perhaps the overall national political climate when they came of age and when their own philosophies were shaped (consider the generational effects of the "dirty thirties," the "silent fifties," or the "activist sixties"). Whatever the causes, it is evident that since about 1940, an increasing proportion of the members of the APHA have come to identify with the American people as a whole, rather than with any of the private health-related professions. There were some ups and downs in this trend during the 1950s as noted earlier, but the general direction has surely been upward. With this has come an enlarging voice in the APHA for changes in the medical care system, for more public as against private initiatives, for greater federal vs. local responsibilities, for wider social vs. individualistic definitions of rights—in a word, for the people in contrast to the elite.

As this progressive voice within the APHA has become stronger, the Association has—in a sort of social equilibrium—responded by exerting larger influences on its environment. By providing a national forum for discussing activities, research, and viewpoints on medical care, it has added to understanding and disseminated knowledge in the field. Its formal policy statements have established professional criteria and standards on various aspects of medical care organization. Equally or even more important, the full and free discussion of medical care questions in the Association has given reassurance to workers in this field, who must still often face tough obstacles in their local settings. APHA's hospitality for medical care debate has lent dignity and respectability to a critically important aspect of human welfare which, for decades, had been considered too controversial for polite discussion.

In some ways, APHA's voice on medical care issues has perhaps influenced specific actions within government. The stronger place occupied by the medical care field in the U.S. Department of Health, Education, and Welfare is at least partly due to the influence of individuals tutored in the APHA environment. Testimony of APHA spokesmen on various legislative proposals has added to the support for certain innovations in medical care, such as the RMP or CHP programs or the amendments to Medicare. In state and local governments, the technical advice of APHA field services, most recently through CHAPS (Community Health Action Planning Service), has led to improvements in the public organization of medical care. In a general way, moreover, the medical care constituency in APHA—predominantly "left of center" as it proudly is—has added force to the pressures for social improvement in other fields as well, like family planning, prevention of lung cancer, anti-pollution measures, and the whole wave of consumerism in the health services.

Yet, in one important sector, APHA has failed to exert an influence which might have been possible. Deriving its original membership strength from workers in official public health agencies—health officers, nurses, sanitarians, statisticians, health educators, and others—the Association was theoretically in a position to channelize new public functions for improved medical care organization into the jurisdiction of these agencies. The important policy statement of 1944 on "Medical Care in a National Health Program" urged that:

> The public health agencies—federal, state and local—should carry major responsibilities in administering the health services of the future. . . . The existing public health agencies . . . may not be ready . . . to assume [these functions, but they] should be training themselves and their staffs. . . .

Now almost 30 years later, we cannot say that the important new programs for medical care have been lodged in Health Departments, even though public health vistas have widened. Whether this has been due to the lack of initiative by public health agencies, the more energetic voices of alternative bodies, or other factors, the result has been a further fragmentation of health service organization in the nation. The major spokesmen for prevention working in the state and local health departments have been largely divorced from the expanding programs of health insurance, medical care for the poor, health service regionalization, expanded primary and emergency care, and other facets of the medical care world.[21]

Was this a failure, or at least an unrealized opportunity, of the APHA? Can the development of most medical care programs in America outside of the Health Department's jurisdiction be attributed to the growth of a Medical Care Section in the Association separate from the Health Officers Section? Hardly so. The forces at play in the nation—in the medical profession, the hospitals, the universities, the different branches of government—were probably the main determinants of all the fragmentation. Yet, if the APHA had served as an arena in which Health Department spokesmen had become inspired to give more aggressive leadership on medical care issues, might the outcomes have been different? If medical care concepts had become absorbed within the Health Officers Section, might the posture of Health Departments toward these new programs have been different? I must leave this question for the reader to ponder.

A final note about medical care in the APHA—the very prominence achieved by the field in the last two or three decades has led many health leaders to reaffirm the primacy of prevention. One can only agree with this emphasis, but it does not follow that efforts to improve the financing and delivery of medical care are inconsistent with or contradictory to it. The importance of medical care stems basically from the inadequacy or failures of prevention. The fight for better medical care in the APHA and elsewhere has always been a fight for prevention as well, for the earliest intervention in a disease which has not been averted, for a personal health service delivery system which would integrate prevention and treatment.

There are, as we all know, plenty of unfinished battles in the American medical care scene. To press them is not to ignore the enormous importance of a better physical and social environment, an economy that provides full employment, decent housing, civil rights, and a world at peace. In fact, the fight for better medical care is a part of the whole social struggle for attaining all these larger goals, and a challenge that will continue to face the American Public Health Association in its next 100 years.

References

1. American Public Health Association: A national program for personal health services. *Am. J. Public Health* 61:191, 1971.
2. ———: Guidelines for organizing state and area-wide community health planning. *Am. J. Public Health* 56:2139, 1966.
3. ———: Health maintenance organizations: A policy paper. *Am. J. Public Health* 61:2528, 1971.
4. ———: Medical care in a national health program. *Am. J. Public Health* 34:1252, 1944.
5. ———: Planning for the chronically ill. *Am. J. Public Health* 37:1256, 1947.
6. ———: Policy statement: A medical program for the nation. *Am. J. Public Health* 60:189, 1970.
7. ———: Policy statement: Public health role in medical care. *Am. J. Public Health* 49:1702, 1959.
8. ———: Policy statement: The local health department—services and responsibilities. *Am. J. Public Health* 54:131, 1964.
9. ———: The organization of medical care and the health of the nation. *Am. J. Public Health* 54:147, 1964.
10. ———: Policy statement: The state public health agency. *Am. J. Public Health* 55:2011, 1965.
11. Chapman, C. B., and Talmadge, J. M.: The evolution of the right to health concept in the United States. *The Pharos of Alpha Omega Alpha* 34:30, 1971.
12. Committee on Medical Care Teaching: Readings in Medical Care. Chapel Hill, University of North Carolina Press, 1958.
13. Cray, E.; In Failing Health: The Medical Crisis and the A.M.A. New York, Bobbs-Merrill Co., 1970.

14. Donabedian, A.: A Guide to Medical Care Administration: Medical Care Appraisal—Quality and Utilization. New York, American Public Health Association, Program Area Committee on Medical Care Administration, 1969.
15. Health Insurance: Report of Standing Committee Adopted by the Conference of State and Territorial Health Authorities with the United States Public Health Service. Washington, D. C., May 13, 1916, *Public Health Rep.* July 21, 1916; pp. 1919–1925.
16. Myers, B. A.: A Guide to Medical Care Administration: Concepts and Principles. New York, American Public Health Association, Program Area Committee on Medical Care Administration, 1965; revised 1969.
17. Roemer, M. I.: The Medical Care Section Completes Its Tenth Year. *In* Medical Care Section News Letter (American Public Health Association, New York), December 1957; p. 3.
18. Roemer, M. I., Anzel, D. M.: Medical care administrative positions in the United States: Analysis of the positions and agencies represented by the membership of the Medical Care Section of the American Public Health Association, 1967. *Med. Care* 6:78, 1968.
19. Rosen, G.: A History of Public Health. New York, MD Publications, 1958; pp. 248–249.
20. ———: The Sociological Section of the American Public Health Association, 1910–1922. *Am. J. Public Health* 12:2515, 1971.
21. Somers, Anne R.: Health Care in Transition: Directions for the Future. Chicago, Hospital Research and Educational Trust, 1971.
22. U. S. Public Health Service: Medical Care in Transition, vols. 1–3. Washington, Government Printing Office, 1964–1967.
23. Vaughan, H. F.: Local health services in the United States: The story of the CAP. *Am. J. Public Health* 62:95, 1972.
24. Viseltear, A. J.: Emergence of the Medical Care Section of the American Public Health Association, 1926–1948: A Chapter in the History of Medical Care in the United States, Washington: APHA, 1972.
25. *Ibid.*
26. Winslow, C.-E. A.: Public health at the crossroads. *Am. J. Public Health* 16:1075, 1926.

4

The Widening Scope of Governmental Health Programs

For a variety of reasons government has become more active in an increasing number of sectors of family life, including the health services. To acquire an overview of these trends, the Russell Sage Foundation supported a series of studies in 1966. Among these was the chapter presented below.

Seen from the perspective of the American family, one can identify public programs oriented to certain types of family, to families with certain disorders, or families needing certain types of services. But changes in American family life have their impacts on the nature of delivery of much health service. The net effect of these trends has been to increase both the quantity and quality of services available to families, in spite of the persistence of many unsolved problems and much unmet need.

ALL GOVERNMENTAL HEALTH programs in the United States affect the American family directly or indirectly and, since the general role of government in the health services has been expanding, the direction of the influence has been widening and deepening. The task is to examine these influences more closely, to analyze them into their component parts, to note the force and direction of each, and to estimate the nature of their impacts on family life.

We shall try to tackle this large task in ten sections as follows:

1. Introduction: The Role of Government
2. Programs Affecting the Entire Community
3. Programs Affecting Certain Types of Families
4. Programs Focused on Certain Diseases
5. Programs for Certain Modes of Service
6. Health Insurance
7. Important New Governmental Programs
8. Trends in Family Life Influencing Health Service
9. Broad Effects of Government on Family Health Services
10. Problems and Issues

Since the wide sweep of government has so many facets, it is evident that each of them will have to be treated rather superficially. It is hoped, however, that there will be no significant blind spots in the landscape.

Chapter 4 originally appeared as "Governmental Health Programs Affecting the American Family" in the *Journal of Marriage and the Family,* 29:40–63, February, 1967.

Introduction: The Role of Government

As in the meeting of other social needs, governmental agencies have tended to tackle health problems that were not being effectively solved by private or voluntary group efforts. This has entailed a changing spectrum of actions at the local (city or county), state, and federal levels, with the trend being increasingly toward greater responsibilities at the higher governmental levels.

The overall role of government in the health services, which has applied to preventive and therapeutic functions alike, has been to promote their social organization. (While this may seem too obvious to state, one of the harsh realities of social debate about government's role has been a view held by some that the "proper" role of government should be restricted to the preventive services, leaving the curative services entirely to private enterprise.) The nature of this organizing role is of four general sorts:

a. the direct, systematic provision of certain technical services, for example, the chlorination of a water supply or the provision of comprehensive medical care to military personnel;
b. the financial support for certain health services or related functions (like professional education or medical research) through use of tax funds, for example, purchasing medical care for the needy or granting money for the construction of hospitals;
c. the setting and enforcing of qualitative standards on the delivery of health services to populations, for example, requirements on the pasteurization of milk or the licensure of physicians to practice medicine;
d. the planning, coordinating, or technical consulting on health services offered or to be offered to people; for example, state-wide planning of hospital construction or giving advice to an industrial plant on the ventilation of toxic fumes.

It may be noted that all but the first of these four governmental roles involve relationships between governmental and nongovernmental health entities. This interplay of sources of power and control is one of the most striking features of government's role in American life. While such interplay is found to some extent in all modern nations, it is clearly an especially marked feature of the United States in the second half of the twentieth century.

This is not to say that the relationships between government and private or voluntary entities are always harmonious. Authority and controls are always somewhat difficult to bear, and when they are applied by government over nongovernmental actions, the irritations may be great. Voluntary health programs are often started with the avowed intent of forestalling governmental measures. In general, private agencies espouse a preference for local or state as against federal governmental controls. Yet the relationships of private to official sectors have steadily increased, and the overall vitality of entities like voluntary hospitals or visiting nurse agencies has actually been strengthened by reason of governmental economic support and standards.

Focusing more particularly on the family side of the question posed in this chapter, one can identify various channels through which government has an impact on families. These channels are of four types:

1. programs affecting all or virtually all families in a community;
2. programs affecting only certain types of families, defined by specific demographic or social rules;
3. programs affecting directly only families with certain specific diseases (although the indirect benefits may, of course, fan out to entire populations);
4. programs affecting only families in need of certain technical modalities of service.

There is inevitably a certain intermingling of these channels, but this classification will help us examine the panorama of governmental health programs influencing families in the pages that follow.

Programs Affecting the Entire Community (All Families)

Unless one takes an artificial and detached view of "the family," the many governmental health activities which affect entire populations must be recognized first of all. Four such types of activity may be described.

Mass-oriented Preventive Services

The main thrust of governmental programs usually defined as "public health" is toward prevention of disease in total populations. Historically, the oldest of such actions involves the sanitation of the physical environment.

Millions of American families may take for granted the clean water coming from the kitchen or bathroom tap, but one need only pause for a moment on the problems of water haulage in a Latin American or Asian village to realize the effect on family life of public water systems. Without a public water system, delivering pure water into homes, a major share of family time—especially that of mothers and older children—must be spent in carrying water in jugs from a stream or spring, sometimes boiling it for potability, going long distances to a watering place for bathing or laundry, and so on. This is quite aside from the question of water treatment, filtration, chlorination, and so on to assure its freedom from pathogenic organisms.

Environmental sanitation in the modern community, of course, involves much beyond water supplies. Safe and effective sewage disposal is a central feature of a satisfactory standard of living for the great majority of American families. The gradually increasing urbanization of the nation has made this task technically easier, simply because it is feasible to operate a vast sewerage system more successfully through government than to enforce standards on the operation of thousands of separate family excreta-disposal units (septic tanks, pit privies, etc.)

among a dispersed rural population. Today the problems of urban waste disposal have entered a larger sphere of concern: pollution of streams and other bodies of water.

While urbanization and city governmental health actions have helped to improve water supply and excreta disposal enormously, city life has created other environmental problems for American families. Pollution of the atmosphere has become a major intrusion on both physical and mental health in metropolitan centers, even though the precise consequences are not yet fully understood. Because of atmospheric pollution, government is imposing increasing controls on industry, home incineration, and the automobile. Radiation hazards are also leading to new governmental surveillance and controls.

Large cities and industrialization have bred slums since the early nineteenth century. At that time the disease and misery among slum families of London, Paris, Berlin, and other European cities generated the impetus to the whole public health movement. In recent years, with the general affluence and satisfactory housing of the majority of American families, the deficiencies of blighted neighborhoods in the larger cities have become the more glaring. Aside from "urban renewal" projects, public health agencies have given new attention to housing inspections and enforcement of minimal housing standards. Control of rats, insects, and other disease-vectors is involved, as well as adequate ventilation, proper garbage disposal, and also minimum space per person in a dwelling. Sanitary control of restaurants, food stores, abattoirs, and other food establishments is another governmental activity in the modern city.

Urban life has also led to a high toll of accidents, which has summoned a great variety of governmental preventive efforts. While the automobile on the highway and the machine in the factory are the subjects of control by police authorities and departments of labor, accidents in the home are a source of concern to public health agencies. Infections and other fatal diseases have been so greatly reduced by public health and medical efforts that the chief cause of death in all American families today for individuals between the ages of one and 35 years is accidents. Doubtless, far greater efforts are needed by government both through control of the hazards of the environment and education of the fallible human being (especially the young) about safe behavior.

Health education on a wide spectrum of problems is another activity of government affecting virtually all families. Of course, many voluntary agencies offer such education also, often on one specific disease or another, but public health departments have an overriding responsibility. In recent years the discovery of cancer-producing effects of cigarette-smoking has led to governmental educational campaigns which, unfortunately, must buck the enticements of multimillion-dollar advertising by the private industrial sector. Most public school systems include elementary health education as a requirement in the curriculum.

School health services also include medical examination of children at intervals for the detection of physical or mental defects. These preventive services reach the 90-plus percentage of children attending schools (even parochial schools are often served by local health departments, while the public schools are covered by health sections of departments of education) and give clues to families on needed corrective treatments. While the usual technique is for the school authorities to simply notify families, many of which do not act on the advice because of ignorance or poverty, government has a wide sweep at early case-finding in the school-age groups.

Similar case-finding among adults is much less extensively carried out by governmental agencies, but here and there health departments offer "multiple screening" programs. The basic principle is use of a battery of laboratory and X-ray tests which may "screen out" possible cases of previously unrecognized disease (like diabetes, glaucoma, heart disease, kidney disease, anemia, etc.) without requiring a physician's time; positive cases are referred to physicians for definitive diagnosis and treatment. Other elements of chronic disease detection and treatment by governmental agencies will be discussed below.

Sound nutrition is, of course, a basic factor in good health, and the resources of government play varied roles in its promotion in families. Nutritional education is part of the program of public health, agricultural, and educational agencies. School lunch programs have a very wide impact, although it is greater on children from low-income families. Almost every family is affected, however, by legislation requiring the iodization of salt (for prevention of goiter) or the enrichment of flour with vitamin B, which is technically removed in the milling process.

A contentious public issue in recent years has surrounded another essential nutrient important in the formation of tooth enamel and, therefore, the prevention of dental caries. Flourine occurs naturally in the water supplies of many localities and in several foods but, like iodine, it is often in insufficient quantities to yield decay-resistant enamel. The most practical expedient to correct this lack has been to fluoridate (1 part of sodium fluoride per 1,000,000 parts of water) public water supplies. About one-quarter of the U.S. population have this benefit but, unfortunately, in many cities it has been made a matter of political debate (like vaccination or pasteurization decades before) and public referenda, in which grotesque arguments have been marshalled against this sound disease-preventive measure. There is also an important economic dimension to the issue, since families must now spend millions of dollars on dental care which could be used for other purposes if dental decay were prevented. Nevertheless, slow progress has been made, and, through governmental action, an increasing proportion of American families are being protected by water fluoridation from this hygienic and economic wastage. (The cost of water fluoridation in public systems is less than 50 cents per family per year.)

Another protective action of government, required unfortunately in a free enterprise medical economy, is control over the production, labeling, advertising, and distribution of drugs. The series of laws on this problem, beginning with the first federal Pure Food and Drug Law of 1906 and evolving through various amendments to the major ones of 1963 (following the Kefauver hearings and the "thalidomide" tragedies), constitute a saga of emerging social controls over the abuses of private commerce and profiteering. In spite of persistent claims that the pharmaceutical industry would "regulate itself," repeated mass human tragedies had to occur to convince legislators (both federal and state) that legal restraints were necessary. Current legislation at the federal level, regulating drugs in interstate commerce (the vast majority), gives families much greater protection against fraudulent or misleading claims than ever before, although a heavy burden of responsibility remains on the prescribing doctor insofar as drug costs are concerned. The new law not only places much more stringent controls on drug safety but also on the "efficacy" of drugs for particular diseases.

One of the bright trends in drug consumption in the United States is the gradual relative decline in purchase of self-prescribed patent medicines, compared with medically prescribed items. This is doubtless a function not only of federal and state regulatory laws, but also greatly heightened access of families to physicians' care, along with more discriminating behavior due to education. For low-income families, meagerly protected by health insurance, however, self-prescribed potions are still all too often a cheap substitute for proper medical attention.

Finally, among the mass-oriented preventive services affecting all families is the whole gamut of governmental programs on the control of communicable diseases. Compulsory vaccination laws and quasi-compulsory requirements on diphtheria, tetanus, and even poliomyelitis immunization (making this a requirement for school attendance, which is, in turn, compulsory) have undoubtedly been responsible for the great reduction (almost eradication) of these diseases which once decimated families, especially their children. The ordinary public health agency requirements on reporting, isolating, and quarantining specific infectious diseases benefit, of course, the entire community. Most of these governmental regulations are on a local or state basis, but national "model codes" have made them nearly uniform across the country. In some governmental programs (to be reviewed below) the prevention of specific communicable diseases through isolation or immunization is done directly by units of government for certain populations, but the legal requirements cited here have their impact on the total population of the nation.

Health Facility Construction

Less dramatic perhaps among the governmental health programs affecting all families are those concerned with the construction of health facilities. The general hospital has increasingly become a center for medical care in a community, not only for the bed care of the seriously sick, but for the complex diagnosis and treatment of even ambulatory patients. It is also an important center for professional education in the health field (physicians, nurses, technicians, etc.) and medical research as well as preventive case-finding services. The construction of general hospitals in some reasonable relation to population needs, therefore, is a basic necessity for modern family health protection, and government has played an increasing role in this task.

Quite aside from special hospitals for the poor (to be considered below) or special hospitals for designated diseases like psychoses or tuberculosis (also reviewed below), hundreds of counties or cities have constructed general hopsitals to serve the entire local population. The great majority of general hopsitals in America, it is true (contrary to Europe), have been built by church groups or other voluntary bodies, but in the less affluent rural counties—especially in the South and Midwest—the only unit with economic resources sufficient to build and operate a general hospital has often been local government. In some states, like Kansas or California, special "hospital districts" have been authorized by law, with taxing powers to raise the money necessary to build needed general hopsitals serving everyone.

More sweeping in its impact on all families has been the federal governmental program, starting in 1946, for subsidy of construction of nonprofit general and allied types of hospitals throughout the nation. The national Hospital Survey and Construction Act (Hill-Burton) has facilitated construction or expansion of hundreds of general short-term hospitals, long-term hospitals, health centers, and other facilities serving total populations in areas of previous hospital-bed deficiency. Top priority has gone to localities of greatest bed shortage, which has meant mainly rural counties and newly settled suburbias. The federal law provides one-third of the construction costs, according to specified minimal standards; but about a dozen states have matched this with a second third from state tax funds, so that the local sponsoring group need only finance the residual one-third of the hospital building costs. The effect of this program has been to equalize access to hospital beds among rich and poor areas, and it does not take much imagination to appreciate how this has benefited American families.

A corollary of this governmental program has been the requirement that each state agency (usually the state health department) must first develop a state-wide "master plan" indicating where there are relative bed shortages in relation to defined standards, i.e., bed-population ratios. This legal proviso has stimulated the entire field of "area-wide hospital planning" with overflow influences on voluntary nongovernmental hospital planning—so that, with or without governmental subsidy, hospitals are being more intelligently planned in relation to family needs. The whole field of area-wide hospital planning is now in great ferment because of increasing community costs of hospitalization, the possibilities of abuse under widespread insurance support, and the increasing realization that the supply of beds in an area is the ultimate determinant of the hospital utilization rate (and therefore expenditures) by a population. We are currently in a national debate between the advocates of "voluntary planning" and governmental franchising of all hospitals. The straws in the wind point to the latter eventual solution, as we approach the time when virtually all hospital operating costs are supported by varied forms of social financing.

Health Profession Standards

Another health function of government affecting all families is in the field of licensure of personnel and facilities. Although the function of professional licensure is sometimes confused between the competitive craft interests of the practitioner and the safety of the patient, there can be no doubt that the latter is its ultimate objective and legal justification.

In the United States (unlike most other countries), the licensure of physicians, nurses, and other members of the "healing arts" is a responsibility of state rather than national government. The policies of the hundreds of state licensure boards (usually separate ones for each of the occupations) are seldom before the public eye, but they obviously provide a quiet underpinning to protect the quality of medical care available to families. Unfortunately, sometimes these authorities have been used to reduce the inflow of physicians or dentists into a state (for the competitive advantage of the local practitioners) rather than to uphold technical standards, but on the whole the latter purpose has been served. Another problem involves the licensure of outright cultists, like chiropractors or naturopaths, or complex professions-in-transition like osteopathy. We are still emerging from a period of nineteenth-century "liberalism" when the law looked upon almost every brand of healing as entitled to sell its wares (the courts often saying that they would not take sides in a scientific squabble). The trend, however, seems to be toward more rigorous protective standards in which lawmakers are recognizing science as a single set of principles rather than one of several competing doctrines.

The methods of achieving these higher standards for protection of people against poor-quality or harmful healing practices have been varied. In some states there are "basic science examinations" which must be passed by candidates for licensure in *any* of the medical arts, and many of the most poorly educated cultists have been obstructed by these. In other states the general severity of the examinations has been increased. In California an important move was made in 1962 with the absorption into "regular" medicine of the entire field of osteopathy, thereby raising its future licensure requirements to those of holders of the M.D. degree. Hand in hand with these governmental quality screenings have been numerous voluntary programs, like that of the National Board of Medical Examiners, Inc., or the more recent special program for testing graduates of foreign medical schools who come to American hospitals for internship or residency training. Up to now, the entire field of "certification" of the medical and surgical specialties has been left entirely to nongovernmental initiative. But the interplay of governmental and private sectors is well illustrated by this field, in that numerous governmental programs, e.g., crippled children's services or workmen's compensation, adopt among their requirements certification by these nongovernmental "specialty boards."

While licensure of physicians, dentists, and other primary healers has the longest history, as the years pass an increasing number of types of health practitioners is brought under the umbrella of state government surveillance. Nurses, pharmacists, optometrists, podiatrists, and other paramedical professions are also subject to state licensure. Newer health occupations, like physical and occupational therapists or laboratory and X-ray technicians, are licensed by some states and not others, leaving much of the social control to nongovernmental bodies. In the nursing field, in addition to the "registered nurse" (R.N.), there is state licensure for less thoroughly trained "vocational" or "practical" nurses. All these governmental programs help to set a minimum standard for the quality of practitioners serving families. The complexities of the 50 separate sets of state laws are reduced somewhat by extensive reciprocity among the states, but many would argue that the time has arrived for uniform national standards in all of the health disciplines.

The protection of public safety and health with respect to the work of the group-oriented health professions like hospital administrators or public health officers, in contrast to client-oriented health professions, is handled in other ways. Only one state now licenses hospital administrators (Minnesota), but reliance is usually placed on Civil Service merit systems for governmental posts and on citizen boards for voluntary agency posts. Organizations and agencies, moreover, do have more built-in checks and balances than the independent health practitioner in a private office.

Licensure authorities, nevertheless, have been applied increasingly to health facilities: to hospitals, nursing homes, laboratories, pharmacies, and so on. Every state now has a system of inspection and approval (often the word "licensure" is avoided) for hospitals and nursing homes, usually under the state department of public health. The principal requirements of these codes concern physical features—sanitation, space, fire hazards, etc.—although increasing attention is paid to functional matters, such as surgical operating rooms, laboratories, and even the organization of the medical staff. Unfortunately, most state agencies are not very well staffed with personnel skilled and effective at implementing the regulations. The new federal legislation on health insurance of the aged (see below) will doubtless lead to further strengthening of these quality-protecting programs as to both technical standards and their enforcement.

Medical Education and Research

Finally, among the governmental health programs having an impact on all families are the indirect but extremely important functions promotive of professional education and medical research.

Approximately half the schools of medicine in the United States are parts of state universities which are, of course, governmental entities. This use of state revenues has been an essential ingredient in the high quality of medical education in the United States, not to mention the quantitative output of doctors. The supply of doctors, in relation to population growth, has been almost stable or slightly downward in the United States over the last 50 years, so that the greatly increased demand for and provision of health services has been met mainly by vast increases in paramedical and auxiliary personnel. Nevertheless, a national shortage of doctors (once seriously debated) is now generally recognized to exist, and it would obviously be more severe without state governmental aid. Medical school operation is a very expensive undertaking; in New York State, for example, three private medical schools were saved from collapse in the last dozen years by conversion to governmental institutions. The training of dentists, pharmacists, and optometrists is also in large part carried out through state universities.

Nurses are the most numerous class of health personnel, and about 40 percent of the approximately 1,100 schools training them are entirely or partially governmental. The great majority of nurses are educated in hospital-based schools, which have numerous deficiencies. It is of interest that the movement to transfer nurse education to universities and junior colleges has been largely undertaken by governmental institutions.

With respect to both governmental and private schools of professional education, general subsidy from governmental grants has been steadily increasing. Starting with federal grants for the construction of research buildings in medical schools, this legislation has evolved toward subsidy of construction specifically for teaching purposes. In 1965 it came to include direct subsidy of teaching, i.e., faculty salaries, and student scholarships. The 1965 law also gives substantial federal support to schools of dentistry, optometry, and pharmacy. Nursing education is being supported through loans to nursing students (R.N. candidates) and full scholarships to candidates for master's degrees in nursing specialties. The graduate schools of public health, training various classes of community-oriented health personnel, are also being supported by increasing federal grants for both faculty salaries and student scholarships. This governmental support, it may be noted, not only serves to strengthen the whole system of health manpower production, but it also specifically fosters entrance of students from low-income families into the medical and paramedical professions.

Governmental support of medical and allied research has been expanding at an even greater tempo. The various National Institutes of Health in the United States Public Health Service have conducted their own internal research programs since about 1905, but since 1945 they have also sponsored research grants to universities, hospitals, and other local organizations throughout the country. By 1965 these research subsidies reached a level of about $1,000,000,000 a year in support of investigations on cancer, heart disease, mental disorder, arthritis, blindness, and virtually every other significant health problem. The proportionate emphases of this research subsidy have reflected the public will (as expressed through Congressional decisions), which may be expected in a democracy. Aside from this selection of priorities for support, among the infinite range of health problems on which research might be conducted, governmental grants have scrupulously avoided restriction of the methodological freedom of the investigator.

A point has now been reached where over half of the medical research being conducted in the nation's universities is supported by federal government grants or contracts. Not only does this advance knowledge, which may be eventually applied to the health service of families, but it supports indirectly the overall operation of the universities. The line between teaching and research in professional schools is increasingly difficult to draw, and the extension of research efforts through governmental aid enhances the quality of professional teachers and their teaching.

Programs Affecting Certain Types of Families

More specific in their impact on American families are a number of programs of organized health services sponsored by government for earmarked types of persons. Some of these programs have a distinctly "family" flavor, like that for medical care of the *dependents* of military personnel, but all of them influence family life directly or indirectly.

Medical Care for the Poor

The story of public responsibility for the survival of the poor, including their health care, is long and fascinating; only the highlights can be touched on. Evolving from succor by the Medieval Church, through town or county responsibility under the Elizabethan Poor Laws, toward the current policies of welfare department programs, agencies of government have taken increasing responsibility for the health protection of poor families. In the United States, the evolution of policy has been toward increasing support from higher levels of government (state and federal as against local), increasing objectivity in determination of eligibility of a person for public assistance, and increasing support for medical care. Responsibility is being shifted from the extended family (that is, relatives of the poor) to the total community through government.

The medical and related services financed by welfare agencies for indigent persons depend on their "category." Since the Social Security Act of 1935 and its numerous amendments over the years, federal grants to the states for public assistance are based on the identifiability of a needy person in one of four major classes: 1. over 65 years of age (old age assistance—OAA); 2. families with children and a lacking or unemployed breadwinner (aid to families with dependent children—AFDC); 3. blind persons (aid to the blind—AB); or 4. persons with "total and permanent" disability (aid to the totally disabled—ATD). This is an oversimplified classification, since there are many special qualifications of each category; but these definitions suggest the approach taken under current social policy. Needy persons who do not fit into one of these categories may be eligible for "general assistance" (GA) which must be supported entirely from state and local government funds. In 1960 a special new federal category, "medical assistance to the aged" (MAA), was added for support of medical services to low-income persons over 65 years who were still not poor enough to qualify for OAA status.

The range of medical services supported by government for these indigent persons varies among the categories and also varies greatly among the states and among local jurisdictions within a state. Generally speaking, the provision of hospital care is the largest sector in terms of expenditures. To some extent this reflects a policy of restricted benefits for the care of minor illness, so that the indigent person gets his first attention all too often only when his illness has reached a critical stage requiring hospital admission. Since medical as well as cash benefits require matching of federal grants from state funds, the scope of health services offered tends to be lowest in states of lower per capita income.

The application of tests of eligibility for public assistance is up to the states, and the definitions are relatively strict. In 1962, about 7,500,000 persons or only about 4 percent of the national population were receiving some form of public assistance. We know that there is a much larger percentage of the population who are of very low income and hard-pressed to finance proper medical care personally. Some of these so-called medically indigent persons may qualify for "general assistance," in fact, largely because of the high expense of a serious illness (especially when requiring hospitalization). Yet there is no doubt that the governmental welfare programs support a vast volume of medical care for the benefit of needy families. In the AFDC programs, reaching about 3,600,000 persons in 1962, the help to families and especially children is quite obvious. But even under the other categories, family health may also be protected either because the eligible person is a family member or because the support of medical expenses by government relieves relatives of a financial output required for other purposes.

Medical and hospital services for the poor are provided under three general patterns: 1. the indigent person may be seen by a personally chosen physician and hospitalized in an ordinary community hospital, with the expenses (fees or hospital charges) being paid by the welfare department; 2. he may be seen in a clinic of a voluntary hospital and hospitalized in a special ward for the poor in such a hospital, with complete or partial reimbursement of the hospital by the welfare agency; 3. he may be served in special governmental clinics and hospitals intended exclusively for the poor and often operated by special governmental authorities (separately from welfare departments). California and Louisiana are states which operate such special hospitals-for-the-indigent, on a state-wide basis; many large cities like New York or Chicago do likewise on a municipal basis.

There are special human and technical qualities to each of these patterns of medical care for the poor. The public clinics and public hospitals are typically crowded places, with little sensitivity to personal comfort or convenience, but often with a high quality of technical supervision. Many of these institutions are affiliated with medical schools and have highly trained physicians in charge. The private arrangements, on the other hand, may be more satisfactory on the human side and less on the scientific side. Some private physicians, with busy private practices, choose not to see welfare clients at all or, if they do, treat them in a perfunctory way. One of the challenges in the sector of organized health services is to retain the technical advantages of large specialized medical clinics and hospitals while, at the same time, recognizing the humanistic needs of patients. To some extent, this is simply a function of adequate financial support and staffing, so that doctors and other personnel will have enough time to devote to each patient.

Care for Mothers and Children

Aside from the children and mothers provided medical care through public assistance programs, these family members are protected by other special governmental services. A major feature of nearly every state and local public health agency program is the "maternal and child health" or MCH component. Great impetus has been given to these services by the dedicated leadership of the United States Children's Bureau, originally in the federal Department of Labor and now in the Department of Health, Education, and Welfare.

The typical local health department operates a series of "well-child conferences" or "well-baby clinics" in its area. Infants and preschool children are brought to these sessions for general examinations and immunizations, and their parents are given preventive health counseling, advice on child-feeding and child-rearing, and so on. The service seldom includes treatment of sickness, for which the mother is referred to a private physician or hospital clinic. While strict means tests are not usually applied for attendance at these clinics, their services are mainly sought by families of low or moderate income. In the nation as a whole, it is probable that no more than about 15 or 20 percent of newborn babies are reached through these programs, but their operation has helped to set a pattern for preventively oriented private pediatric care as well. Child health is also promoted by the home-visiting of public health nurses, devoted largely to instruction of mothers.

Prenatal and postpartum clinics are also held by public health agencies to protect the woman in pregnancy and lay the groundwork for a normal delivery. These tend to be less well developed services than those for children and more heavily concentrated among the poorest segment of families. Since the childbirth will ordinarily take place in a hospital, there is unfortunately a separation in most cases between the prenatal and obstetrical care, as to both doctor and location. Nevertheless, this preventive care of the pregnant woman has been associated with reduction of maternal mortality to very low levels in the United States (about 4 maternal deaths per 10,000 births). Through these clinics also, public health agencies in several states are offering advice on family planning, including contraceptive information and supplies. Further expansion of such birth control programs, under both governmental and voluntary auspices, may doubtless be expected, in response particularly to the needs of low-income families.

One aspect of maternal health in which government plays another role is the enforcement of laws regarding abortion. Medical interruption of pregnancy in nearly all states is illegal except to save the *life* of the mother. Yet hundreds of thousands of unwanted pregnancies occur each year in the United States, and it is estimated that at least 1,000,000 of them end in criminal abortions. The clandestine and sordid circumstances of these actions, not to mention their extortionist costs, lead to many cases of infection and hemorrhage and are responsible for a large portion of the maternal deaths that still occur. A few state laws permit therapeutic abortions in hospitals, with proper medical consultation, in order to preserve the *health* of the mother; but no American state permits interruption of pregnancy for the social well-being of the family. (Note: In 1973, a landmark decision of the U.S. Supreme Court legalized abortions nationally.)

School children are also entitled to certain health services throughout the United States, under the wing of government. It is usually the local boards of education that operate systems of health examination of pupils and first aid during school hours; sometimes local health departments operate these programs in the public schools as well as the parochial schools. While usually limited to case-detection rather than treatment, an occasional school health program includes special clinics for treatment of children from low-income families. These clinics may focus on conditions of vision or hearing which would directly impair classroom learning. The schools, of course, also offer instruction in healthful living, some of which may reach the parents through the child.

Care for Veterans and Military Dependents

One of the most extensive governmental health programs is that developed over the years for veterans of military service. A father served by this program can obviously be helped both medically and economically, with resultant benefits for his family.

This federal program operates through a system of special hospitals and clinics which are open to veterans with disabilities either connected or non-connected with military service. The latter conditions are treated only if hospitalization is required and only if the veteran states that private care would cause financial hardship, but this criterion is liberally interpreted. As a result, a substantial majority of patients in the 175 Veterans Administration hospitals on the average day are there for non-service-connected conditions. Many veteran patients are unattached men for whom the VA facility provides a kind of protective home in the absence of families. A high proportion also are men in the later years of life, who might otherwise be an economic and emotional burden on their children.

Military personnel on active duty are, of course, also entitled to medical services through a comprehensive governmental program that comes closer to full-scale "socialized medicine" than anything else in American life. The young men who return home from military service have been educated, in a sense, about sound preventive and therapeutic medicine in ways that may help them play their role as heads of families.

Since 1956, moreover, the United States Department of Defense provides a wide range of medical services for the family dependents of military personnel on active duty. This is an extension of the program of Emergency Maternity and Infant Care (EMIC) which was developed for military servicemen's wives and infants during World War II. The serviceman's family today may get care either at a military installation, if they live close by, or through free choice of private doctor and hospital, if they live elsewhere. This private care is paid by the Department of Defense, which uses local health insurance carriers as fiscal agents. The whole program is a valuable support for the military family, as well as a morale-booster for the men in uniform.

Care for Other Special Families

There are many other governmental health programs affecting special types of family. American Indians living in or close to reservations are served by a network of hospitals and clinics operated formerly by the U.S. Department of the Interior and now by the U.S. Public Health Service. While these free services may be small compensation for the land seizures and other injustices suffered by the ancestors of today's 500,000 Indians, they clearly help to improve the lot of these generally impoverished and isolated families.

Migrant agricultural workers and families are also beneficiaries of federal health assistance, through special grants to state and local agencies. During World War II, an entirely federal service was conducted for these families, but it was terminated in 1946. Then in 1960 when the plight of the migrant family was "rediscovered," the current program was launched through the grant-in-aid mechanism. Many of the local projects are of limited preventive scope, but some of them provide comprehensive physician's care and drugs through what the federal law defines as "family health clinics." State health departments also may give special attention to these families, beyond the scope of the federal subsidies.

Merchant seamen have been entitled to medical care, financed initially by wage deductions and now by federal tax funds, under a law passed in 1798. While his dependents are not covered, the seaman who is a breadwinner has the benefit of this care at all the major American ports as well as on board ship and overseas.

Most civilian employees of the federal government are now enrolled in health insurance plans, in which about half the premiums are paid by the government as employer. The Federal Employees Health Benefit program has established interesting administrative patterns, allowing each employee a choice of membership in a series of approved voluntary health insurance plans operating in his locality. Each federal agency pays the government share of the premium for its employees, but not for their dependents. While most of the medical care provided to these families is through regular local doctors and hospitals, the involvement of the government in the system has exerted a standard-setting effect on the operation of the many local insurance plans.

Programs Focused on Certain Diseases

Just as special types of persons may provide a basis for governmental health programs, special diseases may also lead to social action. The motives vary from fear to humanitarianism, but in all instances there are economic considerations. The diseases which have summoned governmental programs tend to be long-term and expensive, so that private initiative could not be counted on to cope with them.

Mental Illness

The impact of mental disorder on the individual and family can, of course, be totally disruptive, and psychiatric care is inherently a family-oriented health service. Here it need only be pointed out that governmental programs play an enormous role in coping with this problem. Over 90 percent of the 790,000 mental hospital beds in the United States are under governmental auspices, primarily in large state institutions. In recent years the character of these facilities has been changing from custodial to therapeutic in purpose, although there is still a long way to go. Governmental support—federal, state, and local—for ambulatory care of mental and emotional disorders has also been rapidly expanded, through a variety of special clinics for child guidance, adult crises, alcoholism, and general psychiatric service. The organization of governmental units for mental hygiene either within state departments of public health or separately has promoted both preventive and therapeutic approaches to mental problems in the schools, industry, courts, and everywhere that such problems can be identified.

Tuberculosis

In 1900 tuberculosis was the second cause of death in the United States, so that the stimulus for organized social action was great. Chronic and serious, with a high case-fatality rate, communicable, and destructive of family welfare, this disease of the lungs (though sometimes affecting other organs as well) led to social programs for treatment and prevention more intensive than for any other affliction in America. The initiative was taken by voluntary societies, but the size of the problem soon outstripped the capacities of "Christmas seal" sales campaigns. The major responsibilities came to be assumed by government.

The most expensive task was long-term hospitalization—for both treatment and isolation purposes—of persons with tuberculosis in an active stage, and hundreds of sanatoria were established and operated by state and local governments for this purpose. Later clinics for follow-up of discharged patients, epidemiological tracing of contacts, and general diagnostic work-ups were established by local health departments. With the perfection of the tuberculin test and the miniature chest X-ray, case-finding campaigns were launched among various susceptible population groups. Rehabilitation of the recovered patient was another activity. All these programs were still conducted to some extent by voluntary tuberculosis associations, but the proportionate role of government became increasingly great.

The general improvement of standards of living in the United States, along with these corrective measures, led to a gradual decline in the rate of death from tuberculosis after 1900. With the discovery of streptomycin and other drugs effective against the disease around 1950, the further decline in both deaths and cases became dramatic. The death rate declined to less than 5 per 100,000 persons per year, although the rate of diagnosed cases declined at a slower pace. Tuberculosis now is heavily concentrated among the very poor, where living conditions are wretched and medical diagnosis is often delayed. Yet, the overall problem has been so effectively reduced that virtual eradication of the disease begins to be a practical goal in the United States. Almost everywhere large tuberculosis sanatoria have declined greatly in occupancy levels, while a decade ago there were waiting lists of patients. Many sanatoria have closed down completely, and others have been converted to institutions for different purposes, such as general chronic disease hospitals. In fact, the rise of the problem of diversified long-term illness in the aged, coincident with the decline of tuberculosis in the young, has permitted an intelligent reallocation of social energies in most communities.

Venereal Disease

Diseases acquired through sexual contact are bound to be hidden, especially if the exposure is outside of marital relations. Yet the impact on family life can be profound, not only in the way that any disease may be disruptive, but especially because of the emotional overtones of syphilis and gonorrhea, the serious hazards to a marital partner of extramaritally acquired infection, the production of sterility by gonorrhea, and even the tragic affliction of congenital syphilis in a newborn baby. While voluntary agencies, like the American Social Hygiene Association (the euphemistic name of which reflected the practical problems of community action), tried to tackle these diseases for years, solid progress was not made until government entered the scene in the 1930s.

The United States Public Health Service took the initiative and brought the problems of syphilis and gonorrhea into the open. Through federal grants to the state health departments and technical advice, it promoted the organization of a vast network of clinics for diagnosis and treatment of venereal diseases, examination of contacts, health education, and so on. Improved methods of treatment were also promoted in the offices of private medical practitioners. Case-finding campaigns, through serological tests, were launched in industry. There were movements to suppress prostitution and to educate young people, mainly financed and conducted by governmental health agencies.

Evidence of improvement in the first decade of this effort was slight, because along with many cures came a parallel detection of new cases, concealing a decline of the morbidity rates. Prior to 1945 the therapy of both syphilis and gonorrhea was long, expensive, and not always effective. With the advent of penicillin in 1945, the morbidity picture changed radically. The reported cases of active syphilis fell sharply: from 180 per 100,000 population per year in 1943 to 13.7 in 1958. Federal government appropriations for tackling the problem had begun to decline in 1951, partly because of the success in reducing the disease and partly because of the smaller cost of penicillin therapy. In fact, many venereal disease clinics closed down, since the simplicity of penicillin therapy made the problem manageable both technically and economically in the usual private practitioner's office.

After 1958, however, the rate of reported cases of syphilis and gonorrhea began to rise again, and the problem was viewed with alarm. By 1963, the rate of new syphilis cases had climbed back up to 22.0 per 100,000, which was still far lower than the figures of the 1940s but a reminder that the problem was not yet beaten. As in the past, the cases are heavily concentrated in the nonwhite races, although this may be to some degree an artifact of non-reporting by doctors for white patients seen in private offices. Public health agencies are now taking renewed interest in the venereal infections, and federal appropriations are up again. The reasons for the resurgence of the infections are not entirely clear, but they are believed related both to the biological development of bacterial resistance to the antibiotic drugs and to changed patterns of sexual behavior. In any event, the role of government—principally public health agencies—in venereal disease control is currently an active one again, especially in urban slums with congested Negro populations.

Physical Handicaps

The crippled child or adult has long provoked reactions combining pity and aversion. Families are obviously affected deeply by either a handicapped child or parent, and social measures are geared to reduce the problems. As for tuberculosis and venereal disease, organized programs emanated originally from voluntary agencies. While these continue, the major current programs are under the wing of government.

Programs for diagnosis, treatment, and rehabilitation of crippled children now operate in every state government, with subsidy from the U.S. Children's Bureau. Usually the state health department is responsible (sometimes other agencies), and it often delegates functions to local health agencies. The state defines the precise diagnoses eligible for aid; for example, one state will include hare-lip and another will not. The state also defines criteria for economic entitlement; but, since the cost of treating serious disabling conditions in children is high, few families that apply are excluded. Actual care is given either through private physicians and hospitals or through governmental clinics and institutions. In 1960 about 350,000 children were treated under these programs, which put great emphasis on high-quality standards for personnel and facilities. It is evident that effective treatment of a seriously disabled child not only prepares him for a better adult life but preserves his family from many emotional and economic burdens.

For disabled adults, the rationale of governmental action has been related more to pragmatic than to humanitarian considerations. The federal-state program of "vocational rehabilitation" was given impetus in two wartime periods, partially on the ground of tackling manpower shortages. The U.S. Vocational Rehabilitation Administration gives grants to state agencies, usually departments of education (because of the important job-training aspects), for medical correction of disabilities in employable adults. The treatment is usually given through private resources, including ordinary community hospitals and sometimes rehabilitation centers. The selection of cases for help depends on the state's definition of medical and financial eligibility, within broad limits of employability laid down in federal regulations. Each client is helped through the medical, educational, and employment phases of the rehabilitation process by a VR counselor from the state agency. The tax-support of this program has been steadily expanding, and in 1965 it received a major new boost through a shift of the federal-state matching formula from 50-50 to 75-25 percent.

Industrial Injuries

Another diagnostic category for which major public responsibility has been taken in the United States is trauma arising through the course of employment. Since 1910, state laws have been passed (reaching the last of the states, Mississippi, in

1948) requiring employers to carry insurance which would compensate workers for the wage-loss and medical expenses incurred because of injuries on the job. Occupational diseases are now also covered in nearly all states. Most workers are insured through private insurance carriers, but in many states there are also supplemental (and in five states exclusive) state government funds to carry the risks. In either arrangement, the medical care of the injured worker is typically rendered by private personnel and facilities and paid for on a fee basis by the insurance company under regulations of a state agency.

The workmen's compensation field has been beset with problems relating to insurance company profiteering and abuses by employers, workers, doctors, and lawyers. With money at stake, there is sometimes a tendency for workers (and their legal counsels) to exaggerate the extent of a disability or its relation to a work-accident. Likewise, insurance companies and employers may argue excessively in the opposite direction. Despite the difficulties, there is no question about the benefits to workers and their families from the workmen's compensation laws, especially compared with the earlier period of courtroom litigation in which the worker or his widow was seldom awarded anything. Improvements are certainly required in these state laws, especially with respect to adjudication of claims and rehabilitation aspects; but, even in their current imperfect status, they help to protect the integrity of the injured worker's family in a substantial way.

Programs for Certain Modes of Service

Cutting across the lines of several of the government programs already described are other public activities based on a type of medical service, rather than a particular class of person or illness. Since these have been touched on tangentially above, they will be discussed here very briefly.

General hospital care is provided by governmental hospitals for all types of persons and all types of illness. Aside from the public hospitals for the indigent mentioned above, there are hundreds of general community hospitals—especially in rural counties—built and controlled by local government and open to everyone. These hospitals may have special wards for the poor, but the majority of their patients are privately attended, as in a voluntary hospital, and financed by personal or insurance funds. Local government has, in effect, borne the burden of initial construction of such hospitals, rather than the more usual philanthropy or church resources. Without government initiative these communities might have been quite lacking in local hospital service. In California, special local "hospital districts," cutting across county lines, have been established for the purpose of raising tax funds for hospital construction and operating the hospital when it is built.

General hospitals for chronic illness of all types have been built by local governments in recent years with increasing frequency. While oriented to low-income patients, the costs of long-term care are so high that the majority of cases tend to qualify for admission. In these institutions, the level of rehabilitation service tends to be much higher than in private nursing homes which cater to the same type of patient.

All types of physician's services are usually offered in the out-patient departments of governmental general hospitals for low-income persons. We do not have in the United States, however, separate governmental health centers for the general treatment of ambulatory illness, as found in many other nations of lesser affluence. The new anti-poverty program of 1965 (see below) has begun to sponsor a few such centers in blighted rural villages (such as in Appalachia) or in large city slums.

Dental care in government clinics is sometimes provided for low-income children in the school system or for pregnant women and children in local health departments. Dentists are in such short supply, in relation to effective demand, however, that it is often difficult to get proper staffing for these clinics. Yet the development of auxiliary personnel to extend the arm of the dentist has been very modest.

Laboratories are a standard component of the program of all state health departments and many of the larger local health departments. Their examinations are largely related to environmental sanitation specimens (like water or milk samples), but they also deal with communicable diseases. Tests for syphilis, for example, or for diphtheria or typhoid fever are typically done by public health laboratories for any physician sending a specimen, regardless of the income of his patient. Some of these laboratories also do clinical pathological tests for non-communicable diseases, like diabetes or uterine cancer (Papanicolaou smears). Forensic pathology tests involved in crime detection are also sometimes done. These diagnostic services are, of course, supported by tax funds and, in this sense, represent a government contribution to family welfare.

Nursing services in the home are another standard feature of health department programs, and they are theoretically available to entire populations. While the main focus of these services has been preventive instruction for mothers with newborn babies or for families with a communicable disease, the emphasis in recent years has been shifting to "bedside nursing" in the home for patients with chronic illness. A few public health agencies have even launched generalized "home care" programs providing the services of technicians, rehabilitation therapists, social workers, etc., as well as nurses, to home-bound patients with chronic illness.

The role of government along this dimension of "types of professional service" is obviously less developed in the United States than along the dimensions of "persons" or "illnesses" reviewed earlier. In various ways, however, these programs help to meet the health needs of families.

Health Insurance

While the purpose of this chapter is to explore governmental impacts on the American family in the health field, the nongovernmental health insurance movement has such close relationships to the authority and actions of government that it must be discussed briefly.

In a sense one can regard voluntary health insurance as a social movement to collectivize the financial support of medical care costs not being met by other social devices like government or charity. It has concentrated in the United States on elements of medical care that strike catastrophically, like general hospital care and the services of physicians (especially for surgery) in hospitalized illness. It has been built largely on enrollment of employed groups in industry and has specifically excluded from benefits those services which are available from governmental programs, like the care of tuberculosis, mental disorder, venereal disease, or compensable injuries.

This complementarity between insurance and governmental health programs is seen in other ways. The Depression and then the post-World War II years led to a series of national governmental proposals for universal health insurance under law. The United States was being urged to follow in the path taken by Europe years before. The first such legislative bill was introduced in 1939, four years after the Social Security Act, and then modified versions were introduced and debated in Congressional committees from 1943 to 1952. None of these proposals was enacted, but their introduction had an enormous effect in two ways: in the governmental sector and the private sector.

In the governmental sector, the political "leverage" produced by universal health insurance proposals led to enactment of many other health measures of substantial importance but less sweeping social implications. The Hill-Burton Hospital Survey and Construction Act of 1946 was a direct outcome of the social insurance debates; it was argued that the nation lacked facilities to hospitalize all the patients who would be covered by a national medical care program and that additional hospitals had to be built first. Moreover, the American Medical Association, which spearheaded the opposition to national health insurance, could not effectively oppose *every* proposal, so that it favored this measure which would subsidize construction of voluntary hospitals, with numerous safeguards against governmental "intervention." Somewhat similar political dynamics led to the enactment of other relatively nonthreatening measures, like expanded governmental support for cancer control programs, mental health services, vocational rehabilitation, industrial hygiene, and a vast multi-faceted program of medical research.

In the private sector, the "threat" of national health insurance had even wider effects by stimulating an extremely energetic movement for voluntary insurance. The cliché that unified dissident private groupings and pushed them ahead was, "If we don't do this ourselves, government will do it for us." As a result, soon after the first serious post-war (1945) debates on national health insurance, the state medical societies went into high gear in the development of Blue Shield plans for physician's care insurance. Blue Cross plans for hospitalization insurance, which had started in 1930, took a great spurt ahead. Most important, the commercial insurance giants, which had been skeptical of the fiscal soundness of the whole field of insurance for medical expenses, moved into group enrollment of industrial workers on a large scale. A number of localized consumer-sponsored plans, like the Health Insurance Plan of Greater New York (HIP) and the Kaiser Health Plan of California, also got under way in this period.

The momentum gained by the voluntary health insurance movement under the threat of governmental action has continued to the present time. Enrollment has grown to a coverage of over 70 percent of the national population, with respect to general hospital expenses, although less for other benefits. The largest sector of enrollment is under commercial insurance plans (about 35 percent of the national population), the second largest (about 30 percent) is under provider-sponsored Blue Cross or Blue Shield plans, and the smallest (about 5 percent) is under consumer-sponsored or "independent" plans. The range of precise benefits and limitations on these health insurance programs is wide and endlessly complicated, but their net effect has clearly been to enhance access of people to medical care. The great bulk of enrollment is through employment groups, and the vast majority of persons so covered elect to include coverage of their dependents. Voluntary health insurance has been a substantial boon for the medical protection of families.

As in Europe before America, both the successes and failures of voluntary health insurance have led to further action by government. The successful operation of voluntary plans has proved the soundness of the basic idea, while the failure to enroll enough persons of certain categories—the aged, the poor, and the rural population—has underscored the need for supplementary governmental action. There can be little doubt that the important legislation on health insurance of the aged, enacted in 1965 (discussed below), is largely an outgrowth of this social process.

Government has had another relationship to voluntary health insurance, which has fostered its development and its protective effect on families. Social control over insurance companies, designed to protect the insured person, has been largely through state insurance laws. State insurance departments require various safeguards on maintenance of fiscal reserves to cover unanticipated claims, on investment practices, on announcement of benefits to the buyer (the issue of the offerings in the large print and the subtractions in the fine print), and so on. Commercial carriers selling health insurance come under these laws. The provider-sponsored or consumer-sponsored plans, primarily nonprofit, however, provide mainly "service-benefits" rather than "indemnity" or monetary benefits, so that legal controls over them required special new state legislation. This was enacted in the great majority of states, and these "health insurance enabling acts" have helped to assure the solvency and general integrity of the Blue Cross and Blue Shield plans. Hearings on proposed premium increases, under these laws, have facilitated public review (especially by consumer groups and labor unions) of plan operations. An important decision of the Pennsylvania Insurance Commissioner in 1958, the Smyth Adjudication of the Blue Cross request for a premium increase, drew national attention to the whole question of "over-utilization" of hospital beds by insured persons and the need for some organized surveillance of individual doctor decisions by medical staffs in hospitals. Unwarranted use of a hospital bed by one person, of course, may prevent admission of another person in serious need, so that the "abuse" of insurance—actual or potential—has inevitably summoned greater social controls.

Government has articulated with the voluntary health insurance movement in still another way: through enrollment of federal and state civil servants in existing plans. Many such individual employees and their families, of course, have long been enrolled in medical care plans, but the Federal Employees Health Benefit Act of 1960 established the principle of government as the "employer" and the contributor of about 50 percent of premium costs. Not only did this give a further boost to voluntary health insurance enrollments, but the requirement of plan approval by the U.S. Civil Service Commission promoted a set of national standards with long-term influence for elevating quality. State government employees, like those in New York or California, have likewise become enrolled in voluntary insurance programs with subsidy of their premiums from public funds. These governmental programs have also advanced the principle of "multiple choice" among various health insurance plans by each employee, a feature which has promoted sensible competition and upgrading of benefits.

The ultimate effects of the health insurance movement on family welfare must be expressed both in medical and economic values. There is abundant evidence that insured families are enabled to make much higher use of hospital and physician services, about 50 percent higher on an age-adjusted basis. Some of this utilization (especially elective surgery) may be unnecessary or even harmful, but the general facilitation of patient-doctor contact may be presumed to be more beneficial than noncontact. Moreover, the cushioning of hospital expenses, much the greatest insured benefit, facilitates family expenditures for other non-insured benefits like prescribed drugs or dental care. On the economic dimension, family budgets have been protected with respect to all other living needs; the oft-quoted tragedy of a patient's major illness obstructing a child's college education can be averted. Perhaps the chief disappointment has been the very modest impact of health insurance on the quality of the medical care that is finally delivered; the payment of hospital and doctor bills has been too little associated with surveillance over the content of the services actually given.

Related to insurance for medical expenses is insurance against loss of earnings due to sickness, about which only a word may be said. Disability insurance, as it is usually called, has evolved through voluntary organizations—mainly commercial carriers—and has served to protect families against the whole economic impact of inability to work and earn. It has been extended both through group insurance enrollment and "sick leave" provisions in employment. Since 1943 four state governments (Rhode Island, California, New York, and New Jersey) have established such programs for workers covered by public unemployment insurance for periods of short-term disability, i.e., up to six months. For long-term total disability, the federal old-age insurance program has been extended by a series of Social Security Act amendments since 1954 to provide some basic economic protection to individuals and families. All these forms of disability insurance, which are expanding under diverse auspices, have a direct bearing on family health, both by facilitating access to needed medical care and by helping to meet the overall expenses of living.

Important New Governmental Health Programs

All of the spheres of governmental action affecting family health reviewed above are in continuous ferment and evolution. In the last year or two, however, largely as a result of national political trends, the pace of developments has been especially rapid. From the end of World War II until the Presidential election of 1960, the prevailing political winds in the United States were conservative, with the effect of keeping governmental influence on health affairs (as in other domestic matters) to a minimum. Then, with the election of John Kennedy followed by Lyndon Johnson, the direction of the winds changed. Needs which had been accumulating all the while came to be more sharply defined, and the appropriateness of governmental programs to meet them came to be more widely recognized. A wave of new federal legislation came in 1965, the force of which was unprecedented, and its highlights may be briefly reviewed.

Health Insurance for the Aged

The gaps in health insurance protection for retired persons over 65 years of age have been mentioned, and the passage of the Kerr-Mills Act (medical assistance for the aged) in 1960 did not solve the problem. Meanwhile the proportion of persons over 65 years in the population and the costs of their medical care continued to rise. After a complex series of compromises, therefore, there was enacted in July, 1965, a set of major amendments to the Social Security Act, popularly known as the "Medicare Law," which have vast implications for family welfare.

The most important feature of the new law is social insurance support for hospital and related services to virtually all persons in the nation 65 years and over, whether they are entitled to Social Security old-age pensions or not. The "related services" include those of extended care facilities (such as nursing homes or rehabilitation centers), home health care agencies, and hospital out-patient departments (for diagnostic examinations). There are various limitations in the extent of these benefits supported, but the overall effect will surely be to enlarge the access of old people to health facilities for the treatment of their high burden of both acute and chronic illness.

Supplementary to the above is a national program of so-called voluntary medical insurance, with heavy governmental subsidy. Each aged person decides whether he wishes to pay a small partial monthly premium ($3 in 1966) for insurance against physician's bills for service in the office, home, or hospital and for various ancillary benefits (laboratory examinations, certain appliances, ambulance transportation, etc.). If he so decides, then the federal government will contribute an equal amount toward the total premium. The limitations on this protection are, however, more serious than those in the hospital insurance part (a $50 deductible amount per year and 20 percent cost-sharing by the individual after that). Nevertheless, there is little doubt that this quasi-social insurance will greatly ease the access of old people to physician's care.

The effects of this program on families may be speculated on, even though the effective date for its operation comes after this writing. Aside from the obvious benefits to aged persons as family members, the social support of the costs of medical care will relieve adult children of an economic burden they now must often bear. The institutional and home health services for aged persons will also lighten physical and emotional burdens on families now taking care of an ailing parent.

Families may also be expected to benefit from the impact of the new law on the medical care system itself. The expanded financial support, along with upgraded federal standards for hospitals and related facilities, will doubtless strengthen the basic medical care resources of the nation, which serve everyone. These effects will probably be especially felt in nursing homes, where standards have been notoriously weak. Home health care programs, deficient in quantity rather than quality, will doubtless be expanded. Certain innovative features of the new law may foster great changes in the degree of group-discipline within the medical staffs of hospitals, especially the requirements for a "utilization review" procedure and for "transfer agreements" between extended care facilities and general hospitals. The removal of the aged population, moreover, from the risk-load of the voluntary health insurance plans ought to permit those plans to expand benefits or hold the line on costs for younger members. Indeed, the use of existing voluntary plans as "fiscal intermediaries" for the administration of the "Medicare" provisions will further strengthen those plans by giving them a key involvement in a vast public system.

The new law is far from perfect, from the viewpoint of family welfare. The limitations in benefits are serious, and the administrative tasks are very complicated. But it is an important first step in national health insurance, which will doubtless lead to amendments in administration, coverage, and benefits. If worldwide experience can serve as a guide, the direction of future amendments will be toward broadening the scope of the law.

Expanded Health Services for the Poor

Another important feature of the Social Security Amendments of 1965 is the program of expanded medical care for public assistance recipients of all types, i.e., including families with dependent children and others under 65 years, and also for medically indigent persons. Federal grants will be made to the states on a more generous basis than ever before, on condition that the states develop uniform services of a wider range than now prevails for low-income persons and families.

As mentioned earlier, organized medical care for the poor has variable benefits among the special categories and between states and localities within a state. The new amendments provide a substantial financial incentive to uniformity among these populations and toward a minimum range of benefits for all. By 1967 this minimum must include physician services, hospital care (in-patient and out-patient), skilled nursing-home care, and laboratory and X-ray services. Many of the deficiencies of welfare medical services, mentioned earlier, will doubtless be reduced under this law. Highly important is the availability of federal funds for the medically indigent under age 65 who are not receiving cash assistance. This may be expected to help families facing chronic unemployment, like migratory agricultural families or racial minorities in the metropolitan slums.

Another federal law of 1964 is providing support for expanded health services to low-income families identified geographically. The Office of Economic Opportunity, set up on the "war on poverty" theme, provides grants for "community action programs" in localities marked by great poverty and deprivation. In these "pockets of poverty"—rural or urban—grants are made directly from the federal level to assist in various social improvements, including health service. Relatively well developed is "Operation Headstart" which is providing cultural enrichment—along with corrective medical services—to preschool children from depressed families in the larger cities. Other projects involve the expansion of conventional well-child clinics operated by health departments in blighted localities to include comprehensive medical services, treatment services for school children, and the development of generalized out-patient clinics in rural hospitals.

The emphasis of the anti-poverty program is distinctly on helping youth from disadvantaged families. Because of this focus, as well as because these families are not a significant part of the usual market for private medical service, organizational innovations are possible with less opposition from conservative forces than is usually found.

Regional Programs for Heart Disease, Cancer, and Stroke

An interesting illustration of the dynamics of medico-social progress in the United States is seen in the enactment of the "Heart Disease, Cancer, and Stroke Amendments of 1965." While drawing public and Congressional support by focusing on the serious diseases constituting the three top causes of death in the nation, the legislation has the underlying purpose and probably impact of promoting the vitalized regionalization of all health services in order to improve their scientific quality.

The Hill-Burton Act, reviewed earlier, promoted the regionalized concept through support for hospital construction. The functional operation of networks of hospitals in geographic regions, however, has hardly been achieved except in a few localities where philanthropic foundations have supported special inter-hospital councils. The new amendments approach the same goal of establishing "regional cooperative arrangements among medical schools, research institutions, and hospitals" by defining the objective of these arrangements as research, training, and "demonstrations of patient care in the fields of heart disease, cancer, stroke, and related diseases." In other words, the intent is to extend the scientific influence of high quality medical centers to the hospitals and doctors around them. Grants are to be made by the federal government directly to medical schools, research institutions, and other public and non-profit agencies to develop regional medical programs for this purpose.

Much will depend on the amount of government money appropriated for this program as well as the diligence with which it is executed by national and local agencies. If present hopes are realized, the impact will be to upgrade the quality of medical care for serious illness received by families, especially those depressed and poorly educated families who might not, through their own resources and knowledge, gain access to the best service.

Other Federal and State Developments

The recent flood of national health legislation includes many other measures which widen the role of government and increase its ultimate impact on the family. Aside from child-focused provisions mentioned above, there are expanded funds for the long-established programs of maternal and child health services and crippled children's services under state and local public agencies. There are increased federal funds for immunizations. Federal controls over certain drugs subject to widespread abuse—especially the amphetamines and barbiturates—are tightened. Support for local programs to serve the mentally ill and mentally retarded is increased; mental health centers to treat patients on an ambulatory basis are to receive subsidy of their staffing, as well as the previously enacted subsidy of their construction. The huge problem of lung cancer was accorded a modest blow by a provision that cigarette packages be labeled with a cautionary statement that they "may be hazardous to health" (although controls over cigarette advertising are specifically prohibited for a further three-year period). Other legislation will strengthen medical schools, medical libraries, and medical research programs. Vocational rehabilitation of the disabled is to get more generous federal support. Grants for helping provide health services to migrant families are increased.

On the state government level, there have been numerous other health developments, only a few of which can be mentioned. New York state enacted in 1964 the first state law in the nation granting governmental control over all new hospital construction, regardless of whether or not public subsidies are received. This is an important step in establishment of the concept of the hospital as a "public utility," even if its sponsorship is by a voluntary body. It is a recognition of the ultimate influence of the supply of beds in a region on the utilization rate of hospitals and therefore on the costs which are eventually borne by the whole population through health insurance and other social programs. Voluntary "hospital planning councils" are studying the New York State experience with great interest, and it is a fair guess that the approach will be applied elsewhere.

Connecticut broke the ice in 1965 as the first state to enact a state-wide law on fluoridation of water supplies (in towns of over a certain population). This basic dental health measure has been badly obstructed in many cities by the hesitations of local government in the face of misguided popular objections. While the constitutionality of the Connecticut statute will doubtless be challenged, the trend of previous court decisions on this subject suggests that it will probably be upheld in the long run.

The federal "Medicare Law" has stimulated many governmental moves on the state level, so that full advantage could be taken of the provisions for medical assistance of the poor. In California a 1965 law will probably revolutionize the whole pattern of care for the indigent in that state, with important influences on family welfare. The effect of the new law will be to enable indigent and medically indigent persons to receive care in the mainstream of modern medicine, that is, through regular community hospitals and physicians, instead of in separate county institutions or clinics as in the past. The administrative mechanism is to be through enrollment of these impoverished families in existent health insurance plans, with premiums paid from government funds.

These are only a few highlights of recent developments in governmental health services at federal and state levels. There is ferment in numerous other fields: increased rehabilitation emphasis in workmen's compensation legislation, promotion of group medical practice clinics, extension of birth control information and liberalization of laws prohibiting therapeutic abortions, control over air and water pollution, modification of commitment procedures for mental patients toward more medical (as against legalistic) procedures, and so on. It is not difficult to appreciate how these changes in laws or new program developments will influence family well-being in the future. For those programs requiring governmental monies, however, a great deal will depend on competing demands of appropriations for highly expensive alternative purposes, like wars overseas.

Trends in Family Life Influencing Health Service

The vantage point of this chapter has viewed the family on the receiving end of influences exerted by governmental health programs. But a few words may be said from the opposite side, that is, the influence of trends in American family life upon the patterns of health service. Sociologists of family life analyze more carefully the nature of these trends, so that here one may examine briefly some of their effects in terms of health service.

The smaller average size of the American family in recent decades, due to birth control and other factors, has various implications for health service. With fewer children, on the average, each child can receive more attention to meet his health needs along with other needs. The very low infant and child mortality rates today doubtless reflect not only the advances of medicine and public health but the more solicitous care families can offer their children in day-to-day life.

At the same time, smaller families mean smaller households and fewer persons at home to take care of a sick member. This may well contribute to the much greater use of hospitals and nursing homes than in the past, though there are other causes of these higher institutionalization rates. The family with a retarded child or a disabled grandparent today will seek institutional relief from the burden, and this creates a demand for facilities under governmental or other auspices. Fifty years ago such facilities were much less available, and the family had no choice but to shelter the handicapped member.

The higher proportion of working mothers than in past decades has effects of the same sort. The person most suitable to nurse a sick child or husband or grandparent is likely to be out in a job herself, further heightening the pressure for institutional services. Many compensatory movements have arisen to provide organized visiting nurse services in the home, but the volume of these services has hardly kept up with the growth of population. "Home care" programs emanating from hospitals have hardly scratched the surface of the problem, so that the rate of hospital and nursing home utilization continues to rise.

The greater longevity of adults, of course, is probably the most important pressure for increasing use of nursing homes and all the governmental programs designed to finance these services. Even though an adult son or daughter might be as willing today to take care of an ailing parent as a century ago, the proportion of parents surviving into the seventies and eighties is much higher; the aggregate pressures to provide shelter for the aged are, therefore, greater today than in the past, and many of these pressures demand release through institutionalization.

With greater economic independence of women and the spiritual independence that goes with it, there is less use of a single family doctor. The wife may see her doctor, while the husband sees his, and still another doctor takes care of the children. Of course, specialization in medicine makes this possible, but family dynamics doubtless contribute to it. This segmentation of family medical care is sometimes facilitated by the coverage of the wife under a health insurance plan at her place of work, while the husband is covered through his job. (Premium payment by employers eliminates any double expenditures by the family itself.)

The various organized health programs in different settings also obviously contribute to this segmentation. First-aid services in a factory, diagnostic services in a school, and child health services in a neighborhood public health clinic offer convenient access to different family members. Thus, it is not only the changes in family dynamics but also the organization of health services in the social environment that lead to segmentation of the health care of different family members. One should not jump to the conclusion, however, that this trend is entirely deleterious to family welfare. A coordinating family medical advisor may well be needed, but the enormous proliferation of medical knowledge does, indeed, demand specialization for its sound application.

The relative ease of transportation today contributes also to the individualization of medical care to family members. Home calls by the physician have become a steadily declining proportion of his service; instead, the patient makes his way by automobile or common carrier to the doctor's office or clinic. Thus, the doctor sees one family member at a time in his office, instead of all of them together in the home. This pattern also saves the doctor's time, so that he can see many more patients in a day than he could 30 years ago when he spent hours on the road.

Divorce rates are higher than a generation ago, but remarriage rates are also higher. Whether or not "broken families" yield a higher rate of mental and emotional problems than families staying united but unhappy and turbulent is a difficult question. There is no question, however, about the increased *recognition* of mental health problems by families today and the increased demand for psychiatric and social-work service. The demand is expressed through mental health societies, through legislative channels, and in other ways. The social response has been expressed through a great expansion and improvement of organized mental health services, both institutional and ambulatory.

Greater freedom and permissiveness in child-rearing are another attribute of modern family life that has its consequences for health services. Perhaps the ranking of accidents as the chief cause of childhood death is a partial price paid for this reduction in restraints, although there are, obviously, environmental factors as well. In any event, the prominence of accidents in the morbidity and mortality picture of children and youths has led to many organized programs for promoting safety. Perhaps this is another instance of social processes replacing functions formerly assumed by the family.

Permissiveness for adolescents, along with other influences in the social environment, is associated with easier and earlier relations between the sexes. Earlier marriages create family responsibilities (including medical care) sooner. The unmarried mother in high school and the rise of teen-age venereal disease are other medical consequences of these family trends. Along with them come social programs to cope with the problem, such as sex hygiene education and organized youth recreational activities. The great mobility of American families between neighborhoods, cities, and states increases the exposure of their children to a variety of community settings, which probably heightens their general interpersonal sophistication.

The changed character of the family, viewed here as a causative force, is itself a product of numerous social influences. These influences—urbanization, industrialization, higher per capita income, greater education—also have their bearing on the way families make use of health services. They have greater health consciousness, which can be expressed in economic demand for care. They are more sophisticated about science, and they expect more from doctors and hospitals. If they are dissatisfied they express grievances more openly, and, when a grievance is extreme, they more readily initiate a malpractice suit. These pressures from people exert a constant influence on the medical care system, inducing more organization and professional controls to meet the demands expressed.

In a word, just as the shape and functions of the family are a product of social forces, this modified family exerts its influences on the structure of the health services. The net effect would seem to be the creation of pressures for further organization of both curative and preventive measures. Many of these pressures are expressed eventually through government, and they account to some degree for the panorama of organized programs that we have reviewed.

Broad Effects of Government on Family Health Services

In summary, what are some of the overall influences of government on the health services received by the American family? It is obvious from the previous pages that there are great differences for different types of family. Government plays a greater role in the life of families which are socially dependent (like the poor) or socially important (like the military) than in the life of other families struck by certain types of serious disease (like psychoses) or needing certain types of service (like hospitalization).

But for all families there are some pervasive impacts of government in the health sphere. The control of health hazards in the environment and the promotion of increased disease-resistance in the individual are major benefits of governmental health efforts. Government has increasingly protected the consumer against the incompetence of healers (via licensure laws) or the abuses of commerce (by drug control legislation). Government has increased the output of needed health manpower and the construction of needed facilities. It has advanced medical research and accelerated its application.

In a broad sense, government has increased the financial accessibility of families to medical care. It has established public programs and stimulated voluntary ones which have yielded a much higher utilization of medical care. This has been accomplished with a reduction of economic stress on the total family budget in any one year. On the national economic scale, governmental expenditures and indirect pressures have resulted in a higher proportion of gross national product being allocated to health services. In the last 30 years this has risen from under 4 to over 6 percent, an increase of over 50 percent of an enlarged national output. Greater relative contributions from federal, as against state and local, revenue sources have yielded a more equitable distribution of health services among rich and poor states.

Government has promoted far-reaching improvements in the technical quality of health services. It has contributed to the heightened use of hospitals, clinics, laboratories, rehabilitation centers, and other facilities where a wide range of specialized skills are mobilized. It has fostered group discipline and surveillance in the delivery of medical services. It has increased communications through health records and other measures which can simplify and improve the care of the patient. In spite of general resistance to organization by the individual physician, there can be little doubt that the increased overall organization of health services has yielded an advancement of their quality.

The payoff of these governmental actions, of course, must be measured in a higher level of health in families. The evidence reflected in reduced mortality at all age levels (even among the aged) and increased longevity is clear, although the benefits obviously cannot be attributed solely to government nor even to the entire health service system. Many features of life influence health, aside from preventive and curative medicine. One can claim, however, that the overall organization of health services is associated with improvement of health status. The whole vast literature of clinical medicine provides evidence for the value of scientific therapy, and social organization certainly mediates the application of that therapy.

Reduced mortality rates, however, have not yielded a corresponding reduction in morbidity. With increased longevity, people live to an age level when they are biologically susceptible to more disease. We also keep alive today many persons with diseases, like diabetes or asthma, which require long-continuing care. Moreover, our whole definition of illness has become extended, so that disorders which might have been stoically accepted in the past are now regarded as subjects for medical attention, especially in the sphere of psychiatry and rehabilitation. All these factors contribute to a continuously high level of recognized illness in the population, in spite of great reductions in mortality rates. With this and with rising economic potential and rising expectations comes a steadily increasing demand for medical care.

It has been part of our national mythology that social organization reduces the freedom of the individual. Large systems of health care are alleged to depersonalize attention to the patient. Yet the evidence is that organization has made more services available to more people with more concern for quality performance. The paradox is explained by continuously rising expectations. People want better and better health care not only on a scientific level but on a humanistic level as well. The huge, sordid wards of a public hospital in 1900 produced fewer outcries of indignation than the delay in a nurse's answer to the call button from a semiprivate hospital room today. The ultimate effect of health service organization has really been to protect the well-being and dignity of the majority of individuals and families.

Problems and Issues

This generally positive appraisal of governmental impacts on the health of the family should not be construed to mean that there are no problems. The gaps are numerous, and the problems are many.

While health improvements characterize the experience of most families, there is a disadvantaged minority for which—despite many governmental programs—the deficiencies are serious. The poor still receive generally less medical care than the affluent, in spite of the governmental measures and in spite of their greater burden of illness. The quality of care received by the poor and the uneducated also tends to be low: greater use of general practitioners rather than specialists, patent medicines rather than prescribed drugs, and so on.

The substantial development of health insurance has been largely concentrated on the expenses of hospitalized illness. Insurance for the earlier care of the physician in the office and home is only meager, not to mention that for the cost of drugs, dental care, and other ancillary services. Of all family expenditures for personal health service, only about 25 percent are now covered by insurance. Obviously there is a long way to go before the costs of comprehensive medical care for families are thoroughly buttressed by insurance or other forms of social financing.

Aside from economic support, there are serious deficiencies in the pattern by which individuals receive care. The segmentation of care to different members of a family was mentioned earlier; but, even for any single individual, care is commonly fragmented among several different doctors and places. A supervising personal physician is all too often lacking, and the prevailing pattern of private, solo medical practice does little to promote teamwork. Group medical practice is the pattern for less than 10 percent of physicians. Periodic health examinations, so important for prevention, are received by only a small percentage of people.

Hospitals have steadily improved, but there are still many small, poorly organized units without reliable quality controls. The deficiencies in nursing homes for the chronically ill are notorious. Regionalized relationships among institutions are continually advocated but seldom realized today. Yet every patient ought to have access to the type of hospital that can best handle his case, regardless of where he happens to live or whatever may be his socio-economic pedigree.

Basic public health services are still far from fully developed. The staffs of health departments for public health nursing, sanitary supervision, health education, and so on are far below needs. Serious environmental problems like water and air pollution are still not solved. The mental health services are woefully understaffed both in hospitals and clinics. Mental facilities are still not able to claim from governmental resources anything like enough funds to match the level of care provided in private facilities.

The pluralism of organized health services in the United States, as we have noted, yields a great deal of duplicated administration in spite of the many gaps mentioned. There are different laws and different organized entities coping with scores of separately defined health needs. The lack of coordination means overcrowded conditions in one setting while there may be unused capacity in another. Time and money may be squandered by both patients and personnel in travel to multiple locations. Scarce administrative staff may be duplicated and expensive equipment insufficiently used.

A frequent solution proposed is to bring the care of special groups, like the indigent or veterans, into the "mainstream of American medicine." It is assumed that the services of private doctors and local voluntary hospitals are better in quality and more democratic in spirit than the services of isolated special programs. This argument may be valid for certain classes of special programs, such as the care of the poor in overcrowded and understaffed public clinics. But there are some specialized programs, like those for vocational rehabilitation clients or crippled children, where very high standards—probably higher than the average in the mainstream—have been achieved. This mainstream, moreover, is not a uniform current; parts of it are first-rate; but, as in most human affairs, there is a range down to some very poor levels of care.

The solution would seem to be gradual modification of the central stream of American health service, so that high standards are applied throughout it. Then, the care of special persons or special diseases could be subject to varying fiscal arrangements, while the final delivery of the technical service would be through a unified system. In that system would be an integrated network of hospitals and health centers. The latter could evolve from private group practice clinics, as they are now understood. Every family would have its primary attachment to a health center nearby but would be entitled to referral to any other center or hospital that is best equipped to serve its needs. All medical and related personnel in the system would work as a team, without inhibitions against referral (such as loss of a fee) or toward unnecessary surgery.

The general hospital is the logical technical core of such a pattern of health service; it houses the full range of skilled personnel and has developed effective intramural organization. In larger political units like counties or states, however, administrative coordination and supervision belong in a public agency, like the department of health. Unfortunately, the current scope of such departments is far narrower than this plan would imply, but agency roles can grow.

Whatever may evolve, the solution to current deficiencies in health services for the family will require more social organization rather than less. The weaknesses within existing public programs cannot be solved by a return to individual initiative but rather by an enhancement of social planning and responsibility. This social initiative may be taken by agencies both in the voluntary sphere and in government. Past experience suggests that both forms of organization will grow together, but the major long-term responsibilities in a democracy will be assigned to government.

A widening role for government in the health services may be safely predicted for another reason as well. Aside from the administrative advantages, governmental health programs have many political attractions. Few issues are closer to people's hearts than their health, a fact appreciated by Bismarck in introducing the first social insurance programs for medical care in 1883. The elaborate medical program of the Veterans Administration has obvious political purposes, as have the health insurance amendments of 1965, favoring the aged. Yet there can be no objection to the fashioning of governmental programs to attract votes, if those programs lead to genuine expansion and improvement of services. In the last few decades, such have clearly been the effects of governmental actions, despite their shortcomings, in the movement to close the gaps between medical science and health needs.

References

Anderson, O. W., and J. Feldman. *National Family Survey of Medical Costs and Voluntary Health Insurance*. New York: Health Information Foundation, 1954.

Bressler, M., ed. "Meeting Health Needs by Social Action," *The Annals of the American Academy of Political and Social Science*, 337 (September, 1961).

Brown, E. L. *Newer Dimensions of Patient Care*. New York: Russell Sage Foundation, 1965.

Clausen, J. A., and R. Straus, eds. "Medicine and Society," *The Annals of the American Academy of Political and Social Science*, 346 (March, 1963).

Commission on Chronic Illness. *Care of the Long-term Patient*. Cambridge: Harvard University Press, 1956.

Commission on the Survey of Dentistry in the United States. *The Survey of Dentistry*. Chicago: University of Chicago Press, 1961.
Committee on Medical Care Teaching. *Readings in Medical Care*. Chapel Hill: University of North Carolina Press, 1958.
Davis, M. M. *Medical Care for Tomorrow*. New York: Harper and Brothers, 1955.
Emerson, Haven, ed. *Administrative Medicine*. Baltimore: Williams and Wilkins, 1951.
Freeman, H. E., S. Levine, and L. G. Reeder, *Handbook of Medical Sociology*. Englewood Cliffs, N.J.: Prentice-Hall, 1963.
Friedson, E., ed. *The Hospital in Modern Society*. New York: Macmillan, 1963.
Goldmann, F. *Public Medical Care: Principles and Problems*. New York: Columbia University Press, 1945.
———, and H. R. Leavell, eds. "Medical Care for Americans," *The Annals of the American Academy of Political and Social Science*, 273 (January, 1951).
Greenfield, M. *Providing for Mental Illness*. Berkeley: University of California, Institute of Governmental Studies, 1964.
Harris, Seymour. *The Economics of American Medicine*. New York: Macmillan, 1964.
Jaco, E. G., ed. *Patients, Physicians, and Illness*. New York: The Free Press, a division of the Macmillan Co., 1958.
Joint Commission on Mental Illness and Health. *Action for Mental Health*. New York: Basic Books, 1962.
Katz, A. H., and J. S. Felton, eds. *Health and the Community: Readings in the Philosophy and Sciences of Public Health*. New York: The Free Press, a division of the Macmillan Co., 1965.
Kessler, Henry H., *et al. Principles and Practices of Rehabilitation*. Philadelphia: Lea and Febiger, 1950.
Koos, E. J. *The Health of Regionville*. New York. Columbia University Press, 1954.
Leavell, H. R., and E. G. Clark. *Preventive Medicine for the Doctor in His Community*. New York: McGraw Hill Book Co., third edition, 1965.
Lerner, M., and O. W. Anderson. *Health Progress in the United States*. Chicago: University of Chicago Press, 1963.
Littauer, David, *et al. Home Care*. Chicago: American Hospital Association, Monograph Series No. 9, 1961.
Mott, F. D., and M. I. Roemer. *Rural Health and Medical Care*. New York: McGraw-Hill, 1948.
Mountin, J. W. *Collected Papers*. Washington: Mountin Memorial Committee, 1956.
———, and E. Flook. *Guide to Health Organization in the United States*. Public Health Service Publication No. 196. Washington, D.C.: Government Printing Office, 1953.
Owen, J. K., *Modern Concepts of Hospital Administration*. Philadelphia: Saunders, 1961.
Paul, B. J., ed. *Health, Culture, and Community: Case Studies of Public Reactions to Health Programs*. New York: Russell Sage Foundation, 1955.
President's Commission on Heart Disease, Cancer, and Stroke. *A National Program to Conquer Heart Disease, Cancer, and Stroke,* Volumes I and II. Washington, D.C.: Government Printing Office, 1964.
Roemer, M. I., and E. A. Wilson. *Organized Health Services in a County of the United States*, Public Health Service Publication No. 197. Washington, D. C.: Government Printing Office, 1952.
Rosen, George. *A History of Public Health,* New York: M D Publications, 1958.
Sand, Rene. *The Advance to Social Medicine*. London: Staples Press, 1952.
Shryock, R. H. *The Development of Modern Medicine*. New York: Alfred A. Knopf, 1947.
Sigerist, H. E. *American Medicine*. New York: W. W. Norton, 1932.
———. *Medicine and Human Welfare*. New Haven: Yale University Press, 1941.
Silver, G. A. *Family Medical Care: A Report of the Family Health Maintenance Demonstration*. Cambridge, Mass.: Harvard University Press, 1963.
Somers, H. M. and A. R. *Doctors, Patients, and Health Insurance*. Washington: Brookings Institution, 1961.
———. *Workmen's Compensation: Prevention, Insurance and Rehabilitation of Occupational Disability*. New York: John Wiley, 1954.
Stern, B. J. *Medical Services by Government: Local, State, and Federal*. New York: Commonwealth Fund, 1946.
———. *Medicine in Industry*. New York: Commonwealth Fund, 1946.

Straus, R. *Medical Care for Seamen: The Origin of Public Medical Service in the United States*. New Haven: Yale University Press, 1950.

Talalay, Paul, ed. *Drugs in Our Society*. Baltimore: Johns Hopkins Press, 1964.

U.S. Public Health Service. *Health Services for American Indians*. Public Health Service Publication No. 531. Washington, D.C.: Government Printing Office, 1957.

———. *Medical Care in Transition* (Reprint from the *American Journal of Public Health* 1949-62). Public Health Service Publication No. 1128, Volumes I and II. Washington, D.C.: Government Printing Office, 1964.

U.S. Social Security Administration. *Health Care of the Aged*. Washington, D.C.: Government Printing Office, 1962.

Part Two

Poverty and the Problems of Health Care

Much of the organization applied to health services has been motivated by the existence of poverty, which has stimulated ameliorative social actions. While the ostensible objective of these actions has been to improve the access of the poor to medical care, countless problems are associated with these efforts, and in the American culture a piecemeal approach has caused even further complexities.

Chapter 5 reviews the main features of organized medical care programs for the poor in the United States, with special discussion of the issue of how this care should be provided–in the mainstream of American medicine, as intended by the Social Security Act Amendments of 1965 (Title XIX or Medicaid) or by special mechanisms. In Chapter 6, an overview analysis is given of the health resources and services in a slum district of an American metropolis, Los Angeles, where an urban riot had occurred in 1965. Chapter 7 analyzes one aspect of the medical care of the poor–the all-too-frequent tendency of voluntary hospitals to "dump" on public hospitals impoverished patients coming to their out-patient department clinics. The special programs of health care developed in America for the poor, for other special population groups, and for selected populations have created complexity and fragmentation in our health care system, which are analyzed in Chapter 8. In financing medical services for the poor under the Medicaid mainstream philosophy, state and federal governments have been faced with mounting costs; to reduce these costs one strategy has been to impose co-payment requirements on the poor, but Chapter 9 demonstrates the folly of this device. A further adjustment to a mounting problem of the American health care system–the shortage of general practitioners for primary care–has been the training of various types of "physician extender" (really, doctor substitutes); in Chapter 10, through international comparisons, we see the discriminatory effects of this policy on the poor.

5

Needs and Organized Health Programs for the Poor

The urbanization of America, like that of most industrialized nations, brought problems as well as benefits. Concentrations of poverty, which made social and individual distress highly visible, gave rise to crime, disease, and violence. These social problems have focused increasing attention on urban policy and the need for corrective social actions.

Among these actions have been organized health services to ameliorate the conditions of poverty. Numerous studies have been stimulated by urban riots in the 1960s and a variety of legislation enacted. As part of one comprehensive urban analysis, this overview of special health needs and organized programs of health care for the poor was prepared. It was co-authored with Arnold I. Kisch and gave special attention to a contentious issue of then and now: is health service to the poor better when it is organized specifically for them or when it is given as part of the mainstream of community medicine?

OF THE MANY deprivations of the poor, deficiencies in medical service to heal their ailments and promote their health can be the most distressing. Adequate health service is important not only to cope with pain and suffering, but also to permit work and maintain productivity for the individual and community. It has, moreover, come to be an expected feature of modern civilization. Inaccessiblity to medical care can yield resentment toward the whole society in which deprived persons live and further their alienation from its norms and values.

In this chapter we will examine briefly the heavier burden of mortality and morbidity among the poor as compared to higher income groups. We will explore the lower level of medical services that they receive and their behavior with respect to such services. Over the centuries, numerous social programs have been launched to provide the poor with services which they would not otherwise get in the open medical market place. These will be briefly described, along with a closer look at several important new governmental health programs inaugurated in the last few years. The net outcome of the operations of both public and private health sectors will be considered. Finally we will look ahead at the direction of current trends and consider the meaning of the issue emerging on care of the poor inside or outside the mainstream of American medicine.

Chapter 5 originally appeared as a chapter on "Health, Poverty, and the Medical Mainstream" by Milton I. Roemer and Arnold I. Kisch in *Power, Poverty, and Urban Policy*, Urban Affairs Annual Reviews, vol. 2, ed. Warner Bloomberg, Jr., and Henry J. Schmandt. Copyright © 1968, pp. 181–202, and reprinted by permission of the Publisher, Sage Publications, Inc. (Beverly Hills/London).

Morbidity and Mortality Among the Poor

The heavier burden of sickness and death among the poor has been observed for centuries. In 1842, when Edwin Chadwick was arguing for public health services in the large cities, he collected data from Liverpool showing the average age at death among families of the gentry to be 35 years, among merchants 22 years, and among laborers 15 years. In the United States, a study of infant mortality (deaths under one year of age) in 1925 disclosed a rate of 59 deaths per 1,000 live births in higher income families (over $1,250 annual income), compared with 167 deaths per 1,000 in lower income families (under $450 annual income) (Stern, 1941).

The higher mortality among the poor is found in all age groups, but the differential is greatest among the young. In the younger years, the hazards of a hostile environment in causing fatal infectious disease and injuries are greater.

The causes of disease are many and complex, but in aggregate they affect the poor more seriously than the well-to-do. The United States National Health Survey conducts periodic interviews on a sample of approximately 42,000 households throughout the nation, and produces a wealth of data on disease and disability. For bouts of acute illness, there is little distinction in the frequency *reported* among different income groups, although it is probable that families of lower income are less likely to remember such events (and report them to an interviewer) simply because they are not so often identified through medical attention. For chronic conditions, however, the heavier burden among the poor is striking. In 1962–1963, chronic disorders, sufficiently serious to cause limitation of normal activity, affected 7.9 percent of persons in families of $7,000 and over annual income; among poor families of under $2,000 annual income the percentage was 28.6 so disabled (U.S. Public Health Service, 1964).

In terms of aggregate disability, the loss of days from normal activity is greater for the poor by all available measures. Among school chidren, the upper income families ($7,000 and over) show loss of school days at a rate of 5.9 per child per year, compared with 6.5 days in lower income families (under $2,000). The more solicitous care of the upper income child doubtless reduces the net differnetial between these figures. In terms of work lost due to sickness, upper income persons suffer 5.4 days per person per year, compared with 8.9 days among the poor. As measured by periods of disability spent in bed, the upper income person has a rate of 5.2 days per year, compared with 12.0 in the poor person. In terms of all types of "restricted activity," the higher income person loses 13.1 days per year, compared with 29.1 days for the poor person.

The diagnoses of diseases causing these various forms of disability are numerous, and they may be classified in different ways. Using broad categories, the National Health Survey found the six leading diagnostic groups to be: heart disease, arthritis and rheumatism, mental and nervous conditions, high blood pressure, visual impairments, and orthopedic impairments (excluding paralyses or amputations, which fit into another rubric). For all six of these leading causes of chronic disorder, the load among the poor is heavier. The common notion that heart disease is a special affliction of the rich is borne out by neither morbidity nor mortality data in the United States. As for mental disorder, the intensive New Haven Study by Hollingshead and Redlich suggested not only a higher total prevalence among the poor, but also a greater proportion of the more severe diagnoses leading to hospitalization (Hollingshead and Redlich, 1958).

The hard statistics on mortality and morbidity are necessary to establish the basic disadvantages of the poor, but they tell only a part of the story. Disease means not only pain and distress, but also fear and anxiety. The patient in a poor family is not so often reassured by a doctor, since he has less access to him, and the family may harbor its worries in silence. On the other hand, illness—being a common experience—may be casually regarded and neglected until its progress produces critical symptoms. The loss of time from work caused by disabling disease usually means loss of earnings; in the lowest paid jobs, such absence from work is seldom compensated by disability insurance benefits or "sick-pay" provisions.

The reasons for a greater burden of illness and death among the poor are multiple and complex. The elaboration, disease by disease, constitutes the vast discipline of epidemiology (MacMahon, Pugh, and Ipsen, 1960). This is not to imply that each and every disease is more prevalent among the poor. Cancer of the lung, for example, is far more common in persons who smoke a great many cigarettes, and the mere cost of the habit reduces this liability among the very poorest persons. But the aggregate impact of the physical and social environment of the poor, including their housing, nutrition, occupations, and whole style of life, contributes to a burden of disease and death that blights their lives much more than among the well-to-do.

The health handicaps of poverty apply to all places, rural and urban. In the urban slum, however, congested living, air pollution, lack of recreational space, and the general squalor are not mitigated even by sunshine and grass. It is true that access to medical care for rich and poor alike is greater in the cities than in rural areas. The urban poor, however, receive much less medical treatment for their illness than the well-to-do, so that a given sickness is more likely to become advanced, disabling, and even fatal. For the Negro and other ethnic minorities, the problems of poverty and ignorance are compounded by the barriers of prejudice and discrimination. The character of the health services received by the poor will be examined below, but first we must consider the organized social programs that have evolved to cope with their sicknesses and ameliorate their hardships.

Basic Programs for Health Care of the Poor

The serious handicaps of the urban poor, both in the occurrence of disease and the receipt of medical care, have long summoned corrective social actions. Were it not for numerous organized health service programs, health conditions would be far worse. One need only look at the mortality and morbidity of the impoverished masses in underdeveloped countries to see the effects of abject poverty, unalleviated by socio-medical efforts.

Organized health protection of the urban poor has been launched along many paths. Some programs are focused specifically on the poor and others, while offered theoretically to everyone, are especially useful for the poor. Some programs are directed to certain specific diseases occurring more commonly among the deprived. In all these programs, there are achievements to report and improvements that have benefited the poor; there are also weaknesses and deficiencies that persist, particularly in comparison with the health services available to the more affluent sections of the population. To record the benefits must not be interpreted as glossing over the defects and gaps.

The modern public health movement had its beginnings in nineteenth-century Europe largely in response to the sordid conditions in big-city slums. The rich in their country manors could, in large degree, take care of themselves, but environmental sanitation to assure clean water and proper sewage disposal was a matter of life-or-death for the urban poor. Up to the present day, the task of the public health sanitarian is heavily concentrated in the tenements of the poor. Health departments throughout the United States operate clinics for prevention of disease in infants and pregnant women. While these "maternal and child health programs" are theoretically open to everyone, in practice they are used—and sometimes deliberately restricted to—families of low income. Higher income families are expected to consult private physicians for preventive as well as curative service. In these clinics, infants receive immunizations and advice is given on diet and child-rearing. Although these programs have demonstrably reduced infant and maternal mortality, they seldom succeed in reaching all the poor and rarely assure the level of service enjoyed by the well-to-do. The funds allocated from general revenues to support such public health clinics are far less than the expenditures made by comfortable families for comparable private care (Hanlon, 1960).

Public health agencies operate other services of special value to the poor. There are clinics for the treatment of venereal disease and tuberculosis. Dental clinics are held for children. Sometimes there are clinics, operated in conjunction with the schools, for treatment of heart conditions, deafness, or other disorders in children. The fact that such public clinics usually lack the gracious setting of a private doctor's office, are often overcrowded and understaffed, and may sometimes give perfunctory attention to patients, does not negate the benefits they do offer. The task is to expand the resources going into such services and to improve their effectiveness.

Public health nurses visit the homes of the poor in connection with communicable disease, advice on newborn baby care, and even bedside service to the chronically ill. The education efforts of health departments are largely directed toward influencing the hygienic behavior of the poor. Screening tests to detect chronic diseases such as diabetes, glaucoma, cancer, or hypertension are offered by various agencies, and these have special value for lower income groups who lack regular family doctor contacts. One of the frustrating realities, however, is that the very poorest families—alienated by ignorance or apathy—often do not take advantage of such services even when they are made conveniently available (Anderson, 1963).

While public health agency services are, in practice, devoted largely to the poor, welfare department medical services are legally restricted to the poor. The historic development of these services from the Elizabethan Poor Laws, with their sanctimonious distinction between the provident and improvident poor, to the current welfare programs is a saga of evolution in social responsibility, a saga which is still in process. In relation to the past, today's urban slum-dweller is very fortunate, but in relation to the level of services that our current medical resources could provide, the deficiencies remain serious.

The medical and related services financed by welfare agencies for the poor depend on their legal "category." Since the Social Security Act of 1935 and its numerous amendments, federal grants to the states for public assistance are based on a needy person's identification in one of four classes: 1. over 65 years of age; 2. families with children and a lacking or unemployed breadwinner; 3. blind persons; and 4. persons with "total and permanent" disability. Poor persons who do not fit into one of these classes may be eligible for "general assistance," which must be financed entirely from state and local funds, typically meager. In 1962, about 7,500,000 persons received assistance under these programs, constituting about 4 percent of the national population. These persons are concentrated heavily in the urban slums.

The precise range of medical services available to the poor under public assistance programs varies with their "category," with the state or county in which they live, and with the year under discussion. Recent changes in the Social Security Act, to be discussed below ("Medicaid"), have altered these entitlements greatly. In general, however, medical and hospital services for the "indigent" and the "medically indigent" (see below) are provided under three patterns: 1. the poor person may be seen by a personally chosen physician and hospitalized in an ordinary community hospital, with the expenses being paid by the welfare department; 2. he may be seen in an out-patient clinic of a voluntary hospital and hospitalized in a special ward for the poor in such a hospital; or 3. he may be served in special governmental clinics and hospitals intended exclusively for the poor, and usually operated by special governmental authorities (U.S. Welfare Administration, 1964).

There are special human and technical qualities to each of these patterns of medical care for the urban poor. The public clinics and hospitals are typically crowded places, often badly maintained because of frugal financial support. They have little sensitivity to personal comfort and convenience (long travel time, waiting periods, etc.) although they may give a high technical quality of service—especially if the institution is affiliated with a medical school. The private doctor arrangements, on the other hand, may be more satisfactory on the human side and less on the scientific side. Some busy physicians, however, choose not to see welfare patients at all, so that the poor tend to consult mainly general practitioners in depressed neighborhoods. Here they tend to receive a style of medical care that is deficient both technically and humanistically.

Aside from the governmental hospitals—usually municipal or county—oriented to the poor, there are also state hospitals for mental disorders and tuberculosis, whose patients are largely from the lower income groups. Generally improved living conditions in the United States and effective new drugs (especially streptomycin) have resulted in a great reduction in the census of tuberculosis sanatoria in recent years. These institutions are being converted into facilities for general chronic diseases, predominantly serving the poor. Mental hospitals, on the other hand, are still crowded with patients, mostly from the lower income groups, although there has been a recent slight decline in census due to more effective methods of psychiatric therapy. While mental hospitals have improved their quality of care in recent years, they are still far below the level of maintenance in general hospitals which are supported mainly by the private sector. The large and semi-isolated mental institution remains an unhappy last resort for many senile paupers who, if they had the money, would be cared for at home or in a comfortable local nursing home.

Other special programs of medical care help the urban poor who qualify by reason of certain diagnoses. Crippled children, as defined by various state laws, may obtain service through special clinics or private doctors at governmental expense. Disabled adults may get "vocational rehabilitation," including corrective medical care, if treatment and training would render them employable. These programs typically have a means test, so that they are concentrated in their effects among the poor. They are financed by federal and state funds and maintain high standards of quality for the participating doctors and hospitals. Their quantitative impact, however, is small, because of the restricted medical definitions for eligibility and the relatively meager level of public financial support (Roemer, 1967).

Those urban poor who happen to be dependents of military personnel (wives and children) or veterans of past military service may be the beneficiaries of special governmental medical programs. The dependents can receive care from any physician or hospital, with the bill being paid by the U.S. Department of Defense. Veterans receive care in special governmental hospitals, even for non-service-connected conditions if they are persons of low income. In contrast to the local governmental administration of programs for welfare clients, the federal administration of these servcies is associated with higher standards of medical performance as well as with preservation of the patient's personal dignity (I. J. Cohen, 1966.)

Numerous voluntary health agencies also may serve the urban poor in such fields as home nursing ("visiting nurse associations"); personal assistance to crippled children; treatment of cancer, multiple sclerosis, muscular dystrophy, or other grave diseases; and emergency care after disasters such as floods or fires (Red Cross). Alcoholics may be helped by Alcoholics Anonymous and drug addicts by other bodies. Family planning advice and provisions may be offered in clinics of the Planned Parenthood Association. All these social services help, but they tend to have an impact far below the extent of the need among the poor.

Procurement of medical care by the self-supporting population of the United States has been greatly advanced by the extension of voluntary health insurance. There are many types, under the sponsorship of hospitals (Blue Cross), medical societies (Blue Shield), commercial insurance carriers, and employers or consumer organizations. The principal benefits of this insurance relate to hospitalization and the doctor's services in hospitalized illness, although the range of benefits has been widening. Typically, these programs ease the economic access of persons to private doctors and local hospitals and indirectly they have promoted the quality of care provided. While about 80 percent of the national population is now protected, at least partially, by hospitalization insurance, the non-protected 20 percent are heavily concentrated among the unemployed, the casually employed, the migrant, and other persons who make up the urban slum population (Somers and Somers, 1961).

The foregoing provides only a sketchy review of the principal organized social programs involving certain health services for the urban poor. In a nutshell, they all help. They tend to be improvements over the past, but none of them goes far enough. In terms of our medical potentialities, and our democratic expectations, they are generally deficient. The net impact of all these social programs, as well as the effects of actions derived from their own limited private resources, on the health services received by the poor may now be reviewed.

Health Services Received by the Poor

In spite of the variety of health service programs available to help the urban poor, the net volume of health care they receive is lower than that received by the higher income groups in both quantity and quality. This situation exists in the face of the heavier burden of disease and disability which, as we observed earlier, afflicts the poor.

The basic element in medical care is the service of a physician. From an initial contact with the doctor, other services that may be necessary follow, such as prescribed drugs, nursing care, laboratory or X-ray examinations, physical therapy, and hospitalization. Using the basic measure of "physician visits," the average American receives 5.0 such services per person per year (1959 data). For persons in families earning $7,000 or more, however, the rate is 5.7 physician visits, and it declines steadily to 4.5 visits in families earning under $2,000 annually. This relationship characterizes each age group observed separately (U.S. Public Health Service, 1964).

Table 5-1
Physician Contacts

Locale of Physician Contacts	*Family Income* *$7,000 & Over*	*Under $2,000*
Doctor's office	3.8	2.8
Patient's home	0.6	0.5
Telephone	0.7	0.3
Hospital clinic	0.3	0.7
Other	0.3	0.2
All places	5.7	4.5

The locales of these physician services reflect the character of medical services received by the affluent and the poor. For both groups, the bulk of services are obtained in the office of a private physician, but the proportions at different sites are revealing. As indicated in Table 5-1, within the lesser overall rate of doctor's services received by the poor, the rate is lower for all locales of contact, except in hospital clinics, where it is much higher. In such clinics, the time allotted per patient is typically much shorter than in a private office.

In spite of conventional notions that the poor are bountifully served in public clinics, it is evident that over 60 percent of their physician's care is obtained in private offices. Those offices, however, usually belong to general practitioners rather than specialists. Among high income families, for example, a pediatrician was consulted during the year by 29.4 percent of children (under 15 years of age), compared with 9.6 percent of low income children. An obstetrician or gynecologist was consulted by 17.1 percent of women in higher income families, compared with 3.5 percent of low income women. General physical examinations are a keystone of preventive medicine, but these too are rare among the poor. In 1963, among higher income families ($10,000 and over annually) 54 percent of youth under 17 years had such check-ups, compared with only 16 percent of youth from poor families (under $2,000) (U.S. Public Health Service, 1965).

The handicaps for dental service to the poor are even greater than for physician's service. Persons in higher income families ($7,000 and over) have 2.3 dental visits per person per year, compared with 0.7 visits among the poor (under $2,000). The dental services for the higher income groups, moreover, are more likely to consist of fillings and cleanings—preventive in effect—while for the poor they are much more likely to be extractions—the end result of neglect.

Prescribed drugs are also received at lower rates by the poor. Of the total drug consumption of the lower income groups, moreover, a higher proportion consists of self-prescribed or patent medicines. The corner druggist, it has been said, is often the poor man's doctor, offering across-the-counter pills which may only serve to alleviate pains and mask symptoms, thus delaying the procurement of needed diagnosis and therapy (Consumers Union, 1963).

It is only for hospitalization that the record of health services among various income groups shows a different relationship. When prevention has failed, and when early ambulatory medical care has not halted a disease process, admission to a hospital becomes necessary. The basic findings for 1959 are set out in Table 5-2, but more recent data show the same relationships. As the table demonstrates, the poorest families have admissions to hospitals less than middle-income families, but almost as frequently as the highest income families. Once admitted, however, the average length-of-stay of the poor is much longer, so that the aggregate days of hospital service received by the poor is significantly *higher* than among the well-to-do.

These data reflect a great deal about the disease patterns of the poor and the way in which our society has reponded to the general problems of medical care. In a word, our ameliorative social measures have followed a crisis strategy. When health problems get bad enough, we move on them. Thus, the social programs for providing hospitalization are relatively well developed. As noted earlier, there are many municipal and county hospitals for the poor. The extensive Veterans Administration hospital network will serve low income veterans even for non-military disabilities, but such resources are not eligible for ambulatory treatment. Examining the budgets of welfare departments, we find that about two-thirds of the expenditures go for hospital care of the indigent and one-third for out-of-hospital services; among self-supporting persons, the allocations are almost exactly the opposite. In New York State, the expenditures for welfare medical services in 1963 were $184 million of which nearly $160 million or 87 percent were for institutional (hospital and nursing home) services (Yerby, 1966).

Once admitted to a hospital, the low income person stays on a longer time than his more affluent counterpart. This differential is due to several reasons. His illness is more likely to be at a far advanced stage, when recovery takes longer. Having a poorer nutritional state, his rate of recovery from surgery or his response to other therapy is likely to be slower. In public hospitals, the actual man-

Table 5-2
Hospital Discharges and Stay, 1959

Family Income	*Hospital Discharges per 1,000 Persons*	*Average Stay (Days)*	*Aggregate Days per 1,000 Persons*
Under $2,000	92.8	11.7	1,086
$2,000–$3,999	103.5	8.5	840
$4,000–$6,999	101.3	7.2	729
$7,000 and over	97.9	7.9	773

agement of his care is more likely to be assigned to a young resident or intern, whose skills are less than those of a fully trained physician. The non-paying patient is more likely to be "teaching material" in a medical school—kept longer for the education of medical students. On top of all this, the indigent person's home conditions are known to be meager, so that the conscientious physician cannot discharge him as rapidly as he would release the middle-class patient, with a pleasant home in which to convalesce.

All these characteristics of the health services received by the poor are ultimately consequences of their poverty, but this is not to say that lack of money is the total explanation. As we have seen, many programs of financial support have developed over the years and these have compensated to varying degrees for the inability to purchase medical service in the private market. But beyond low purchasing power, as such, the poor suffer other handicaps that obstruct their proper use of modern medical care and their maintenance of health. Having lower levels of education, they are less likely to recognize significant symptoms and seek care. The repeated physical and emotional traumas of poverty make them fatalistic and even apathetic; delays and neglect in seeking care are the result. Even when services for mothers and infants are provided by a public health clinic in a slum neighborhood, it is common for the utilization rate to be low. Initial response to a symptom of illness is more likely to be communication with a neighbor than consultation with a doctor (King, 1962).

Compounding fatalistic attitudes are many practical impediments to medical care like time and transportation. As noted earlier, the low-income worker, unlike the white-collar employee, seldom has "sick-leave" provisions in his job, and a day lost waiting at a public clinic or even seeing a private doctor often means loss of a day's wages. The slum tenement mother cannot take a sick baby to the clinic without making provision for her other small children or dragging them along. Transportation is another problem. Dependence on buses and street cars, rather than a family automobile, is time-consuming, uncomfortable, and often irritating. On top of all this are the insensitivities and long waits in public clinics and even in the private offices of doctors serving a large proportion of the poor.

In the big-city slums, the physicians and dentists located close to the poor are likely to be the least well trained. The Watts area of Los Angeles, for example, has only one-third the doctor-population ratio of the county as a whole and only a handful of specialists. Among the smaller supply of doctors in the Watts area, only 16 percent are specialists, compared with about 55 percent in the nation as a whole. Two-thirds of the 16 percent, morever, are self-declared specialists, rather than doctors certified by the appropriate American Specialty Boards (Roemer, 1966).

Chiropractors, herbalists, and other cultist practitioners are more likely to be located in the central-city slum than in the fashionable professional sections of a city. They are used more frequently by the poor, not only because they are close at hand, but also because they are less expensive and often more reassuring than scientific physicians. They promise quick cures, about which the unsophisticated or desperate slum-dweller may be gullible. Slick patent medicine and food faddist advertising compound the fraudulence perpetrated on the poor by various profiteers (Deutsch, 1960).

New Health Programs for the Poor

The deficiencies in health services received by the poor have been recognized by socially minded health leaders for some time. In spite of the numerous categorical programs reviewed earlier, especially the medical services of welfare departments directed to the needs of the indigent, the heavier volume of morbidity among the poor has been far from adequately served. Because of this patent deficiency, a number of new health programs have been launched in recent years by federal legislation. These programs may represent a turning point in America's approach to health services for all the people, poor and affluent (Forgotson, 1967).

Most important of the legislative output were the Social Security Act amendments of 1965 which established the first nationwide social insurance program in the United States for medical care. Known popularly as "Medicare," Title XVIII of the Act provides a series of hospital, medical, and related benefits to virtually all persons in the country 65 years of age and over, whether or not they are entitled to a Social Security old-age pension. The significant point is that there is no means test for these benefits; every aged person receives the same hospital services and related care in an "extended care facility" (nursing home) or at home ("home health services"). For physician's care and certain ancillary services, the aged person must pay (or he may choose to forego these benefits) a small "voluntary" monthly premium ($3 in 1967), which is more than matched by federal subsidy. Moreover, Social Security cash benefits were elevated by over $3 per month to cover this added expenditure (Cohen and Ball, 1965).

Since a major share of the urban poor, especially in slum boarding houses, are over 65 years of age, Medicare will doubtless be of great value to the poor as a social class. As statistics also show, the burden of illness among the aged in all income groups is much greater than in the young, and the aged parent's children must often foot the bills. Voluntary health insurance, as noted earlier, had its least impact among the aged, especially those of low income, so that the Medicare legislation has obviously been a great step forward in social welfare.

The precise benefits of Medicare are far from comprehensive. There are limitations on the number of hospital days payable (90 days in a "spell of illness"), there are cost-sharing requirements (e.g. $40 on hospital admissions and $10 per day after the sixtieth day), and important items are not covered at all, like dental care and out-of-hospital drugs. Limitations on the "voluntary insurance" benefits for physician's care are greater, with a $50 per year deductible and 20 percent cost-sharing for all services.

In spite of these limitations, imposed in the interests of reducing the total social insurance budget and thereby gaining Congressional approval, Medicare has clearly ushered in a new era for medical care of the poor. For those poor who are aged, the law facilitates access to the same mainstream of community medical care—the private physician and the voluntary general hospital—that serves the well-to-do. In part, even the administration of the law makes use of the existing framework of private insurance plans as "fiscal intermediaries" between the central Social Security Administration and the providers of service. The mainstream entitlements, of course, apply only to those poor who are aged. If any lesson can be learned from the history of social insurance for medical care in other countries, however, it is that with time and experience both population coverage and medical benefits are expanded. There is little doubt that the same will happen to Medicare.

Although Medicare is mainly a "bill-paying" mechanism and accepts the existing framework of private medical practice, it has introduced certain modest influences on the quality of care. Hospitals, to receive payments, must be "certified," and this requires meeting various technical standards. "Utilization review" of cases is one of the most important of these requirements—a measure which should heighten the self-discipline among physicians on hospital staffs. Nursing homes, to be certified, must have a "transfer agreement" with a general hospital, a device which can reduce the previous isolation of these units from professional stimulation. Perhaps most important, the very public visibility of medical care costs—already produced by Medicare—will induce a closer examination of the whole social structure of American medicine. Soaring costs can highlight much of the extravagance and inefficiency of private, solo medical practice, and this publicity in turn can lead to corrective innovations in the patterns of organization. These innovations can have special meaning for the poor.

Along with Medicare for the aged, the Social Security amendments of 1965 also added Title XIX, which involves radical alterations in the whole pattern of medical services for the poor under age 65. "Medicaid," as it has come to be called, is a modification of the long-established public assistance medical care legislation, reviewed earlier, which rests on the principle of federal grants to the states for help to certain demographic categories. Title XIX liberalizes the basis of these federal grants—allowing substantially open-ended matching of state appropriations—and authorizes the states to include among their medical beneficiaries not only the recipients of cash assistance, but also similar persons who are "medically indigent." The latter would include a family with a missing or unemployed breadwinner and dependent children (AFDC) which was not poor enough to qualify for cash assistance but still could not afford private medical care. Theoretically, this provision could reach a substantial proportion of urban slum-dwellers who were not previously receiving medical care. Medicaid also provides that, to receive federal grants, a state must assure a minimum range of five professional and hospitalization benefits to all categorical recipients. Moreover, it must gradually expand its coverage, so that, by 1975, virtually all poor people in the state—whether or not "categorically linked"—must be entitled to financial support for essential medical services (Greenfield, 1966). (Note: In 1972 Congress unfortunately rescinded this requirement.)

How successful Medicaid will actually be in extending good medical care to the nation's poor is a serious question. For one thing, the state government must agree to the federal conditions and, as of this writing two years after enactment of the law, 24 states have still not done so. For another, the definition of indigency and medical indigency is still left up to each state; many of the poorest states with large numbers of impoverished people draw these lines at very low thresholds. Third, the definitions of health services, even within the federal schedule of five benefits, are subject to varying interpretations; drugs and dental care, moreover, are not even among them. Fourth, the whole Medicaid program, like Medicare, accepts the mainstream approach as unreservedly desirable; it incorporates no provisions that might modify organizational patterns to better suit the needs of the poor or, for that matter, others.

The neutrality of Medicare and Medicaid on the critical issue of patterns of health service organization in America lends special significance to two other pieces of health legislation enacted by the Eighty-ninth (1965–1966) Congress. These are the "Heart Disease, Cancer, and Stroke Amendments of 1965" (PL 89-239) and the "Comprehensive Health Planning and Public Health Service Amendments of 1966" (PL 89-749). Neither of these laws is focused specifically on the poor, but their long-term significance for those in this category may be as great as the milestone of social insurance.

The Heart-Cancer-Stroke law is based on an effort to attack the three leading causes of death in the United States by encouraging improvements in the quality of care for these diseases at the grass roots and in the average urban neighborhood. It provides federal grants for developing "regional medical programs" to improve the diagnosis and treatment of these and related diseases. The regional programs are intended to establish active professional connections between the great medical centers and peripheral hospitals around them. So far, these ties have been largely limited to the organization of postgraduate instruction for practicing physicians, but there is hope that they might be extended to include active consultation and referral services. The goal is to enable every person to receive the best scientific care for his disease, regardless of his geographic location or socioeconomic status. The regionalization concept, embodied in this law, has been applied throughout the world as a mechanism for systematizing medical care and elevating its quality. Whether the Heart-Cancer-Stroke law will evolve into such a full-dress regionalization pattern depends on other political developments in the coming years (Russell, 1966).

The Comprehensive Health Planning amendments have even a broader potential influence on medical care patterns, although the terms of the law are relatively modest. Its immediate purpose is to consolidate federal grants to the states in formerly earmarked fields, such as venereal disease control, chronic illness and aging programs, and "general public health," in order to permit each state to allocate the funds flexibly according to a "state plan" based on its own particular needs. The long-term purpose is much broader; it provides grants to the states for overall planning of health facilities, personnel, and services—in the private as well as the public sector—to best meet the total health needs of the population. If this purpose is taken seriously, the implications are great for improvement of health services to the poor. Any objective description and assessment of our current patterns of medical care, the chaotic multiplicity of agencies, the sovereignty of private, solo medical practice and small autonomous hospitals, and the irrational separation of prevention and therapy can only help to set us on the road to their correction (Stewart, 1967).

Still another federal program, with clear impacts on the health of the urban poor, is the so-called war on poverty administered by the Office of Economic Opportunity (OEO). Several projects of this agency, including "Operation Head Start" for preschool youngsters and the Youth Job Corps for unemployed teenagers, have an indirect bearing on health. Most direct and daring of the OEO projects, from the viewpoint of health needs, are the "neighborhood health centers." These are centers for comprehensive ambulatory medical care located in the heart of the slums and open 24 hours a day. In contrast to the out-patient departments of the big municipal hospitals, the neighborhood centers emphasize a personal doctor relationship for each patient and stress participation of the local people in the management of the program and as auxiliary health workers. With such involvement, it is hoped that the poor will make fuller use of the services, instead of distrusting them as the reluctant charity of "the establishment." At this writing, only a half-dozen such centers are in operation, in the central ghettos (mainly Negro) of large cities, but some 40 are being planned. Doctors are engaged in the centers on full-time or part-time salaries, and overall direction is under medical schools, medical societies, local health departments, or other bodies. The neighborhood centers are clearly a deviation from the mainstream concept of medical care for the poor, and it remains to be seen how their character takes shape (Geiger, 1966).

Several other established governmental health programs were expanded or liberalized in 1965–1966 to improve services for the poor. The traditional "maternal and child health" grants to the states were amended to permit comprehensive maternal and child *care* in "high risk" families, meaning essentially families of the poor. The Community Mental Health Amendments of 1965 (PL 89-105) support wider funding of both construction and operation of psychiatric centers oriented mainly to the needs of the poor. The Vocational Rehabilitation Amendments of 1965 (PL 89-290) enlarge the federal share of these grants which, as we noted earlier, help principally low income persons who are disabled but employable. These and other new laws of the last few years, at both federal and state levels, mark an apparent turning point in social concern for the provision of health services to the nation's poor.

The View Ahead

Improvement in the health of the urban poor depends, first of all, on their living conditions. Two hundred years ago Johann Peter Frank wrote that "poverty is the mother of disease." Although there are other progenitors of sickness as well, Frank's axiom is still true. Not only does an insanitary and congested environment contribute to the causation of disease, but the alienation and apathy of poverty discourage behavior that could protect health. Racial and ethnic discriminations compound the difficulties for millions of dwellers in the urban ghetto. The most basic approach to the health of the poor, therefore, must emphasize improvement of their whole standard of living. Adequate employment is obviously essential, associated with proper education, good housing, balanced nutrition, ample recreation, and above all, equal opportunity.

There are two somewhat competing philosophies at play in the current American scene with respect to health services for the indigent. One is to set up special organized facilities for the poor—municipal hospitals and clinics, specially appointed doctors, public health clinics for children, and so on. The latest implementation of this approach is the OEO "neighborhood health center" discussed above. The other philosophy has been called the "mainstream approach"—that is, arrangement for medical care of the poor through existing resources serving the general population, these being principally private physicians and voluntary hospitals. This latter philosophy is embodied in the important Medicare Law of 1965. In either case a public agency pays the costs, but the mainstream approach is thought to have a more democratic quality, because it does not segregate the poor in separate places. And as already noted, the conditions in those separate facilities—whether in massive municipal hospitals or in public health clinics located in the basement of a county courthouse—are often conducive to perfunctory and insensitive medical care (Strauss, 1967).

The issue is not so simple, however, because the quality and accessibility of medical service in the medical mainstream may also be very deficient. Free choice of private doctor, which results in assembly-line treatment in a poorly staffed office of a slum general practitioner is no blessing. Welfare department tabulations reveal shocking mediocrities and abuses of both patients and public moneys in such private practices. In the voluntary community hospital, moreover, the poor may still be segregated in second-class wards, where they do not receive the physician's care, the nursing care, and various amenities accorded to private patients (Rogatz, 1967). On the other hand, the quality and even the human sensitivity of medical care in a special facility may be excellent. The level achieved in most "segregated" Veterans Administration hospitals demonstrates this, as do the standards now being applied in several new OEO neighborhood health centers. Separate facilities for the poor, in other words, may appear to have undemocratic overtones, but they are good or bad depending on the quantity of resources put into them and the policies of management applied.

The root problem is that the mainstream of American medicine has inherent deficiencies that compromise the accessibility and quality of medical care for the affluent as well as the poor. The predominance of solo medical practice, uncoordinated hospitals, self-prescribed drugs, and similar factors represent a heritage from earlier centuries, a heritage which blocks the realization of the full potential of modern medical science. The task, therefore, is to modify the patterns and direction of "mainstream medicine," so that it becomes appropriate to the true requirements of science and the needs of people. This is a long and complex challenge to explain, but it involves essentially *organization* of both preventive and curative health services economically, technologically, and geographically.

If the character of the mainstream in American medical care is appropriately modified—with more imaginative use of comprehensive group practice, with regionalization of hospitals, and with better integration of prevention and treatment—then the care of the poor should certainly be provided within it. In a word, this would mean that certain patterns of health service organization, now applied in a faltering way in the segregated streams, would be improved in their application—through more generous financial support and competent leadership—and incorporated within the mainstream of medicine. The issue posed earlier would then disappear, and all persons, rich and poor, would receive one uniformly high quality of medical care, regardless of the source of financing.

The new legislation for "comprehensive health planning," along with several other developments reviewed above, may help to promote such a better future. If it does, one more blow may be struck against the sordid cycles of poverty and disease that now enchain the dwellers in urban slums.

References

Anderson, Odin W. "The Utilization of Health Services," in H. E. Freeman, S. Levine, and L. G. Reeder (eds.), *Handbook of Medical Sociology* (New York: Prentice-Hall, 1963), pp. 349–67.

Cohen, I. J. "The Veterans Administration Medical Care Program," in L. J. DeGroot (ed.), *Medical Care: Social and Organizational Aspects* (Springfield, Ill.: Charles C. Thomas, 1966), pp. 425–36.

Cohen, Wilbur J. and Robert M. Ball. "Social Security Amendments of 1965: Summary and Legislative History," *Social Security Bulletin*, 28, No. 9 (September, 1965), pp. 3–21.

Deutsch, R. M. "Nutritional Nonsense and Food Fanatics," in *Proceedings, Third National Congress on Medical Quackery* (Chicago: American Medical Association, 1960), pp. 15–24.

Editors of Consumer Reports. *The Medicine Show: Some Plain Truths about Popular Remedies for Common Ailments* (Mount Vernon, N.Y.: Consumers Union, 1963).

Forgotson, E. H. "1965: The Turning Point in Health Law—1966 Reflections," *American Journal of Public Health*, 57 (June, 1967), pp. 934–46.

Geiger, H. Jack. "The Poor and the Professional: Who Takes the Handle Off the Broad Street Pump?" paper presented at the Annual Meeting of the American Public Health Association, San Francisco, California, November 1, 1966.

Greenfield, Margaret. "Title XIX and Medi-Cal," *Public Affairs Report* (Bulletin of the Institute of Governmental Studies, University of California, Berkeley), Vol. 7, No. 4, August, 1966.

Hanlon, John J. *Principles of Public Health Administration* (St. Louis: C. V. Mosby Company, 1960), "Maternal and Child Health Activities," pp. 470–92.

Hollingshead, August B. and Frederick C. Redlich. *Social Class and Mental Illness* (New York: John Wiley, 1958).

King, Stanley H. *Perceptions of Illness and Medical Practice* (New York: Russell Sage Foundation, 1962).

MacMahon, Brian, Thomas F. Pugh, and Johannes Ipsen. *Epidemiologic Methods* (Boston: Little, Brown and Company, 1960).

Roemer, Milton I. "Health Resources and Services in the Watts Area of Los Angeles," *California's Health*, 23, Nos. 8–9 (February–March 1966), pp. 123–43.

———. "Governmental Health Programs Affecting the American Family," *Journal of Marriage and the Family*, 29 (February, 1967), pp. 40–63.

Rogatz, Peter. "Our Care of the Poor is a Failure," *Medical Economics*, 29 (May, 1967), pp. 209–17.

Russell, J. M. "New Federal Regional Medical Programs." *New England Journal of Medicine*, 275 (August 11, 1966), pp. 309–12.

Somers, Herman M. and Anne R. Somers. *Doctors, Patients, and Health Insurance* (Washington: The Brookings Institution, 1961).

Stern, Bernhard J. *Society and Medical Progress* (Princeton: Princeton University Press, 1941), "Income and Health," pp. 126–41.

Stewart, William H. *New Dimensions of Health Planning* (The 1967 Michael M. Davis lecture) (Chicago: University of Chicago, Center for Health Administration Studies, 1967).

Strauss, Anselm L. "Medical Ghettos," *Trans-Action*, 4 (May, 1967), pp. 7–15, 62.

U.S. Public Health Service, National Center for Health Statistics. *Medical Care, Health Status, and Family Income*. Series 10, No. 9 (Washington, May, 1964), pp. 52–74.

U.S. Public Health Service, National Center for Health Statistics. *Physician Visits–Interval of Visits and Children's Routine Checkups, United States, July 1963–June 1964*. Series 10, No. 19 (Washington, June, 1965).

U.S. Welfare Administration. *Characteristics of State Public Assistance Plans under the Social Security Act: Provisions for Medical and Remedial Care*. Public Assistance Report, No. 49 (Washington, 1964).

Yerby, Alonzo S. "Public Medical Care for the Needy in the United States," in L. J. DeGroot (ed.), *Medical Care: Social and Organizational Aspects* (Springfield, Ill.: Charles C. Thomas, 1966), pp. 382–401.

6

Organized Health Services in the Area of an Urban Riot

Since the Civil War (1861–65), "race riots" have been a feature of American urban development. In the 1960s a series of such riots shook larger cities with ghettoes of black and other minority families. The first and perhaps the most tragic of such riots occurred in Los Angeles in August, 1965. In response, the Governor of California appointed a "blue ribbon committee" to investigate the causes of the riot and recommend measures to correct them.

As part of this investigation, the health conditions and programs of the riot area would be analyzed and I was appointed to make this study. The result was the following report on "Health Resources and Services in the Watts Area of Los Angeles." Several of the recommendations of the report were implemented, especially the construction of a large public general hospital in the heart of the riot area, an impressive neighborhood health center for organized ambulatory health care, and the strengthening of basic health services of the County Health Department. These events illustrate very well the initiation of organized health programs in response to social crises.

THE MEDICAL CIRCUMSTANCES of the Los Angeles Riot Area bear all the usual stigmata of poverty. Relative to the prevailing standards of the American life in general or Los Angeles in particular, they are seriously deficient in both quantity and quality. While various social programs have helped to ameliorate the worst consequences of laissez-faire inequities, their impact has been far below the measure of human need. As President Harry Truman said, the old saw about the rich and poor getting good health care—while the middle groups suffer—is half true. All the evidence suggests that the untrue half of this cliché applies to the Los Angeles Riot Area.

Population and Background

This report will focus its main attention on the health resources and services of the geographic sections defined by the Los Angeles County Health Department as the *South District* and the *Southeast District*. This territory is not exactly coter-

Chapter 6 originally appeared in *California's Health* (the official periodical of the California State Department of Public Health), pp. 123–143, February–March, 1966.

minous with the Riot Area, as defined by the National Guard Curfew imposed at the height of the riots. It is almost entirely included, however, within this larger zone. These two Health Department districts contain the highest concentration of Negro families and individuals in Los Angeles County, living under the kind of social conditions which bred the August Riots. Their residents, therefore, may be considered the central core of the population in the larger zone where some violence occurred—and where a military curfew was imposed.

The total population of South and Southeast Districts of the Los Angeles County Health Department recorded by the 1960 Census was 251,221. The South Health District contains 143,524 people, of whom 53.8 percent are Negro, 1.8 percent are other non-white races, and 44.3 percent are white. This district contains the community customarily described as Watts, with an estimated population of 34,000 persons, of whom 87.0 percent are Negro. The Southeast Health District has a population of 107,697 (as of the 1960 Census), of whom 82.1 percent are Negro, 1.8 percent other non-white races, and 16.1 percent white. This district contains the community of Avalon with a population of 52,500, of whom 94.8 percent are Negro.

Because of varying methods of subdividing the county for different social and administrative purposes, not all the statistical data even within the sphere of health services fit neatly into the jurisdictions just outlined. For certain purposes it was necessary to accept other geographic boundaries and other population figures. These statistical short-cuts do not introduce serious errors, however, in light of the general similarity of demographic and social conditions characterizing the depressed people in the territory immediately adjacent to the South and Southeast Districts.

A few other characteristics of the South and Southeast District populations shed some further light on their health needs. By California standards, it is a crowded population. The density is over 10,000 persons per square mile—the highest in Los Angeles County. The in-migration to these districts in recent years has been enormous. The influx of Negroes, mostly from the Southern states, has been great in many Northern cities since 1940. In Los Angeles the new settlers have increased eight times in this span of years, compared with 2½ times in New York City or three times in Detroit. Most of these people have settled in the South and Southeast Districts, and they bring with them the educational, social, and health handicaps of generations of segregated living the South.

The proportion of children in these districts is high. In the South District 14 percent of the population is under five years of age, compared with 10.7 percent in Los Angeles County as a whole. There are relatively fewer aged persons—7.4 percent of the South District population being 65 years or over, compared with 9.2 percent in the County. There are relatively more women, since men move out, and many more broken families. Educational attainments are lower; the median school year completed is 10.2 grades in the South District and 9.0 in the Southeast District, compared with 12.1 grades in the County as a whole.

Overcasting the whole social description of the Riot Area people, of course, is poverty. In the South District 5.8 percent of families have annual incomes of under $1,000, and in the Southeast District 7.4 percent. The median family income in the South District, as of 1960, was $5,424, and in the Southeast District $4,225, compared with $7,046 in Los Angeles County as a whole. All these basic features of life have an obvious bearing on the health status of this population as well as its access to health services.

By all the usual indices of medical need, the population of the South-Southeast Districts suffers a heavier burden than that of the rest of Los Angeles County's 6,700,000 people. Infant and maternal mortalities are higher. Life expectancies, as a whole, are lower. (Another section of this Report summarizes the available data on the mortality and morbidity of the Riot Area population.)

Medical and Related Personnel

The keystone of day-to-day medical care is the personal physician, but the Riot Area is sparsely provided with such essential personnel. In the Southeast District (108,000 population) there are 41 physicians, a ratio of 38 per 100,000 population; in the South District (144,000) there are 65 physicians, 45 per 100,000. These figures may be compared with a Los Angeles County ratio of 127 physicians per 100,000—about three times as many.

Of course, not every neighborhood in a metropolitan city needs to be supplied with *all* the doctors required to serve its local population. People can ordinarily be expected to travel out of their immediate environs for certain elements of medical care. The fact is, however, that Los Angeles County—with its great geographic sprawl—is remarkably well covered by neighborhood doctors. In most of the county, there is a reasonable distribution of doctor's offices, medical arts buildings, and private medical clinics in relation to the scatter of population. In spite of some concentration of medical and surgical specialists along Wilshire Boulevard, the great majority of local communities in the county do have a good supply of private physicians close at hand. They are relatively convenient and accessible without long travel. Even the large prepaid medical care plans (Kaiser-Permanente and Ross-Loos) have established networks of neighborhood clinics relatively close to where their subscribers live.

In the Riot Area, however, this adjustment of physician resources to population needs has been only poorly attained. The explanation is not mysterious. The free market has held only limited financial rewards for doctors settling in this locale of poverty. There are no Kaiser or Ross-Loos branch clinics in the South or Southeast Districts, nor any private group practice clinics. A major share of the general medical care required by the 251,000 people in these two districts, therefore, must be obtained outside their borders, and principally at the Outpatient Department of the Los Angeles County General Hospital. Yet resources for transportation are limited, time-consuming, and relatively expensive.

The professional qualifications of the restricted supply of physicians in the Riot Area cast further light on the probable quality of care received by their patients. Of the 106 practitioners in the South and Southeast Districts, only 17 are specialists; this 16 percent of specialization compares with about 55 percent of physicians nationally. Not all of the 17 specialists, moreover, are certified by their respective American Specialty Boards; according to the 1964–65 edition of the *American Directory of Medical Specialists*, only five are so qualified. These include only one each in obstetrics-gynecology, surgery, pediatrics, ophthalmology, and pathology. Four of these five certified specialists are Negro physicians, and one is white. Of the total number of 106 physicians in both districts, 62 are Negro and 44 are white. There are also eight chiropractors in the South-Southeast Districts.

Dentists are no more plentiful in the Riot Area than physicians. In the combined South-Southeast Districts there are 47 dentists, but nine of them are reported to be professionally inactive. The balance of 38 dentists serving 251,000 people yields a ratio of 15.1 per 100,000, compared with a California statewide ratio of 67 per 100,000—4½ times greater. Not only is this relative discrepancy greater than that for physicians, but it must be realized that resources for dental care available outside the Riot Area are much fewer. In the Los Angeles County General Hospital, dental service is available only for emergency extractions, not for restorative care. There are limited other resources available in the area for low-income children and pregnant women, which are reviewed below.

Hospitals and Related Facilites

The center for scientific modern medicine has increasingly become the community general hospital. Not only is it properly a place for the bed care of the seriously sick, but it has become a major resource for elaborate diagnosis of the ambulatory patient, for professional education, research, and even for disease prevention. Its impact is important on the quality and style of medical practice outside its walls, through influence on its medical staff. This role has come to be played in American medicine by general hospitals under the auspices of nonprofit associations (religious or otherwise) or governmental agencies.

In the Riot Area the principal institutional resources are small proprietary hospitals. Data based on the Curfew Area (which is larger than the South-Southeast Districts, although not entirely inclusive of them) show eight such hospitals in this Area, ranging from 22 to 136 beds in capacity, with a total of 454 beds. Only two of these hospitals are approved by the Joint Commission on Hospital Accreditation, indicating that they fail to meet minimum standards of professional quality.

On the northern edge of the Curfew Area, there are two specialized hospitals which meet accreditation standards but do not serve general medical purposes, the nonprofit Orthopedic Hospital having 162 beds, and John Wesley Hospital (under Los Angeles County government) having 259 beds. The Orthopedic Hospital provides care for serious bone and joint disorders to the entire Los Angeles metropolitan area. Despite its location, it is not a major resource for the population of the Riot Area. The John Wesley Hospital does serve the low-income population of the South and Southeast Districts, but its services are predominantly maternity cases (almost two-thirds of the admissions)—the balance for medical (i.e. nonsurgical) patients.

The generally poor quality of patient-care in the South-Southeast Districts hospitals has been noted in hospital licensing reports by the California State Department of Public Health. Space permits only a few examples: In one 43-bed hospital, the 1964 report ordered the kitchen to be cleaned, mice-droppings to be removed, infected dressings to be incinerated, a registered nurse to be on duty for the 11 P.M. to 7 A.M. shift, the doctors to sign medication orders, and several other actions reflecting serious deficiencies. In another hospital of 67 beds, the official report called for disposal of garbage in proper containers, the storage of drugs and poisons separately from foods, the recording of infant formulas on charts, etc. In a 49-bed hospital, the report indicated cockroach infestation near the coffee urns, torn or missing screens, no written manual of maternity nursing procedures, inoperative nurse-call signals. Medical staff organization in these hospitals is so casual as to be almost nonexistent, which accounts for their nonaccreditation.

It is only reasonable, of course, to expect people to travel a certain distance for hospital care, so that one must count as resources for the Riot Area population the general hospitals near to, though not within, the South-Southeast Districts. The most important is probably the St. Fancis Hospital of Lynwood, an accredited 530-bed institution located about one mile west of Watts. While non-profit, this hospital does not operate an organized outpatient service, but only receives emergencies or private patients referred by its staff doctors for diagnostic tests. During the August riots, for example, 73 emergency patients were brought to this hospital, of whom 18 were admitted, 10 sent to the County General Hospital, and three were dead on arrival. On the medical staff of 235 active physicians in the St. Francis Hospital, there are 15 Negro physicians; it is significant that in 1960 there had been 22 Negro doctors on this staff, but seven terminated their connection because, it is reported, their patients could not afford the private costs.

A principal hospital resource for the 251,000 persons in the South-Southeast Districts is the Los Angeles County General Hospital—both for bed-care and for organized outpatient services. This important institution, affiliated with three medical schools, undoubtedly provides high quality medical care along its technical dimension, although, as with many public institutions, there may be widely recognized deficiencies along humanistic lines. In a special one-day census of all patients taken on the night of 13 July 1965, there were 2,287 hospitalized patients, of whom, by direct count, exactly 100 cases resided in the 23 Census tracts (72,000 population) in and around Watts. Applying the average length-of-stay in the County General Hospital (about 9 to 10 days) to these 100 cases, and assuming this one-day count was roughly representative of the year, one can calculate that approximately 42 admissions per 1,000 persons per year come to this hospital from Watts and its immedicate environs. National Health Survey data for low-income people show a nation-wide hospital admission rate of 125 cases per 1,000 persons per year, but other evidence suggests a lower rate in California. By this crude measure, it would appear that about 40 percent of the Watts area patients hospitalized per year go to the Los Angeles County General Hospital.

Other patients from Watts and the remainder of the South-Southeast Districts seek hospitalization at Harbor General Hospital, John Wesley, St. Francis and California Hospitals (also fairly near these districts), the local proprietary hospitals and, to a limited extent, at many other hospitals in the Los Angeles region. It must be pointed out, however, that the hospital resources for the physicians *practicing* within the South-Southeast Districts are not these peripheral institutions of good quality but, in the main, the small proprietary hospitals within the districts reviewed earlier. The institutional influences on their mode of practice would be correspondingly limited.

While an 8- or 10-mile automobile or ambulance trip to the County General Hospital may not be excessive for inpatient admission, this distance by bus—taking, on the average about one hour and costing 68 cents—can provide a serious obstacle to repeated outpatient visits. The problem is compounded when patients must accept long delays in a crowded clinic waiting-room. It is further compounded by the problems of lost time from work for an employed man or woman who is asked to come to the clinic in the daytime hours, or the expense of babysitters for other children at home while the mother is away at the hospital. Yet this constitutes a major resource for ambulatory medical care for thousands of persons in the Riot Area who are unable to afford private physician's care or are not entitled to governmentally financed care from local physicians (see below).

Other health facilities in the Riot Area include a few small institutions for aged or chronically ill patients. The Lynwood Hospital Service Area, the jurisdiction of the California State Plan for Hospitals inclusive of Watts, contains five nursing homes with an aggregate of 305 beds. While four are called "convalescent hospitals," all five are regarded by knowledgeable observers as below the average in quality for this type of facility.

There are also 11 drugstores in the South-Southeast Districts, important as health facilities since many poor people rely on druggists for medical advice and purchase of patent medicines to cope with their symptoms.

Public Health Services

In any modern community the preventively oriented services of a department of public health have become an accepted necessity of life. In an economically depressed community, like the Los Angeles Riot Area, the importance of such services is even greater. Infectious and other preventable diseases are more prevalent among the poor. A given public health effort in impoverished areas, moreover, can yeild greater returns in reduction of disease and death.

The South and Southeast Health Districts are designated by the Los Angeles County Health Department to serve a major portion of what proved to be the Riot Area. They constitute slightly modified versions of districts, of the same names, in the Los Angeles City Health Department, prior to its consolidation into the County Department, July 1, 1964. Activities of these district public health programs are concentrated in well-constructed health centers: at 4290 Avalon Boulevard, Avalon, for Southeast District and at 1522 East 102nd Street, Watts, for South District; a smaller subcenter at 8019 Compton Avenue (the Florence-Firestone Unit) also serves part of South District.

While these centers are well designed, their use has outgrown their capacities, and they are usually cramped and crowded places. There are lacks in basic equipment for efficient administration, like duplicating or dictating machines, and laboratory facilities are quite limited. Various clinic sessions, especially for child health, are also held at other locations (like schools and housing projects) around the districts.

The key personnel in a generalized health program are public health nurses, but these personnel have been in seriously short supply. For the 251,000 people in both districts there have been 48 such nurses, or only one per 5,230 people. In an economically depressed area, a desirable ratio would be one public health nurse to about 2,000 people. The limited corps of nurses are so busy staffing various clinics that they have little time for important field visits to homes. For example, the many broken appointments at tuberculosis or venereal disease clinics properly require follow-up visits, but there is no time to make them. The County Health Department requested funds for 200 additional public health nurses to serve the entire county in fiscal year 1965–66, but the action of the County Government resulted in a reduction of 15 positions.

The Health Officer of South District retired on July 1, 1965 and, at the time of the riots, this position had been vacant for six weeks. The overworked Health Officer of Southeast District was asked to be responsible for South District as well. Only after the August Riots was a medical officer of the U.S. Public Health Service requested and, on an emergency basis, lent to the County to cover South District.

The program of the County Health Department in both districts follows traditional lines. The main emphasis is on the preventive aspects of maternal and child health services. In addition, there are activities in the field of tuberculosis and venereal disease control, general health education, and environmental sanitation. Somewhat more enterprising is a limited program in family planning and a small schedule of bedside home visits to post-hospital patients with hemiplegia and other chronic disorders.

The limitations of a public health program can be illustrated by the practices in the prenatal service. There are four prenatal clinic sessions (about 2½ hours each) held per week in South District and six in Southeast District. The initial visit involves registration, after which the pregnant woman must return for an "eligibility interview." The average waiting-period for this interview by a social worker is reported as 14 days in South and 30 days in Southeast District. A principal purpose of this interview is to ascertain that the woman is, indeed, poor and therefore not a suitable client for private medical attention. After eligibility determination there can be a further waiting-period of one to two weeks, until on the third visit the woman is permitted to see a physician. Since many of these patients do not make their initial contact until well along in pregnancy, it may be shortly before childbirth that the expectant mother has her first examination by a doctor. This examination is typically very brief, since the clinics average 19 or 20 patients per session.

It is important to record that after the August Riots this policy in prenatal clinics changed; a pregnant woman is now seen by a physician on her initial visit. Eligibility and other social data are collected by the social worker at subsequent visits.

As everywhere in California, there is an unfortunate separation between the prenatal care of expectant mothers and their hospital deliveries. Recent data show that 48 percent of the childbirths from South District and 59 percent from Southeast District take place in one of the Los Angeles County Hospitals. But as a County Health Department medical officer has written, the care in these institutions "is characterized by anonymity, endless waiting, overcrowding, and lack of continuity." It is perhaps small wonder that the maternal mortality rate in Southeast dstrict is 5.2 per 10,000 live births and in South District 8.9, compared with 3.5 in Los Angeles County as a whole. The differentials are equally dismal for the rate of premature babies (12.4 per 1,000 live births in South District compared to 7.5 in the County), fetal deaths (17.8 per 1,000 versus 13.6), and in general infant mortality (38.7 per 1,000 versus 23.2).

One family planning clinic session per week is held at both South and Southeast District Health Centers, supplemented by another weekly session at the Florence-Firestone Subcenter under the auspices of a voluntary agency (Planned Parenthood and World Population, Inc.). Since the advent of the contraceptive pill, attendance at these clinics has increased (40–45 per session in South District). Service is available to any woman who has had a pregnancy.

Child health conferences are held nine times per week in South District, six times per week in the Southeast District. There is no financial eligibility test for these services and they are heavily utilized. Patients are seen by appointment, however, and the pressure is so great that in the South District there is typically a waiting-period of six weeks for a new case. Babies must be under one year of age for admission, and they are seen only until their second birthday. The routine involves an interview and weighing by a public health nurse, and examination, with immunizations, by a doctor. Initial visits offer about ten minutes with the doctor, subsequent visits only about five minutes. The impact of these clinics is fairly large: about 45 percent of newborn babies in South District and 50 percent in Southeast District visit a clinic at least once in their first year of life (compared with about 10 percent in California as a whole—many of the balance, of course, being seen by private physicians).

The physicians attending these "child health conferences" are typically general practitioners, rarely pediatricians. But no treatment may be given. If a baby is sick, he is referred to a private physician or to a County Hospital out-patient clinic. Such needed treatment may or may not be received, depending on circumstances of time and transportation. There is no significant (general) health service in the County Health Department for children ages two to five except occasional immunizations in generalized "health officer clinics." There is a "child development clinic" for detection of mental retardation held once a month in each of the two districts.

Perhaps the only services of the public health agencies that involve treatment of the sick are the clinics for venereal disease and tuberculosis. Daily sessions are conducted at both District Centers at which examinations for syphilis and gonorrhea are made and treatments given. Each session averages 19 patients, but many appointments are broken. In the six-month period January–June 1965, for example, 2,375 patients were seen at South Center—but 1,304 other appointments were broken or cancelled. The disposition of such cases is not clear since nurses do not have time for follow-up in the community.

Tuberculosis clinic sessions are held twice a week in South District and three times weekly in the Southeast District. These clinics diagnose cases screened through mass chest X-ray surveys or through follow-up contacts of known patients. The health centers have X-ray equipment for this work. Cases of active tuberculosis are usually hospitalized in the county at Olive View Hospital.

Finally, there are the environmental sanitation activities of the County Health Department which, in a sense, are most preventive of all. Since water and sewage control is handled by the Los Angeles City Government, the tasks within South and Southeast Health Districts are largely related to food establishments and housing. Inspections are made of markets and restaurants, where problems are numerous. The greatest portion of sanitarian time, however, is spent inspecting housing. Twenty percent of the housing units are reported to be below very minimal standards, and 75 percent are in need of major structural repairs. Cockroaches and other vermin abound, for which the Health Department gives advice but does not perform extermination. The implementation of various orders given on housing repair, in accordance with the standards of the Los Angeles City Building and Safety Code, is impaired by the fact that most units are tenant-occupied, while the landlord (often absentee) is responsible for maintenance. There are 14 sanitarians on the job in both districts (one per 18,000)—the highest ratio in the county, yet not nearly enough to cope with the problems in the Riot Area.

In summary, the public health program of the South and Southeast Health Districts is an active one, following traditional lines. One must salute the devotion and dedication of most of the medical, nursing, and other personnel (sanitarians, social workers, health educators, technicians, clerks, etc.) who work in these programs. But their effectiveness in protecting and improving the lives of the 251,000 people in these districts is impaired by two factors: a. inadequacy of staff in relation to the enormity of the problems and b. a timid definition of functions deemed appropriate to public health agencies.

School Health Activities

Various health services are provided for children attending public schools throughout the City of Los Angeles, including of course the schools in the Riot Area. This program is supervised by the Los Angeles City School Districts. Comparable services for children in religious or parochial schools are offered by the Los Angeles County Department of Health.

Brief physical examinations by a physician are made on children entering school (kindergarten or first grade), in the fourth, ninth and thirteenth grades, and on all newcomers. There are also dental examinations and tuberculin testing. Certain immunizations are offered, in cooperation with the County Health Department. The educational program includes instruction in health subjects and, of course, school sanitation is supervised. The principal thrust of these efforts is obviously the prevention of disease or early disease detection, so that the child's education will not be impaired.

The correction of physical or mental defects found in children is left, in the main, to family responsibility. The standard routine is to send a note to parents advising them to have the child seen by a personal physician or dentist. In addition, the Health Services Branch of the Los Angeles City School System supervises several special health centers, where treatment is given or prescribed for defects in children whose families are of very low income and unable to afford private medical care. For certain legal reasons (since a school system is not authorized to give medical treatment), these centers are nominally operated by the Parent-Teachers Association of Los Angeles and are known as "P.T.A. School Health Centers."

Two such health centers are located within the South-Southeast Health Districts (21st Street and Florence Avenue) and one is just outside the South District (Gardena). There are 29 physicians serving part-time in these three centers, for the equivalent of about 3.5 full-time doctors per month. In the 1963–64 school year, 6,705 children were sent to these three centers. The bulk of cases are for eye examinations—4,679 in this period—but smaller numbers are for cardiac, skin, ear-nose-throat, orthopedic, or other conditions. In spite of this service and because of problems of communication between school nurses and families, high transiency among these low-income families and other obstacles, it is reported that a high proportion of defects detected in Riot Area children are not properly corrected. This situation, of course, is not unique to the Riot Area, but it is distressing.

There are special centers also for correction of dental defects and for mental-emotional problems in school children. Dental clinics, officially under the auspices of Dr. Robert E. Taylor (also adjusted to legal requirements), are held at the three P.T.A. Health Centers, and at a fourth location on Manchester Avenue. In the latter dental clinic, 295 children were treated during the six-month period of January to June 1965—obviously representing a very small proportion of the local school population (in whom we know the prevalence of dental disease is close to 100 percent).

As mentioned, children in parochial schools are served by the Los Angeles County Health Department. In South Health District, for example, there are about 2,300 such children; in the 1962–63 school year they received 598 initial medical examinations, 161 reexaminations, and 1,104 immunizations. The follow-up of defects for correction is done by public health nurses.

Welfare Medical Services

Unlike the services of public health or school authorities, the welfare agencies of the United States focus their medical efforts on the treatment (rather than the prevention) of disease among their clients. In the nation as a whole, about 4 percent of the population are recipients of public assistance, but in the economically depressed tracts of the Los Angeles Riot Area the proportion is much higher. Organized social welfare programs for medical care are actually more numerous in this Area than elsewhere in the nation or in Los Angeles County.

Space does not permit a full explanation of the complexities of welfare medical services in Los Angeles County, but a few background facts are essential. Hospital care for the poor in California is mainly a county government responsibility, handled through the operation of County Hospitals. These hospitals are operated by the Los Angeles County Department of Charities. For the remainder of medical care, the agency responsible, the source of funds, and the pattern of service depend on the "category" of poor person concerned.

Persons who are designated as "categorical recipients" are entitled to a fairly wide range of ambulatory medical care through the California Public Assistance Medical Care Program (PAMC) which, in turn, receives about half of its funds from the Federal government (U.S. Department of Health, Education and Welfare, Bureau of Family Welfare). Needy recipients include beneficiaries of a. old age security (OAS); b. aid to families with dependent children (AFDC); c. aid to the blind (AB); and d. aid to the totally and permanently disabled (ATD). A fifth, special category was added in 1960: the "medically indigent" aged who may be helped for medical care only (not for financial relief) under the Medical Assistance for the Aged (MAA, Kerr-Mills) program. These cases, in contrast to the other four Federal categories, may have hospitalization supported from Federal and State funds in *any* (i.e., either governmental or voluntary) approved local hospital, after an initial "corridor" of 30 days of care at county government or personal expense. In spite of the Federal and State government financing of these services for "categorical recipients," the administration of the California PAMC program is delegated to a branch of the Los Angeles County Department of Charities—its Bureau of Public Assistance (BPA).

As for *other* poor persons, not definable as "categorical recipients," medical care out-of-hospital is availble through the Outpatient Medical Relief (OMR) program. This is operated by the County Department of Charities, but as an extension of the branch responsible for County Hospitals rather than the BPA branch. This program is sometimes described as "general assistance" (GA), and includes both persons receiving some cash assistance and others whose only aid is in the form of ambulatory medical care. This care is given by a designated panel of private physicians who are paid on a fee-for-service basis by administrative units known as "Medical Aid Districts." Since this program is financed entirely out of county funds, without State or Federal contributions, its volume, both in persons served and scope of services provided, is much smaller than the programs for "categorical recipients."

For *both* "categorical" and "general assistance" cases, the prevailing policy in Los Angeles County is free choice of private physician, dentist, pharmacist, and other providers of care, who are paid on a fee basis for their services (according to an agreed upon fee schedule) by one or another branch of the County Department of Charities. This is the pattern of medical care for the designated indigent population in the Riot Area as well.

The specific medical benefits available have unfortunately not been uniform for the six types of person just described (four Federal-State "categories" plus MAA plus GA cases). Some types of indigent persons have been entitled to more extensive services than others. Children have been favored more than adults. One of the most serious gaps has been the exclusion of treatment to mothers or disabled fathers within AFDC families who have been entitled only to ambulatory medical care available in the outpatient department of a County Hospital or to emergency dental treatment.

In Los Angeles County as a whole, counting all the categories and types of public aid recipient reviewed above, there were (as of August 1965) 351,000 persons entitled to some form of publicly financed medical care—about 5.0 percent of the county population. In the Curfew Area, such persons are concentrated, 92,000 out of 658,000 or 14.0 percent. In the area in and around Watts, with a population of 94,000, there are 22,243 public aid beneficiaries—23.7 percent. It is apparent that in the heart of the Riot Area nearly one-quarter of the population are poor enough to be entitled, under current laws, to a variable range of medical services through local private practitioners or county hospitals.

Unfortunately, data are not avilable on the exact volume of medical, drug, and related services received by these public aid beneficiaries in the Riot Area. We know, however, that a great deal of money is spent for this care. Taking the county as a whole, about $44 is spent each year for each AFDC client eligible, and about $228 for each OAS client, not counting inpatient care costs in county hospitals. Based on U.S. National Health Survey findings for the West Coast, we do know that in spite of this apparently generous public support, needy persons—with a high burden of illness—still receive a lower volume of medical, dental, and related services than the self-supporting population.

For the general assistance or Outpatient Medical Relief (OMR) program, the Riot Area is mainly encompassed in what is known as Medical Aid District No. 6. In fiscal year 1964–65, there were 13,438 patients served by this district, and for their private doctor care and drugs $272,475 was spent by the County Department of Charities (aside from County Hosptial services). This amounts to $20 per person aided per year, which suggests the rather small medical proportions of this program.

With respect to all indigent persons, whatever the precise expenditure and volume of services received, serious questions may be raised about how wisely the money is being spent for quality and medical effectiveness. Sub-standard practices have been observed by a staff of highly qualified physicians who review medical bills submitted to the Bureau of Public Assistance. General practitioners, who render a heavy share of office-and-home care to the indigent, are well below the average qualifications of physicians in Los Angeles County as a whole. Even at best, there are inherent limitations to the quality of medical care that can be rendered in an isolated medical office, especially if that office is located in an area of doctor shortage where the pressures on the doctor's time are great. Laboratory and X-ray facilities, not to mention professional consultation, are seldom available in such a setting.

Persons entitled to welfare medical services are heavily concentrated among the very young and the very old, among whom illness needs are also greatest. Yet it is in the young adult and middle years, when men must earn a living and support a family, that unemployment causes the sharpest frustrations. It was among persons of these age levels, reached only slightly by the welfare medical services, that the August Riots were bred.

One other program administered by the Los Angeles County Department of Charities, though most of the funds come from state and federal sources (the State Department of Public Health and the U.S. Children's Bureau), should be mentioned. The Crippled Children Services finance diagnosis and complete medical care for low-income children with certain serious chronic physical disorders—orthopedic defects, rheumatic heart disease, hare-lip, paralyses, etc. The professional standards in this program are high; only certified specialists and accredited hospitals may be used. The administrative arm of this program in Los Angeles County is the network of Medical Aid Districts. For District No. 6, which has a total population of about 608,000 and contains most of the Riot Area (plus more), there were 420 children served in this program during the 1964–65 fiscal year. This represented 0.69 new or reactivated cases per 1,000 population in District No. 6 during 1964–65, compared with a rate of 0.84 such cases per 1,000 in the County as a whole. These services were rendered both through private physicians and county hospitals. While the quality of care received by these handicapped children is high, it is apparent that their overall population impact is small.

Mental Health Services

The mental and emotional health of a population has importance which has been increasingly recognized in our society, not only because of the suffering involved (often greater than physical pain), but also because of its influence on other aspects of life—on employment, family welfare, crime and delinquency, alcoholism, drug addiction, even life itself (suicide).

Private psychiatric services, at $25 per hour or more, are so expensive that for all practical purposes they may be considered nonexistent for the population of the Riot Area. Resources, therefore, are found only in the sphere of organized social programs, governmental or voluntary.

The care of psychotic patients in mental hospitals is a responsiblity of the California State Department of Mental Hygiene. The rate of admissions to these hospitals from Los Angeles County as a whole in 1964 was 92 per 100,000 population. For the South and Southeast Health Districts, however, it was 163 and 145 per 100,000 respectively. Classical studies in this field (Hollingshead and Redlich, *Social Class and Mental Illness*, 1958) have demonstrated that lower social class persons are frequently admitted to state mental hospitals for conditions which, in a higher class person, would be treated at home or in a voluntary general hospital. In spite of this distortion, the high rate of mental hospital admissions in the Riot Area is doubtless a reflection of social and environmental stresses.

Within the South-Southeast Health Districts, there are three facilities offering ambulatory psychiatric services. The "P.T.A. School Guidance Clinic" has already been mentioned. This unit serves pupils from 269 schools on the east side of Los Angeles; in the school year 1963–64 only 316 children were seen from this large territory, of whom only a small fraction would have been from the South or Southeast Districts. This clinic is served by the equivalent of less than one full-time psychiatrist, so that it is small wonder that the waiting-period for attention is several months long, and relatively few parents have the endurance to seek its services.

A second facility is the Westminster Health Unit, supported by the Presbyterian Church, the United Crusade, and a grant from the National Institute of Mental Health. It concentrates on adolescent patients with severe depression and other serious problems. Its team consists of a psychiatrist, two social workers, and a psychologist, but its net impact is obviously small.

The largest resource in the South-Southeast Districts is the South Central Mental Health Service, which was opened in August 1964 as a unit of the Los Angeles County Department of Mental Health and financed largely from California State (Short-Doyle Act) funds. This clinic is served by two full-time psychiatrists, two psychiatric social workers, and other personnel. It admits about 90 patients per month, usually on referral from agencies, physicians, or other sources. It gives immediate short-term care, including attention to alcoholics, juvenile delinquents, and other tough cases. The clinic has been criticized that none of its key professional staff is Negro, but efforts are being made to expand and improve this critical service, which is sorely needed.

Just outside the South-Southeast Health Districts is another unit of the County Department of Mental Health, the "Agency Service Center" located in Compton. Here, the three full-time psychiatrists are all Negro, as are most of the supporting staff. The chief source of referral is the Bureau of Public Assistance, followed by voluntary social work agencies, ministers, doctors, and others. This unit was established only about ten weeks before the August Riots, and its future impact remains to be observed. At present its services are largely consultative to other agencies, but increased direct therapy is projected.

Mentally disturbed patients from the Riot Area may also be sent, of course, to other facilities in Los Angeles County, including clinics attached to the county hospitals, certain voluntary hospitals, the Youth Authority, the court and prison systems, etc. But the demands on all these resources are great—and staffs very limited. On top of these handicaps are the inherent inhibitions of low-income (and poorly educated) people regarding psychiatric care, the difficulties of communication between such patients and middle-class medical personnel, problems of transportation and waiting-periods, and the whole overlay of pessimism and fatalism that mar the judgment of the poor under the weight of their seemingly endless personal problems.

Other Governmental and Voluntary Health Programs

Federal governmental agencies also provide medical and hospital services to military veterans with either service-connected or nonservice-connected disabilities. Both hospital and ambulatory services are available for service-connected conditions, but for nonservice-connected conditions (the great majority of disorders affecting the average veteran), only hospital inpatient care is available, dependent on financial need. By the latter criterion, veterans in the Riot Area would certainly tend to qualify, and they may secure care at a large Veterans Administration facility in West Los Angeles. In downtown Los Angeles, not far from the

Riot Area (at 1031 South Broadway) there is also a V.A. Clinic for ambulatory care of service-connected disabilities. The key question, of course, is how many residents of the Riot Area are veterans? One may hazard a guess that the high Selective Service rejection rate among low-income Negroes for both physical defects and educational deficiency (well established in previous studies) would mean that a lower proportion of this population are veterans than in the State of California or Los Angeles County as a whole. In the United States, about 13 percent of the population are veterans. Aside from military rejection rates, this proportion is probably further reduced in the Riot Area by the especially high proportion of females and small children.

Another Federal program supports the cost of medical care for the dependants (wife and children) of active military personnel. Doubtless some families in the Riot Area benefit from this program but they probably constitute a smaller proportion than in the population as a whole. In the entire South Health District with a population of 144,000, there were in 1960 only 128 men in the armed forces.

A collaborative Federal-State program for helping employable disabled persons is operated by the California State Department of Rehabilitation. The Riot Area is included within a jurisdiction of this agency known as the "South Gate Area," with a population of about 718,000. The impact of this vocational rehabilitation program, however, is rather small. In the entire South Gate Area, there were 669 medical examinations performed in 1964 to determine eligibility for services. The great majority of even this small number, however, were excluded from the program for non-employability, alcoholism, or other reasons and during 1964 only 57 persons were actually provided physical restoration services. Of this number 14 were provided eyeglasses, nine psychiatric treatment, eight leg prostheses, and lesser numbers were provided other therapies.

Supplementing and often blazing the trail for governmental health services in any community are a variety of organized health programs sponsored by voluntary agencies. These are usually focused on special disease problems or special types of health service. The leadership for such programs in our society tends to come largely from middle-class families—often the non-employed wives of white-collar professional and business men; activity in a particular neighborhood depends a great deal on the local participation of similar persons. It should not be surprising, therefore, that the impact of the voluntary health agencies in the Riot Area, despite great needs, is less than in the Los Angeles region as a whole.

The Visiting Nurse Association (VNA) of Los Angeles, for example, is an important agency providing bedside and other nursing services, under a physician's direction, to patients in their own homes. Services are available to persons of all income, and the charges are made on a sliding scale so that poor families may receive care free (or with payment from the Bureau of Public Assistance). Since services must be authorized by a doctor, however, their receipt by a family depends initially on that family's being under medical attendance.

In the last year of record (March 1, 1964 to February 28, 1965), the VNA made nearly 80,000 home nursing visits to persons (largely chronically ill) in its geographic area of 3,750,000 population. The Riot Area is encompassed largely under what the VNA defines as its "Southeast Area Office" serving a population of 853,217; in this Area 13,558 home visits were made. A simple computation shows that in this economically depressed area there were 16 nursing visits per 1,000 persons per year, compared with 23 visits per 1,000 in the rest of the VNA territory. To paraphrase the explanation of a knowledgeable nurse in this program, the Riot Area people "don't have doctors to authorize VNA visits, and so they just put up with illness. This is true especially of the older people, and the younger people need to be educated."

One of the oldest and most important voluntary health agencies is the Tuberculosis and Health Association. In Los Angeles County, its current program consists largely of screening tests for tuberculosis and other chest diseases (by mobile chest X-rays and tuberculin skin tests) and health education. Examinations are carried out in parochial schools, homes for the aged, nursery schools, and other places. Since 1960 the Association has established four branch offices to serve the great sprawling population of Los Angeles County. None of these offices, however, is in the Riot Area, which is covered from the Association headquarters on Beverly Boulevard; no staff person is specifically assigned to the Riot Area.

The Los Angeles County Heart Association carries out a program of education on heart disease for the general public and health professions. It operates a "work classification unit" which, after medical examination, recommends the level of physical work that a person with an impaired heart may safely do. It also operates an "information and referral service." Careful tabulations of this Association reflect interesting comparisons between the activities in the Riot Area and elsewhere in the County. In the jurisdictional divisions of the Heart Association, the South and Southeast Health districts are encompassed in an area defined as Section III-B, with a population of 491,500. This is 7.7 percent of an overall population of 6,374,000 reached by the Association. Educational activities in 1964 within Section III-B were: five films out of a total of 585 showings (under 1 percent), three public lectures out of a total of 185 (2 percent), three exhibits out of a total of 58 (5 percent), 13,000 pieces of literature out of a total of 250,000 (5 percent). The Work Classification Unit served 11 persons from Section III-B out of a total of 185 (6 percent). The Information and Referral Service answered 141 requests from Section III-B out of a total of 2,694 (5 percent). Thus, by measures of all the Heart Association services, the Riot Area received less than its share of the population. On the other hand, in the "Heart Sunday Drive," Section III-B had participation of 3,500 volunteers out of the county-wide total of 44,500 (8 percent). It is not surprising that the financial yield of this drive was a relatively modest $11,000 of the $343,000 collected in the county (3 percent).

The Los Angeles chapter of the American Cancer Society conducts an educational program to promote early detection of this second cause of death. It also provides housekeeper and home-help services to families with bed-ridden cancer patients. The latter services, however, are offered only to families *not eligible* for services from governmental welfare agencies. For this reason, the Cancer Society reports that it has very few requests for services from the South or Southeast Health Districts.

The American Red Cross is another important voluntary agency which includes certain health services in its varied program. Within the Riot Area a course for training "home aides" was recently offered (18 students) at the Nickerson Gardens Housing Project, and it is intended to offer further instruction in home nursing—under the direction of a well-qualified Negro nurse—in other housing projects of the Area.

The Family Service of Los Angeles offers general social casework to families in trouble. At the time of the August Riots, however, it had no office in or near Watts; the nearest service was at the headquarters office about eight miles away. After the Riots occurred the Family Service Society provided a caseworker to help in a "legal service center" set up by the Los Angeles Welfare Planning Council (with volunteer lawyers) in the Riot Area. The Society has now approached the United Crusade for funds to staff a branch office in Watts.

This account of the activities of voluntary health agencies and certain special governmental programs in the Riot Area is sketchy and incomplete, but it may be enough to suggest the general impact of these programs. It is evident that the influences are generally small and relatively weaker than in other sections of Los Angeles County, in spite of a greater burden of health needs.

Health Insurance

One of the principal social mechanisms for making medical care readily available to the American population has been health insurance in various forms. Unfortunately, time did not permit collection of specific data on the insurance coverage of the population of the Riot Area, but indirect evidence suggests that it is probably much lower than the prevailing national or county average.

In general, it is well known that insurance for hospital or medical care is much less frequently held by families of low income than by the rest of the population. The U.S. National Health Survey found in 1963, for example, that hospitalization insurance (the most extensive type) protected 70.3 percent of the national population. For persons in families of under $2,000 annual income, however, the figure was only 34.1 percent, and for families of $2,000–$4,000 annual income it was only 51.9 percent. Moreover, even for the same income level, the insurance protection of non-white persons is lower than that for white persons. In the $2,000 and under family income group, hospitalization insurance covered 37.8 percent of white persons and 24.5 percent of non-white persons, with similar racial disparities at all income levels.

The reasons for this are probably not only poverty, per se, with inability to afford the insurance premiums, but also the relatively meagre level of employment of lower social class persons in large industrial groupings. Most health insurance coverage in the United States is based on enrollment through place of employment, and the greatest share of this enrollment is through factories or offices with large staffs. Negro and poor white adults, however, are not only more frequently *unemployed*, but when employed it is more typically in service trades (domestic work, gasoline stations, restaurants, etc.) and casual jobs, where the work force tends to be small and the insurance coverage usually low.

Examining the 1960 Census data for South District (containing Watts), for example, of the 143,524 total population, males in the civilian labor force (that is, 14 to 65 years of age and not enrolled in school or military service) numbered 35,221. Of these 90.5 percent were employed, leaving 9.5 percent unemployed—much higher than national or county rates. Counting both sexes, 49,576 persons in South District were employed in 1960, and only 16,033 were in "manufacturing" industries, where large groupings of workers tend to be aggregated in factories or other places readily reached by health insurance programs. A much larger proportion were engaged in industries like "personal service, including households," "retail trade, including eat and drink," "business and repair services," "construction," and similar employment where small aggregations of workers are the rule. In Southeast District, the proportion of the civilian labor force engaged in "manufacturing" industries was even lower—10,216 out of a total of 40,224.

These Census data support the estimate that only a small proportion of persons in the Riot Area are probably covered by health insurance.* Moreover, to the extent that casual workers or workers in small enterprises are medically insured, they tend more often to be enrolled as individuals than as persons in "membership groups." In the insurance business, this is well known to mean relatively higher premiums, lower medical benefits, or both. Health insurance of individual enrollees or even small employment groups, furthermore, is seldom associated with premium payment or premium sharing by employers—a common advantage of enrollment via large industrial establishments (with or without collective bargaining). Membership in unions like the Retail Clerks, Culinary Workers, or Teamsters Union tends to compensate to some extent for these handicaps of isolated or small business employment, but it is not known how many of the workers in the Riot Area are unionized. The special medical protection of the Federal Employees Health Benefit Program and the California State Employees Retirement Service are enjoyed by those families with a Federal or State government

*A separate study, disclosed after this report was completed, tended to further confirm this estimate, with a survey finding that only 16 percent of persons in 1964, with a history of unemployment or currently unemployed in this general area, had any type of health insurance coverage.

worker. In 1960, about 12 percent of the employed persons in the South and Southeast Districts were "government workers," but a large share of these were doubtless employed by city and county (not federal or state) agencies.

Another feature of employment by small establishments, aside from health insurance, is the type of protection available from in-plant health services provided by management. It is well known that small plants offer much less adequate services of this sort than do large. Preventive health examinations, first-aid after accidents, health counseling, etc., are seldom available to casual or small-plant employees. Environmental safeguards against industrial accidents and occupational diseases are usually weaker, and workmen's compensation cash and medical benefits are less available to such workers. Under California law, workers specifically excluded from this industrial injury protection are casual employees (that is, persons engaged for a job to be completed in less than 10 days or involving pay of under $100), newspaper salesmen, household domestic workers, part-time gardeners (that is, employed by one person for less than 44 hours per month), and other such occupations which characterize many workers in locations like the Los Angeles Riot Area.

Conclusions and Recommendations

Conclusions on the health services available to the people of the Riot Area are not difficult to draw. Medical resources—personnel and facilities—are far below American norms in volume and quality. Public programs for general disease prevention, for treatment of the poor, for mental health, for the health of school children are relatively well developed, but their impact is far below the needs, and they are inhibited by the conventional restrictions of governmental action in a free enterprise medical setting. Organized private health actions supported by voluntary donations, insurance, or industry are weak.

One can hardly attribute the August Riots to these health service deficiencies in any major degree. Even the poor health status of the population must probably be blamed less on the inadequacies of services than on the generally low socioeconomic level at which people live. But it is equally true that proper health protection and medical care are essential components of an American standard of living, that they contribute to general social well-being, and that they are important factors in the achievement of maximum potential in every individual. Inadequacies and failures in meeting health needs in the Riot Area undoubtedly have added to the weight of frustration and misery which in Los Angeles, as elsewhere, has so often led to violence. A brighter future for the people of the Riot Area of Los Angeles demands vast improvement, therefore, in the health services available to them.

Approaches to this goal may be suggested at three levels: a. deliberate improvements in existing resources and programs; b. inauguration of new programs in the near future; and c. long-term changes and improvements in the system of health services. Since the August Riots, a medley of proposals has been made by concerned health leaders from Los Angeles and elsewhere in California, to improve health services in and around Watts. The recommendations which follow draw upon these, along with ideas of the author.

A. To improve existing resources and programs, it is recommended that:

1. steps be taken to achieve accreditation of the hospitals in the Riot Area, through active consultation from the California State Department of Public Health, Bureau of Hospitals, the Hospital Council of Southern California, and other agencies;
2. additional physicians be encouraged to settle in the area, through active efforts of the Los Angeles County Medical Association, the Charles Drew Society (of the National Medical Assoication), and other bodies (their financial support can be virtually assured through expanded welfare medical services, discussed below);
3. services of the Los Angeles County Health Department be expanded in the South and Southeast Districts through a. substantial enlargements of the complement of public health nurses, sanitarians, and other personnel; b. widening the role of maternal and child health servcies to include treatment of mothers and children attending clinics, when they are sick; c. addition of multiple screening clinics for detection of numerous diseases in adults; d. appointment of a competent, energetic Health Officer in the South District (with a salary adequate to attract such a person);
4. prompt expansion of the scope of welfare medical services to include a. ambulatory medical care for adults in AFDC families; b. establishment of a comprehensive outpatient department at the John Wesley Hospital;
5. extension of organized health services for school children to include correction of all defects impairing the child's ability to learn;
6. enlargement of the capacity of the local mental health centers providing ambulatory care, through increased support from the Los Angeles County Department of Mental Health;
7. enrichment of the programs of voluntary health agencies in the Riot Area, especially for visiting nurse services, heart disease, cancer, crippled children and adults, planned parenthood, and Red Cross activities.

B. Among new programs, which should be achievable in the near future (two or three years), it is recommended that:

8. a first-class voluntary or governmental hospital, with a teaching and research program, be established in the heart of the South-Southeast Districts. This may be developed through acquisition of one of the existent proprietary hospitals by a nonprofit association or by local government, with grant support for substantial expansion from the California State Hospital Planning and Construction (Hill-Burton) Program. If a new hospital is established by the Los Angeles County government, it should have the benefit of a board of directors representing the local population, and guidance on professional standards from the medical schools in Los Angeles. The geographic lines of the State Plan of Hospitals should be redrawn to take account of current human needs and social realities in this blighted area, so that necessary grant support can be properly provided;

9. the sensible "Pomeroy Plan" of 1933 (proposed by the Los Angeles Health Officer at the time) for public health centers to provide comprehensive medical care to persons of low income should be reactivated. Initially, 3 or 4 such centers, each serving about 20–30,000 people, should be established in locations of greatest poverty. They should be staffed in the main by physicians now practicing or desiring to practice in the area, who should be paid adequately for their time on the basis of part-time or full-time salaries. Supervision should be provided by highly qualified physicians, under contract with the County Health Department, and drawn from medical school faculties in Los Angeles. Financial support for launching these centers should be sought from the Office of Economic Opportunity, Community Action Program;
10. private group practice clinics should be encouraged in the area, with expectation of financial support from welfare medical payments, health insurance, and other sources;
11. all self-supporting persons should be encouraged and enabled to join health insurance plans, as an important mechanism through which their medical services might be financed. Employed persons should be covered through their place of work. Indigent or medically indigent persons should have their plan membership subvented by the welfare agency. There should, however, be a *free choice of plans* by the individual, including "plans" which would give service through the health centers described above. (Such free competition among health insurance plans offering services under different patterns will foster the gradual growth of patterns yielding economy and quality of care.)

C. Among long-term goals, it is recommended that:

12. the California county hospital system be reorganized so that these institutions be open to all patients (indigent or paying) and, correspondingly, all approved non-governmental hospitals be open to all patients—both paying and indigent. Hospital use should be based on the geographic convenience of the patient and doctor, not on social class lines (After this report was prepared, the California Legislature in November 1965 enacted AB-5 [Casey Bill], which paves the way for implementation of this recommendation.);
13. all persons in California should become insured for comprehensive medical care, under State law, with cost-sharing by employers. Recipients of public assistance should be blanketed into the system through welfare payments. As mentioned above, the insured individual should be free to choose the pattern of personal medical care he prefers, as offered by different health insurance plans (This approach would emulate that now followed in the health program of the California State Employees Retirement System.);
14. in each geographic district of 20,000 to 30,000 population, all organized health agencies—governmental and voluntary—should offer their services through a unified health center. The comprehensive health service centers recommended above for three or four locations would naturally serve this purpose, supplemented by others necessary to reach eventually the total population. "One door" in each neighborhood should replace the bewildering jungle of agencies now operating, for the better service of people and also for administrative economy and efficiency. Such unified district health centers should be built where feasible in close connection with general hospitals;

15. more medical, dental, nursing, and other health personnel should be trained to meet overall needs. This education should be subsidized by government, so that qualified persons from low-income families will have ample opportunities. In return for educational support, graduates should have a social obligation to work in designated areas of need for a specified time period;
16. all health services in the Riot Area should be integrated, through regional relationships, with services emanating from the major medical centers in Los Angeles. Difficult cases should be readily referred to those centers, and technical consultation should be continuously offered outwardly from those centers.

To study and possibly implement these or other appropriate recommendations for improved health services in the Riot Area, it is proposed that the California State Department of Public Health designate a technical Task Force, on loan to Los Angeles County.

These 16 recommendations are a greatly oversimplified outline of a very complex program of social reform in health service. It is apparent that most of them would require action at a level much above that of the Riot Area. The basic fact is that the health service problems of this Area—or almost any depressed locality in the United States—spring from social and economic causes with very wide and tortuous roots. The difficulties we see in the Riot Area, in health as in other fields, are only the final excrescence of malfunctions and failures in our whole society. Their correction, therefore, requires action on a very broad scale, including the State of California and the nation as a whole.

Fortunately, we live at a time when such corrective action need no longer be considered utopian. In the health services, the organized resources now available are remarkably large, and they are likely to become larger. In addition to the whole framework of public and voluntary health services built up over the last century, social legislation of the last two years has provided great additional resources.

The new national "Medicare Law" contains many provisions which will facilitate action on the recommendations made above. Title XVIII will, of course, offer substantial support for both institutional and physician services for all persons past 65 years. (It will, incidentally, hasten the integration of the county hospitals into the overall community hospital network as proposed.) Title XIX on the care of the indigent and medically indigent will lead to much more liberal support for medical services to persons of younger age groups, especially in families (AFDC) with dependent children. The operation of health centers and group practice clinics could be, in large part, financed through welfare payments made on behalf of persons covered through this expanded program.

There are other provisions of the new "Medicare" Law directed especially toward helping children. Special grants may be made for expanded maternal and child health services, including treatment, and for improved services to crippled children. These funds also can help in achieving some of the recommendations made.

The "anti-poverty program" administered by the U.S. Office of Economic Opportunity is another important resource provided recently. Localities like the Los Angeles Riot Area are precisely the raison d'être of this program, and a well-conceived plan for providing comprehensive services through health centers could probably expect support from it. The channel for this assistance would be the OEO division on "Community Action Programs," under which active participation of poor people themselves is mandatory. Such participation of local citizens in the Riot Area would be all to the good.

The new legislation on regional complexes for tackling heart disease, cancer, and stroke is still another resource which should help in tying newly launched programs in the Riot Area with the centers of medical teaching and research in Los Angeles. There is room under this legislation for imaginative plans to improve the quality of medical services through regional relationships with the humblest neighborhoods—and funds to back up such arrangements.

Expanded funds are also now available from Federal sources for vocational rehabilitation, ordinary public health services, health facility construction, and for the education of physicians, nurses, and other personnel. New State funds are available to diagnose and treat mentally retarded.

The tasks of linking the 16 specific corrective actions suggested above with these varied channels of financial support are beyond the scope of this report. They require careful administrative exploration by health leaders in Los Angeles County—governmental and voluntary—but the opportunities are great.

The anti-poverty program and many other Federal and State developments, of course, offer resources far beyond the field of health services. Indeed, the impact of external funds on the health of the Riot Area population may well be greater through their support of job-training, education, better housing, and industrial development than through health moneys as such. To be effective, in fact, health services must be part of a much wider program of social and economic improvements.

The philosophy behind these recommendations is that health service be regarded as a basic human right, in the spirit of the United Nations Declaration of Human Rights. To achieve this right in everyday life requires a vast amount of planning and social reform. It is not enough simply to pump money into a static health care system in the hope that dollars will solve the problem merely by bringing poor people into the "mainstream" of American medicine. The *quality* of that stream is not always cool and clear; it is often muddy and contaminated with substandard and wasteful practices. The task is to improve the patterns of health service so as to assure their quality and effectiveness, and this is especially true in the blighted slums of our large cities. Because resources are now so meagre in such areas, the opportunities for improvement are great. Opposition to medico-social reform from commercial and conservative interests may be expected to be less in such areas. Not that these recommendations are radical. In almost every detail, they were expressed at President Johnson's White House

Conference on Health held in early November 1965. The health circumstances of the Los Angeles Riot Area not only cry for help, but they present an opportunity for bold improvements which could offer a demonstration of needed health service reform to similar communities throughout our nation.

7

Inadequacies of Voluntary Agency Health Programs

Since the nineteenth century, American voluntary hospitals have established out-patient departments for the poor in the European tradition. However, these departments have been kept relatively weak because the private physicians who staff these hospitals and admit most of their patients fear competition with their private practices. As a result, a very heavy load of out-patient and emergency services for poor and even moderate-income families has fallen on the relatively few large public hospitals operated by local governments.

These large public hospitals, serving mainly the poor in major cities, have faced increasing difficulties in the 1960s and 1970s, as local tax funds for their support have not been able to keep up with the mounting demands. In 1969, colleagues and I conducted a national study on "Large Urban Public Hospitals" to explore the political and economic basis of their problems. One of the findings was the "dumping" of high risk and low income patients by voluntary hospitals. This chapter reports these findings and their dynamics. It was prepared jointly with Jorge Mera and presented to the American Public Health Association in 1971.

THE SORDID DIFFICULTIES of medical care in urban public hospitals for the poor (UPHP) are widely recognized as a major component of the current crisis in the health services of the United States. The inhumanly crowded wards, the congested clinics, the neglected patients waiting hours for care, the dull food and dirty linen, the perfunctory nursing services, the callous attitudes of many doctors—these and scores of other problems have been documented and exposed again and again. In the last few years especially—along with the rediscovery of poverty in the nation—has come a new recognition of "the plight of the public hospital," as the issue is usually epitomized.[1]

Causes of the UPHP Problems

Numerous investigations have sought the causes of these UPHP problems. Studies have been made in New York, Chicago, Boston, and a dozen other large cities in response to immediate crises—crises such as withdrawal of accredita-

Chapter 7 originally appeared as "Patient-dumping and Other Voluntary Agency Contributions to Public Agency Problems" in *Medical Care*, 11:30–39, January–February, 1973, and is reprinted by permission of that journal.

tion, mass public demonstrations, strikes of house-staff, or impending closure of the hospital for lack of money.[2] National studies have also been made, ranging from some excellent journalistic round-ups in the general press[3] or the medical press[4] to scholarly surveys carried out by academic centers.[5]

Some of these studies perhaps confuse the causes with the symptoms of the problem. Nursing staff vacancies and high turnover, for example, may be defined as a "cause" of poor patient care, when it is quite evident that these are simply part of the problem, and a result of other deficiencies in UPHP financing and management, not to mention the general national shortage of health manpower. From the various accounts, however, one can identify a number of causative factors which, in our view, boil down to three basic determinants. These may be summarized as history, financing, and politics.

By the first of these causes, *history*, we refer to the whole tradition of charity institutions for the poor. Originally, of course, almost all hospitals were devoted exclusively or mainly to the poor. When voluntary hospitals for the self-supporting developed, however, the public general hospitals gradually became stigmatized as places of charity for society's failures and outcasts.[6] The prudent and the self-respecting would see a private doctor and be admitted to a private or voluntary hospital. With this two-class system of hospital care, the energies and resources of affluent citizens naturally went to build up the voluntary facilities.[7] Local governments were left to take care of the beggars, who could not be choosers, and would have to be grateful for any crumbs from the tables of the elite. The social attitudes emerging from this charity tradition affect almost every aspect of UPHP operations, which we need not take time to explore.

The second cause, *financing*, encompasses numerous issues.[8] Originally the financial support of public hospitals came almost exclusively from local revenues. Depending mainly on real estate taxes, the local social power structure naturally forced a modest ceiling on these rates. Movement of middle-class families to the suburbs further reduced the urban tax base. Moreover, there were and are all the other local services—police, education, welfare, etc.—that compete for the local tax dollar. After the 1930s, higher levels of government, first the state, then the federal, came to contribute to the financing of UPHPs. The various amendments to the Social Security Act after 1935 tended to bring increasing shares of federal money into the public hospital budgets. These contributions, however, seemed only to enable public hospitals to barely keep up with the rising costs, associated with advancing medical technology and enlarging population demands.

The greatest impact of federal and state support was through the Medicaid legislation of 1965. It must be appreciated, however, that these funds can only be used for the care of persons in one of the four federal categories (aged, blind, disabled, or families with dependent children), getting cash assistance or for medically indigent who are categorically linked.[9] All the other poor people requiring hospital care remain a financial responsibility of state and local governments. In California, for example, only about 50 percent of the patient load in UPHPs are beneficiaries of Medicaid.[10] It is a complicated fiscal story, but it boils down to the persistent dependence of UPHP's on local revenues as their principal source of support; for many reasons, these revenues are seldom adequate to provide medical care of adequate quantity and quality. And were it not for the compensatory upgrading of the technical (if not human) quality of patient care, brought about by medical school affiliations of many UPHPs, conditions would surely be worse than they are.[11]

The third cause of problems, *politics*, also has a complex dynamics. As sources of jobs and favors, local public hospitals inevitably became vehicles of political patronage and sometimes corruption. To cope with this, civil service merit systems were set up for hiring personnel, and various surveillance procedures were applied to the purchase of supplies and equipment.[12] In time, these policies—designed to assure honesty and social accountability—became more elaborate and bureaucratic. Every UPHP study has described the self-defeating bureaucracy involved in hiring or firing employees or in purchasing aspirin.

Each of these three basic causes of UPHP problems has generated its own sort of solution. The charity tradition has led to the proposal that public hospitals should open their doors to private, middle-class patients (and hence change their image).[13] The financial strictures have led to numerous proposals for enlarged funding—varying from increased local and state taxes of various sorts to national health insurance.[14] The political bureaucracy problem has led to perhaps the commonest "solution" of all in recent years—transfer of the control of UPHPs to non-governmental or at least non-political bodies.[15] These may be medical schools, special quasi-public corporations, or other entities. Along with the transfer of authority, it is also generally expected that financial support will become enhanced.[16]

Deficiencies of the Private Sector

Beyond these three basic causes of the UPHP plight, however, there is a fourth which is seldom mentioned and to which this paper is principally addressed. We would call it the deficiencies of the private sector of hospital care with respect to social responsibility. In one of its crudest forms, the problem has come to be called "patient-dumping."[17] In a nutshell, the "undesirable" patient appearing at the door of the voluntary hospital is simply sent away to the public hospital.

Since the Middle Ages, hospitals have been established for meeting certain social needs, initially the bed care of the seriously sick poor. In the 19th century they acquired other functions: out-patient service for the poor, then medical education and research. All of these are essential functions which must somehow be performed in modern communities. But most U.S. voluntary general hospitals, serving as the doctor's workshop for his private patients, do not carry out these latter tasks very effectively. The majority of voluntary general hospitals in the nation offer no organized out-patient services; emergency rooms have been set up and expanded in recent years only in response to pressing public demands.[18] Educational functions are often meager (e.g., only 15 percent of U.S. hospitals have interns or residents), and research is typically absent. To the extent that these social responsibilities are not carried by voluntary hospitals, urban public hospitals for the poor are left to carry the load.

Since late 1969, we have been conducting at the UCLA School of Public Health a survey of the conditions and problems of large urban public hospitals throughout the nation.[19] The focus has been mainly on the ambulatory services, although almost every aspect of financing, staffing, operations, and community relationships has been examined. In connection with data derived from this study, it was possible to pose a question that might quantify the issue mentioned above. The specific question was: to what extent is the load of out-patient services carried by public hospitals in a community related to the degree of assumption (or non-assumption) of responsibility for such services by voluntary hospitals in the same community? More bluntly, what are the dimensions of patient-dumping with respect to ambulatory care?

To answer this question, we derived and analyzed hospital out-patient data for 1969 from 33 counties. These counties were widely distributed in 21 states and were selected because they contain one or more urban public hospitals for the poor, as well as numerous voluntary hospitals. For each county, data on out-patient services provided were tabulated for urban public hospitals for the poor, and the aggregate of all voluntary general hospitals in the same county. The UPHPs included all state and local (but not federal) government short-term general hospitals; long-term general or special (mental or tuberculosis) public hospitals were excluded. The voluntary general hospitals included those specialized for children, cancer, or the like (but not mental or tuberculosis) institutions. Proprietary hospitals, which seldom offer any out-patient services, were excluded in order to show the non-governmental sector in its best light. Kaiser foundation facilities were omitted because of their atypically large volume of "out-patient" services to nonindigent Kaiser Health Plan members. For each hospital, data were recorded on total out-patient department (OPD) services, defining these as the sum of visits to organized clinics plus emergency room visits. (Since our interest was OPD services for the poor, so-called referral visits of private patients were excluded.)

Conversion of these numbers into rates required, of course, application of proper population denominators. Ideally, we should have liked to relate OPD visits to the populations of hospital service areas, empirically determined; since this was not feasible, we took recourse to county populations (although we realize that many hospitals in a study-county are used by people from elsewhere, and many local residents use hospitals in other counties).

Looking at the nation as a whole, the American Hospital Association reports

(*Hospitals*, August 1, 1970) that, in 1969, all short-term general (and other special) hospitals provided 89,746,885 OPD visits, defining these as the sum of organized clinic and emergency services (but excluding "referred services" to private patients, as done in our study-counties). This amounts to about 450 OPD visits per 1,000 U.S. population. Since there are vastly more non-governmental than governmental general hospital beds in the United States, it is not surprising that more than half of these OPD services were provided in non-governmental hospitals. The relationship of OPD visits to hospital bed capacity, however, shows the load carried by state and local public hospitals to be disproportionately heavier, as follows:

Hospital Sponsorship	*Beds (Percentage)*	*OPD Services (Percentage)*
Voluntary non-profit	61.1	53.9
Proprietary	5.1	2.9
State and local government	20.9	31.5
Federal government	12.9	11.7
All types	100.0	100.0

It should be realized that in the great majority of counties in the nation, no state or local governmental general hospital exists. Thus the 31.5 percent of the total OPD load borne by public hospitals is based on a very high volume of service in only a small fraction of the total of 3,070 counties in the nation.

When we focus on the 33 study-counties which contain large urban public hospitals for the poor, the disparity of loads carried by public and non-public hospitals is found to be more striking. Here the overall rate of OPD visits in short-term general hospitals (excluding both federal and proprietary hospitals, as explained above) is 625 per 1,000 population. Of these visits, 42.5 percent are provided by the local public hospitals with only 21.1 percent of the beds. Ranking the 33 counties into eight sets of four counties each (except for one containing five counties), in order of their aggregate rates of OPD services, the data are given in Table 7-1. It may be noted in this table that in the counties with a higher overall rate of OPD services per 1,000 population, the relative share of the load borne by the voluntary hospitals tends to be greater. Indeed, in the ungrouped series of individual counties, the OPD visit rates in the voluntary hospitals are correlated with the county-wide rates at a coefficient of 0.91.

Further insight regarding the influence of voluntary hospital performance on public hospital tasks may be gathered from comparing rates based on the number of out-patient visits per in-patient admission per year. This measure reflects, we

Table 7-1

Out-patient Department Services in Voluntary and Public Hospitals: Rates of OPD Visits[a] per 1,000 County Population in All Voluntary Hospitals[b] and in Local Public Hospitals[c] of 33 Counties, by Eighths Ranked in Order of Total County OPD Visits per 1,000 Population, 1969

Rank	(N)	Total OPD Visits per 1,000 County Population (ranges)	OPD Visits per 1,000 in: Voluntary Hospitals	Public Hospitals	Percentage of Total OPD Visits in Voluntary Hospitals
1	5	157.6–348.9	126.2	164.2	43.5
2	4	349.0–384.9	153.0	216.2	41.4
3	4	385.0–419.9	141.6	267.1	34.6
4	4	420.0–530.9	215.0	272.3	44.1
5	4	531.0–609.9	362.2	208.3	63.5
6	4	610.0–1049.9	441.5	362.4	54.9
7	4	1050.0–1179.9	543.1	594.1	47.8
8	4	1180.0–2466.1	1107.5	703.6	61.2
Total	33	625.2	359.2	266.0	57.5

a. Sum of visits to organized clinics and emergency rooms.
b. Excludes proprietary hospitals.
c. Excludes federal hospitals.

believe, the degree of attention given by a hospital to OPD service in relation to its total resources—the latter being reasonably well indicated by the volume of in-patient admissions. For the aggregate sets of hospitals in the 33 study-counties, these rates ranged from 2.29 OPD visits per in-patient admission per year in the county with the lowest rate to 8.23 in the county with the highest rate. With simplified ranking of the counties into eight sets, using this measure of performance, the data are presented in Table 7-2.

In all 33 counties, the ratio of OPD services to admissions was much higher for the public hospitals than for the voluntary ones. The overall average for the voluntary hospitals was 2.80 OPD visits per in-patient admission per year, compared with 12.67 visits for the public hospitals.* Thus, it was possible to calculate for each county a percentage by which the voluntary OPD/admission ratio related to the equivalent public hospital ratio. In the individual county with weakest relative voluntary hospital performance, this figure was 3.8 percent, ranging up to 51.0 percent in the county with the strongest voluntary hospital performance. The findings for the eight sets of counties are shown in Table 7-2, where the average for the full series is seen to be 22.1 percent.

From these two tables, taken together, the nature of relationships for OPD services between voluntary and public hospitals would seem to be as follows. Because of their far greater resources in the United States, the voluntary hospitals in aggregate carry more than half of the OPD load—54 percent of the total nationally. In the 33 study-counties, where we focus on voluntary non-profit (excluding proprietary) hospitals and state and local (excluding federal) government hospitals, the voluntary facilities carry 57.5 percent of the load. In the latter urban counties, however, the voluntary hospitals have 78.9 percent of the short-term general beds and undoubtedly a still higher percentage of health manpower and other hospital resources. In relation to their resources, therefore, voluntary hospital assumption of social responsibilities for out-patient services to the poor is far less than that of public hospitals.

In virtually all the counties in our series, the public hospitals were carrying a very heavy load; in only 4 of the 33 counties was the public hospital OPD visit ratio less than 10 per admission. Putting it another way, the lowest ratio in the public hospital series (7.83 visits per admission) among the 33 counties was higher than the highest ratio (6.30:1) in the voluntary hospital series.

The most striking finding by *both* measures of OPD services, that is, rates per 1,000 population and rates per hospital admission, was the great influence of voluntary hospital performance on the overall county volume of out-patient service. The public hospitals seem to be giving OPD services to capacity everywhere. Anyone observing public hospital out-patient departments can confirm this im-

*In another phase of our study, we determined the comparable rates for all voluntary and local public hospitals of 300 beds or more throughout the nation. Even with this exclusion of smaller hospitals, the ratios (for the same year, 1969) were 4.5 OPD visits (including "referred" services) per admission in the voluntary hospitals and 14.0 visits in the public ones.

Table 7-2
Out-patient Department Services in Voluntary and Public Hospitals: Ratios of OPD Visits[a] to In-patient Admissions in All Voluntary Hospitals[b] and in Local Public Hospitals[c] of 33 Counties, by Eighths Ranked in Order of Total County Out-patient Visits per Admission, 1969

Rank	*(N)*	*Total OPD/Adm. Ratio per County (Ranges)*	*Mean OPD/Adm. Ratio*		*Voluntary Hospital Ratio as Percent of Public Hospital Ratio*
			Voluntary Hospitals	*Public Hospitals*	
1	5	2.29–2.79	1.03	12.62	8.16
2	4	2.80–3.17	1.36	12.52	10.86
3	4	3.18–3.48	1.66	15.35	10.81
4	4	3.49–3.74	1.94	13.92	13.94
5	4	3.75–4.24	2.34	11.47	20.40
6	4	4.25–4.39	2.95	12.59	23.43
7	4	4.40–5.49	3.14	13.82	22.72
8	4	5.50–8.23	5.12	16.15	31.70
Total	33	4.18	2.80	12.67	22.10

a. Sum of visits to organized clinics and emergency rooms.
b. Excludes proprietary hospitals.
c. Excludes federal hospitals.

pression. It is only when the voluntary hospitals do more, in relation to their resources, that the total county-wide rate of OPD service rises. By the criterion in Table 7-2 (OPD services per admission), the coefficient of correlation in the ungrouped series of 33 counties between voluntary hospital performance and the county's total OPD visit rate is positive at a level of 0.84. In other words, where the voluntary hospitals are, so to speak, pulling their weight, the total rate of OPD services in the county is greater. Where they are not—that is, where patient-dumping is presumably more frequent—the total county-wide OPD rate is lower. In these counties, one must conclude that many of the poor are getting ambulatory services in some other way or not at all.

We realize that this analysis leaves several questions unanswered. We have not yet investigated the percentage of poor persons in each of the 33 counties, although an inspection suggests that there is no consistent gradient in the series (e.g., the Southern and Northern state counties are all intermingled in the sequence, with no clustering). We also do not know the patient load—paying and indigent—borne by the private doctors in each county. There would seem to be no doubt, nevertheless, that the net volume of OPD services provided in counties containing public hospitals depends almost entirely on the proportion of that total load which is borne by the voluntary hospitals. Inspection of the 33 county sequence, moreover, suggests that those with stronger voluntary hospital performance tend to contain non-governmental university hospitals, where poor patients are needed for teaching purposes.

The story of patient-dumping told over and over again is one of rejection by voluntary community hospitals of out-patients considered to be "undesirable."[20] At one public institution in California, the OPD staff keeps an "Atrocity Book" listing the serious or tragic cases rejected by and transferred from voluntary hospitals. These are the alcoholics (acute and chronic), cases of drug abuse and attempted suicide, serious trauma cases (especially due to personal violence or automobile accidents), psychiatric disorder cases (associated with senility or otherwise), gonorrheal salpingitis, incomplete abortion, infectious tuberculosis, or other communicable diseases. The patients sent from the voluntary to the public hospitals are the poor, the aged, the black, the socially deviant young or old—with almost any diagnosis. These are the patients that constitute the heavy load which public hospitals must bear. These are the patients who must sometimes even be turned away by public hospitals, when their capacities have been reached or exceeded.

A recent study in Chicago, reported by the Assistant Director of the Illinois Regional Medical Program, estimated that 18,000 emergency patients were refused admission to private hospitals in 1970. Typically these cases were transferred to the Cook County Hospital. "Hundreds of these transfers were unsafe," says the report, "and resulted in about 50 deaths."[21]

Thus, the plight of the public hospitals, as reflected in their heavy out-patient burdens, must be traced at least partly to the rejection of social responsibilities by the voluntary hospitals. Perhaps the fault lies more with the predominantly private medical staffs, busy with their private patients, than with the hospital administrations, but the result is the same. Notwithstanding the problems of lean budgets and political bureaucracy, the burdens would be lighter and the problems somewhat alleviated, if the voluntary hospitals put more of their resources into serving the distressed and the poor.

Other Inequities

This influence of voluntary agency behavior on the genesis of public agency problems, in out-patient hospital care, is only one instance of what seems to be a general phenomenon in our society. Similar inequitable burdens are borne by public hospitals in the training of young doctors, in the use of patients as research subjects, and of course in the overall load of in-patient care for the aged and chronic sick. In other sectors of health service, the problems are similar. Public health clinics for babies or mothers, for venereal disease or tuberculosis, serve the poor and the racial minorities who are not very welcome in private medical offices. State mental hospitals must take the senile psychotics and other disturbed patients who cannot afford the private sanatorium nor the psychoanalyst's couch.[22] For migrant farm workers and their families or for impoverished American Indians, the medical care burden rejected by local communities is borne by the federal government.[23]

In the field of workmen's compensation for industrial injuries, the great bulk of the insurance business is carried by private companies.[24] They apply experience-rating in setting their premiums, each carrier thereby competing to attract the lowest risk employment groups. In 11 states, however, there are state government insurance funds as well. Their function is to carry the insurance load for the high-risk industries which private enterprise is not interested in protecting. As a result, the largest relative claims are made against the state funds, so that the private carriers end up with greater profits.

Another form of discriminatory risk selection operated for many years in the California state-wide disability insurance program.[25] The original law of 1946 permitted employers to be insured either through private carriers or through a state government fund. Because of experience-rated premiums and active sales promotion, by 1953 about 51 percent of the business had been attracted to the private carriers, leaving 49 percent—the poorest risk workers—to be insured by the state fund. Then in 1961, the law was amended to require that every insurance carrier must insure a fair share of high risk and low risk workers, reflected by the age, sex, and wage distribution as proxies for sickness experience. Promptly, the private insurance companies lost interest in this line of coverage, and, in 1969, over 92 percent of California workers were insured under the state fund.

The same sort of public-private inequities is found in other fields. In social welfare, it is generally known that the public assistance agencies must carry heavy caseloads of multi-problem families, while being staffed by inadequate numbers of social workers with relatively little training. The private family agencies, on the other hand, carry lighter caseloads of less problem-ridden families, with relatively greater numbers of better trained social workers.[26] The public school–private school nexus is similar. Private schools have more money to attract better teachers, for the education of fewer children. Public schools are just the opposite. Moreover, the energies of articulate upper middle-class parents are channelled to the further improvement of the private schools, where their own children attend. No wonder the public schools are left with overwhelming problems.

One could multiply examples of fields in which government is left to pick up the pieces from private enterprise neglect or failure. Transmission of electricity to farms was of little interest to the private utility companies until subsidies came from the R.E.A. (Rural Electrification Administration). In Great Britain of the 1940s, there was the bankrupt coal industry, saved only by government intervention. In the United States of the 1960s, there were the railroads. And today the issue can be epitomized by just one recently illustrious corporate name: Lockheed.

Solutions

We do not imply that private enterprise or voluntary agencies are incapable of sound socially oriented service. We do mean that in many contexts, private organizations—proprietary or non-profit—are able to do relatively high quality work only because they have in some way rejected the tough problem cases. These cases are pushed onto the backs of public agencies. We also mean to challenge the hackneyed charges about government inefficiencies and private business know-how. It ill behooves the spokesmen of free enterprise, therefore, to criticize government for its failings—when these have been caused or at least aggravated by the buck-passing of the private sector.

With respect to urban public hospitals for the poor, given the current realities, the need for them persists. So long as we have a two-class (or perhaps three-class) system of hospital care, we need facilities where the tough cases will be taken.[27] As John Affeldt, Medical Director of the Los Angeles County Department of Hospitals, has said, "There has to be a hospital which will not shut its doors to a patient regardless of the circumstances. There has to be a hospital of last resort."[28]

One can speculate about long-term solutions in which there would be a single high standard and a single system of health care for everyone. With nationwide, universal health insurance and regionalization of all hospitals and ambulatory care centers, one can visualize a pattern under which the patient's health needs and geographic location would be the only determinants of his hospital care.

But short of the ideal, there are practical steps that can be taken now to reduce the plight of the public hospitals and improve health services for the poor. The paths of increased budgets and transferred control have been mentioned earlier. Beyond these, however, the voluntary hospitals could show more willingness, than they have so far, to assume a greater share of the community burden. It took a crisis in Chicago's Cook County Hospital to lead 45 other hospitals in that turbulent county to recently set aside certain beds for the indigent in their neighborhoods, even when a public agency would pay the costs.[29] In Philadelphia, Los Angeles, and other metropolitan centers, the public hospitals have long had contracts with voluntary hospitals to pay for outpatient emergency services to indigent people. In recent years, money has not been the obstacle, so much as willingness.

The OEO-initiated neighborhood health centers, built in urban ghettos, are another approach to reduce the out-patient load in municipal and county hospitals. They have been an important development, but in relation to the size of the problem their impact has been small. They reach, altogether, less than 2,000,000 out of an estimated 30,000,000 urban poor. Perhaps more could be accomplished by broadening the scope of the traditional district health centers of public health agencies to include generalized primary medical care, as a few metropolitan cities have done.

Existing requirements of state and federal law, on voluntary hospital obligations to serve the poor, ought to be enforced. The tax-exemption of non-profit hospitals is based largely on the legal assumption that they provide charitable services. The Hill-Burton Act requires that any hospital receiving a federal construction subsidy shall "make a reasonable volume of services available at no charge or at reduced cost to persons unable to pay for them."[30] The OEO National Legal Program on Health Problems of the Poor has brought legal action against certain voluntary hospitals (former recipients of Hill-Burton grants) in Louisiana for refusal to accept poor patients, even when they had been turned away from that State's governmental "Charity Hospitals" because these were filled to capacity.

A survey of all the states by this OEO Legal Program yielded 22 responses on Hill-Burton administrative procedures. Of these, only one state reported any administrative mechanisms to monitor the claim—made always at the time of application for a Hill-Burton grant—that the hospital would serve the poor.[31] Only two state agencies indicated that they had ever received complaints about denial of hospital services—a fact that would seem mainly to reflect a lack of awareness among the poor of their entitlements under law. Surely this weakness in state health agency supervision could be remedied.

Studies in New York and elsewhere show that over the years, the load on public hospital out-patient departments has been increasing much more rapidly than that on voluntary OPDs. Between 1950 and 1964, the emergency room visits to voluntary hospitals in Brooklyn doubled, while those in municipal hospitals increased fourfold.[32] Put another way, the voluntary hospitals are carrying a declining share of an enlarging load.

The inequities, therefore, are getting increasingly serious. The milestone judicial decision in the *Darling* case of 1965 may have been an important warning to voluntary hospitals of the critical social responsibilities they are expected to bear.[33] Perhaps the short-run solutions are no longer adequate, and a major recasting of the U.S. system of financial support, organization, and governance of hospitals is overdue.

References

1. "The Plight of the Public Hospital," a series of articles in *Hospitals* (J.A.H.A.), July 1, 1970.
2. For example, Citizens Committee on Cook County Government: Interim Report on Health and Hospital Services. Chicago, Chicago Board of Health, 1967.
3. "The Changing City: A Medical Challenge," *New York Times*, June 2, 1969.
4. "End of the Line for City Hospitals?" *Med. World News*, May 9, 1969.
5. Ellwood, P. M., and Hoagberg, E. J.: Problems of the public hospital. *Hospitals* 44:47, 1970.
6. Sand, René: The Advance to Social Medicine. London, Staples Press, 1952.
7. Faxon, N.: The Hospital in Contemporary Life. Cambridge, Harvard University Press, 1949.
8. Brown, R. E.: The public hospital; Survival depends on financing and reorientation. *Hospitals* 44:40, 1970.
9. Greenfield, Margaret: Title XIX and Medi-Cal. *Public Affairs Rep.* 7:4, 1966.
10. California Department of Health Care Services. County Hospital Quarterly (A One-Day Patient Census Report), Sacramento, April 16, 1969; p. 6.
11. Sheps, C. G., et al.: Medical education and hospitals: Interdependence for education and service. *J. Med. Educ.* 40:1, 1965.
12. Gerdes, J. W.: Anticipated directions for the future of public general hospitals. *Am. J. Public Health* 59:680, 1969.
13. Breslow, L.: The changing role of county hospitals in California. *Calif. Med.* 106:176, 1967.
14. Henderson, W. F.: Tax revenue supports long-term needs. *Hospitals* 42:83, 1968.
15. Coodley, E. L.: Treatment for public hospitals: Medical school takeover. *Hosp. Physician* 5:62, 1969
16. Torrenzio, J. V.: The Evolution of the New York City Health and Hospital Corporation. New York, City of New York Department of Hospitals, 1970.
17. "Doctors Ask: Is This Equal Care?" *Med. World News* 11:17, 1970.
18. Sanford, G. A.: The outpatient explosion. *Md. State Med. J.* 16:44, 1967.
19. "Large Urban Public Hospital—Ambulatory Services Project," James P. Cooney (Principal Investigator), Milton I. Roemer (Co-Principal Investigator), and Martin B. Ross (Project Director), University of California, Los Angeles, 1970–71.
20. Lerner, R. C., and Kirchner, C.: Social and economic characteristics of municipal hospital outpatients. *Am. J. Public Health* 59:29, 1969.
21. de Vise, P.: Cook County Hospital: Bulwark of Chicago's apartheid health system. *The New Physician* 20:394, 1971.
22. Hollinghead, A. B., and Redlich, F. C.: Social Class and Mental Illness. New York, John Wiley, 1958.
23. Roemer, M. I., and Anzel, D.: Health needs and services of the rural poor. *Med. Care Rev.* 25:371, 461, 1968.
24. Skolnik, A. M., and Price, D. N.: Another look at workmen's compensation. *Social Security Bull.*, October 1970; pp. 3–25.

25. California Unemployment Compensation Disability Fund, Statistical Handbook on Disability Insurance 1969. Sacramento, Dept. of Human Resources, 1970; pp. 20, 30.
26. Burns, Eveline: The role of government in health services. *Bull. N. Y. Acad. Med.* 41:753, 1965.
27. International Health Advisory Council (Booz, Allen, & Hamilton, Inc.): The Organization, Administration, and Financing of Public Hospitals and Public Health Facilities. Oak Brook, Ill., 1970.
28. *Op. cit.*, ref. 4.
29. "Hospitals' Plan Eases Overcrowding," *AMA News* March 16, 1970.
30. "Court Cases Filed to Test 'Right to Health Services,' " *Hosp. Pract.* June 1971; p. 148.
31. Marilyn Rose, Esq. provided these questionnaire returns.
32. Hospital Review and Planning Council of Southern New York: The General Hospital Needs of Brooklyn, May 1966; p. 11.
33. Southwick, A. F., Jr.: Legal aspects of medical staff function. *In* The Medical Staff in the Modern Hospital, C. W. Eisele, Ed. New York, McGraw-Hill Book Co., 1967; pp. 65–83.

8

Fragmentation of Organized Health Care Programs

The laissez-faire development of American health services for the poor and other special population groups or diseases has led to a highly complicated system, often described as "pluralistic." It is seldom realized that for this freedom of local and voluntary initiative, we pay a hidden price–in overlapping administration and noncoordination of services.

This chapter examines these hidden costs in fields such as visiting nurse services, medical care for the poor, hospital services, health care insurance, drug distribution, and general ambulatory care. It explores how both economies and greater effectiveness could be achieved by coordination of services. The paper was presented at a meeting of Medical-Social Consultants in California, in May, 1964.

A FEATURE OF the democratic process is the free exercise of local initiative and voluntary action to accomplish various social purposes. In no field of human need is this seen more vividly than in coping with disease—either its treatment or its prevention. Especially in America, where the very size and diversity of the country have raised localism and voluntarism to the level of high national principles, do we see this approach to problems of health and medical care.

We all know the great achievements that have followed from these freedoms to develop health services. Quite aside from the private procurement of medical care—the ultimate, perhaps, in local and voluntary responsibility—the development of organized programs to tackle particular health problems in the United States has been astonishing. No one has ever made a full national count of the discrete organizations concerned with health service. In the field of voluntary health agencies oriented to a specific disease, Dr. Robert Hamlin estimated about 100,000 definable units—but this says nothing about governmental programs nor about voluntary programs of other categories.[1] In 1948, I attempted to describe the total universe of organized health programs operating in one rural county of only 60,000 population, considering both preventive and curative services, voluntary and governmental sponsorship, and actions originating outside as well as inside the county (so long as they had impact within the county). Health service was defined strictly, to include only specific technical functions—excluding, for example, educational, housing, recreational, or welfare programs, which surely influence health indirectly.[2]

Chapter 8 appeared in *Tuberkuloza* (a Yugoslavian journal), 18:213–219, 1966. It has not been previously published in English.

By this conservative definition, we found 155 different *types* of agency concerned with health services for the population of this small county. The separate discrete organizations—for example, counting each chapter of the Red Cross in the county or each insurance company carrying a prepaid health plan—numbered 640. This was 16 years ago and the situation is undoubtedly more complex today. Moreover, in an urban center, the multiplicities are manifestly greater. One can imagine what might be the findings of such an analysis on a national scale.

America has certainly made progress in meeting health needs in spite of the bewildering diversities of our medical culture. Specific population groups have been served—the indigent, the veteran, the child, the industrial worker, the Indian, and others—in some response to their special needs. Special diseases have been tackled with great effectiveness—tuberculosis, poliomyelitis, diphtheria, lead poisoning, industrial accidents, and others—both through prevention and treatment. Specific technical skills have also been made more widely available through organized action—laboratory tests, nursing services, physician's care in clinics, dental services, and hospital care. Programs definable along all three of these dimensions have been launched under both governmental and private auspices. They have been financed by different types of taxation, by insurance, or by philanthropy. There can be no doubt that the highly focused approaches of these hundreds, or rather thousands, of discrete health programs have paid dividends. They have conquered diseases, helped people cope with costs, and met many specific human needs.

Hidden Costs of Fragmentation

But there is another side to the story to which our attention must be directed. There is a price we pay for all the fragmentation. The price is both economic and human waste, and it is none the less real for its often being hidden. One may examine a few instances of such waste.

In the field of *home-nursing service*, the folly of separatism has been recognized for a long time. Instead of having one corps of nurses for child health visits, another for tuberculosis, and another for acute communicable diseases, health departments have developed "generalized" public health nursing services in geographic districts; the savings in travel expense and effort were obvious and the improved relationships with families were equally clear. The sacrifice of some specialized skills was a small price to pay for the benefits of a coordinated nursing service—at least within a single health agency.

But the wisdom of coordination is not so readily acted upon when multiple agencies are involved. The controversies between voluntary VNAs and the nursing division of the health departments are an all-too-old story. Peace is often kept by a division of the bailiwick—the health department doing preventive nursing while the visiting nurse agency does the bedside care. In Los Angeles there was a minor crisis not long ago because the Health Department crossed the line and attempted to offer some bedside nursing care to low income chronic patients (though both agencies together could hardly scratch the surface of the unmet need).

The whole program of *medical care for welfare recipients* is full of difficulties from its separatism. In California, virtually all hospitalization of indigent persons must be done in designated county governmental hospitals. As a result, needy persons, to whom transportation costs are a major item, often have to travel long distances for in-patient or out-patient hospital care, instead of going to the community hospital that might be right down the street. The same disparity characterizes ambulatory medical care in many states and counties, where only designated out-patient clinics may be attended by the poor. Even where a panel of private physicians has been established to serve the indigent there are other wastages, like the time lost and administrative overhead involved in requiring prior authorizations—a concomitant of categorical programs with limited funds.

The medical care of indigent beneficiaries in separate hospitals—not only in whole states like California or Louisiana, but in most metropolitan areas—exacts a price from the private paying patient as well. A staff of interns and residents has become almost essential to the provision of top-quality medical service in hospitals. Yet the majority of hospitals in the United States that cater only to private patients are unable to attract any of such doctors-in-training. They are concentrated in the hospitals serving the poor, where training programs are so much stronger. The private patient, especially in the *small* voluntary or proprietary hospital, pays a price for this segregation policy, in the lesser thoroughness and comprehensiveness with which his case is diagnosed and treated.

In the total world of *hospital care*, there are other hidden extravagances, springing from the proud sovereignty of thousands of separate institutions. Regionalized teamwork among hospitals has been preached for a good many years in the United States, but has been little effectuated—either with respect to construction or operation of facilities. In the absence of coordinated regional systems, it is commonplace for new hospitals to be built in a city or county, while established hospitals have 30 or 40 or even 50 percent of empty beds. Many sectarian factors or professional competitiveness and sometimes simply cliquishness or snobbery lie in back of these wasteful decisions, but they follow nevertheless from lack of true community planning and teamwork, and they create inevitably costs which must ultimately be borne by the whole population.

Sacrifices of quality follow also from the separate sovereignty of thousands of institutions caring for the chronic sick. There are today some 600,000 beds in nursing homes and other long-term care facilities in the United States. This is almost as many beds as exist in all general hospitals. Yet only a handful of the 23,000 long-term care units have any ties to the mainstream of medical activity in the community, found in the general hospital.[3] The result is usually mediocre quality medical care, with little if any attention to rehabilitation concepts. With respect to the care of the mentally ill, the enormity of the problem of the large, isolated, custodial facility has been increasingly dawning on our national consciousness. On the whole, the standards tolerated in our mental hospitals are like those characterizing our general hospitals a century before. Improvements would, of course, cost money, but it is essentially the separateness of our approach to mental illness that has permitted the evolution of this double standard.

Just one more example from the hospital sphere, which is, after all, the most critical and certainly the most expensive sector of total medical care. Consider the highly developed system of Veterans Administration hospitals and clinics, devoted to the care of about 25,000,000 Americans who, usually through no decision of their own, came to serve in the nation's military forces. This is no criticism of veterans and the VA benefit program which has helped millions. But there is no question that this elaborate and quite high-level, though separate, system of federal medical care is a result of our lack of a nationwide health service. The vast majority of patients in the VA hospital network are there for nonservice-connected conditions. No country with a national health insurance program has anything like this. How much more sensible it would be to serve veterans and nonveterans alike in the 7,000 community general hospitals, instead of the 172 special VA facilities. The manipulation of money to pay for the care, along lines that the Congress may decide, would then be simply a bookkeeping task.

In the vast field of *medical care insurance*, there are manifold prices we pay for fragmentation. Local initiative and voluntarism have led to the creation of well over 1,000 competing plans, most of them under commercial profit-making auspices. The private carriers have 36,000,000 persons insured through individual (as distinguished from group) enrollment policies, which paid benefits in 1958 of 48 cents from each premium dollar.[4] The rest of the consumer's dollar—and these policies are held mainly by the aged and the poor—goes to sales commissions, overhead, and profits. This is only the most glaring waste of voluntary health insurance, but there are many other forms. The forces of competition have led inevitably to so-called experience-rating not only by the proprietary companies but by the nonprofit plans as well. Under this principle, persons with the highest sickness risk, and usually the leanest resources, pay the highest premiums. The commonest form taken by voluntary insurance today is indemnification rather than health service benefits. Thus, the patient receives a cash allowance for a particular surgical operation, hospital experience, or other item of care, but the provider of service has no obligation to limit his charges to this amount. The result has been a general inflation of medical and related fees, and a substantial rise in the share of the national income going to health purposes.

Other hidden costs result from our fragmentation of medical care need into different classes of health insurance. There is insurance for the hospital bill, other insurance for the doctor's bill in hospitalized illness, other insurance for physician's care in the office and home, and still other prepayment programs for drugs or dental care. What is the effect on patient and professional behavior of these segmental benefits? Inevitably the patient and his doctor will try to fit a particular diagnostic or treatment problem into the arrangement for which there is insurance coverage. Thus, thousands of patients are now being hospitalized for procedures that could be carried out just as well and much more economically on an ambulatory, though non-insured, basis. Fee incentives aggravate these wastages, as has been amply demonstrated by comparative studies in New York and elsewhere. Thus, comprehensive benefits under health insurance, while at first glance more costly, are actually more economical when one considers the total economic burden on families and communities.

Medical care under the workmen's compensation laws has long faced similar difficulties. These segmental programs of compulsory health insurance for industrial injuries antedate the voluntary health insurance coverage of most workers. It was only natural for the worker—and his lawyer and often his doctor—to attempt to attribute as many of his injuries and illnesses as possible to the work situation. Endless litigation results from these claims, the cost of which is ultimately borne by all consumers, since management derives the money for its workmen's compensation premiums from the sale of its commodities. The solution is not more laws and lawyers, but simply wider medical care and general disability benefits—whether or not the ailment is work-connected. There are many other wastages in this field referable to insurance carrier profiteering, documented by numerous studies and state investigations.

Profiteering in the *drug industry* reached the point of a national scandal a few years ago. The 1962 amendments to the Food and Drug Control Law may help cope with some of the most flagrant abuses, but there is no sign that they will stem the avalanche of drug advertising which all of us must pay for as consumers. About 20 percent of our total health care expenditures now go to drugs—about $5,000,000,000 a year. The Kefauver Committee Hearings in the U.S. Senate brought out that roughly 25 percent of "ethical" or prescribed drug sales income is spent on advertising and other forms of promotion (though one hears much more about the 5 or 10 percent spent on research).[5] This is aside from the sale of patent medicines. This handsome cost is one of the prices we all pay for the entrepreneurial competition among hundreds of drug manufacturing firms, vying for the favor of the prescribing doctor or the self-prescribing patient.

Finally, the very separation of the world of ambulatory care from the world of hospital care—aside from insurance factors mentioned earlier—leads to duplication and waste. Laboratory and X-ray procedures done on patients in the doctor's office or clinic are endlessly repeated in the hospital, simply because the two sectors are not tied together administratively. The same duplication occurs among the offices of medical practitioners, who are not integrated in a group practice team. And consider the human fragmentation of our standard policy in health department well-child conferences, where the baby is seen at any time *except* when he is sick. At this point he is expected to see his "family doctor." This separation of preventive from curative medicine is a testimony to our respect for the private sector of the medical economy more than for the proper needs of children.

Toward Future Coordination

These examples of some of the human and economic prices we pay for fragmentation of health services—and one could cite many more—may be enough to tell the other side of the story of America's health progress. The piecemeal approach has certainly moved us forward, but the price of this strategy has been high. Is there anything to be done about it?

One must not be so naive as to expect that coordination of the myriad of health service programs, public and private, could be achieved in America overnight. Even the enactment of so sweeping a social reform as the British National Health Service did not achieve more than partial coordination—as the Porritt Commission and several other British studies have shown. But if efforts at coordination are to be fruitful, to move us forward, it is essential to have at least an approximate picture of the ultimate goal.

In this picture, one can envisage a health service system in which access to care is based primarily on where a person lives—"regionalization" is the usual way of epitomizing the idea. Thus, the receipt of care would not depend on the category of the person—whether he is a veteran or an indigent client or an industrial worker or some other category for which isolated social programs now operate. Likewise it would not depend on the class of his illness—whether cancer or an infectious disease (like syphilis) or whether a "crippling" condition or a mental disorder or some other diagnosis for which still other isolated social programs now exist. Access to health service would depend simply on residing in a geographic area or region.

In that region, the medical services would be provided through an integrated network of health facilities, with a multi-purpose hospital at the core. Nursing homes and other special facilities for the long-term patient should be affiliated with this general hospital, as should any institutions for the mentally ill. Around this base-facility would be smaller hospitals and health centers, close to where people live. The physician's office can be conceived as the most peripheral of such "health centers," or better, the group practice medical clinic. But the doctors and other personnel in the neighborhoods would be professionally affiliated with the nearest hospital. In their offices or clinics people would receive personal preventive services (like periodic health examinations and immunizations) as well as diagnosis and treatment of overt disease. Necessary drugs would be provided according to proper scientific standards at reasonable prices.

The payment for these services might or might not be from a single source, as in Great Britain. There might be multiple sources, depending on economic and political considerations (like public assistance status, veteran's eligibility, industrial injury compensability, etc.), but the financial mechanism should not interfere with the pattern for effective delivery of services. If special financial support is available for hospital care of the aged or of military veterans, for the treatment of industrial injuries or crippling disorders in children, or for any sort of service to the poor, let it be used and contributed to the maintenance of the integrated system. For the large balance of medical needs, not encompassed under some special financial program, health insurance ought to be the prevailing method of economic support. On a non-profit basis with maximum population coverage, all but a few cents (used for administration) of every insurance dollar would be devoted to health care costs.

This ultimate goal of an integrated health service system, in which the wastages of fragmentation were eliminated, can help to guide day-to-day policy decisions. But it must be approached realistically, little by little. Efforts must be made in the sphere of welfare medical services, such as we see in the movement to integrate California's county hospitals into an overall hospital system. Efforts must be made in the health insurance sphere, such as the movement for comprehensive non-profit prepayment plans or the movement for social security coverage of hospital costs of the aged. Efforts must be made in the sphere of drugs through effective legislation or in the mental illness sphere through offering psychiatric services in general hospitals.

At the local community level, there are many blueprints to define the configuration of health agencies which might work together toward a coordinated goal. One philosophy puts the hospital in the pivotal position; another, the medical society; another, the health insurance plan. The American Public Health Association sees the health department as carrying the major responsibility for coordinating health services at the local level.[6] Its reasons are compelling, even though the reality in this agency is often a far cry from the ideal. The local health department should be as concerned about the efficient use and management of hospitals in the future as it has been about milk pasteurization plants in the past. Coordination, however, requires decisions beyond the local level, for funds and authority in many programs flow from state and national jurisdictions (in voluntary no less than governmental spheres).

The path to intelligent health service organization, even with a modest piece-by-piece approach, is not an easy one. Vested interests are involved and conflicts must be expected. But the process is nevertheless a constructive one, for it is directed to the wise and effective use of scarce resources. Even a rich country like ours does not have money to burn. The waste of money—or the personnel and facilities that money buys—in one sector of the economy means that it cannot be used in another sector where there are unmet needs. When we achieve a condition in which every American receives not only top-quality health service for all his physical and mental ills, but also the good life in terms of housing, education, and all his other needs, then we can rest in our efforts at eliminating waste.

References

1. Robert Hamlin, *Voluntary Health and Welfare Agencies in the United States*. New York: Schoolmaster's Press, 1961.
2. Milton I. Roemer and Ethel A. Wilson, *Organized Health Services in a County of the United States*. Washington: U.S. Public Health Service, Pub. No. 197, 1952.
3. A. Stageman and A. M. Baney, *Hospital-Nursing Home Relationships: Selected References Annotated*. Washington: U.S. Public Health Service, Pub. No. 930-G-2, 1962.
4. H. M. Somers and A. R. Somers, *Doctors, Patients, and Health Insurance*. Washington: Brookings Institution, 1961, p. 272.
5. D. C. Coyle, *How to Get Safe Drugs and Cut Their Cost*. Washington: Public Affairs Institute, 1960.
6. American Public Health Association, "The Local Health Department—Services and Responsibilities," *American Journal of Public Health*, 54:131–139, January 1964.

9

Medical Care of the Poor: The False Economy of Co-payment

When federal Medicaid legislation was enacted in 1965 to pay medical bills for the poor in the mainstream of private delivery, the many abuses of fee-for-service medical practice were exposed; doctors and hospitals provided countless unjustified services and program costs spiralled. This induced state governments, responsible for about half the costs, to introduce various controls on utilization of services.

Among these controls was a "deterrent fee" or co-payment of one dollar imposed on beneficiaries in California for the first two doctor visits each month. Our university health services research group was asked to evaluate the effects of this experiment, and the principal findings are reported in this chapter. The co-payment requirement did, indeed, lead to reduction in the rate of use of ambulatory services (saving the state government some money), but this was followed by a relative increase in the use of costly hospital services (compared with a "control population" receiving care without co-payments), more than outweighing the savings on ambulatory care costs. The paper was, therefore, entitled "Co-payments for Ambulatory Care: Penny-wise and Pound-foolish." It was co-authored with Carl E. Hopkins, Lockwood Carr, and Foline Gartside. A debate ensued on the statistical methods employed, but the criticisms were readily rebutted. An independent statistical analysis by personnel of the RAND Corporation in 1977 confirmed our original findings.

Note: The following paper was prepared and submitted before the publication of "California's Medi-Cal Co-payment Experiment" by Earl W. Brian and Stephen F. Gibbens as a special Supplement to the December 1974 issue of *Medical Care*. Although examining the same medical care program, our study is based on a cohort analysis over time—before and after the imposition of co-payment requirements—and applies statistical techniques which adjust for the critical differences in "test" and "control" populations, not done in the previous report. Moreover, it examines hospitalization experience not only because of its costliness but especially because of its value as a reflection of the long-term effects of the demonstrated reduction in ambulatory services. As a result, our conclusions on the ultimate consequences of copayment fees for ambulatory services in a low-income population are very different from those of Brian and Gibbens.

Chapter 9 originally appeared in *Medical Care*, 13:457–466, June, 1975, and is reprinted by permission of that journal.

One of the persistent subjects of debate in planning health insurance or other financial support programs for medical care is the effect of co-payment or deductible requirements. Applied in many programs, both private and governmental, the general assumption has been that these cost-sharing charges would inhibit "unnecessary" or "frivolous" demands for medical care, and therefore reduce the burden on the fiscal source and available health manpower.[2]

Co-payment as a Deterrent to Use of Medical Care

Much research has been done on the question of co-payment as deterrent, with conflicting findings. Obviously the effects of cost-sharing on utilization or demand depend on the amount of money involved—either in fixed dollars or percentage of charges, on the income level of the insured, on whether the co-payment applies to a service ordered by the doctor (like hospitalization) or to one initiated by the patient (like an ambulatory visit), and on other factors. The weight of evidence seems to suggest that for services decided upon by the doctor, if the cost-sharing requirement is small, the effects are transitory or virtually nil.[5] For patient-initiated services, on the other hand, the inhibiting effect of co-payments on utilization may be substantial, but especially so for lower income families.[1]

A depressing effect of co-payments on consumer demand obviously reduces medical care expenditures in the short run, even if one counts both personal outlays and payments from a social (insurance or revenue-derived) fund. For the social fund, moreover, the saving results from two mechanisms: 1. the reduction in numbers of medical claims, and 2. the nonpayment by the fund of the co-payment amount itself. These fiscal effects, however, tell us nothing about the medical or health consequences of the co-payments. It certainly cannot be inferred that a patient's failure to see or delay in seeing a doctor for a symptom means that the ambulatory visit was unnecessary or frivolous. It means only that the co-payment obligation effectively inhibited the procurement of care, whether it was medically advisable or not. A recent review paper by researchers from the RAND Corporation, for example, draws the conclusion that co-payments reduce ambulatory care demand, thereby saving health insurance funds; it does not consider, however, the possible effects on health.[6] Nor does it consider the later demands for care that these health effects might generate, perhaps more than offsetting any initial savings.

An investigation of the so-called California Copayment Experiment (hereafter called COPE) which operated under the Medicaid program from January 1972 until July 1973 provided us with an opportunity to probe this question—that is, the longer term effects on health and costs of a small co-payment obligation imposed on Medicaid beneficiaries as a condition for visiting a doctor and for having a prescription filled. Examining the experience of the California COPE program before its start and for 12 months after permitted some inferences on both these matters.

The California "Experiment" and Its Assessment

In brief, the California State Department of Health Care Services imposed a co-payment charge of $1 on certain Medicaid beneficiaries for the first two visits to a doctor each month after January 1, 1972. The doctor or his assistant was expected to collect the dollar and, whether he did or not, the State deducted one dollar from the fee payable under the program. Similarly, a 50 cent co-payment was imposed for the first two drug prescriptions each month, this amount to be collected by the pharmacist. A survey of providers showed that over 80 percent of the doctors and 90 percent of the pharmacists collected the COPE charges.

Under the original Medicaid law (which barred states from imposing any payment obligations on the indigent beneficiary for statutorily required medical services), this California measure could be approved by the federal Department of Health, Education and Welfare, only if it was considered an "experiment." Our research group at UCLA, which was called upon by the federal Department to evaluate the results, was not involved in the experimental design. Had we been we would have much preferred to establish two randomly chosen or matched populations of Medicaid beneficiaries, one of which was required to co-pay while the other was not. Instead, the State—perhaps in the intersts of compassion—decided to impose the co-payment obligation only on those Medicaid beneficiaries who had some additional financial resources outside their statutory cash benefits, while not imposing it on the rest of the eligible persons.

Thus the two populations, with respect to "co-pay" or "no-pay" status, were not basically alike. The co-pay groups, constituting families with some resources, tended to be a decidedly older-age population. Even though our evaluative study was confined to AFDC (Aid to Families with Dependent Children) beneficiaries, the children in the co-pay families tended to be older. Moreover, the very existence of some extra resources in these families meant that their standard of living and perhaps other cultural characteristics were likely to differ from those in the more impoverished no-pay AFDC population. These differing sociodemographic characteristics would inevitably influence tendencies to seek medical care and meant, unfortunately, that our evaluative research could not be based on a simple comparison of the trend lines of the medical care demand rates of the two populations.

Instead, it was necessary to establish two cohorts of co-pay and no-pay populations, to follow their demand rates for a reasonable length of time both *before* and *after* the imposition of the co-payment charge, and then to compare not the absolute rates but the *relative* levels of utilization of various types of medical care by the two populations. This could be achieved by establishing a base period, prior to co-payment, at which the actual utilization rates of the two populations were converted to a common *index* figure of 100. Then one could follow the trend lines for the indices of the two cohorts to determine whether, after the imposition of co-payment in one cohort, a difference was observable in the demand or utilization trends followed by each.

Since California is a large state, and our research funds were limited, we could not examine the total experience of the State's over 2,000,000 Medicaid beneficiaries. We chose instead the AFDC universe within three counties (San Francisco, Tulare, and Ventura) believed to be fairly representative of the State as a whole, both in urban-rural distribution and in ethnic or racial composition of Medicaid persons.* In these three counties, the co-pay cohort population throughout the observations numbered 10,687 and the no-pay cohort numbered 29,975, or a ratio of roughly 1:3. This ratio was also characteristic of the Medicaid population in the State as a whole.

To establish the basis for these two trend lines, as noted above, a time span was studied beginning six months before the co-payment charge was imposed and ending 12 months after. Computerized data were examined for medical and related claims paid for services actually rendered during six quarterly (three-month) periods over this 18-month span. The exact quarters for which service data (from paid claims data tapes) were collected are shown in Table 9-1.

Table 9-1
Service Data Collection Quarters

Quarter	*Time Period*	*Status*
1	July–September 1971	Before co-payment
2	October–December 1971	Before co-payment
3	January–March 1972	Co-payment started (Jan. 1)
4	April–June 1972	Co-payment in effect
5	July–September 1972	Co-payment in effect
6	October–December 1972	Co-payment in effect

Findings

In Table 9-2 are presented the actual rates of doctor's office visits per 100 eligible AFDC Medicaid beneficiaries over the 18-month study period. Also presented in this table are the same rates, adjusted to an index figure of 100 for the first quarter, as explained above. Graphic presentation of the index figures from Table 9-2 appear in Figure 9-1.

*Originally, information had been obtained on seven counties, but examination showed so many serious gaps and problems in the claims and eligibility data in four of the counties that we felt compelled to reduce the sample to three counties; in these, the data were satisfactory for analysis.

Table 9-2
Doctor's Office Visit Rates for AFDC Families, by Co-payment Status in California Medicaid Program, July 1971–December 1972: Number per 100 Eligibles per Quarter-Year, and Indices of Rates Based on Quarter 1 = 100

Quarter	*Doctor's Office Visits per 100 Eligibles*		*Index of Office Visit Rates (Quarter 1 = 100)*	
	No-pay	*Co-pay*	*No-pay*	*Co-pay*
1	79.54	75.47	100	100
2	66.79	59.98	84	79
Co-payment Started				
3	79.09	69.13	99	92
4	71.24	64.77	90	86
5	67.46	59.55	85	79
6	73.18	66.31	92	88

Note: Illustrated graphically in Figure 9-1.

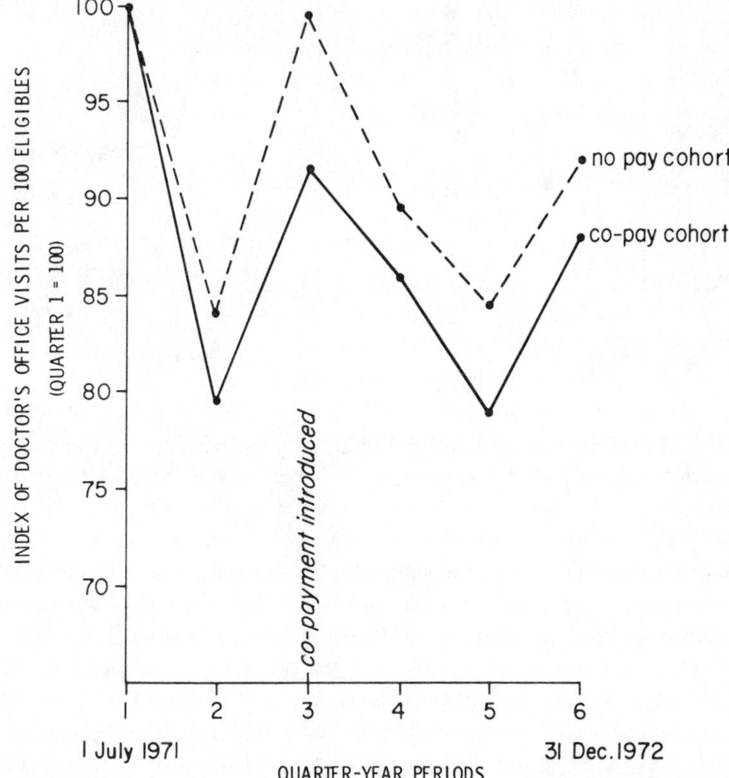

Figure 9-1. Doctor's Office Visit Rates for AFDC Families (by co-payment status in California Medicaid program, July 1971–December 1972: indices of rates based on Quarter 1 = 100)

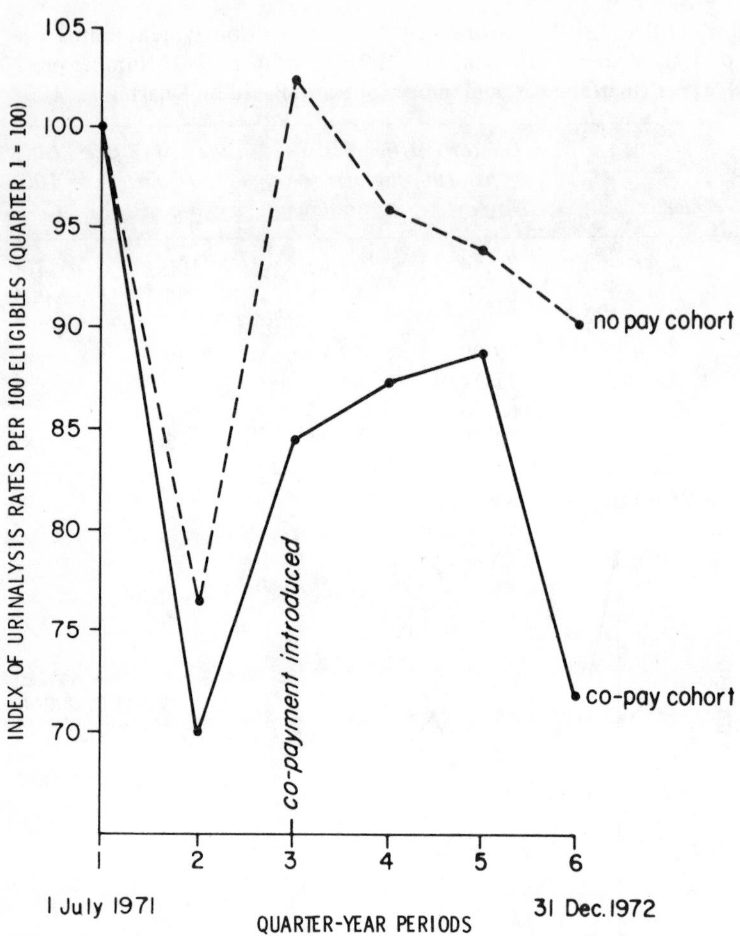

Figure 9-2. Urinalysis Rates for AFDC Families (by co-payment status in California Medicaid program, July 1971–December 1972: indices of rates based on Quarter 1 = 100)

Interpretation of this table (and subsequent tables and figures) requires further explanation about the course of events in California's Medicaid program over this 18-month period. In October 1971, at the start of Quarter 2, a number of administrative changes were introduced in the program; most important among these was a requirement of prior authorization from a State Medicaid Consultant for more than two ambulatory services or more than two prescriptions in any month. It is evident that this requirement was associated with a sharp decline in utilization rates of *both* the no-pay and co-pay cohorts for Quarter 2, even before

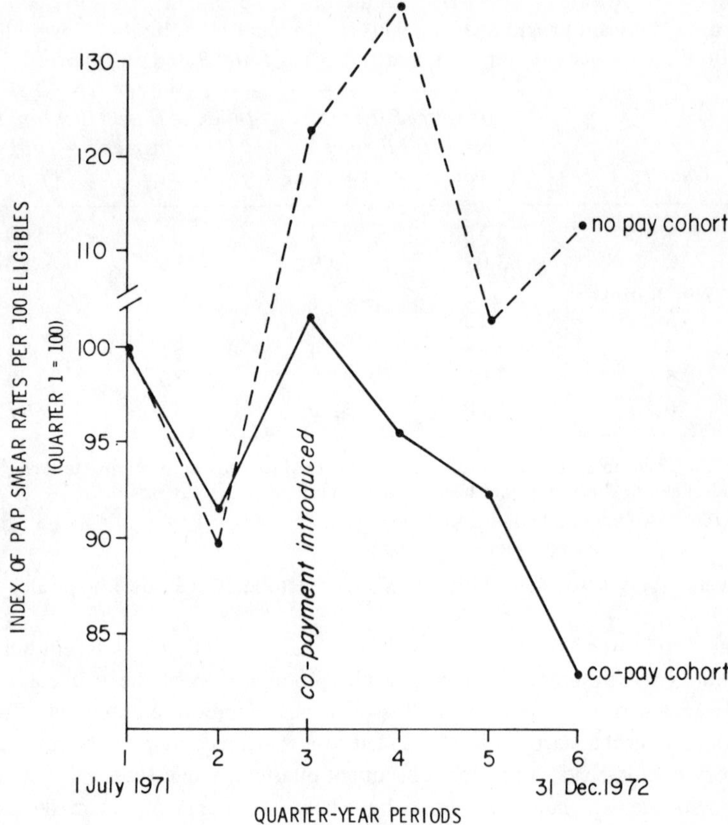

Figure 9-3. Pap Smear Rates for AFDC Families (by co-payment status in California Medicaid program, July 1971–December 1972: indices of rates based on Quarter 1 = 100)

co-payment was introduced.[3] Prior authorization for ambulatory services beyond two per month, for nonemergency hospital admissions,† and for certain other services was a continuous requirement for both cohorts throughout the remainder of these observations. It is not possible to disentangle the inhibitory effect of this requirement from the co-payment obligation in the co-pay cohort, but its substantial effect may be estimated from the trend line for the no-pay cohort. Probably seasonality also had some effect on both trend curves—for example, the rise in doctor's office visits and drug prescriptions in the sixth quarter for both groups

†This restriction had, in fact, been operative since April 1968. Such prior authorizations, of course, have been used to restrict medical care use in welfare program for centuries.

Table 9-3
Hospital Patient Rates* for AFDC Families, by Co-payment Status in California Medicaid Program, July 1971–December 1972: Number Hospitalized per 100 Eligibles per Quarter-Year, and Indices of Rates Based on Quarter 1 = 100

	Hospital Patients per 100 Eligibles		*Index of Hospitalization Rates (Quarter 1 = 100)*	
Quarter	*No-pay*	*Co-pay*	*No-pay*	*Co-pay*
1	3.56	2.54	100	100
2	3.07	2.09	86	82
Co-payment Started				
3	3.12	2.37	88	93
4	2.88	2.14	81	84
5	3.05	2.29	86	90
6	2.70	1.71	76	67

*Data are based on an unduplicated count of hospital *patients* during a quarter year, rather than admissions, which may have been more than one for some patients.
Note: Illustrated graphically in Figure 9-5.

was very likely associated with fall-winter (October-December) respiratory disease.

Keeping in mind the combined effect of the prior authorization requirement, as well as the different sociodemographic composition of the two cohorts, it would appear from these data that the prior authorization requirement, after its introduction at the start of Quarter 2, led to a sharp reduction in the rate of ambulatory doctor visits. Then for subsequent quarters, while seasonality and disease incidence associated with it may have been exerting an influence, the co-pay cohort had a rate of doctor's office visits—relative to the base period for the index—substantially below that of the no-pay cohort throughout the study span. There would seem to be little doubt that this differential was due to the co-payment requirement.

Continuing, for the sake of simplicity, with the data simply in graphic form, we can consider a common diagnostic laboratory test, urinalysis, in Figure 9-2, and a common preventive screening test, the Pap smear, in Figure 9-3. By both of these trend lines, it is apparent that the co-pay cohort had substantially lower utilization indices than the no-pay cohort. In Figure 9-4, the use of prescription drugs, with a 50-cent co-pay requirement, shows similar relationships. All three of these types of service were associated with ambulatory doctor's visits, for which co-payments were usually required.

Table 9-3, however, presents data for the two cohorts, with an important distinction. It applies to the hospital patients, and—while showing rates and indices separately for both cohorts—no actual co-payment was required from either

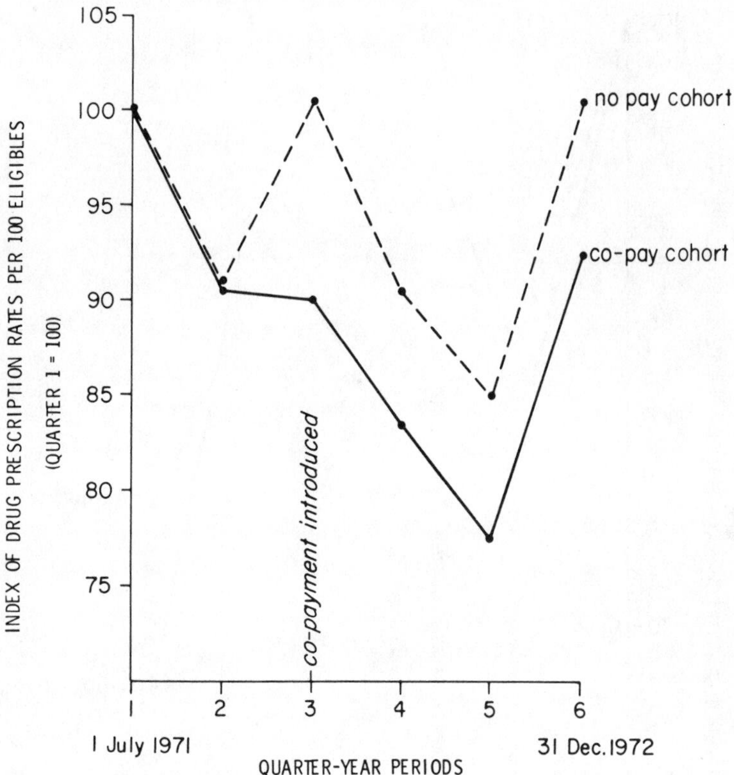

Figure 9-4. Drug Prescription Rates for AFDC Families (by co-payment status in California Medicaid program, July 1971–December 1972: indices of rates based on Quarter 1 = 100)

population, and the decision on hospitalization was made by the doctor.** The same data are shown in graphic form in Figure 9-5. The data in Table 9-3 and Figure 9-5, in sharp contrast to trends in all previous tables, show that after introduction of co-payment in January 1972 the index figures for the co-pay cohort leaped up to a *higher* level than those for the no-pay cohort. They remained at a higher level for three of the four co-payment quarters. The drop in the final quarter may simply reflect the completion of hospitalizations in the previous three quarters for persons needing such care, as well as the usual overall drop in hospital use around the Christmas holiday season.

**Our data are based on an unduplicated count of hospital *patients*, rather than admissions, which may have amounted to more than one for some patients.

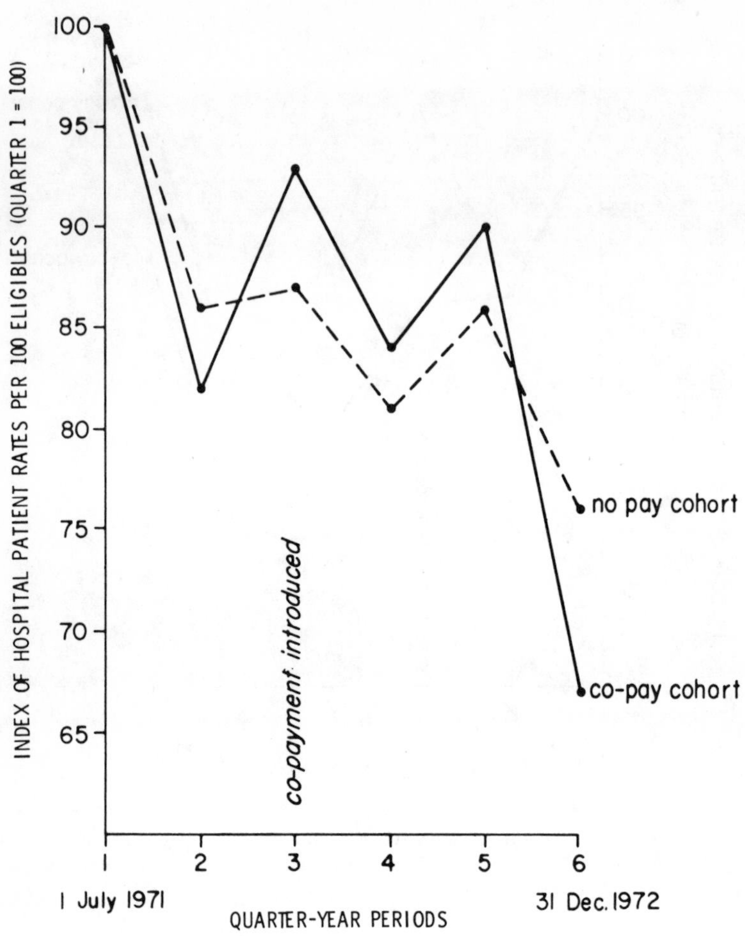

Figure 9-5. Hospital Patient Rates for AFDC Families (by co-payment status in California Medicaid program, July 1971–December 1972: indices of rates based on Quarter 1 = 100)

Figure 9-6 presents the hospitalization rates on another basis. It shows the trend of indices for all diagnoses except those related to pregnancy. The latter may be regarded as "nature-generated" and relatively independent of a doctor's judgment in modern American society. With these cases removed, it is apparent that the differentially higher indices of hospital use for the co-pay cohort are even greater in three out of the four co-payment quarters than for the total of hospital patients shown in Figure 9-5.

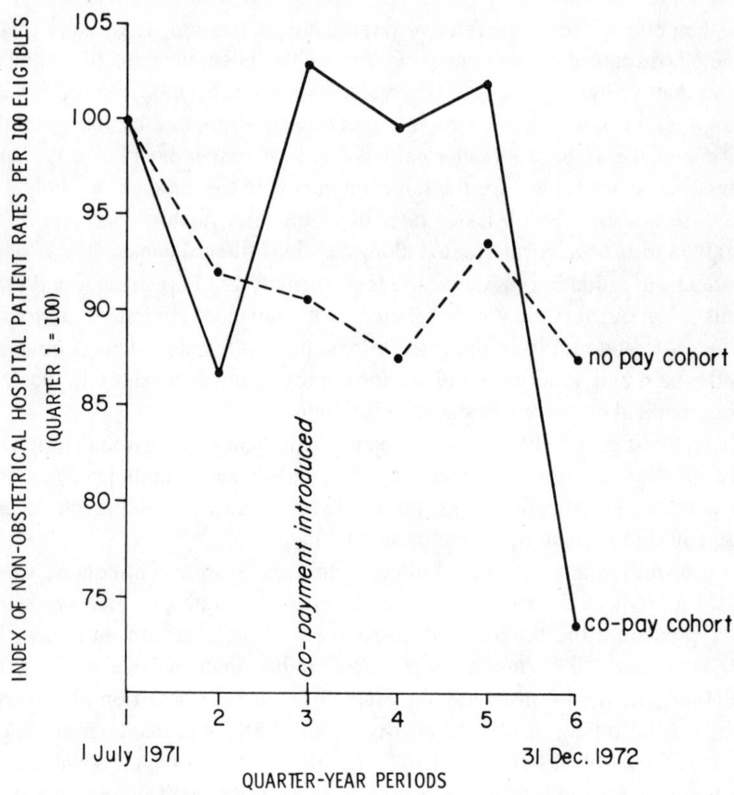

Figure 9-6. Hospital Patient Rates for All Non-obstetrical Admissions in AFDC Families (by co-payment status in California Medicaid program, July 1971–December 1972: indices of rates based on Quarter 1 = 100)

Discussion

These findings suggest that the effects of co-payment requirements for ambulatory services (and prescriptions) in a medical care program for low-income families were to exert a deterrent effect on demand or utilization. The inhibiting effect applied to office visits—the bedrock of general medical care—and also to typical diagnostic tests (urinalyses), to preventive procedures (Pap smears), and to drug prescriptions. Easy access to and use of general ambulatory doctors' services are widely considered to have preventive value, by permitting prompt diagnosis and treatment of an illness before it becomes more serious.

When such ambulatory services are inhibited, it would seem that a price is paid—namely, a rise in the relative rate of hospitalization. It is likely that this elevated hospitalization rate index is due to the postponement of ambulatory care, so that when the patient finally seeks assistance, his case is more advanced and requires in-patient care. This interpretation is supported by the general observation in the U.S. National Health Survey of longer hospital stays among low-income persons, even for the same diagnosis, in the nation as a whole.[8] This is likewise associated with lesser rates of ambulatory doctor's care by the poor generally and is usually interpreted along the lines offered above.

A clear-cut reduction in diagnostic tests (urinalyses, Pap smears, and others) as well as ambulatory treatment (doctor visits and prescriptions)—as found in our study—could hardly be expected to benefit health status. This is quite aside from the pain and suffering involved for the low-income patient who postpones seeking medical care at early stages of his illness.

These findings also have serious financial implications. Hospitalization is by far the costliest sector of medical care. A reduced rate of ambulatory care may yield short-term financial savings, but a subsequent increase in the rate of hospital use could more than outweigh these amounts.

To determine the net financial effect within the co-payment cohort, we may estimate an expected cost to the State, based on the rate of office visits in the quarter preceding the initiation of co-payment, which was on an annual basis 2,400 visits per 1,000 (much lower, incidentally, than the rate in the general population, and hardly justifying the State government's assertion of "overutilization"). Multiplying this by the cost-per-visit of $8.79 in that quarter yields an "expected" cost of $21,096 per 1,000 eligibles. After co-payment was initiated the actual cost for the year was $21,008 or a theoretical net saving to the state of just $88 per 1,000.‡

Turning to the hospitalization experience, the "expected" expenditure would be based on the base-period rate of 83.6 patients per 1,000 per year at a cost of $623 per patient (the annual cost per patient in the co-payment period) or a total of $52,082 per 1,000. Actually, the expenditure in the co-payment period was $53,017 or a net excess of $935 per 1,000. (It should be noted that this excess was due entirely to the increased hospitalization rate; if one took account of actual inflation of hospital costs over the pre-co-payment period, the difference would be much greater.) Subtracting the estimated saving for ambulatory services of $88 per 1,000, the net *excess cost* to the State was $1,228,150. (It is noteworthy that California discontinued the entire co-payment procedure June 30, 1973, even though federal P.L. 92-603, effective January 1, 1973, officially permitted such co-payment under certain circumstances.)

‡In spite of the lower indices of office visit rates for the co-pay cohort, compared with the no-pay cohort (shown in Table 2 and Figure 1), it may be noted that the actual rate of visits of both cohorts (for epidemiological or other possible reasons) exceeded the pre-co-payment rate during three out of the four co-payment quarters. Thus, despite the $1 saving to the State for most visits, this explains the small differential in total expenditures.

In a word, it would appear from this study of the California Copayment Experiment with Medicaid beneficiaries that the State government's strategy was penny-wise and pound-foolish. Short-term savings for lower ambulatory care use were followed by relative increases in costly hospital use. It is of interest to note that this general course of events was predicted in a legal brief submitted in opposition to the co-pay program before it was instituted.[4] As the experience of many "health maintenance organizations" has repeatedly demonstrated, comprehensive medical care, without cost-sharing deterrents, is probably not only the best way to maintain a person's health, but is also most economical in the long run.[7]

References

1. Beck, R. G.: The effects of copayment on the poor. J. Human Resources, publication pending.
2. Brian, Earl W.: The Medi-Cal Reform law. California's Health, April 1972, p. 3.
3. ———: Government control of hospital utilization: a California experience. N. Engl. J. Med. 286:1340, 1972.
4. Butler, Patricia, *et al.*: Attorneys for California Welfare Rights Organization: California's Copayment Waiver Proposal. Los Angeles, August 17, 1971.
5. Hall, Charles P., Jr.: Deductibles in health insurance: an evaluation. J. Risk Insurance 23:253, 1966.
6. Newhouse, Joseph P., Phelps, Charles E., and Schwartz, William B.: Policy options and the impact of national health insurance. N. Engl. J. Med. 290:1345, 1974.
7. Roemer, Milton I., and Shonick, William: HMO performance: the recent evidence. Health and Society, Summer 1973, p. 271.
8. U.S. National Center for Health Statistics: Medical Care, Health Status, and Family Income. Public Health Service, Washington, 1964.

10

Physician Extenders for Primary Care in Affluent Countries

Another response to rising medical care costs in the United States developed in the 1960s was to train allied or auxiliary personnel to render primary care in the place of doctors. First, former military medical corpsmen (from the Vietnam War) were given brief courses to serve as "medical assistants." Later, nurses were given supplemental training in the diagnosis and treatment of common disorders to serve as "nurse practitioners." Both types came to be known as "physician extenders."

In 1973, along with my wife, Ruth, I was awarded a contract to study this and other health manpower policies and practices in Australia, Belgium, Canada, Norway, and Poland–all industrialized countries, and somewhat comparable to the United States, with differing national health care systems. We found that none of these countries had adopted the "physician extender" idea for primary care, although auxiliary personnel were used for many procedures, *such as midwifery and anaesthesia, under medical direction; instead, greater support was given to general medical practitioners. We also observed that U.S. physician extenders were used mainly for primary care of the poor, thus relieving overspecialized physicians of this social responsibility. The dynamics of this health manpower policy are explored in the following chapter.*

AFTER A WORLDWIDE swing to specialization in medicine—beginning around 1910, gaining great momentum after World War II, and reaching a crescendo around 1960—a reaction has set in. Since 1960, the importance of the medical generalist has been rediscovered. Many influences have doubtless contributed to this reversal of trends in medical manpower: a fresh recognition of the need for "wholistic medicine" or understanding the patient as a whole person, the power of antibiotics and other effective therapies that did not require a specialist for their proper use, the increasing demands of patients for prompt and comprehensive health service. These and other factors are responsible for a worldwide movement to increase the access of people to primary health care.

Chapter 10 originally appeared as "Primary Care and Physician Extenders in Affluent Countries" in the *International Journal of Health Services*, 7:545–555, Fall 1977, and is reprinted by permission of that journal.

Demands for Primary Health Care in America

It is not surprising that a mounting unmet need for primary health care should have been recognized early and prominently in the United States. This was the country where specialization had been growing most rapidly. In 1931, of all American physicians actively engaged in clinical practice (117 per 100,000 population), only 17 percent (or 20 per 100,000) were full-time in a specialty, and 83 percent (or 97 per 100,000) were general practitioners or only partially specialized. By 1969, these relationships had reversed so that 77 percent (96 per 100,000) were in a full-time specialty and only 23 percent (or 29 per 100,000) remained in general practice or with limited specialization.[1] By 1973, the overall supply of clinically active U.S. doctors had risen to about 140 per 100,000, but those devoted to general practice had declined to under 15 percent of the total.[2]

The consequences of these changes for the type of medical care available to the population were obviously great. On the positive side, they meant of course that a major share of the health service provided was given by highly skilled specialists. But such care might often be technically inappropriate and economically extravagant; it might have been well within the competence of a generalist at lower cost. Because specialist service was relatively expensive and often available only on referral from a generalist, the trend meant that low-income people became increasingly dependent on a shrinking supply of general practitioners. Access to a doctor became more and more difficult for the less affluent families, general practitioners faced increasing pressures, home calls declined steeply to save scarce medical time, and even in the doctor's office the time available per patient became shorter and shorter. These problems were particularly acute in the slum areas of larger cities, where poor people were concentrated.

One of the major adjustments to the problem of reduced access to individual doctors was a rapidly mounting use of hospital out-patient departments (OPD). Between 1962 and 1971, for example, when the size of the U.S. population increased by about 10 percent, the number of visits to hospital OPDs—for both emergency and organized clinic care—rose from 54 to 133 million, or by 146 percent.[3] As a secondary reaction to the extremely crowded out-patient departments, especially in large public hospitals, there was developed in the mid-1960s a new type of "neighborhood health center" for the ambulatory care of the poor.[4] While comprehensive health centers for ambulatory service were long established in many other countries, in the United States they had been effectively resisted by private doctors until the load of patient demands could no longer be met.[5] In addition to about 100 such centers, there were developed another 150 special comprehensive care facilities for mothers and infants and for children and youth, also located in poverty districts.[6]

Another important adjustment to the unsatisfied demands for primary health care in the United States was the development of so-called innovative uses of health manpower.[7] In the early 1960s, the United States had intervened in a civil war occurring in Vietnam. As soldiers returned from the distant battlegrounds, American doctors conceived of the same idea as did Russian doctors a century before: why not use medical corpsmen discharged from the military services for civilian medical care?[8] The American "physician assistant" took shape as almost the exact analogue of the Russian "feldsher."

With the higher standards of a later era, the American ex-soldier was given somewhat more training than his nineteenth-century Russian counterpart.[9] His role, however, was regarded along essentially the same lines as that of the Russian feldsher—namely, to provide health care for the poor, particularly in localities where fully qualified physicians were scarce or totally lacking. In Czarist Russia this was mainly in the rural districts; in twentieth-century America this was principally in the ghettos of large cities and to a lesser extent in impoverished rural areas. State laws were rapidly passed to authorize this new form of "physician extender," as he was called.[10] In practice, however, he became not an assistant to the physician but mainly a substitute in areas of doctor shortage and principally for the low-income patients in such areas (see discussion of this below).

At first, the nursing profession of the United States resisted the pressure to modify its role along similar lines. Nurses, it was claimed, offered "caring" and not "curing" skills; they wanted to give superior nursing service, it was argued, and not "second-class medical service."[11] But as the flood of interest in "physician extenders" swelled, and as the earnings of these male auxiliaries were seen to exceed nurse salaries, attitudes changed. The movement for women's equality added to the ferment, and there emerged by the late 1960s the concept of the "extended role nurse" or the "nurse practitioner."[12] Almost overnight, there sprang up scores of special educational programs for training nurse practitioners.

The scope of functions of the registered nurse in America, as in most other countries, had been gradually broadening over the years.[13] In hospitals, nurses were being delegated an increasing variety of tasks, from giving intravenous injections or changing surgical dressings to monitoring the sophisticated equipment in "intensive care units." In well-baby clinics, as doctors became less available, public health nurses contributed more to the routine examination of infants; in addition, visiting nurses had long been given much latitude in the bedside care of chronically ill patients at home.[14]

But the newly formulated functions for which both nurse practitioners and physician assistants were being prepared were quite different. While the content of different training programs varied, none of them was restricted to preparing the student only to carry out technical procedures; instead, they aimed to prepare him or her for *decision making in the primary care* of patients. While all sorts of semantics were used to avoid conflict with the medical licensure laws, these new health personnel were trained to carry out the diagnosis and treatment of so-called common diseases.[15]

Space does not permit exploration of the full implications of this American development, but we may acquire some perspective on it by examining equivalent health manpower developments in certain other countries. Opportunity for such observations has been provided by an international study I have been doing since 1973, a discussion of which follows.

Primary Health Care in Other Countries

Studies of the health care system and health manpower policies have been made in Australia,[16] Canada,[17] Belgium,[18] and Norway.[19] In this work, special attention has been given to the provision of primary health care and the use of allied health personnel for this purpose.

In all four of these countries, a conspicuous contrast from the United States is the much greater proportion of physicians engaged in general practice. Among doctors in active clinical work, 40 to 50 percent are generalists compared to less than 20 percent in America. Even so, the trend everywhere over the last 50 years has been toward an increase in specialization. As a result, efforts have recently been made everywhere to reinforce or strengthen primary health care. This has taken several forms, which may be briefly reviewed.

Medical Schools

A basic approach in all countries studied has been through the medical schools, where greater attention is being given to instruction in general practice. Almost all schools have developed formal courses in the field, using a variety of methods. There are model "family medicine clinics," preceptorships with community practitioners, and lectures and demonstrations given by academic departments of family medicine; even admission policies have been altered in some schools to give greater priority to applicants strong in the humanities, on the premise that such students are more likely to enter family practice.

Continuing Education

A second approach in all four countries is to increase and enrich programs of continuing education for doctors in general practice. These have also followed a variety of formats. Hospitals hold periodic clinical conferences, courses of several weeks' duration are given, instruction is presented by closed-circuit television, and so on. In Australia, national government grants are used to support these educational efforts, and in both Norway and Belgium regular subsidies come from the health insurance systems. To encourage attendance at postgraduate courses, general practitioners attending a certain number of hours may earn a certification that carries prestige and also entitles them to collect higher insurance payments. In addition, the structure of official fee-schedules may be modified to elevate the compensation for general practitioner services, relative to that for specialist services.

Specialist Training

Third, a planned approach to the training of specialists indirectly influences the supply and proportion of doctors in general practice. This is very deliberate in Norway, where virtually all specialists must have appointments on the staffs of hospitals (full-time or part-time) and the number of such positions is determined by the supply of hospital beds, which, in turn, depends on a hospital regionalization plan under government control. The rest of the doctors are available for general practice. Although such fully salaried medical staffs are not customary in Australia and Belgium, hospital appointments are limited to specialists, so that general practitioners naturally spend almost all their time on service in the community.

All four of these countries, moreover, are expanding the total output of doctors. The United States has done likewise, but an even greater expansion has occurred in the residency programs training specialists;[20] as a result, the proportion of generalists and their ratio to population keep declining. But when the training of specialists is constrained as it is in Norway, Belgium, and Australia, while total medical manpower expands, the supply of generalists inevitably increases.

Promotion of Community General Practice

Direct actions to enhance the attractiveness of community general practice is a fourth approach. In Canada and Australia, minimum incomes for rural practitioners are guaranteed by certain states or provinces. Norway goes further, with its highly successful system of District Doctors. Almost every square mile of the nation is served by one of some 600 District Doctors, who are appointed and paid a basic salary by the national government. Most of their income is actually earned from insurance fees for private medical care, but they are part of an official network that carries great prestige. If the U.S. had an equivalent number of doctors in its National Health Service Corps, that program for "underserved areas" would be staffed with 30,000 physicians, instead of a few hundred.[21]

Organized Ambulatory Service

A fifth and important approach to strengthening primary health care in the community, not only in the four countries studied but almost everywhere in the world, has been through the promotion of frameworks for organized ambulatory service.[22] To some extent this has been through subsidies of private group practice clinics, as in Great Britain or Norway. More often it has been through the establishment of health centers by national, provincial, or local governments. In the health centers are teams of personnel, including general practitioners along with nurses, technicians, social workers, and others. Primary health care, including both treatment and prevention, is the central purpose of most health centers, and sometimes, for example, in Quebec (Canada) and Norway, social welfare services are provided as well.

These five approaches to expanding or strengthening primary health care do not exhaust the list of strategies in various industrialized countries, but they illustrate the range of principal actions. The noteworthy point is that none of these actions—in countries of social and economic development roughly comparable to the United States—include training "physician assistants" or "nurse practitioners" along American lines. There is perhaps a partial exception in the very thinly settled lands of the Canadian Far North or the Australian "outback," where "outpost" and "bush" nurses serve small populations of Eskimos, Indians, or aborigines. Even these nurses, however, are mainly providers of first aid, and they have continuing radio communication with doctors; more important, they are not serving crowded populations in the slums of large cities, nor the equivalent of impoverished families in the villages of U.S. southern states.*

Doctor-substitutes in Other Countries

It is important to clarify two aspects of the use of allied health personnel in other countries, compared with the United States. The previous account focuses on primary health care, and it applies to several industrialized countries. Regarding narrower aspects of health service in all types of countries, and with respect to total health care in the less-developed agricultural countries, the uses of allied health personnel are very different.

In Australia and Norway, as well as elsewhere in Europe and in many countries of Asia and Africa, extensive use is made of nurses trained for specialized functions that in America are considered the exclusive domain of doctors. Most

*After the above observations were made, field studies were done in a fifth country, Poland. In this socialist nation, the approach to primary care is somewhat different, being divided between "internists" for adults and "pediatricians" for children; both are of course physicians, but with very generalized approaches. They work almost entirely in organized ambulatory care centers, aided by nurses and clerks. There is an active program of continuing education, including periods of rotation in hospitals. The Polish output of physicians has been steadily accelerated, so that the national ratio is currently about 1 doctor to 580 population, or better than the ratio in the United States. In this setting, the former Russian-style "feldsher" is rapidly being phased out; these doctor-substitutes are no longer trained. The more competent among them go to medical school and become physicians; others are retrained as sanitary inspectors, laboratory technicians, ambulance attendants, and the like. Some become nurses or midwives.

important is midwifery, in which thousands of nurses are trained throughout the world. Midwives do obstetrical deliveries both in homes and in hospitals, but in the industrialized countries, they work mainly in hospitals.[23] Another important category is the nurse-anesthetist used widely in Norway. Canada and Australia train psychiatric nurses for mental hospitals and clinics, not after the basic R.N. training, but as a special field in itself. Registered graduate nurses may also be trained for special work in well-baby clinics; these functions include counseling of mothers on infant care and the detection of abnormalities, but not the diagnosis or treatment of sickness. Family planning service is another common function for nurses or even nonnursing allied personnel.[24,25]

These specialized nursing tasks are sharply distinguishable from primary health care. In the main they require manual skills and performance of certain procedures, rather than the type of judgment involved in medical diagnosis and therapy. Some judgment, of course, is required even in taking a pulse, let alone delivering a baby, but it is of a different quality from the decision making necessary in good primary medical care. The scope of knowledge and reasoning required for the proper management of a backache, for example, is of much greater magnitude than that involved in handling a normal obstetrical presentation.

Regarding total health services in the less-developed countries, the uses of allied health personnel should be different and they are. In the recently liberated nations of Africa, medically starved from centuries of European domination, with hardly one doctor (African or expatriate) per 50,000 people, what choice existed for getting some health services to the predominantly rural populations? Village health workers, rapidly trained to recognize common diseases and to carry out vaccinations or other preventive services, were the obvious solution.[26,27] "Hospital assistants" or "medical aides" were likewise a practical adjustment in India and Southeast Asia generally. In China after its 1949 Liberation, a Chinese version of the Russian feldsher was trained, and then after 1966, in the wake of the Cultural Revolution, there arose the "barefoot doctor." Over 1,000,000 of these peasant health workers were briefly trained to meet the primary care needs of the rural 80 percent of China's enormous population of 800,000,000.[28]

But even in these impoverished developing countries, the rapidly trained primary health worker is regarded as a transitional solution to a critical problem. In Malaysia, for example, where the British colonial heritage of "hospital assistants" had been the mainstay of primary care in the rural health centers, a medical school was founded in 1959 and a second one was established recently.[29] As young doctors are produced, they are obligated to go to the rural areas first to supervise and then to replace the auxiliaries. China has developed some 85 medical schools, whose graduates serve in the rural areas and train the barefoot doctors.[30] As the numbers of physicians increase, there can be little doubt that they will eventually replace the village health workers, and the barefoot doctors will become true auxiliaries, helping but not substituting for the physicians.

It is noteworthy that in Russia, where the "feldsher" concept had been born, immediately after the 1917 Revolution it was discarded as "second-class medicine." Then, as the enormity of medical care needs in the Soviet Union was recognized, feldshers were reactivated, but this time with much more systematic training and for work under regular supervision.[31] Today, with the Soviet supply of doctors surpassing a ratio of 1 to 350 population (far more than the United States), and over half of them working as generalists for adults ("therapeutists") or children (pediatricians), the feldsher is again being phased out from his or her traditional role.[32] Feldshers are being used less and less for general primary care in rural or urban areas, but more and more for specialized ancillary functions as sanitary inspectors, vaccinators, laboratory assistants, ambulance attendants, X-ray technicians, feldsher-midwives, or the like. For some years, this has been the policy toward feldshers in Poland and other countries of Eastern Europe.[33]

Perspective on the U.S. "Physician Extender"

In the perspective of these policies toward primary health care and the use of allied health personnel in other countries, how should one view the recent enthusiastic expansion of physician extenders, or more accurately "doctor-substitutes," in the United States? Recognizing the enormous swing to specialization in America, with a resultant decline in generalists to less than 20 percent of all clinical doctors, one must regard this "innovation" with much concern. It is a hasty expedient for adjusting to the serious shortage of primary care doctors. Even the semantic sleight of hand, which defines internists (including endocrinologists and cardiologists), pediatricians, and also obstetrician-gynecologists as "primary physicians," does not solve the problem, nor reduce the flood of patients coming to hospital OPDs in search of primary care.[34]

But the doctor-substitute adjustment tends to be very selective with respect to the populations served. With the seemingly worthy objective of tackling unmet needs where they are greatest, physician extenders work predominantly among the poor, such as black residents of urban ghettos, Indians on rural reservations, or low-income chronic patients in public hospital clinics. Precise documentation of this widely evident impression is difficult to offer, since the studies so far conducted have not formulated their analyses along these lines. As a major 1975 survey put it:[35]

> The main benefit of physician extenders (PE) may well be to relieve the problems of service maldistribution. But to date, where PEs practice and who they serve are perhaps areas *least* researched [italics in the original].

One might even suspect that the lack of quantitative data on this issue is not merely a research oversight; its clarification might expose various inequities which would prove embarrassing in a presumably democratic society.

The classification of work settings for physician extenders (both nurse practitioners and physician assistants) in the largest nationwide study conducted so far yields the distribution shown in Table 10-1.[36] One may infer that the 56.7 percent of nurse practitioners working in hospital out-patient departments (18.9 percent) and clinics or health centers (37.8 percent) are essentially serving poor patients. The types of patients, however, served by the 50.5 percent of physician assistants in solo (28.3) or group (22.2) medical practices can only be a matter of speculation. Other data showing a heavy concentration of physician assistants in rural locations, and also in the southeastern states, would suggest that these personnel, even in private settings, are probably serving mainly patients of limited education or medical sophistication.

Specific evidence of this relationship is found in unpublished data on the deployment of the first 136 graduates of the Medex Physician's Assistant Program of the Charles R. Drew Postgraduate Medical School in Los Angeles. Of these, 71 percent are engaged in "primary care practice," the balance being in other forms of work or unemployed. Among those in primary care practice (97 persons), 87 percent are reported to be located in settings with disadvantaged populations; the latter are defined as a high proportion of racial or ethnic minorities, and dwellers in rural locations.[37]

At a national conference in 1974, a Dartmouth Medical School professor of community medicine observed (without, alas, offering data): "We found that the patient's age, social class, and access to medical services are significantly correlated with certain attitudes toward physician assistants."[38] Studies reporting high patient satisfaction with nurse practitioners have been carried out in public charity clinics, where the rushed attention of young residents or busy visiting physicians, applied to one series of patients, is compared with the solicitous care of seasoned nurses, applied to another series. Small wonder that patients have preferred the sympathetic care of the nurses, and even shown greater improvement from such care—especially when the diagnosis and therapeutic regime had been medically established beforehand for both series.[39]

In the few situations where nurse practitioners have been evaluated in a private practice setting, as in the Ontario clinical trial of 1971–1972, the dice have also (perhaps unwittingly) been loaded.[40] While patients were randomly assigned to the nurse or the doctor, the nurses had *twice* the time per patient; moreover, the doctor was on hand for prompt consultation—which was sought, indeed, in 33 percent of the cases. Small wonder again that the two patient series showed equivalent satisfaction and outcomes. At the Kaiser-Permanente Health Plan in Los Angeles, where nurse practitioners are also being used experimentally in some "walk-in" clinics, patients likewise seem to be well satisfied. "Why not," says one participating Permanente physician, "when a doctor is nearby to give advice and the nurse sees two patients per hour, while the doctor must see six."[41]

On the American scene, where greater per capita expenditures are made for medical care than in any other nation, the resort to nurse practitioners or physi-

Table 10-1
Work Settings of Physician Extenders: Percentage Distributions of 1,070 Nurse Practitioners and 451 Physician Assistants, United States, 1976[a]

Work Setting	*Nurse Practitioners*	*Physician Assistants*
Solo physician's office	8.1	28.3
Medical partnership or group	6.0	22.2
Hospital outpatient department	18.9	8.9
Hospital inpatient service	4.2	9.8
Clinic or health center	37.8	18.6
Community and home health agency	13.8	0.9
Other	11.2	11.3
All settings	100.0	100.0

a. Source, reference 36.

cian assistants for providing primary health care must be interpreted as an abdication of social responsibility by doctors. It is an easy way out for a private entrepreneurial profession that prefers to devote its time to surgical specialties in the suburbs much more than to primary health care in the inner-city slums. It goes along with staunch opposition to national health manpower legislation, which would require new medical graduates to settle for a time in underserved areas. One can hear the echo of the Czarist aristocrats, "let the feldshers take care of the peasants with their 'simpler' diseases." Let the physician assistants or the nurse practitioner take care of the urban blacks or the Appalachian poor whites. Besides, it can be shown to be less expensive.[42]

Nations in which universal health insurance programs have established medical care as a human right view it differently. They see many values to ancillary health personnel for selected procedures, but not for all-important primary care. For this crucial function a fully educated physician is necessary, not only to apply sophisticated judgment to distinguish the backache due to arthritic vertebrae from that due to emotional tension, but also to achieve continuity of care. This is the essential role of the European general practitioner, who derives his strength from enduring ties not to hospitals but to families.[43] He or she (a rapidly mounting proportion of doctors are women) is glad to make a home call for flu or to incise an infected hangnail in the office, not because these actions require seven or eight years of university training, but because they help him to understand his patients better. This has been the role, after all, of the good physician from Hippocrates to Osler.[44]

Countless procedures in health service are, of course, and should be assigned to auxiliary personnel in all countries. General primary medical care, however, should be delegated to others only in impoverished countries, as a temporary expedient until economic development yields an adequate supply of doctors. The rationale in developing countries is manifestly linked to weak economic resources. In the "welfare states" or the industrialized and socialist countries of Eastern Europe, the doctor-substitute has been clearly rejected on principles of equity.

In the world's most affluent nation, there would hardly seem to be economic justification for the use of physician extenders for primary care. Current American policies can only be attributed to an unwillingness to impose social obligations on the physician (e.g., location in areas of need) and to train adequate numbers of primary care doctors. Such policies are an unfortunate acknowledgment of failure by medicine to fulfill its social mission and of failure by society to achieve equity in the health services.

References

1. Stevens, R. *American Medicine and the Public Interest*, p. 181. Yale University Press, New Haven, 1971.
2. Silver, G. A. *A Spy in the House of Medicine*, p. 93. Aspen Systems Corporation, Germantown, Md., 1976.
3. *Health Resources Statistics 1972–73*, p. 483. U.S. National Center for Health Statistics, Washington, D.C., 1973.
4. Schorr, L., and English, J. Background, context, and significant issues in neighborhood health center programs. *Milbank Mem. Fund Q*. 46:239, July 1968.
5. Roemer, M. I. *Evaluation of Community Health Centers*. Public Health Paper No. 48. World Health Organization, Geneva, 1972.
6. Stewart, W. H. The unmet needs of children. *Pediatrics* 39:157–160, February 1967.
7. Stead, Jr., E.A. Training and use of paramedical personnel. *N. Engl. J. Med.* 277:800–801, 1967.
8. Sigerist, H. E. *Socialized Medicine in the Soviet Union*, pp. 143–144. W. W. Norton & Company, New York, 1937.
9. Coye, R. D., and Hansen, M. F. The "doctor's assistant"—A survey of physicians' expectations. *JAMA* 209:259, 1969.
10. Curran, W. J. New paramedical personnel—To license or not to license. *N. Engl. J. Med.* 282:1085–1086, 1970.
11. Bullough, B., editor. *The Law and the Expanding Nursing Role*, pp. 53–61. Appleton-Century-Crofts, New York, 1975.
12. Baker, A. S. Primary care by the nurse. *N. Engl. J. Med.* 290: 282–283, January 31, 1974.
13. Bullough, V.L., and Bullough, B. *The Emergence of Modern Nursing*, Macmillan Company, New York, 1969.
14. Davis, F., editor. *The Nursing Profession: Five Sociological Essays*. John Wiley & Sons, New York, 1966.
15. Secretary's Committee to Study Extended Roles of Nurses. *Expanding the Scope of Nursing Practice*. U.S. Department of Health, Education, and Welfare, Washington, D.C., November 1971.
16. Roemer, R., and Roemer, M. I. *Health Manpower in the Changing Australian Health Services Scene*. DHEW Pub. (HRA) 75-58. U.S. Health Resources Administration, Washington, D.C., 1976.
17. Roemer, M. I., and Roemer, R. *Health Manpower under National Health Insurance. The Canadian Experience*. U.S. Health Resources Administration, Washington. D.C., in press.

18. Roemer, R., and Roemer, M. I. *Health Manpower Policies in the Belgian Health Care System*. U.S. Health Resources addministration, Washington, D.C., publication pending.
19. Roemer, M. I., and Roemer, R. *Manpower in the Health Care System of Norway*. U.S. Health Resources Administration, Washington, D.C., publication pending.
20. *Directory of Approved Residencies 1974–75*. American Medical Association, Chicago, 1975.
21. Health personnel will be assigned to critical manpower-lacking areas. *Medical Tribune*, June 28, 1972.
22. Roemer, M. I. Organized ambulatory health service in international perspective. *Int. J. Health Serv.* 1(1): 18–27, 1971.
23. Williams, C. D., and Jelliffe, D. B. *Mother and Child Health: Delivering the Services*. Oxford University Press, London, 1972.
24. Non-physicians trained to provide medical family planning care. *Family Planning Digest* 2(4): 1–6, July 1973.
25. Morehead, J., editor. *Paramedical Personnel in Family Planning*. Pathfinder Fund, Boston, 1974.
26. Fendall, N. R. E. Auxiliary health personnel: Training and use. *Public Health Rep*. 82: 471–479, June 1967.
27. Jensen, R. T. The primary medical care worker in developing countries. *Med. Care* 5: 382–400, November–December 1967.
28. Sidel, V. W. The barefoot doctors of the People's Republic of China. *N. Engl. J. Med.* 286: 1292–1300, 1972.
29. Roemer, M. I. Strengthening of Health Services and Training of Health Personnel in Malaysia; General Overview and Analysis. World Health Organization, Western Pacific Region, Manila, February 1969 (processed report).
30. Hsu, R.C. The barefoot doctors of the People's Republic of China—Some problems. *N. Engl. J. Med*. 291:124–127, 1974.
31. Sidel, V. W. Feldshers and feldsherism: The role and training of the feldsher in the U.S.S.R. *N. Engl. J. Med*. 278: 934–940, 981–992, 1968.
32. Terris, M. Strategies for primary care: False starts and lesser alternatives. *Bull. N. Y. Acad. Med.*, in press.
33. Weinerman, E. R. *Social Medicine in Eastern Europe: Organization of Health Services and Education of Medical Personnel in Czechoslovakia, Hungary, and Poland*. Harvard University Press, Cambridge, 1969.
34. American Society of Internal Medicine. Primary care: A function, not a discipline. *Internist* 17: 10, March 1976.
35. Appel, G. L., and Lowin, A. *Physician Extenders: An Evaluation of Policy-Related Research*, p. XIX. InterStudy, Minneapolis, 1975.
36. Nurse Practitioner and Physician Assistant Training and Deployment Study, pp. VI–18, 19. System Sciences, Inc., Bethesda, Md., July 1976 (processed).
37. Kivel, R. M., Program Director of the Charles R. Drew Postgraduate Medical School, Medex Physician's Assistant Program, personal communication, February 8, 1977.
38. Jacobs, A. R. in *New Health Practitioners—Partners in Patient Care*, p. 45. Institute of Medicine of Chicago (1974 Workshop), 1975.
39. Lewis, C. E., Resnick, B. A., Schmidt, G., and Waxman, D. Activities, events, and outcomes in ambulatory patient care. *N. Engl. J. Med.* 280: 645–649, March 20, 1969.
40. Spitzer, W. O., et al. The Burlington randomized trial of the nurse practitioner. *N. Engl. J. Med.* 290: 251–256, January 31, 1974.
41. Personal communication from a Permanente Medical Group physician, July 1976.
42. Garfield, S., Collen, M. F., Feldman, R., Soghikian, K., Richart, R. H., and Duncan, J. H. Evaluation of an ambulatory medical-care system. *N. Engl. J. Med.* 294: 426–431, February 19, 1976.
43. *The Role of the Primary Physician in Health Services*. World Health Organization, Regional Office for Europe, Copenhagen 1971.
44. Sigerist, H. E. *Medicine and Human Welfare*, pp. 105–145. Yale University Press, New Haven, 1941.

Part Three

Health Insurance and Payment Methods

One of the major worldwide strategies for improving access to needed medical care has been insurance–both voluntary programs of many types and mandatory programs established under law. Along with this collective form of financing, there occur many influences on the patterns of delivery of the services.

In Chapter 11, we review briefly the evolution of the health insurance movement in the United States. Chapter 12 reports the results of a study analyzing the effects–in utilization rates, costs, attitudes, etc.–of different types of health insurance plan which have grown up in America. Under insurance, or without it, doctors may be paid in various ways; Chapter 13 explores the consequences of these diverse methods. Health insurance is primarily intended to ease the costs to individuals and therefore improve the access to medical care, but preventive services may also be fostered through insurance programs; how this is done is examined in Chapter 14. For some years the rising overall costs of medical care in the United States and elsewhere have been attributed in part to the extension of health insurance, with its removal of economic constraints on the procurement of services; Chapter 15, however, explores how national (governmental) health insurance has acted in many countries as a device for stemming the tide of rising expenditures.

11

The Evolution of National Health Insurance in America

In the 1970s, only five years after enactment of Medicare insurance for the aged, numerous legislative proposals were introduced in the United States Congress to extend health insurance protection to all or nearly all of the population, but the origins of this movement dated back many decades before. It was traceable to European experience and was related closely to the growth of voluntary or nongovernmental health insurance from the 1930s.

In May, 1975, a Symposium on "National Health Insurance" was held in Los Angeles, California, and the text that follows was the opening address.

RECENTLY I HAD the opportunity to spend two months in Canada, a country very similar to our own. One could see there the full scenario of what might have happened in the United States, except for a few votes in the New York State Legislature in 1917. For Canada started its movement toward national health insurance at the provincial (or state) level, as the United States also did, but with different results.

Beginnings of Social Insurance in the United States

A proper tracing of the evolution of national health insurance in the United States would start with the medieval guilds, then the German Krankenkassen, Chancellor Bismarck's 1883 law initiating the social insurance concept, the British health insurance law of 1911, and many other significant events which later influenced the United States. But, in the interests of brevity, let us start with the first extensive social insurance legislation here—the industrial injury compensation field pioneered by New York State in 1911.

Perhaps note should be taken, parenthetically, of a much earlier piece of social insurance legislation in America, but one confined to a special kind of worker—the merchant seaman. In 1798, Congress had mandated wage deductions to finance medical care for these men, essential for trade with Europe. With these funds, a network of marine hospitals was built in the nineteenth century at the main ports. By 1884, the voice of the working man had become sufficiently strong for the financing to be shifted to the shipowners through a ship tonnage tax. And by 1906, the system had become so well established that its cost was shifted to general revenues, and the program was renamed the Marine Hospital

Chapter 11 originally appeared in the *Proceedings of the Symposium on National Health Insurance*, ed. R. D. Goodman (Los Angeles: University of California Extension, January, 1976), pp. 5–13.

Service; in 1912, its name was changed again to the United States Public Health Service. It is noteworthy, however, that this idea of legally mandated general health care insurance did not spread beyond the merchant mariners. It was an isolated current in a social stream dominated by other forces.

Returning to the industrial injury problem, the original New York State law had been enacted in 1910. It required employers in certain hazardous industries to insure their workers against the loss of wages and medical costs arising out of job-related accidents, but the law was found unconstitutional by the State Supreme Court, under the "due process" clause of the Fourteenth Amendment. Abraham Lincoln might have turned over in his grave had he known that the Constitutional amendment barring slavery after the Civil War ("no one shall be deprived of life, liberty, or property without due process of law") was invoked to strike down a law requiring employers to bear the responsibility for accidents occurring under their employment. Then came the horrendous Triangle fire, in which scores of women garment workers were burned to death. Popular outrage was so great that a few months later, when a slightly modified law was passed, the judges changed their minds, and soon state after state passed similar social insurance legislation—Mississippi being the last in 1950.

Encouraged by this victory for humane legislation, and influenced by the 1911 enactment in Great Britain of national health insurance for low-paid workers (it provided only for general practitioner care and drugs, and did not cover dependents), in 1915 legislatures in a dozen states considered bills for general health care insurance. These bills would have required insurance of manual workers, earning under $100 per month, for the costs of any type of illness—costs due both to wage loss from disability and the need for medical care. The insurance would be carried by mutual benefit associations, trade unions, or other non-profit bodies, and payment of the premiums would be shared by the workers themselves, employers, and state governments. These bills were modeled after the original German legislation of 30 years before, maintaining a key administrative role for local non-governmental protective organizations that had already been operating in the large cities. With a few more votes, the New York State bill might have passed, but in the end none of some 15 state bills was enacted. Opposition came not so much from the doctors (several state medical societies supported the idea, in order to get paid for treating low income patients whom they were previously serving free), but from the employers, commercial insurance companies, and even from some organized labor groups who objected on grounds of "paternalism." By 1920, in the conservative atmosphere following World War I, state health insurance became a dead issue.

The Voluntary Health Insurance Movement

Meanwhile, the health insurance idea under voluntary sponsorship did not disappear. Small mutual aid societies providing insured sickness benefits for workers in particular establishments had been operating since the mid-nineteenth century.

Fraternal orders, composed of ethnic minority immigrants from Europe, working for different companies, were another approach, sometimes paying their "lodge doctors" on a periodic per capita basis. Isolated industries in mining, lumbering, or railroad construction found that only through paying "contract doctors" a salary, derived from wage deductions or "check-offs," could medical service be assured in out-of-the way places. In the timber country of Washington and Oregon, the county medical societies organized "medical bureaus" that collected their funds from periodic wage deductions, but allowed free choice of local doctors who were then paid on a fee basis. Here and there private insurance companies sold policies for general sickness or accident wage-loss compensation, first to individual workers and later, at lower rates, to groups of workers, in a factory.

The post-war decade of the 1920s, however, was full of confidence in America, with an expanding economy and a devil-may-care spirit of individual freedom. This was not the atmosphere for planning ahead nor for benevolent governmental concern about the health needs of the poor. Even the modest Sheppard-Towner Act, giving small federal grants to the states for preventive maternal and child health services, was staunchly opposed by the American Medical Association, and allowed to die a few years after its enactment in 1921. Then in 1929, the balloon burst with the stock market crash, ushering in the Great Depression of the 1930s.

That same year, 1929, a group of school teachers in Dallas, Texas, conceived the idea of paying small periodic dues to the Baylor University Hospital, which would build up a fund to pay for any future hospitalization that any teacher needed. The same basic concept, incidentally, had been implemented 15 years before in Grinnell, Iowa, and some other small one-hospital towns, but the time was not ripe and the idea didn't spread. With the economic adversity of the 1930s, the response of the hospitals was totally different. In Essex County, New Jersey, faced with half-empty beds and near bankruptcy, a group of hospitals got together offering to contract on a similar basis with groups of people. Then, Detroit, Michigan, and other areas followed suit. In 1934, the American Hospital Association decided to promote the idea nationally, establish minimum standards, and give the movement a symbol, the Blue Cross. Despite opposition from the A.M.A. as another "entering wedge to socialized medicine," voluntary hospitalization insurance grew.

The New Deal and Social Security

By 1935, Franklin Roosevelt's New Deal had been going for three years. Mass suffering had been somewhat alleviated with the Federal Emergency Relief Administration, but it was time for a more basic approach. The Committee on Economic Security had been drawing up plans for a comprehensive social insurance program—one that would cushion not only the adversities of unemployment and old age, but also the costs of medical care. Mr. Roosevelt was aware, however, of the strong opposition of the doctors, and not wishing to jeopardize the cash-benefit provisions, he proposed replacement of general health insurance with reactivation of the Sheppard-Towner grants to the states for MCH services plus federal grants for other public health purposes. Senator Wagner obliged, and thus came Titles V and VI of the Social Security Act of 1935.

This landmark social legislation softened the worst blows of the Depression, but the country was still far from prosperous. By 1939, some doctors realized that Blue Cross wasn't so bad after all, and perhaps the same idea could be applied to payment of doctor's fees in hospitalized cases. The California Medical Association was the first state society to act on this, and it was soon followed by several others, so that Blue Shield was born. With the success of both Blue Cross and Blue Shield, the commercial insurance carriers became convinced of the actuarial soundness of insurance for hospital services—institutional and medical—and they joined the movement.

Also by 1939, Senator Wagner thought the time had come to fill the medical care gap in his Social Security Act. In the preceding years, the Committee on the Costs of Medical Care (1928–33) and the first National Health Survey (1935–37) had demonstrated the great paradox of greater volumes of sickness and lesser amounts of medical service being experienced as one descended the income ladder. The voluntary health insurance plans were growing, but they did not reach the poorest people with the greatest needs. In July, 1939, therefore Mr. Wagner introduced the first National Health Bill. Like Social Security Titles V and VI, however, it had a modest conception, offering grants to those states which wished to develop health insurance programs for their workers; federal subsidy of such plans would be an inducement. A few months later, however, Hitler marched on Poland, World War II had begun, and social legislation took a back seat.

The Wagner-Murray-Dingell Bills

The Second Front in Europe had not yet been opened when the confidence of the Allies was sufficiently great for America to start talking of "post-war planning." The Atlantic Charter of Mr. Churchill and Mr. Roosevelt had declared a goal of the war to be "freedom from want," and in 1942 the British Beveridge Report called for a "national health service" to guarantee complete medical care for everyone. So in 1943, Senator Wagner—with Senator Murray and Congressman Dingell—came forth again with a new National Health Bill, this time more sweeping than the 1939 version. Instead of subsidizing state insurance plans, it would set up a single national health insurance fund, in the model of the old-age pension system; this fund would support the costs of comprehensive services to all working people and their dependents. It would be financed by mandatory contributions from employers and workers and administered through a network of federal offices. At the same time, there would be no change in the pattern of providing or receiving medical care; everyone would have his or her customary free choice of doctor, hospital, and all the rest. The crucial change would be that the bills would be paid not by the sick patient, but by the insurance fund which had been built up while he was well.

The Wagner-Murray-Dingell bills, not surprisingly, engendered a storm of opposition from the private medical profession, the insurance companies, and Chambers of Commerce. Support came from organized labor, social workers, and a handful of socially oriented doctors. As hearings proceeded, the bill went through several versions, though it never came to a vote on the floor of Congress. Nevertheless, the Wagner-Murray-Dingell Bills of the 1940s had an enormous effect; by posing a great threat to the voluntary health insurance movement, they stimulated its growth at a robust rate. By the mid-1950s, some 70 percent of the nation's population were protected with some degree of private health insurance. Meanwhile, in 1952, a conservative General Eisenhower was elected to the Presidency after 20 years of Democratic Party control. The opposition to national health insurance breathed a sigh of relief.

The great majority of voluntarily health insured people, however, were covered through their place of work. This meant that when they became unemployed or retired, they lost the protection. Moreover, the bulk of the protection was for hospital-related illness; ordinary ambulatory services, which might help to prevent more serious illness were not covered. Most serious was doubtless the problem of the aged, for not only were they unlikely to have insurance but, for biological reasons, their volume of serious sickness was greater than ever. Here was the Achilles heel of the voluntary health insurance movement and it was only to be expected that government would attempt to step in to fill the gap.

Medicare for the Aged

The logical step was taken by Congressman Forand of Rhode Island, who in 1957 introduced a bill to amend the Social Security Act so as to supplement pensions for the insured aged with assumption of the costs of their hospital and in-hospital doctor's care. Once again a storm of opposition broke loose, and once again a series of hearings and modified bills came along to offer financial protection for medical care to the aged. In response to the pressure, in 1960 there was enacted the Kerr-Mills amendment on Medical Assistance to the Aged—essentially broadening the definition of neediness to include old people who were not getting cash relief but could not afford the costs of medical care. The MAA program helped a little, but by no means solved the problem, and the issue remained alive into the election campaign of 1964.

When Lyndon Johnson won for the Democrats a landslide victory, the first bill introduced into the Senate, S.1., was to provide medical care insurance for the aged. By July 1965, just 30 years after passage of the original Social Security Act, a bill—soon dubbed by the newspapers "Medicare," was signed into law. It provided much wider benefits than the original Forand proposal, and greatly expanded the accessibility of old people to medical care, but still did almost nothing to modify the prevailing system of delivering health service in America.

With more billions of dollars pumped into the medical marketplace, it was only to be expected that medical and hospital prices would take a steep jump upward. Although the former public medical care program for the poor had been greatly expanded under other legislation (Medicaid), accessibility to service for the poor, the near poor, and even the middle classes became gradually more difficult. Enactment in late 1965 of the Regional Medical Programs for Heart Disease, Cancer, and Stroke (RMP) and in 1966 of the Comprehensive Health Planning Act had done little to improve the situation. In July, 1969, a conservative White House was led to declare that the nation faced a breakdown in its whole medical care system, and leaders from all points on the political spectrum spoke of a "health care crisis" that required corrective action urgently.

National Health Insurance Proposals of the 1970s

The first move in response was introduction by Senator Kennedy in August, 1970, then in slightly modified form in January, 1971, of a new bill for comprehensive health insurance which would cover the entire national population—the Health Security Bill. In February, 1971, President Nixon sent to Congress a major message on "Building a National Health Strategy." It called not only for mandatory health insurance—the first such proposal by a Republican leader—but for promoting moves to modify the traditional fee-for-service system through encouragement of "health maintenance organizations" or HMOs. So ripe was the time for action that within 18 months a dozen other health insurance bills were introduced in Congress, including measures sponsored by the American Medical Association, the commercial insurance industry, and the Republican administration itself.

Since 1972 the Congressional scene regarding national health insurance has been a boiling cauldron. There are various ingredients in this broth, but I might point out that the crucial differences among the several bills proposed are not their total costs, as is often claimed, but rather what proportion of those costs are channelled through the private sector, compared with the public sector where they are more subject to planning and controls. Separate legislation has been enacted on HMOs, on "professional standard review organizations" or PSROs, on national health planning, and on other aspects of the health service industry. With inflation, unemployment, an energy crisis, the Watergate scandal, and other issues, legislative priorities have changed almost from week to week; as of today national health insurance is not in the front-runner position it was even a year ago. But there is little doubt that some action will be taken soon.

The experience of Medicare for the aged—ten years of it by now—has convinced nearly everyone that more than a financial solution is needed. It has become almost a cliché to point out that the whole system of delivering medical care in America requires basic overhauling. Almost all the dozen or more bills before both houses of Congress would encourage some changes, with varying degrees of sweep. And a fair guess is that the more liberal Congress elected in November, 1974, will settle on some compromise bill to the left of center.

This review of the evolution of national health insurance in the United States has been very sketchy. Political prediction is a hazardous game, but it is safe to say that the costs of medical care, accessibility to it, and the control of its quality have all become political issues. As I stated at the outset, Canada started its movement to national health insurance by action at the level of one prairie province; this was Saskatchewan, where a program launched in 1947 became nationwide by 1958. Rhode Island, incidentally, enacted a social insurance law to cover catastrophic medical costs in 1974. The same year Hawaii enacted a social insurance law for much broader medical care protection of all employees in that island-state. In the state legislature here in California, other more comprehensive bills have recently been introduced. With so much brewing at both state and national levels, one can expect that the United States will soon lose its dubious distinction of being the only industrialized nation on earth whose people lack the protection of a social insurance program for general health service.

12

Diverse Voluntary Health Insurance Plans and Their Comparative Effects

The pluralism of American health services is demonstrated in no sector of the field more vividly than in the many voluntary health insurance programs operating side-by-side. Despite its many problems, this very diversity of financial mechanisms for protection against medical care costs permits comparative research. With the aid of a federal grant in 1964, such research was undertaken at UCLA on the three principal types of health insurance program, as found in Southern California.

The research required several years, and in June, 1972, I was invited by a U.S. Senate Subcommittee investigating monopolistic practices in the insurance industry to summarize our principal findings. The text that follows is drawn from the testimony presented to this Congressional body in 1972 and published later in the Hearings *of the U.S. Senate Subcommittee on Antitrust and Monopoly. A fuller version of the findings in Chapter 12 was co-authored with R.W. Hetherington and Carl E. Hopkins and appeared in monograph form as* Health Insurance Effects: Services, Expenditures, and Attitudes under Three Types of Plan, *Research Series No. 16 (Ann Arbor, Mich.: University of Michigan School of Public Health, Bureau of Public Health Economics, 1972).*

I AM PLEASED to present to the Senate Subcommittee on Antitrust and Monopoly some of the highlights of our findings from seven years of research on health insurance plans. I hope that these findings may have some relevance for your deliberations, to quote from your letter, on "the commercial health insurance industry and its overall role in helping to develop a health-care system responsive to the needs of consumers."

Research on Health Insurance Plans

The three principal types of health insurance program operating in our country today are, in order of their enrollment size, those sponsored by 1. commercial insurance companies; 2. providers of health care—mainly the medical and hospital associations (symbolized commonly as Blue Cross and Blue Shield plans); and 3. consumers, employers, or other groups applying the pattern of prepaid group medical practice. The third of these types have recently come to be called "health maintenance organizations" (HMOs).

It is of some interest that, historically, the development of these programs has been in the reverse order from that just given—that is, the consumer-sponsored plans being oldest, the provider-sponsored plans coming next, and the commercial plans being newest. The market dynamics of sales in the insurance field, however, has resulted in a situation where currently the largest share of the market is held by the commercial insurance companies, followed by the other two types of plan as stated. To simplify my summary of our principal research findings, I shall refer to these three types of health insurance program as: 1. commercial plans, 2. provider plans; and 3. group practice plans.

It would be tedious to explain the detailed methodology of this research, but let me simply indicate that our main strategy was to study the experience and attitudes of representative samples of the persons or families enrolled in each of these three types of plan. To heighten the reliability of our findings, we investigated two examples (believed to be typical) of each of the three plan-types in California, and in each of these six organizations we studied the experience of 300 to 600 (usually 600) enrolled family units, or about 3,000 persons in each plan-type. These samples were randomly chosen with the greatest care, to assure representativeness and eliminate any bias, so that we are confident of the validity of our findings. Our information was collected in 1967 and 1968.

I would like to summarize some of our principal findings under five headings:

1. composition of plan memberships
2. utilization of hospital and doctor services
3. technical content of services provided
4. expenditures incurred
5. attitudes of plan members

Information on these features was gathered through various methods, including carefully designed questionnaires, household interviews, analysis of actual medical records, interviews of health plan administrators and doctors, and examination of the several insurance policies (or benefit-packages) in effect. On the latter point, I cannot take time to describe the various complex provisions of the diverse offerings, but I can state that in each of the three plan-types, the benefit-packages are believed to be representative of those offered to group enrollees as a whole. (We did not study individual enrollment coverage, which is generally more restrictive and expensive.)

Composition of Plan Memberships

It is well known that the sickness experience of a population, and therefore its demands for medical care, will be influenced by its demographic and background characteristics. If an insurance organization can selectively enroll persons with lower risk of illness, it will probably have fewer claims to pay. Evidence of risk is reflected in such factors as age level, previous chronic illness, and the individual's inherent sensitivity to symptoms of disease.

The severity of illness tends to increase with age. In our study the age level of the persons enrolled in the three types of plan was found to be as follows:

Plan-type	*Average Age (Years)*
Commercial plans	31.7
Provider plans	34.0
Group practice plans	34.0

Considering just the persons in the older age brackets, when illness rates are heaviest, we found these proportions:

Plan-type	*Percentage 41 Years and Over*
Commercial plans	24.6
Provider plans	33.8
Group practice plans	35.9

Thus, by either of these measures, the commercial plans are found to have enrollees of the youngest age levels, compared with the other two plan-types. The group practice plans appear to have the highest risk members, as reflected by age level.

With respect to a past history of chronic illness of some sort in the family, our data showed the following percentages:

Plan-type	*None*	*One or More Chronic Illnesses*
Commercial plans	62.6	37.4
Provider plans	53.4	46.6
Group practice plans	39.4	60.6

Even for bouts of acute illness in the most recent three-month period, we found that these had occurred in 17.1 percent of commercial plan families, compared with 23.4 percent and 25.3 percent of families in the other two plan-types.

A third reflection of "risk composition" is a measure we have defined as "symptom sensitivity"—that is, the tendency of an individual with a given problem to seek medical attention. Interpretation of this characteristic is admittedly complex, but our basic findings, in percentages, were:

Plan-type	*Less Sensitive*	*More Sensitive*
Commercial plans	36.1	63.9
Provider plans	33.7	66.3
Group practice plans	29.0	71.0

Thus, by all three measures of sickness risk, contrary to common assertions, our findings indicate that the commercial companies have the lowest proportion of high risk persons, the group practice plans have the highest proportion, with the provider-sponsored plans falling in between. The sales or marketing practices that have resulted in this situation are beyond my competence to explain, but the social implications are clear to anyone: namely, the responsibilities for people with the lightest burden of medical need are being borne by the commercial insurance carriers, the next level by the provider-sponsored plans, and the responsibilities for the heaviest burden of need are being borne by the group practice plans.

Utilization of Hospital and Medical Services

The payoff of risk-selection practices might be expected to show up in the rates of utilization of services by persons enrolled in the different types of health insurance program. These utilization rates, moreover, would naturally be influenced by two other factors: 1. the precise benefit packages or "coverage" of the insurance policies, and 2. the patterns of medical practice and remuneration of the doctors, insofar as these may or may not create incentives toward hospitalizing patients.

Keeping all these influences in mind, our basic findings on hospital admission rates were as follows:

Plan-type	*Admissions/1,000/Year*
Commercial plans	102
Provider plans	150
Group practice plans	107

With respect to the aggregate days of hospitalization, which count most in determining the high costs of modern hospital care, our findings were:

Plan-type	*Hospital Days/1,000/Year*
Commercial plans	864
Provider plans	1,109
Group practice plans	526

Thus, it is clear that the provider-sponsored health insurance plans show the highest rate of both hospital admissions and hospital days. The group practice plans, despite their heavier load of high-risk enrollees, have a hospital admission rate very close to that of the commercial plans, but much the lowest rate of aggregate hospital days. Explanation for this is probably to be found partly in the medical incentive system operating in the salaried group practice or HMO-type plans, and partly in the convenient access to ambulatory care in those plans.

I might add that we have made analyses of these hospitalization data, according to various types of family (large and small), various social class and income groupings, etc. The basic relationships reported above tend to prevail in all these breakdowns; the lesser rate of hospital days in the commercial, compared with the provider, plans, however, is found to be attributable mainly to the experience of lower social class families (as reflected by the occupation and educational background of family heads).

As for ambulatory doctor's care, insured or not, the experience of persons enrolled in the three plan-types was found to be as follows:

Plan-type	*Doctor Visits/1,000/Year*
Commercial plans	3,108
Provider plans	3,984
Group practice plans	3,324

Thus, once again, we see the lowest rate of ambulatory medical services in the enrollees of the commercial plans. It should be realized that most patient-doctor contacts beyond the initial office visit are decided upon by the doctor, but the first contact must be initiated by the patient. In the light of this, it is interesting to note our findings on the percentage of families that had no doctor-visits in a recent three-month period:

Plan-type	*Percentage with No Doctor Contacts*
Commercial plans	49.6
Provider plans	36.1
Group practice plans	33.4

The fact that roughly half of the commercial plan families saw no doctor at all in this time-period—compared with much lower percentages in the other plan-types—seems to confirm the evidence reported earlier about risk selection, as well as to reflect something about the restricted benefit offerings in the commercial plans.

Technical Content of Services Provided

Analysis of the technical content of medical services actually rendered under the different plan-types was a complex process, and I should like only to report two of our principal findings.

Without elaborate explanation of our methodology, we applied certain "value units" to each type of medical service rendered, based upon a well-known "Relative Value Study" done by the California Medical Association. Through this process, we calculated a "doctor's care index" per person per year for the subscribers to each of the three plan-types. The results were as follows:

Plan-type	*Doctor's Care Index/Person/Year*
Commercial plans	71.6
Provider plans	121.6
Group practice plans	87.9

The low index of services furnished under the commercial plans is evident from these figures, in back of which are literally thousands (about 12,000) of pieces of information derived from study of actual medical records. As for the comparative indexes of the provider-sponsored, compared with the group practice, plans, it should be realized that the very low rate of hospital days under the latter would substantially influence this measurement of doctor services given anywhere (office, home, or hospital).

The second finding I should like to report concerns the provision of preventive health services. In our detailed study of medical records, we identified those services which could be considered as probably preventive in purpose—such services as well-child examination, "annual check-ups" of adults, vaginal cytology tests, routine rectal examinations, and immunizations. Summating these items, we derived a measure of preventive service for each type of plan, and these were found to be as follows:

Plan-type	*Preventive Services Index/Person/Year*
Commercial plans	0.384
Provider plans	0.404
Group practice plans	0.452

While the record of preventive service is not impressively high in any of the plans, it is clearly highest in the group practice plans and lowest in the plans sponsored by commercial companies.

Expenditures Incurred

Another important reflection of the operational effects of different types of health insurance plan is the expenditures incurred by families. These are of two types: 1. the premiums levied (which may be paid partly or wholly by employers), and 2. the out-of-pocket expenditures of persons for medical care. The latter may be referrable to the expense of deductibles, co-payment charges, etc., or to the costs of services not covered at all under an insurance policy.

Our data on this question apply to annual expenditures for hospital and physician services (not to family expenses for medications, dental care, or other types of service). The basic findings for family units in the three types of insurance program were as follows:

Plan-type	*Average Premium*	*Out-of-pocket Expenditures*	*Total Costs*
Commercial plans	$208	$156	$364
Provider plans	257	190	447
Group practice plans	271	52	323

These figures, I believe, tell us a great deal about the cost implications of the three types of health insurance plan. Their interpretation should not be oversimplified, for many factors are involved, but it would seem to be essentially as follows: The commercial plans have the lowest average premiums, which probably go along with their strategies for enrollment of low-risk populations and extensive application of cost-sharing (co-payment) requirements. The group practice plans, with their higher risk subscribers, more comprehensive medical benefits, and very modest cost-sharing features, have the highest premiums. The provider-sponsored plan premiums fall in between.

Out-of-pocket expenditures, on the other hand, are clearly lowest in the group practice plans. They are relatively high in both commercial and provider plans, but highest in the latter which, as we saw, have the highest rates of both hospitalization and ambulatory care.

The aggregate or total costs, summating premiums and out-of-pocket expenditures for hospital and physician's care, are the major issue of social concern. These, we see, are highest in the provider-sponsored plans, next highest in the commercial plans, and lowest in the group practice plans. These findings would seem to provide further support for the soundness of the idea of "health maintenance organizations," based on patterns of group medical practice.

Our expenditure findings have also been analyzed according to size-of-family, past illness history, and other characteristics. Without troubling you with recitation of all these statistics, I can report that the lower overall costs of the group practice plans, compared with the other two types, applies to most of the subgroups.

As a crude approach to a cost-benefit analysis of the three types of health insurance plan, one may relate these total cost amounts to the aggregate "doctor's care index" figures reported earlier, insofar as these figures reflect medical services to both ambulatory and hospitalized patients. Such a calculation makes no judgment on the medical necessity of various events, such as hospitalizations, but only on the ratio of total dollars spent (cost) to the doctor's care given (benefit). This calculation comes out as follows:

Plan-type	*Total Costs*	*Doctor's Care Index*	*Cost-Benefit Ratio*
Commercial plans	$364	71.6	5.1
Provider plans	447	121.6	3.7
Group practice plans	323	87.9	3.7

By this analysis, the cost per unit of medical value in the commercial insurance plans is found to be substantially higher than in the other two plan-types.

Attitudes of Plan Members

A final measurement of the effects of different types of health insurance is the attitudes of subscribers toward their plan. Our study solicited these along two dimensions: 1. attitudes toward the medical care received, and 2. attitudes toward the financial protection offered by the plan. We asked subscribers to record their feelings by checking an 8-point scale, ranging from "highly satisfied" to "highly dissatisfied."

With respect to the medical care received, one must keep in mind that both the commercial and the provider plans allow the subscriber free choice of doctors, who are generally in solo medical practice. The group practice plans require persons to use a specific organized clinic for their care. To listen to hostile critics of the latter arrangement, one might expect to find massive dissatisfaction among the families served by the group practice plans. In fact, our findings for the subscribers to the three plan-types, expressed as percentages, were as follows:

Plan-type	*Very Satisfied*	*Moderately Satisfied*	*Dissatisfied*
Commercial plans	46.5	36.2	17.4
Provider plans	44.9	34.8	20.3
Group practice plans	42.6	49.3	8.2

Thus, it would seem that—in spite of the departure from customary and traditional medical care delivery patterns—the group practice plan members show only a slightly lower proportion of high satisfaction with their care than do persons in the free choice or open-market types of plan. Moderate satisfaction is substantially stronger in the group practice plans. Most interesting is the substantially lower proportion of frankly dissatisfied persons in the group practice plans—less than half the percentages found in the commercial or provider plans.

When analyzed by various social sub-groups, these findings continue generally to prevail. One interesting sidelight, however, is the record of satisfaction among single persons of each sex. Focusing on the extreme poles of high satisfaction versus dissatisfaction in the three types of insurance plan, we find the following:

	Men		*Women*	
Plan-type	*Very Satisfied*	*Dissatisfied*	*Very Satisfied*	*Dissatisfied*
Commercial plans	38.4	36.4	52.5	18.7
Provider plans	39.4	32.0	45.3	13.0
Group practice plans	65.1	7.8	45.7	12.6

Perhaps there is a lesson in these findings for the management of group practice plans, with respect to women. Or perhaps, if Henry Higgins's plea—"Why can't a woman be like a man?"—were generally heeded, then the group practice plans might show not only the lowest level of dissatisfaction but also the highest level of top-satisfaction as well.

Another barometer of consumer satisfaction, especially meaningful for the group practice plans, is the percentage of medical services procured outside of these organizations. To listen to hostile medical critics, one might expect that large proportions of the members of these plans go elsewhere for their medical care, even though this means that they must pay privately. Our findings, however, indicate that in the families insured by the group practice plans only 12 percent of specific medical services over the course of a year were obtained outside the framework of the plan. For hospitalizations, the out-of-plan cases were only 7.2 percent of the total. By contrast, in the families insured through commercial carriers, for one reason or another (such as exclusions of certain types of diagnosis, waiting periods for maternity, etc.), the hospitalizations not financed by the plan in one year amounted to 29.1 percent.

Concerning attitudes of subscribers toward the financial coverage offered by each of the plan-types, the findings of our study were clear-cut. Expressed as percentages, these were as follows:

Plan-type	*Very Satisfied*	*Moderately Satisfied*	*Dissatisfied*
Commercial plans	36.5	39.0	24.6
Provider plans	28.1	37.1	34.8
Group practice plans	65.1	26.3	8.6

Obviously, there is an overwhelmingly greater degree of high satisfaction with the financial protection offered by the group practice plans, and much less dissatisfaction, in spite of the higher premiums required for enrollment in those plans. Between the two open-market plan-types, the financial protection offered by the provider plans elicits less satisfaction than that offered by the commercial plans, but one must recall the selectivity of enrollee risks in these plan-types. Moreover, it should be pointed out that competition from the commercial carriers has forced most of the provider-sponsored (Blue Cross and Blue Shield) plans in the United States to introduce indemnification and cost-sharing features, which those plans initially lacked and which tend to be irritating to many consumers.

Analyzed by various social sub-groups, the levels of satisfaction just reported prevail generally for all categories. Considering the attitudes of persons in different social classes, however, the proportions of dissatisfaction are highest among lower class families in the provider plans, and among upper class families in the commercial plans.

Summary

In summary, our research on the operations of different types of health insurance plan indicates that the commercial carriers have enrolled persons of a lower level of sickness risk than the provider-sponsored (Blue Cross and Blue Shield) plans or the HMO-type plans based on group medical practice. The latter plans are serving higher proportions of people with greater sickness needs. The rate of hospital days per 1,000 persons per year is highest in the provider plans and, by far, lowest in the group practice plans. Ambulatory medical service rates are relatively similar in all three plan-types, but are highest in the provider plans, next in the group practice plans, and lowest in the commercial plans. Among the three plan-types the lowest index of doctor's care, by an aggregate measure, is also in the commercial plans, as is the lowest rate of preventive health services.

As for expenditures by families for hospital and physician's care, much the lowest out-of-pocket outlays are made by subscribers to the group practice plans. For their more comprehensive benefits, these plans charge higher premiums, but considering total costs (the sum of premiums and personal outlays), those in the group practice plans are lowest and in the provider plans are highest. When total costs are related to an aggregated measure of in-hospital and out-of-hospital doctor's care, however, the commercial plans show the costliest ratio.

The attitudes of insured persons toward the medical care received under each type of plan show much less dissatisfaction in the group practice plans, despite their departure from conventional delivery patterns. With respect to the financial protection offered by each plan-type, the level of consumer satisfaction is overwhelmingly strongest for the group practice plans. As between the two open-market free choice types of insurance organization, consumer satisfaction is somewhat lower for the provider-sponsored than for the commercial plans. If these organizations, however, wished to tailor their offerings to consumer wishes, as they frequently claim, it would seem appropriate for them to offer more comprehensive benefits than they now do.

I appreciate the opportunity to present these research findings to the Subcommittee, and I hope that they may help in evaluation of the complex variety of health insurance programs now operating in the United States.

13

The Dynamics of Different Methods of Paying for Medical Care

Whether payments for medical care are made directly by patients or indirectly through insurance programs, the methods of remuneration have substantial influences on the behavior of providers. Unfortunately, economic gain or the potential of such gain inevitably influences the decisions not of only physicians, but also hospitals, pharmacies, and other providers of health services.

Since these realities must be considered in planning the methods of organizing medical care systems, the California Office of Comprehensive Health Planning commissioned an analysis of their dynamics. The text of this chapter was prepared in response.

THE FINANCING OF medical care is obviously basic to its availability. Within "financing" are two components which require clarification. One is the method by which monies are derived—their sources and schemes of collection. The other is the method by which money is paid to providers of service for their efforts. It is the latter component that this paper will explore, but first a few words must be said about the former.

Sources of Health Care Financing

Funds for the support of medical care may be derived from several sources. Oldest, of course, is the personal income of the patient or that of a relative or friend who may pay on his behalf. Until recent years this private buy-and-sell mechanism was the predominant one in the United States.[1] Increasingly, however, various collective sources of financing have gained prominence, as the value of medical care has come to be more widely appreciated and the costs of care (when meeting proper standards) have risen. Taxation is the oldest and most ubiquitous of these collective or social mechanisms; a vast variety of taxing devices may be used at local, state, and federal levels. Occasionally there are special taxes earmarked for medical purposes, but more often health appropriations are made from general revenues. Another collective mechanism is social insurance, under which governmental authority is used to raise money for health and

Chapter 13 originally appeared as "Diverse Methods of Paying for Medical Care and Their Effects on the Services Provided" in *Selected Papers on Health Issues in California* (Sacramento, Calif.: California Department of Public Health, May, 1971), pp. 769–786 (processed).

other benefits for designated beneficiaries; this method obviates the need for legislative appropriations.[2] A third social method is voluntary insurance, through which groups of persons voluntarily make periodic contributions (premiums) to a fund which meets future medical expenses (or part of them) of the individual contributors. There are numerous possible sponsorships and organizational schemes for voluntary health insurance.[3] A fourth social method is charity, in which there is no relationship between the donation of money and the receipt of benefits. A final social source for financing medical care is the industrial process, through which certain earnings from the sale of products may be used for supporting health services to the workers involved.[4]

Each of these individual or social methods of deriving funds may be used for a variety of health purposes—for medical care to certain persons, for treatment or prevention of certain diseases, or for provision of certain classes of technical services. They may also be used for furnishing the underlying requirements of a health service system, such as training of health personnel, construction of facilities, or the conduct of medical research.

With respect to personal health service, each of these mechanisms may apply a variety of methods for paying the providers of service for their efforts. It is these diverse methods, and their consequences, which will now be explored.

Regardless of the mechanism by which the monies are derived, they may be paid to the providers of service by several methods:

1. fee-for-service
2. fee-per-case
3. capitation
4. salary (time basis)
5. combinations of the above.

While these five methods of payment have been traditionally applied most often to the remuneration of doctors, they may be applied in principle, with some modifications, to remuneration of other types of personnel as well as hospitals.

Each of these methods has important consequences for the volume and quality of services provided and the aggregate costs to the community. These diverse consequences are not merely conjectural, but have been empirically demonstrated at numerous times and places. In the text that follows, the attributes and some consequences of each method will be briefly considered, first as applied to the physician (on which the data are most abundant) and then as applied to other providers of health service.

Fee-for-Service and Fee-per-Case Payment

When physicians or other providers of health care are paid a fee for each unit of service, there is inevitably an incentive to maximize the numbers of units provided.[5] This is true whether the patient pays the fee directly or through the mediation of a health insurance plan (of either the "service-benefit" or "indemnification'' pattern). Under insurance or other ''third-party'' support, however, the maximizing tendency is undoubtedly aggravated.

It must be recognized that the great majority of services rendered in a medical care program are decided upon by the physician and not the patient. The initial medical contact is the patient's decision, but almost every other service after this—subsequent visits, hospitalization, prescribed drugs, laboratory or X-ray examinations, physiotherapy, etc.—is ordered by the doctor. For most of these services, especially hospitalization (in the American setting, though not in Europe), the physician stands to gain additional earnings. In terms of total costs, the services which are patient-decided probably account for about 10 percent, while the doctor-decided services account for 90 percent. It follows that various cost-sharing or ''co-insurance'' devices used to inhibit patient demand for medical care in organized programs exert only small impact on total expenditures.[6]

The effect of fee-for-service payment methods in maximizing services has been demonstrated in many contexts. A critical experience occurred in Baltimore, Maryland, for example, when the program of medical care for the indigent was modified in 1963 from a capitation to a fee-for-service pattern of remunerating general practitioners (specialty services were given throughout by salaried physicians in hospital clinics).[7] The rate of general physician services per person per year jumped promptly from 2.6 to 3.2. Other studies have shown significantly higher rates of hospitalization, especially for elective surgery (tonsillectomy, hysterectomy, etc.), when physicians are paid by fee-for-service, compared with salaries.[8] A study of Blue Shield fees has demonstrated that supplemental charges tend to be higher for surgeons who do fewer operations–evidently in the effort to maintain a certain level of professional income.[9] In Germany and New Zealand, studies of general practitioner services under health insurance have shown the same basic dynamics; that is, doctors seeing fewer cases in a month tend to furnish more visits per case (each visit, of course, yielding a fee).[10]

One cannot be dogmatic about the effect on the patient's welfare of a higher or lower volume of service. To some extent, maximization of service may be beneficial, especially if it is compared with a situation in which patients get perfunctory care. Medical audits in hospitals, however, have long disclosed a great deal of unnecessary surgery under fee-for-service patterns[11] and claims review of ambulatory services in public assistance medical care programs paying fees have shown indefensibly multiplied numbers of office visits and house calls.[12] As for the effects of multiplied services on patient health, two important studies of the Health Insurance Plan of Greater New York—in which doctors in group practice clinics are paid by salary—have shown lower mortality rates among infants and among aged persons (65 years and over) served by this plan than among comparable populations served by fee-for-service private doctors in that city.[13]

While the maximization of services, associated with fee-for-service payment, may conceivably have some good as well as bad effects for the patient's health, there can be no question that it tends to elevate costs. The evidence for this in the national Medicare program, in which there have not even been fixed fee schedules, is overwhelming.[14] Escalation of costs can be slowed by use of fee-schedules, but most state medical societies in the United States (through their Blue Shield plans) have insisted on the doctor's right to charge moderate-income patients supplemental amounts beyond the scheduled fees. Another device—proration of fees within an annual allotment per person covered by an insurance plan—is used under the German social insurance program, under some provincial plans in Canada, and formerly under the U.S. Farm Security Administration health program for low-income farm families, but has not found wide favor in the United States.[15]

Without specifically prorating fee payments within a fixed annual per capita sum, a system of rigorous medical claims review may help to control costs in a fee-for-service program. This has been well demonstrated in the Medical Care Foundation of San Joaquin County, California, sponsored by the medical society of that county.[16] Such review can identify extreme irregularities—and perhaps the very knowledge of the review process induces a higher level of self-discipline among doctors—but it could hardly be expected to control minor abuses and it is an administratively costly process. Fee-for-service payments, with the various control procedures required, inevitably impose a higher load of "paperwork" and bureaucratic surveillance on the doctor than do other methods. While the incentives are toward maximizing services, furthermore, they do not operate to encourage referral of patients to other doctors who may be better qualified to handle special problems; in fact, fee-for-service may discourage referrals to specialists, since these may mean loss of both the fee and the patient.

A variant of the fee-for-service method of paying doctors is the fee-per-case. This is often applied in surgery or obstetrics, where a flat fee is charged for the case as a whole, rather than for each medical visit or medical act. In the old German health insurance program, fees were once paid per case of illness, but the method led to abuses (e.g., the multiplication of diagnoses during a single bout of illness) and was dropped. In current German health insurance operations, a "case of illness" is defined administratively as a period of 3 months from the onset, as a device for preventing wasteful "shopping around" among different doctors during the same illness (after 3 months the doctor can be readily changed, or before then if it can be justified).[17] In effect, the fee-per-case method is no longer used in health insurance programs outside of setting charges for surgical or obstetrical cases.

These comments about fee payment methods for physician's care apply substantially to dental care. In treating disorders of the teeth, there are often alternative procedures of different cost and the incentives naturally tend to favor the more costly options.[18] On the other hand, these incentives may yield painstaking work to preserve teeth, which might simply be extracted under other payment methods if there were not proper quality controls (see below).

Fee-for-service methods are also applicable to prescribed drugs, with the pharmacist receiving a fee based upon the wholesale drug costs plus various "mark-up" amounts for dispensing, overhead, etc.[19] The cost question for drugs involves the whole pattern of operation of small independent pharmacies, as against larger dispensaries enjoying economies of scale. It also relates to the whole issue of the type of drugs prescribed—especially brand-name compared with generic compounds—a topic fully discussed elsewhere and not really germane here.[20]

With respect to hospital payments, the fee-for-service method has many ramifications.[21] A charge for each item of hospital service (drugs prescribed, laboratory tests, use of the operating room, etc.) naturally creates incentives to multiply such services in order to maximize hospital income; the amounts of these charges, moreover, may bear little relation to the true accounted costs but rather are often designed to yield the highest feasible revenue. Even when hospital services are paid for according to an all-inclusive patient-day rate (as is done under various insurance plans), the incentives operate to maximize the number of days per case, since an empty bed means lost hospital income.[22] The effect of such incentives has been dramatically demonstrated in the hospital insurance plan of Saskatchewan: after a period of payment to hospitals based on per diem rates, the system was changed to one of flat monthly payments calculated through a prospective budget, with only small increments paid for each patient-day of care.[23] Promptly the hospital utilization rate (patient-days per 1,000 persons per year), which had previously been steadily rising, levelled off. The new payment system gave the hospitals their full costs, but yielded no additional income for superfluous days of care.

Fee-for-service payments have been justified in the past as a device which enabled the provider to adjust charges to the income level of the patient (the "sliding scale of fees"), thereby helping the poor at the expense of the rich. Careful economic analysis, however, discloses that this practice was essentially "price discrimination," motivated largely by the well-known commercial principle of "charging what the traffic will bear" and accomplishing very little in the way of assuring services to the poor.[24] Another adjustment of the fee system—to changing price levels in the business cycle—is by use of "relative value scales" for an inventory of medical procedures, with the dollar value of one unit being modified from time to time.[25] This RVS device, of course, does little to modify the behavioral incentives of the fee system.

Because of the general incentives of fee-for-service payments to maximize services and costs—whether applied to physician, hospital, or other types of care—all sorts of surveillance procedures are needed to detect and reduce abuses.[26] The operation of these procedures is onerous and commonly generates controversies. Moreover, at best they tend to succeed in stopping only the most extreme abuses. In any event, the surveillance process adds to the administrative costs of the program. Whatever advantages may be credited to the fee system, it is obvious that the price paid—in terms of dollar costs, quality, and administrative complexities—is quite high.

Capitation Payment

Because of the difficulties of the fee system, the capitation system of paying for medical services has been developed. In its usual form, the provider of service receives a flat monthly sum for each person who has chosen that provider for care, whether or not services are actually rendered. The best known application of the system is in Great Britain, where general practitioners are so remunerated under the National Health Service, although the idea dates to the earlier National Health Insurance program.[27] It is worth recording that at the outset of the original program in 1911, fee-for-service was also used, but it led to so much abuse that the British doctors themselves voted for exclusive use of the capitation method.

The amount of periodic capitation payments obviously depends on the law of averages. This can be readily applied to general practitioner services, which are relatively frequently furnished in a population; to calculate a dependable average load of services for specialists of various types (surgeons, ophthalmologists, psychiatrists, etc.) requires a much larger population base and longer time periods, because the rate of use of any one type of specialist is less frequent. The consumer, moreover, is seldom competent to select a battery of specialists in advance of illness. As a practical matter, therefore, capitation payment has been applied only to the services of general practitioners or family doctors.

In the hospital field, a few instances have occurred in the United States where capitation payment has been applied. In college towns, like Grinnel, Iowa, where there was only one hospital to serve the whole community, an insurance plan was developed as long ago as 1921. Through this plan, each member paid an annual sum to the hospital, this fund covering the costs of any hospitalization that occurred.[28] The same idea was applied by school teachers in Dallas, Texas, in 1929 with respect to the Baylor University Hospital—an event that is often given credit for the origin of the Blue Cross movement.[29] Actually, Blue Cross and other insurance plans collect *premiums* on a capitation basis, so to speak, but pay the money out to hospitals or doctors on a fee-for-service basis. If only a single hospital is involved, however, and the premium goes directly to the hospital, the arrangement is, in effect, capitation remuneration.

The capitation payment method eliminates the problem of over-servicing associated with the fee-for-service pattern, but it generates other problems. Because he is paid nothing extra for more service, the doctor or other provider may give perfunctory care; he may refer excessively to other resources (hospital outpatients departments, public health clinics, or private specialists) cases that he could properly handle himself.[30] The protection against these tendencies is the liability of losing the patient to another doctor's capitation "panel"; in other words, the general practitioner is constrained to keep his patients satisfied. Yet many persons are doubtless unable to detect inadequate care, so that there are limits to this compensatory mechanism.[31]

Abuses of the capitation method would tend to increase with the total number of persons on a doctor's list. Therefore, in the British National Health Service, a maximum limit is set on the size of a general practitioner's panel; moreover, the monthly amount paid for each person decreases gradually as the panel enlarges, to discourage very long lists. Theoretically, the capitation method is supposed to encourage preventive service, since the doctor can save himself work by preventing disease, but in practice there is no real evidence for this.[32] Indeed, in Great Britain the capitation doctors have had to be offered special supplemental fees for performance of immunizations or prenatal examinations (to reduce their referrals of patients to public health clinics for these services).

In the Health Insurance Plan of Greater New York, the group practice clinics are paid periodic amounts for each person choosing to get his care from a particular clinic.[33] While this has been called "capitation" payment, the word is used in a different sense; the individual doctors in H.I.P. clinics are actually paid by salary, and their behavior is affected by salary mechanisms to be discussed below. The group clinic as a whole, however, may be influenced by the incentives of capitation remuneration which yields no additional rewards for extra services; as noted earlier, this seems to result in a lower rate of elective surgery than the fee-for-service method.

Salary Remuneration

Considering health personnel as a whole, payment on a time basis is actually the commonest method applied, although it is a minority pattern for physicians and dentists. The tradition of independence, as small entrepreneurial providers of medical care, has run deep in the medical profession, so that even under health insurance programs in the United States and Western Continental Europe, the fee-for-service system has remained the commonest pattern. For nurses, technicians, physiotherapists, and most other types of health manpower, however, salaries are the usual mode of compensation.

Salaried remuneration exerts a different set of behavioral influences than the other methods. By paying for the time of the health professional, it attempts to place a value on that time, not in terms of the marketplace of patients but in terms of the judgment of peers. Salary levels are ordinarily based on the richness of training of the person, his skills, his seniority, and the level of responsibility he bears. Virtually always, salaries imply that the work is done in some sort of organized framework, in which there is a hierarchy of authority and delegation of responsibility.[34] Advancements of pay or other special awards are usually based on the review and judgment of colleagues.

The hazards of salaries lie in the frailties of social organization. Judgments on individual merit may be faulty or biased, so that inequities may result. Supervision may be poor, so that work performance may deteriorate. If the leadership in an organization is poor, the quality of work of all persons in it may decline.

Despite these hazards, mankind has been learning more about the ways to make organizations work effectively.[35] In every aspect of social life—in industry, agriculture, religion, government, education, transportation, health services—the degree of organization has been increasing. In health care, the complexities of technology have required more and more organizational solutions.[36] An increasing variety and mixture of health personnel have been necessary to furnish modern health service—curative and preventive. These health workers—nurses, technicians, pharmacists, physiotherapists, etc.—can be coordinated properly only in organized settings. It is not surprising, therefore, that an increasing proportion of doctors in the United States are found to be engaged on full-time salaries each year.[37] While it is hard to draw an exact line between salaried and non-salaried employment, my analysis of the most recent national inventory by the American Medical Association suggests that in 1966 over 40 percent of American physicians depended more on organized employment than on fee payments for their income.[38] Salaried doctors are increasing not only because of the growth of positions in medical research, education, and strictly administrative work but also due to the increasingly organized delivery of clinical services in hospitals and clinics, both governmental and voluntary. On a world scale, the trends are even more striking than in America.

Salaries may be full-time or part-time. A vast variety of positions in public health clinics, in industrial or school health services, in hospitals or other institutions call for less than full-time duty. Thousands of doctors are able to respond to these demands for part-time salaried service, while retaining their independent private practices, and the experience tends to be educational for them. At the same time, it permits the organizational process in medicine to continue.

There has been a common notion in America (though seldom elsewhere) that salaried remuneration leads to a deterioration in the quality of medical care.[39] It is understandable how such a notion should develop in an era when the most lucrative rewards went to the independent practitioner and only the doctor who "failed" in this free market was attracted into a salaried position. But as medical schools and medical centers have grown, as hospitals have become more organized and group practice has expanded, the falseness of this notion has become generally apparent. The highest excellence in medicine, found in the medical schools, in the Mayo Clinic and other such centers, is indeed associated with salaried employment.[40] In Europe and most other continents, specialty practice is predominantly based on salaried posts in hospitals, and only the less fully qualified doctors must rely on fee-for-service earnings for their income.

It is, moreover, a subtle slander to the integrity of the medical profession to imply—as is all too often done—that only with specific monetary awards for each act can the doctor be expected to do his best work. University professors, clergymen, and other persons of high occupational ethics do not need such financial inducements, and there is no good reason to expect doctors to require them.

From the viewpoint of costs, salaried remuneration has many advantages. For one thing, there are no incentives to give superfluous or unnecessary services. Second, the costs are predictable in advance, so that in an organized program annual budgets can be prepared and relied upon. Third, the assurance of stable income seems to induce physicians and others to work for lesser hourly awards than they expect under the uncertain conditions of entrepreneurial practice. Most important, the organizational setting of salaried medical work can yield many economies of structure and scale; maximal use of auxiliary health personnel in such settings and various forms of automation of diagnostic procedures can usually produce greater medical output per dollar of input.[41] Because of these economies and enhanced productivity, American doctors in group practice—usually on salary—actually earn higher incomes than solo practitioners of comparable age and specialty.

The salary method is so basically satisfactory for all health personnel outside of physicians or dentists that it is seldom even questioned. The issues concern the *level* of salaries and this, of course, may be the subject of much debate and negotiation. Market considerations, in terms of the supply-and-demand of health manpower, inevitably influence salary levels, such as the sharp rise in nurses' salaries that came after augmentation of hospital incomes by the Medicare law.[42] But this is a different sort of market dynamics than that involving the determination of fees for specific services. The latter mechanism can operate to limit certain services, or the services of certain doctors, to the well-to-do who can pay the price. Bargaining for salaries, on the other hand, establishes rewards for a whole category of personnel in the light of manpower supply in the health field compared with other occupations.

Salaries in organized settings can also do much to improve the availability of health personnel in relation to social needs—defined both geographically and functionally. The free market for medical care has resulted in serious disparities in the physical distribution of doctors—between rural and urban areas, and between the depressed and affluent neighborhoods of the cities.[43] It has also resulted in disproportionately high supplies of doctors in lucrative fields like surgery, which in turn leads easily to the performance of many surgical operations of dubious justification.[44] Under salaried arrangements, however, physicians can be attracted to under-doctored localities in rural sections or urban slums (for example, in the "neighborhood health centers" of the U.S. Office of Economic Opportunity). As for specialist proportions, it is significant that a comprehensive prepayment plan, like the Kaiser-Permanente system, gets along with a much lower ratio of surgeons on salary than is found in the free market of private medicine.[45]

The equivalent of salaries (i.e., payments for time) in the field of hospital remuneration would be paying for the institution's "readiness to serve" on the basis of a flat monthly amount calculated to meet overall costs. Such payment through "prospective budgeting" in Saskatchewan was noted above, and it has obvious advantages for economy and managerial efficiency. The method depends, however, on a diligent and objective prior review of hospital budgets. This necessitates submission of all hospital budgets in advance to some agency, presumably in government, where reasonable standards of review would be applied objectively.[46] Such review might sometimes lead to a reduction in the proposed expenditures (for example, there might be excessive kitchen staff in relation to a standard range of figures), or it might lead to suggestions for increased expenditures (for example, an enlargement of the physiotherapy department). Many hospitals might object to this process, although the value and general acceptability of standard-setting has been well demonstrated in the hospital field by the Joint Commission on Accreditation of Hospitals, not to mention the state hospital licensure laws.[47] A somewhat similar system of budgetary financing is now used in the hospital network of the Veterans Administration, and it would be feasible for general application only under circumstances in which the majority of hospital costs were payable from a single source.

Implications of the Payment Method for the Future

The objective of any method of payment for health care is to encourage services in the most effective and efficient manner. "Effectiveness" implies maximum quality, and "efficiency" implies optimal economy. As a practical matter, one hopes to achieve an optimal mix of quality and economy in any system of medical care.

By these criteria, one can consider the implications of the different payment methods reviewed above. Perhaps one should add a third criterion from the point of view of the provider of care—namely equitable remuneration in relation to his merit and his labors. We thus would have three criteria which may be epitomized as:

- effectiveness (quality)
- economy
- equity (to the provider)

With respect to effectiveness of medical care, the principal lesson of the current era is the need for rational organization to apply properly the numerous specialties of medicine and the ever-increasing number of para-medical disciplines involved. This is obvious within the walls of hospitals, but it is equally true for ambulatory care, especially if an integrated approach is taken to preventive and curative service. Within an organization, the personnel must work as a team, and the most practical method of remuneration is on the basis of the time of each team-member, taking account of the overall value of his contribution to the team effort.

As for economy, the method of remuneration should give no incentives toward maximizing services beyond the proper needs of the patient. Protection against negligence or perfunctory service should depend on colleagial review or group discipline. (Ultimately, the respect of one's colleagues becomes translated into monetary awards through personal advancement in an organization.) Thus, payment for time, rather than by piecework, favors economy as well.

Equitable remuneration depends on the application of reasonable criteria in assessing the value of a person's work. The mercantile philosophy calls for these judgments to be made in the marketplace of supply and demand. In the world of professional service, where subtle skills and knowledge are involved, one might hope that the judgment can establish the value of a person's time and yield a scale of increments according to training, experience, seniority, skills, and responsibility.

Thus, by all three criteria, the salary method of remuneration makes most sense in the current world of medical care. It is small wonder that this is the method which has come to prevail for the great majority of health workers and has been growing most rapidly for physicians and dentists. On a world scale, of course, salaried remuneration predominates for doctors and dentists as well.

While this conclusion follows from the focus of this paper on "methods of paying for medical care," it constitutes a tangential approach to the more basic issues of *how* medical care should be delivered. In essence, our conclusion means that considerations of effectiveness, economy, and equity dictate the wisdom of providing medical services through organized teams of personnel; the salaried remuneration is simply a concomitant of organizational structure.

Essentially the same reasoning has been applied by the U.S. Department of Health, Education and Welfare in its recent advocacy of "health maintenance organizations" as an important new approach to the delivery of medical care. The highly significant statement of Secretary Robert Finch on 25 March 1970 called for contracts between government agencies (such as the administrations of Medicare and Medicaid) and these HMOs for provision of comprehensive health service to people.[48] The HMO would be paid a fixed per capita amount for comprehensive medical services to each person whose health it was undertaking to maintain per month or per year. Such contracts would only be made, however, at per capita rates no higher than 95 percent of the average cost of such comprehensive care (i.e., at least 5 percent lower than the average cost) in the open medical market. If economies of greater than 5 percent can be achieved, the balance would be retained by the HMO as a "profit" or "bonus," presumably to be distributed among its personnel.

It follows that "health maintenance organizations" could achieve such economies—while assuring adequate quality of service—principally through the type of systematic organization described above. Theoretically, economies might also be achieved within the framework of independent medical practice through a system of rigorous review of medical performance and claims (such as under the

San Joaquin Foundation for Medical Care). The evidence for this, however, is not clear; it suggests that claims review may lead to savings in ambulatory care, but they are counterbalanced by an actual excessive expenditure for hospital care.[49] As a practical matter, the HMO concept would mean mainly the type of health care organization illustrated by the existing prepaid comprehensive medical care plans based on group practice, such as the Kaiser-Permanente Health Plan and the Health Insurance Plan of Greater New York.

In these organized programs, it is important to appreciate that the advantages (in effectiveness, economy, and equity) depend on a consideration of the total care provided—that is, including hospital care—rather than physician services alone. Physician salaries in these plans are competitively high, in comparison with average earnings of private solo practice, and the volume of ambulatory service given, especially including laboratory and X-ray examinations, is also high.[50] Preventive examinations are considerably more frequent than under conventional medical arrangements. The financial savings are principally referrable to the lower rate of hospitalization of persons served by these programs. Because of the high cost of a day of hospital care, small reductions in this sector lead to relatively large savings. Thus, it is important that a health maintenance organization include hospitalization among its services.

Thus, consideration of payment methods in medical care leads us to appreciate the value of the Kaiser and H.I.P. patterns as a solution to some of our pressing problems in American health service. To be relevant for health planning in California, or any other state, however, more than this must be said. It is not likely that the federal or any state government in the United States would institute such a pattern of medical care organization by law, no matter how convincing were the evidence of its value. American culture calls for a far more gradualistic approach.

In terms of state health planning in California, it may be proposed that every encouragement should be given to the establishment of health maintenance organizations. Such programs might be sponsored by groups of consumers (including co-ops, labor unions, clubs, etc.), groups of providers (including medical group clinics, medical societies, medical staffs of hospitals, etc.), or by middlemen. If middlemen are involved, there are, of course, hazards of profiteering at the expense of both patient and doctor, which must be cautiously watched.

The establishment of an HMO is not easy and requires an organizational staff which can work out the administrative structure patiently. To facilitate such exploratory efforts, the state government might give seed grants. (It may be recalled that the Kaiser-Permanente Health Plan was started only after substantial subsidy, later repaid, from the Kaiser Corporation, and the H.I.P. program depended for its initiation on subsidy from the Rockefeller Foundation.) Loans might also be given, at low interest rates, for the construction of necessary facilities; the resources of the Hill-Burton hospital construction program can properly be applied for this purpose.

Enrollment of persons in health maintenance organizations is another task. In the past, each health insurance plan has had to mount its own sales force for this purpose. Recently, however, a new pattern has developed, in which Blue Cross and Blue Shield plans have come to use their enrollment machinery for soliciting memberships in other medical care organizations. This was done in Boston by the Massachusetts Blue Cross with respect to a new comprehenesive plan developed by the Harvard Medical School, and it is being considered now in Los Angeles between the Southern California Blue Cross and the UCLA Medical School.[51] The cost of the enrollment process would be recovered from future premium income.

Besides public grants and loans for organizational or capital financing purposes, health maintenance organizations should be encouraged through widespread discussion in both professional and lay circles. Fortunately, there are no legal restrictions against group practice or consumer sponsorship of health insurance plans in California, as exist in some other states.[52] But the idea will not grow without deliberate educational efforts. There are still many apprehensions among both doctors and patients that organization of health services leads inevitably to a deterioration of the personal doctor-patient relationship. The problems are real in this sphere, but they are not inevitable, and the rapid growth of membership in the Kaiser-Permanente Health Plan in California demonstrates that, whatever humanistic deficiencies result from bureaucratic structuring, they are more than overcome by the advantages of the pattern. (Indeed, the Kaiser Plan would grow still more than it has, if it could recruit more doctors; it has actually put a stop on new enrollments.) In any event, the doctor-patient relationship can be perfectly satisfactory in an organized setting, if the health manpower supply is adequate and the performance standards are proper. All these issues require discussion and education.

Finally, the encouragement of health maintenance organizations can be made a matter of social policy by the California State Health Planning Council and other state health agencies. State and local health departments should become informed on the subject and be prepared to answer questions and spread the word. By concerted effort, the pattern of health service embodied in the HMO concept could evolve from its current embryonic status into the predominant pattern for health care in the state and nation.

References

1. Seymour E. Harris, *The Economics of American Medicine*, New York: Macmillan, 1964, pp. 31–48.
2. Milton I. Roemer, *The Organization of Medical Care under Social Security*, Geneva: International Labour Office, 1969.

3. Herman M. Somers and Anne R. Somers, *Doctors, Patients, and Health Insurance*, Washington: The Brookings Institution, 1961.
4. Bernhard J. Stern, *Medicine in Industry*, New York: Commonwealth Fund, 1946.
5. James Hogarth, *The Payment of the Physician: Some European Comparisons*, New York: Macmillan, 1963.
6. Charles P. Hall, "Deductibles in Health Insurance: An Evaluation," *Journal of Risk and Insurance,* 33:253–263, June 1966.
7. C. A. Alexander, "The Effects of Change in Method of Paying Physicians: The Baltimore Experience," *American Journal of Public Health,* 57:1278–1289, August 1967.
8. Paul Densen, E. Balamuth, and S. Shapiro, *Prepaid Medical Care and Hospital Utilization,* Chicago: American Hospital Association, Monograph No. 3, 1958.
9. United Steel Workers of America, Insurance, Pension and Unemployment Benefits Department, *Special Study on the Medical Care Program for Steel Workers and Their Families*, Pittsburgh, Pa., 1960. Reported in: University of Michigan, *Medical Care Chart Book*, Ann Arbor, 1968, p. 43.
10. G. M. Emery, "New Zealand Medical Care," *Medical Care (London),* 4:159–170, July–Sept. 1966.
11. Paul A. Lembcke, "Evolution of the Medical Audit," *Journal of the American Medical Association*, 199:543–550, 20 February 1969.
12. Henry Anderson, "Statistical Surveillance of a Title XIX Program," *American Journal of Public Health,* 59:275–289, February 1969.
13. Sam Shapiro, "End Result Measurements of Quality of Medical Care," *Milband Memorial Fund Quarterly,* 45:7–40, Winter 1967.
14. Herman M. Somers and Anne R. Somers, *Medicare and the Hospitals: Issues and Prospects*, Washington: The Brookings Institution, 1967.
15. F. D. Mott and M. I. Roemer, *Rural Health and Medical Care*, New York: McGraw-Hill, 1948, pp. 392–400.
16. Richard Sasuly and Carl E. Hopkins, "A Medical Society-Sponsored Comprehensive Medical Care Plan: The Foundation for Medical Care of San Joaquin County, California," *Medical Care* (New Haven) 5:234–248, July–August 1967.
17. William A. Glaser, *Paying the Doctor: Systems of Remuneration and Their Effects,* Baltimore: Johns Hopkins Press, 1970.
18. Helen H. Avnet and M. K. Nikias, *Insured Dental Care*, New York: Group Health Dental Insurance, 1967.
19. J. F. Follmann, Jr., *Drugs, Their Cost, and Health Insurance*, New York: Health Insurance Association of America, 1960.
20. Raymond R. Clapp, *Study of Drug Purchase Problems and Policies,* Washington: U.S. Welfare Adminstration, Welfare Research Report No. 2, March 1966.
21. L. V. Seawell, *Principles of Hospital Accounting*, Berwyn, Illinois: Physicians' Record Co., 1960.
22. Columbia University, School of Public Health and Administrative Medicine, *Prepayment for Hospital Care in New York State*, New York, 1960.
23. F.B. Roth, G. W. Myers, F. D. Mott, and L.S. Rosenfeld, "The Saskatchewan Experience in Payment for Hospital Care," *American Journal of Public Health,* 43:752–756, June 1953.
24. Reuben A. Kessel, "Price Discrimination in Medicine," *Journal of Law and Economics,* 1:20–53, October 1958.
25. California Medical Association, *Relative Value Studies,* San Francisco, 1964.
26. C. A. Metzner, S. J. Axelrod, and J. H. Sloss, "Statistical Analysis as a Basis for Control of Fee-for-Service Plans," *American Journal of Public Health,* 43:1162–1170, September 1953.
27. Almost Lindsey, *Socialized Medicine in England and Wales: The National Health Service 1948–1961,* Chapel Hill: University of North Carolina Press, 1962.
28. I. S. Falk, C. R. Rorem, and M. D. Ring, *The Costs of Medical Care*, Chicago: University of Chicago Press, 1933, p. 478.
29. Louis J. Reed, *Blue Cross and Medical Service Plans*, Washington: Public Health Service, 1947.
30. J. S. Collings, "General Practice in England Today," *The Lancet,* 1:555–585, 1950.
31. Franz Goldmann, "Methods of Payment for Physicians' Services in Medical Care Programs," *American Journal of Public Health,* Vol. 42, No. 2, 1952.

32. Milton I. Roemer, "On Paying the Doctor and the Implications of Different Methods," *Journal of Health and Human Behavior,* 3:4–14, Spring 1962.
33. George Baehr, "Professional Services under Medical Care Insurance," *American Journal of Public Health,* February 1951, pp. 91–98.
34. James G. March (Editor), *Handbook of Organizations*, Chicago: Rand McNally and Co., 1965.
35. Peter M. Blau and W. R. Scott, *Formal Organizations: A Comparative Approach*, San Francisco: Chandler Publishing Co., 1962.
36. Leslie J. DeGroot (Editor), *Medical Care: Social and Organizational Aspects,* Springfield, Illinois: Charles C. Thomas, 1966.
37. Arthur Owens, "Report of a Nation-wide Survey of Full-time Hospital Staff Physicians," *Medical Economics,* 25 January 1965, pp. 73–89.
38. J. N. Haug and G. A. Roback, *Distribution of Physicians, Hospitals, and Hospital Beds in the U.S., 1967*, Chicago: American Medical Association, 1968.
39. For example, Arthur Kemp, "Economics and the Practice of Medicine," in R. B. Robins (Editor), *The Environment of Medical Practice,* Chicago: Yearbook Medical Publishers, 1963, pp. 261–293.
40. See John H. Knowles (Editor), *Hospitals, Doctors, and the Public Interest*, Cambridge, Mass.: Harvard University Press, 1965.
41. Milton I. Roemer and Donald M. DuBois, "Medical Costs in Relation to the Organization of Ambulatory Care," *New England Journal of Medicine* 280:988–993, 1 May 1969.
42. William F. Berry and J. C. Daugherty, "A Closer Look at Rising Medical Costs," *Monthly Labor Review,* 91:1–8, November 1968.
43. Milton I. Roemer and D. M. Anzel, "Health Needs and Services of the Rural Poor," *Medical Care Review,* 25:371–390, 461–491, May and June 1968.
44. John P. Bunker, "Surgical Manpower: A Comparison of Operations and Surgeons in the United States and in England and Wales," *New England Journal of Medicine,* 282:135–144, 1970.
45. D.M. DuBois, "Group Medical Practice—An Analytic Study" (prepared for the National Advisory Commission on Health Manpower), Los Angeles: University of California, School of Public Health, 1967 (processed), Appendix A.
46. Glyn W. Myers, "Hospital Budgeting Under Government Health Insurance," *The Canadian Chartered Accountant,* May 1956.
47. American Hospital Association, *Hospital Accreditation References,* Chicago: the Association, 1965.
48. Robert H. Finch, "Statement on Medicare and Medicaid Reforms," Washington: Department of Health, Education, and Welfare (processed), 25 March 1970.
49. Foline Gartside and Donald M. Procter, *Medicaid Services in California under Different Orgainzational Modes: Physician Participation in the San Joaquin Prepayment Project,* Los Angeles: University of California (School of Public Health), January 1970.
50. Bryan Gerstel and D. M. DuBois, "The Medical Care Program of the Kaiser Foundation Health Plan," in *Health Insurance Plans: Studies in Organizational Diversity,* Edited by M. I. Roemer, D. M. DuBois, and S. W. Rich, Los Angeles: University of California, School of Public Health (processed), 1970, pp. 292–317.
51. D. M. DuBois (University of California, Los Angeles), personal communication.

14

Preventive Services in Health Insurance

While health insurance has traditionally been developed to pool the costs of medical care over groups of people and over time, it can also serve to promote prevention of disease. Easy and rapid access to medical service, facilitated by insurance, is itself preventive, insofar as early treatment of an illness is more likely to be effective than late treatment. Health insurance may also pay for distinctly preventive measures such as immunizations or prenatal examinations. Screening tests for detection of pre-symptomatic chronic disease are further forms of prevention that health insurance may finance.

Health insurance programs developed from labor-management negotiations have shown increasing interest in including such preventive services among plan benefits. A review of potentialities in this field was presented at the 1974 Annual Conference of the International Foundation of Employee Benefit Plans and constitutes the chapter that follows.

Traditional Approaches

The traditional approach to the health service component of fringe benefits in industry has been to cover the costs of the most expensive sectors of medical care. Hospital bills and the costs of surgeons or physicians in hospitalized illness, while striking relatively infrequently, tend to be very costly or even catastrophic blows to family budgets. From an economic point of view, it was perfectly reasonable to try to soften the impact of these medical expenses that hit hardest. Moreover, insurance for hospital-based service was, for many reasons, the type which insurance carriers—both the commercial companies and the non-profit "Blue" plans—offered most readily. In fact, for some years, it was hard to find an insurance plan that even offered coverage for ambulatory medical care, let alone preventive services.[1]

Another consideration was the thought that ambulatory medical care costs, being relatively small, could be easily met out of the regular family budget and did not require the buffering of insurance. Preventive services, furthermore, were historically looked upon as something in the sphere of public agencies—health departments or sanitation agencies—not the normal responsibility of workers or

Chapter 14 originally appeared in *Textbook for Employee Benefit Plan Trustees, Administrators, and Advisors*, the proceedings of the International Foundation of Employee Benefit Plans (Toronto, Canada, 1975), pp. 76–81, and is reprinted by permission.

employers. As the costs of curative hospital-based medicine have risen, however, and even sky-rocketed compared with other costs of living, there has dawned on many health and welfare trust funds, as well as health insurance legislators, a kind of rediscovery of an old maxim; "an ounce of prevention is worth a pound of cure." The problem faced has been how to operationalize this principle in health benefit programs. Furthermore, some have asked, is the old maxim really true, after all?

Comprehensive Approach to Prevention

In fact, depending on the way one defines "prevention," it is not necessarily so easy to show that it is always cheaper than cure. With the infectious diseases, like diphtheria or smallpox, it could quite easily be proved that the immunization of, let us say, 1,000 children, was less expensive than the treatment—often unsuccessful—of five or six cases.

With the very great reduction of most of the acute communicable diseases, however, the economies of prevention have not been so simple to prove. As we shall see, for some non-communicable diseases and under certain circumstances, savings can be and have been proved. More important, however, is to consider whether the question of economies is the only question or the crucial one to ask. If we are interested in the total welfare of human beings, perhaps the first question we should ask should be, is prevention *better* than cure? Then, secondly, we can consider, how much does it cost?

With today's spectrum of diseases and 20th century health science, we must first of all take a broader view of prevention than that which was identified with the fight against infectious diseases. For some years now, public health specialists have come to recognize four levels of prevention.[2] I don't mean to give a classroom lecture, but let me try to summarize these levels.

Primary Prevention

This most basic type of prevention has been called "health promotion." It involves strengthening a person's physical or mental health so that he is more resistant to disease or, to put it positively, more likely to enjoy good health and effective living. Maintenance of good nutritional status through proper diet is a classical example of primary prevention. Engaging in regular exercise, avoiding clearly harmful habits like cigarette smoking or excessive alcohol consumption are other examples. These health promotional measures, it may be noted, involve the behavior of individuals, and the whole professional field of *health education* is devoted to this task of influencing human behavior in a sound direction. Regular access to a diligent primary care doctor is also a way to get this sort of health education or counselling.

Secondary Prevention

This involves protection of the individual against specific diseases or other hazards of the environment. Immunization against several communicable diseases is the classical example of this level of prevention. If certain forms of cancer are found to be caused by viruses, as some scientists suspect, we may some day have an immunization to offer against this major cause of suffering and death. A worker wearing protective goggles or gloves in an occupation with hazards of injury to his eyes or skin is another implementation of secondary prevention. It might well be best to guard the machinery so that particles cannot fly into a worker's eye, but even if this is not done adequately, the protective goggles can prevent injury.

Tertiary Prevention

It is at this third level of prevention that special interest has grown in the last 20 or 30 years; this involves the early detection of disease, when it may still be causing no symptoms that induce the person to seek medical care. The great importance of this level of prevention is that it may help us identify a *chronic* disorder, which has not been prevented by any action at the primary or secondary levels or, indeed, which medical science does not really know how to prevent anyway. If so identified, many—though not necessarily all—such disorders can be more effectively treated and often cured than if the first attention to the condition depended on the patient feeling some distinct pain or other symptom. The particularly practical aspect of this third level of prevention is that, with modern technology, much of it can be conducted without the expensive services of doctors and in a rather simple automated way. Known as "multiphasic screening" or "automated health testing," this important procedure will be discussed further below.

Fourth-level Prevention

Finally, if all first three levels of prevention have failed to stop the onset of a disease, there remains the fourth level at which action can be taken. This involves the prompt treatment of illness, after its presence has become manifest but before it has become serious or disabling. For many, if not most, diseases, early treatment is more effective in preventing disability or even death than neglected or late treatment. Middle ear infection promptly treated to prevent deafness and early excision of a cancer before it has hopelessly spread are just two out of scores of examples that could be cited. The essential requirement for this fourth level of prevention is to have ready access to medical care, while the patient is still up and about and before the condition has become so advanced as to necessitate hospitalization.

Implementing Prevention in Health Benefit Programs

This brief theoretical background may be enough to move to the practical question of how any or all these levels of prevention could be incorporated in health benefit programs.

In its simplest form, I think the answer is to provide *comprehensive* health services to all eligible persons. By "comprehensive" I mean not only all curative services inside and outside of hospitals, but all four levels of prevention. To do the latter means making doctors and allied health personnel readily available to all eligible persons when they feel the need—essentially what has been called the fourth level of prevention. But much more than this, it means reaching people regularly when they do not have an obvious complaint—the first three levels of prevention.

To implement the first two levels—health promotion and specific protection—health education, personal health counselling, and aggressive outreach efforts of many types are needed. Regarding the third level—early disease detection—as noted earlier, particular interest has grown in recent years throughout the world, as simple and relatively low cost automated procedures have been developed for screening out an increasing number of diseases.[3] At the same time, as the number of these procedures has multiplied, some skepticism has arisen on the value—both in terms of health achievement and in terms of cost-effectiveness—of all these recommended tests. With commercial companies entering the field of automated multiphasic screening, eager to market their services to union groups and to health fund trustees, some natural "sales resistance" has grown up and also some eagerness to find out what screening tests really "pay off" and which ones are not worth the time and money.

If we had the time, I could recite to you a list of 50 or more health screening tests that have been advocated for application to population groups over the years. It might start with: *chest X-rays, urinalyses, electrocardiograms, Pap smears in women, serum cholesterols, blood pressures* and go on to dozens of additional physical, chemical, immunological, or simply pencil-and-paper tests which, in combination, could theoretically identify the possible presence of a hundred or more common or rare pathological states. Rather than attempting this, I think it would be more useful to confine my remarks to a few basic principles about health screening tests in relation to prevention of disease.

First of all, the absolutely final answers on the value—in health gains or money—are not yet available on the great majority of tests. All over the world, research is being done on these tests, and there are disagreements among scientific investigators. The British scientists, for example, tend to be more skeptical than the American.[4]

Second, it is not necessary, in my opinion, to have incontrovertibly conclusive evidence of a positive cost-benefit ratio for a particular test before offering it in a multiphasic screening program. We are not so demanding of proof of the value of countless surgical or other curative procedures—for example, tonsillectomies, cholecystectomies, hysterectomies and appendectomies—which are regularly done by the thousands. If there is *presumptive* value for a test, and if it can be done easily and inexpensively, it ought to be offered until the research scientists prove to us that it is not of any value.

My reason for this somewhat unorthodox view is that I believe there is value in the very concept of screening tests that is achieved, even if what the rigorous scientist calls a "controlled clinical trial" has not finally proved its value. My point is that screening tests embody and emphasize a preventive approach to health, as distinguished from what Dr. Lester Breslow has epitomized as the "complaint-response approach," which has characterized medicine for centuries.[5]

If we cannot prove with absolute certainty, for example, that the early detection of elevated blood glucose will enable a patient to live a longer and happier life than if this condition is discovered only after frank symptoms of diabetes show up, there is still probably more value in knowing this physiological fact than not knowing it. The patient who has this abnormal condition can be advised earlier rather than later to eat and live in a way that can reduce the many risks associated with diabetes. And while the crucial scientific experiment to prove this point may not be conducted for many years, there are good presumptive reasons, in the opinion of numerous diabetes experts, why such early disease detection is of value.

Third, when evidence is still tentative, it is wise to concentrate screening tests on the detection of diseases that are known to be of high severity and importance in the population. There are chemical tests for Tay-Sachs disease or phenylketonuria or other disorders that are extremely rare. Eventually these tests may prove to be worth doing on a mass basis, but for the present it makes better sense to confine our efforts to tests for the detection of heart disease, different forms of cancer, hypertension, diverse conditions of the liver or kidneys, anemia, tuberculosis, hearing impairments, obesity, or other conditions that directly or indirectly lead to the major causes of death or disability in our society.

A fourth principle, I would suggest, is that certain tests should be done with discretion in relation to various age, sex, and racial or ethnic groups. There is little point in doing chest X-rays today on persons under 20 years of age, nor is red cell sickling worth seeking in white persons. In general, more chronic disorders develop with aging, and the various signs of heart disease, cancer, or glaucoma should be sought more diligently in the older age groups.[6]

Fifth, screening tests are worth doing only if they are properly followed up with full medical examinations, definitive diagnoses, and treatment or health counselling. Experience shows that it is not enough to leave this essential action to the individual; it requires not only letters to the patient and his doctor but also personal follow-up by public health or visiting nurses in many cases.

Sixth, health screening should not be regarded as a one-shot affair. To be effective, it should be repeated at reasonable intervals (increasing in frequency with aging) throughout life.[7]

Seventh, automated health testing is bound to be most successful if it is part of a general program of comprehensive preventive and treatment services. In this way, its educational value, its practical implementation, and its proper follow-up can be best assured.

Some Hard Evidence

Having offered some general principles and perhaps leaned over backwards to avoid dogmatism, what can we say about the proven value of various screening tests? In my opinion and that of many specialists in preventive medicine, there can be little doubt about the value of certain tests, where widespread performance in certain regions has been associated with sharp declines in mortality. Among these I would include:

- chest X-rays and the decline of tuberculosis
- serological tests and the decline of syphilis
- Pap smears and the decline of uterine cancer

One may grant that other factors have also contributed to the decline of these diseases—just as the virtual disappearance of diphtheria has been due to many things outside of immunizations—without denying the contributory effects of early detection of unrecognized cases.

Beyond these observations, there has been impressive evidence from studies in New York of the value of a routine X-ray procedure known as "mammography" in saving the lives of women with breast cancer. Evidence has been mounting that early detection and treatment of high blood pressure can reduce the occurrence of paralytic strokes and death from this cause. It has also been getting increasingly clear—especially from some recent Finnish research—that high blood cholesterol (detectable by a screening test) can be reduced by diet, and that such reduction leads to a lower occurrence of heart attacks and cardiac death rates.[8]

Hundreds of scientific papers have been published on the results of automated multiphasic health testing.[9] While the findings of different surveys obviously vary, one may conclude roughly that when adult populations are screened with a battery of about 10 or more procedures, somewhere between 25 percent and 33 percent of positives (i.e., possible evidence of disease) will be identified. Of these, roughly half, or 12 percent to 16 percent, are conditions of which the person was previously unaware. These findings will differ with the age level of the persons screened (higher yields coming with older age groups) and with the standards of normality applied in judging the results of certain tests. In any event, a detection of previously unrecognized disease in roughly one person out of seven tested would seem to be a good start in applying the third level of preventive service.

Of the many scientific investigations that have attempted to evaluate the consequences of multiphasic health screening, probably the most careful and long term has been that by Dr. Morris Collen and his colleagues at the Kaiser-Permanente Health Plan in Oakland, California. We cannot take the time to review all the details of Dr. Collen's work, which has been reported in the professional literature, but I can assure you he has applied unassailable scientific techniques in studying the effects of a battery of screening tests on a series of some 5,000 people, compared with another 5,000 people similar in all respects except for the lack of screening examinations.[10] Starting in 1964, the test group received periodic health questionnaires, electrocardiograms, blood pressure readings, chest X-rays, vision and hearing tests, lung capacity tests, a series of blood chemistry determinations, and so on. After seven years—which, after all, may not be long enough to show the full effects—it was found that the screened population compared with the others showed:

1. no significant difference in the use of ambulatory medical services (aside from the screening tests themselves),
2. a higher rate of diagnoses established,
3. a lower rate of days of sickness-disability, especially for males entering the study in the 45–54 year age group,
4. after a small initial rise in the first years, a hospitalization rate in the later years that declined to consistently lower levels,
5. and, most important, a significantly lower mortality rate (35.6 per 1,000, compared with 39.2 in the others), referrable mainly to fewer deaths from cancer and cardiovascular disease.[11]

It is important to realize that *both* of these comparison populations were equally accessible to complete curative health service, and the only difference between them was the availability of health screening tests to the first group. In my opinion, this crucial investigation gives very powerful proof of the value of numerous health screening tests for the improvement of health and the reduction of mortality. It is reasonable to expect that with a period of observation longer than seven years, the differentials will prove to be even greater.

For those who wish a dollar-and-cents value placed on the benefits of health screening, Collen and his colleagues computed the costs of the screening tests, plus the costs of all the medical care obtained by both screened and unscreened populations. The costs of disability and death were computed on the basis of the lost wages of the persons affected. For women, who were often not in the labor market, it was difficult to make proper calculations of all the costs involved (such as lost time from work), but for men, it was found that over the seven year period there was a net saving of about $800 per man in the screened, compared with the unscreened population, or about $115 per man per year. This was in spite of the additional cost of about $22 per person per year for the screening examinations themselves.

Conclusion

This has been a very sketchy review of some of the principles and the findings involved in multiphasic health testing, as an approach to health maintenance, at the third level of prevention. In closing these remarks on the place of preventive and diagnostic services in health benefit programs, I should like to return to the concept of all four levels of prevention with which we started. The point is that health screening by itself is not likely to do much good. It must be backed up by prompt access to ambulatory medical care for proper medical diagnosis and prompt treatment of any disorders found or health counselling (for example advice on diet, exercise, and smoking to a patient found to have high serum cholesterol) with respect to any of the important risk factors that have been detected.

Furthermore, the whole worldwide experience of medicine suggests that if prevention at the first and second levels—health promotion and protection—is aggressively pursued, the rate of persons in whom signs of disease are detected, at the third level, or requiring treatment at the fourth level, will be reduced.

Multiphasic health screening, thus, should be viewed as one sector of a general program of prevention and medical care. To make such comprehensive services available to workers in employee benefit programs is a much bigger order than to launch an isolated screening program. Some 20 or 30 organizations have grown up in the United States, prepared to move a large, elaborately equipped and staffed testing van to the factory gates, and for about $30 or $40 per head per year—which I guess comes to about two cents per hour in an average worker's wages—do a large battery of tests on several thousand workers. There are economies in larger scale operations, of course, but the important economies and the real benefits depend on the provision of all the services at the other three levels of prevention, plus the further components of curative medical care.

This kind of comprehensive health service is a far cry from the typical health benefit program now being offered in American industry either through trust funds or unilaterally. Realistically, it requires organization not only of the financing but also the delivery of total health care. It requires a *system* of health service which traditional private fee-for-service medical practice is hardly capable of offering.

The answer, in my view, can be best found in the pattern of the "health maintenance organization" (the HMO), an idea which has been tested and has proved itself in America for at least the last 50 years, although only recently recognized by the federal government.[12] Happily, the HMO idea is now being promoted by government grants, and it obviously relates closely to the objective of mobilizing preventive and diagnostic services in health benefit programs.

I hope that the several thousand labor-management trust funds in North America will recognize the opportunity now before them to modify their current hospital-oriented benefit programs into comprehensive HMOs, designed on a medical teamwork model. This is no easy task, but there is much reason to believe it is the wave of the future. In so doing, the benefits of all levels of prevention—benefits both in health and in economies—can be best achieved for employees and their families.

References

1. Herman M. Somers and Anne R. Somers, *Doctors, Patients, and Health Insurance*, Washington: Brookings Institution, 1961.
2. Hugh R. Leavell and E. Gurney Clark (Editors), *Preventive Medicine for the Doctor in His Community*, New York: McGraw-Hill Book Co., 1958.
3. J. M. G. Wilson and G. Jungner, *The Principles and Practice of Screening*, Geneva: World Health Organization, 1966.
4. Thomas McKeown et al., *Screening in Medical Care: Reviewing the Evidence*, London: Oxford University Press, 1968.
5. Lester Breslow, "Incorporation of Preventive Medical Services into National Health Insurance," Washington: Association of Schools of Public Health (processed), November 1973.
6. Milton I. Roemer, "A Program of Preventive Medicine for the Individual," *Milbank Memorial Fund Quarterly*, 23:209–226, 1945.
7. A. Yedidia, M. A. Bunow, and M. Muldavin, "Mobile Multiphasic Screening in an Industrial Setting: The California Cannery Workers Program," *Journal of Occupational Medicine* 11:601–662, November 1969.
8. Matti Miettinen et al., "Effect of Cholesterol—Lowering Diet on Mortality from Coronary Heart Disease and Other Causes," *The Lancet*, 21 October 1972, 835–838.
9. Anna C. Gelman, *Multiphasic Health Testing Systems: Reviews and Annotations,* Washington: National Center for Health Services Research and Development, March 1971.
10. John C. Cutler et al., "Multiphasic Checkup Evaluation Study," *Preventive Medicine*, 2:197–206, June 1973.
11. L. G. Dales, G. D. Friedman, and M. F. Collen, "Evaluation of a Periodic Multiphasic Health Checkup," *Meth. Inform. Med.*, 13:140–146, 1974.
12. Milton I. Roemer and William Shonick, "HMO Performance: The Recent Evidence," *Health and Society*, Summer 1973, pp. 271–317.

15

National Health Insurance as a Means of Cost Control

The impact of health insurance, whether voluntary or governmental, in increasing the rates of use of health services by removing financial barriers, is well known. Less well appreciated are the many ways that a governmental health insurance program can contain costs by introducing various regulations in the free market of medical care.

With medical costs increasing rapidly in the United States at the same time as pressure for national health insurance, debate has been active on the probable effects of such legislation on costs. In this chapter, the various ways that health insurance operations can be used to limit costs are explored, based on policies and practices in other countries. Strategies have been applied to control the cost of physician services, hospitalization, drugs, and other services. While costs may rise with increased utilization, the expenditures can be directed toward needed and not unjustified services. The very rise of costs stimulates greater controls and also modification of the delivery of health care toward more efficient patterns. The text that follows was presented at the New York Academy of Medicine Conference on "Health Policy: Realistic Expectations and Reasonable Priorities" in April, 1977.

BEFORE DISCUSSING NATIONAL health insurance as a means of containing or controlling health care costs, may I offer a basic premise. From the viewpoint of human welfare, there is no good reason to attempt containment of *all* health care costs or, more accurately, expenditures. The problem is to constrain or eliminate those expenditures that are not beneficial to health, or not beneficial enough to justify the costs. The distinction between beneficial and non-beneficial health care expenditure is not always easy to make, but it is important. It obviously requires judgments and actions quite outside the sphere of programs of financing.

Health Care Expenditures

In recent years it has become fashionable to question the soundness of all medical care expenditures—especially in the light of their escalation—in contrast to the value of prevention, health promotion, and life style.[1] While we cannot now discuss this basic issue, I would urge that you not regard medical care, or national

Chapter 15 originally appeared as "National Health Insurance as an Agent in Containing Health Care Costs" in *The Bulletin of the New York Academy of Medicine*, 54: 102–112, January, 1978, and is reprinted by permission of that journal.

health insurance to finance it, as competitive or obstructive to disease prevention or health promotion. Medical care should be—if not always so in practice—supportive of preventive strategies; it can and does help people also when prevention has failed.

The rising expenditures for health services, both preventive and therapeutic, are a worldwide phenomenon—with or without national health insurance. The increases are both absolute, in amounts of money spent, and relative to the national wealth or gross national product (GNP) of countries.[2] In general, the proportions of GNP spent on health service are higher in the more technologically advanced countries, where life expectancies are indeed higher, age-specific death rates lower, and the quality of life far better than in the impoverished less-developed countries.[3] The reasons for rising costs are too complex to analyze here, but they include advances in the capabilities of medicine, increases in utilization rates, reduction of economic barriers through social financing, and many other changes. We must not decry all these increased expenditures any more than we should regret the worldwide escalating outlays for public education. Harmful expenditures, such as for cigarette production and advertising, should be condemned and these monies used for socially sound purposes. But in health service, the task is to discriminate between beneficial expenditures and wasteful or even harmful ones, and direct our containment efforts at the latter.

National Health Insurance as a Regulatory Force

About 70 nations have, over the last century, developed systems of social insurance which include, with various ranges of population coverage and health care benefits, support for medical and related services. This mechanism of social financing has extended rapidly on all six continents because it combines a relatively conservative method of fund raising, acceptable to conservative political parties, with a remarkably stable source of support over the years, demanded by more left-wing political groups.[4] Where national health insurance (NHI) has been introduced in countries with a flourishing private medical profession, it has initially been designed mainly to pay the bills of doctors and other health care providers along traditional lines. In poorer countries, with a weak private medical market, even the initial pattern of NHI programs has usually departed sharply from conventional private sector delivery patterns; the doctors and other health care providers have typically been appointed to work on salaries in facilities owned and controlled by the insuring organization.[5] Even in the former type of country (as in Western Europe), however, under NHI conventional patterns of medical care delivery are soon subjected to various forms of social intervention.

The reasons for social intervention are many. National health insurance inevitably leads to increased rates of provision of health services, particularly among lower income families previously deprived. Expenditures rise and, being socially visible, they are subject to political debate. The money paid to providers, by whatever method, must be raised through various forms of tax on all consumers. Thus political pressures mount, to assure that the money is wisely spent. This leads typically to intervention first into the fiscal aspects of the medical care process, and eventually into the content and pattern of provision of the health services themselves. These interventions usually involve controls on both the quality and costs of health service. Our focus here is on cost containment, and in the brief space available we may note some of its principal strategies with respect to the main components of medical care: physician's services, hospitalization, and drugs.

Costs of Physician's Care

Broadly speaking, NHI programs have applied either or both of two approaches to limit expenditures for physician's care: constraint on the patient or controls on the doctor. The usual constraint on patients is one or another form of cost-sharing—most commonly payment of a percentage of the doctor's fee. Such co-payment is intended to contain costs in two ways: by deterring so-called unnecessary utilization and by reducing the money payable from the insurance fund for each unit of service.

It is noteworthy that in Germany, where social insurance for medical care was first launched, cost-sharing has never been imposed.[6] In the Scandinavian countries, France, Belgium, and most of western continental Europe it has been applied. There is evidence that co-payments selectively reduce the doctor's care utilization rate of low-income families, but not of others;[7] for this reason it is often waived for pensioners or other presumably poor persons. Cost-sharing, moreover, is seldom applied to hospitalization or referred consultations, for which the primary physician, rather than the patient, makes the decision.

Since most health care expenditures result, indeed, from the decisions of doctors, not of patients, the second cost-containment approach—controls on the doctor—is much more widely used. In countries paying doctors on a fee-for-service basis, with or without cost-sharing by the patient, there are almost always negotiated schedules of fees for specific procedures. The U.S. Medicare approach of paying flexible "usual and customary" fees under a governmental health insurance program is unknown elsewhere, because of its obvious inflationary effects. Even so, physicians in Western Europe, Japan, Australia and elsewhere seem to be as adept as certain American doctors in defining the services rendered under a fee-schedule in ways that maximize their financial return. To cope with this problem, a variety of methods have been developed to monitor the patterns of practice of individual doctors, in order to detect deviance from reasonable norms.[8]

Thus, most Western European health insurance programs have long engaged "advisory" or "control doctors" to help monitor deviant medical performance, especially excessive servicing. In recent years, computerized records have simplified the screening out of doctors whose fee claims warrant investigation. A sequence of, first, written communication, then discussion, warnings, professional hearings, fiscal penalties, and ultimately exclusion from an NHI system is applied to exercise these controls. In my view, the very existence of this surveillance in NHI programs is probably more important than the occasional detection of definite abuse or fraud, in encouraging self-discipline among physicians.

Other control devices under fee-for-service insurance patterns include: prior approval required for elective surgery (Holland), authorization of hospital stays beyond seven days (Belgium), payment of higher specialist fees for ambulatory care only when the patient has been referred by a general practitioner or another specialist (some provinces of Canada and all states of Australia), and so on. In Germany, the operation of the fee system is particularly complex, involving the intervention of a physician's association between the sickness insurance funds and the individual doctor; since this medical association takes financial responsibility for the total volume of services rendered by its members to insured persons during each quarter-year, it has strong interest in monitoring professional performance. If services have been excessive, the association may have to prorate fee payments below the scheduled level to stay within the quarterly allotment.

Less onerous and far simpler administratively has been the modification of fee-for-service remuneration for general practitioner services in the NHI systems of a few countries.[9] In Great Britain since 1911 (well before the National Health Service) and the Netherlands, general practitioners are paid primarily by the capitation method—that is, a fixed per capita amount per month for each person choosing to be on a G.P.'s list. In Denmark, the capitation method is used in Copenhagen and to some extent elsewhere. There are various levels of capitation payment to discourage excessively long visits, and also supplemental fees for certain services (e.g., home calls), but the capitation method obviously avoids the cost-inflating effects of fee-for-service, even though it entails certain other problems.

A more important cost control is the policy of paying for the in-hospital services of specialists by salary, full-time or part-time. This is true in virtually all hospitals of the Scandinavian countries, in many hospitals of Germany and France, and in some hospitals of every country with NHI legislation. The surgeon or other specialist in these setttings has no *financial* incentive to operate upon or give other in-hospital treatment to a patient; professional judgment and the availability of hospital beds are the only determinants, and group medical discipline is the protection against under-servicing of patients. There seems little doubt that this pattern of specialist remuneration is a major factor in explaining the substantially lower rate of elective surgery in most European countries than in the United States.[10]

Finally, there are the economies of health centers, with salaried teams of doctors and ancillary personnel, serving as the conventional pattern for ambulatory care in the NHI systems of Latin America, the Middle East, and other developing regions.[11] Perhaps more salient to the United States is the gradual but definite extension of this health center pattern in the NHI programs of Western Europe, Canada, Australia, New Zealand, and even in highly entrepreneurial Japan. There can be no doubt that this method of delivering ambulatory care under NHI programs promotes both economy and quality.

Hospitalization Costs

Health insurance financing—whether governmental or voluntary—has clearly led to the expansion of hospital resources and improvement in the quality of hospital care. With this economic support, hospitals, which were previously dependent on inadequate funds from charity, general revenues, or personal payments, have been enabled to enlarge their staffs and improve their equipment in scores of countries. Relative to preventive and ambulatory services, of course, hospitalization is costly and has probably been over-supported. As expenditures have risen, however, cost-containment strategies have been stimulated.

One such strategy in countries with NHI has been the establishment of controls over hospital construction and the level of bed-population ratios. Before 1945, hospitals were constructed or enlarged throughout the non-socialist world without any overall plan. In the industrialized countries, the decisions were simply based on local initiative. As the rate of hospital days per 1,000 increased under NHI support, and the dependence of this rate on the bed supply became clear, constraints have been put on hospital construction. This has been most deliberate in countries such as Canada, Japan, or Belgium, where fee-for-service incentives strongly influence hospital admissions. As we know, the same dynamics have occurred through "certificate of need" legislation in the United States, when voluntary hospitalization insurance and Medicare came to cover the large majority of the population.

Related to the constraints on the hospital bed supply has been the extension of the regionalization concept. This aims, of course, to rationalize the provision of expensive hospital services over large geographic areas, so that needs can be equitably met without the wasteful duplication of facilities in a free market.[12] Along with regionalization of hospitals, there has arisen in many countries a new recognition of the importance of primary health care and ambulatory services, in general, so that the out-patient departments of hospitals and also free-standing polyclinics have been strengthened. When fee incentives prevail and hospital beds are abundant, insurance for ambulatory care—at least under U.S. conditions—has not led to reduction in hospital utilization, as some had hoped.[13] But with constraints on the bed supply and elimination of fee incentives, effective ambulatory service can reduce hospital use and expenditures, as has been repeatedly demonstrated by the "health maintenance organization" (HMO) experience in the United States.[14] In the American setting, NHI legislation could doubtless promote extension of the HMO pattern, with its many cost-containment features.

Mechanisms of paying hospitals under NHI programs can and do include numerous constraints on expenditures. Many NHI systems, that pay for hospital services on a per diem basis, set a limit on the percentage of increase in these rates which will be accepted annually. Naturally this constrains the numbers of hospital personnel engaged, their salaries, and other components of hospital costs, but it controls the level of expenditures.

In Canada, Great Britain, New Zealand, and elsewhere, the strategy of prospective budgeting has been applied. I do not mean "prospective reimbursement rates," which simply "hold the line" on per diem payments for a year but do nothing to avoid superfluous days of hospital care. "Prospective budgeting" pays the hospital a global sum each month for its total operations, based on budget review, application of sound standards of staffing, and a reasonable occupancy level. In several provinces of Canada, where this method is used, there is no financial incentive to "keep beds filled" unjustifiably;[15] yet if a deficit can be reasonably explained by a hospital, the insurance system gives an extra grant. If the hospital can operate at less than the global budgetary allotment, it keeps the balance. This is an over-simplification of the prospective budgeting mechanism, but, in a word, the Canadian hospitals are basically happy with the system and their costs have risen less than those in the United States. It would be very difficult, however, to implement this cost-containment strategy except in an NHI system with a single source of financing for all or nearly all hospital services.

Drug Expenditures

Expenditures for prescribed drugs have risen sharply under most NHI programs offering such benefits, but time permits only brief mention of the methods of control developed in response. In Germany, Sweden, and elsewhere the prescribing habits of doctors are monitored, and disciplinary actions taken where necessary. In Belgium, an approved list of drugs is prepared by nationally respected experts, and the extent of co-payment required from the patient is lower when the doctor prescribes items on this list.

Several NHI systems send periodic bulletins to all doctors on the relative prices of pharmacologically equivalent drugs with different brand names. Some Canadian provinces go so far as to require the pharmacist to dispense the least expensive preparation of a prescribed medicament, unless the physician gives specific instructions to the contrary. In Norway, where most drugs are imported, those authorized in the country are a carefully selected 2,000, compared with the bewildering tens of thousands sold in the United States.

Where the organized health center pattern of health care delivery characterizes NHI systems, as in Latin America and the Middle East, drugs are purchased in bulk by the program and dispensed directly to patients without middleman profits. The choice of preparations purchased is naturally governed by considerations of both economy and quality.

Other cost-containment strategies under NHI systems involve dental care, physiotherapy, eyeglasses, diagnostic tests, prosthetic appliances, and so on. The methods entail prior authorization of services applying reasonable criteria, surveillance of the prescribing habits of individual doctors, wholesale purchase and dispensing, and similar approaches. The expenditures for these ancillary services, however, are usually small compared with those for hospitalization, physician's care, and medications.

The Overall Effect on Expenditures

In conclusion, there can be no doubt that national health insurance leads to increased rates of provision of health services, largely by increasing the access of patients to doctors who order the hospitalizations, tests, operations, drugs, and other components of comprehensive health care. This is bound to mean greater expenditures, but one must realize that the same process occurs under voluntary health insurance, and even without any insurance for persons who can afford the costs. The point is to channel more spending through the public sector where it can be reasonably controlled. It is noteworthy that the United States, with the weakest social insurance program for health care of any industrialized nation in the world, spends the highest share of its GNP—about 8.6 percent—on health purposes. In other nations, spending less—but a greater share through the public sector—the people are getting more for their money.

In today's world, where health care has come to be regarded as a human right, it is pointless to decry the principle of social financing of some sort to achieve equity. The task is to prevent extravagance or corruption in the use of a people's money. Given the operation of an American-style open market for health care, in which the provider makes most of the decisions, but neither he nor the patient is (nor should be) constrained by price, social regulation of many sorts becomes necessary. Under a national health insurance system, such regulation becomes not only more feasible, but social and political dynamics are generated to extend it.

The ultimate issue is not which system of health service is least costly. It is rather which system promotes health most effectively, with least waste and inefficiency. World experience suggests that national health insurance, in varying formats determined by political forces, provides a foundation for evolution toward more efficient and effective patterns of health service.

References

1. Ivan Illich, *Medical Nemesis: The Expropriation of Health*, New York: Pantheon Books, 1976. See also: Rick Carlson, *The End of Medicine*, New York: John Wiley, 1975.
2. Teh-wei Hu, *International Health Costs and Expenditures*, Washington: Fogarty International Center for Advanced Study in the Health Sciences, 1976.
3. Brian Abel-Smith, *An International Study of Health Expenditure*, Geneva: World Health Organization, 1967.
4. Eveline M. Burns, *Social Security and Public Policy*, New York: McGraw-Hill, 1956.
5. Milton I. Roemer, *The Organisation of Medical Care under Social Security*, Geneva: International Labour Office, 1969.
6. Fritz Kastnev, *Monograph on the Organisation of Medical Care within the Framework of Social Security in the Federal Republic of Germany*, Geneva: International Labour Office, 1968.
7. R. G. Beck, "The Effects of Co-Payment on the Poor," *Journal of Human Resources*, 9: 129–142, Winter 1974.
8. Derick Fulcher, *Medical Care Systems: Public and Private Health Coverage in Selected Industrialised Countries*, Geneva: International Labour Office, 1974.
9. William A. Glaser, *Paying the Doctor: Systems of Remuneration and Their Effects*, Baltimore: Johns Hopkins Press, 1970.
10. John P. Bunker, "Surgical Manpower: Comparisons of Operations and Surgeons in the U.S. and England," *New England Journal of Medicine*, 281: 880–884, 16 October 1969.
11. Milton I. Roemer, *Evaluation of Community Health Centres*, Geneva: World Health Organization, 1973.
12. Arthur Engel, *The Swedish Regionalized Hospital System*, Stockholm: National Board of Health, 1967.
13. Daniel B. Hill and James E. Veney, "Kansas Blue Cross/Blue Shield Out-Patient Benefits Experiment," *Medical Care*, 8: 143–158, March–April 1970.
14. Milton I. Roemer and William Shonick, "HMO Performance: The Recent Evidence," *Health and Society* (Milbank Memorial Fund Quarterly), 51: 271–317, Summer 1973.
15. Maurice LeClair, "The Canadian Health Care System," in *National Health Insurance: Dan We Learn from Canada?* (Spiro Andreopoulos, Editor), New York: John Wiley, 1975, pp. 11–96.

Part Four

Organized Ambulatory Services

Another form of growing organization in the health field has been the manner of delivery of services to the ambulatory person. After a long history of one-to-one relationships between patient and healer, the provision of ambulatory health care has gradually become increasingly organized.

In Chapter 16, we review several streams of development of organized ambulatory health services, under various sponsorships and for different purposes, in the United States. One of the more important of these forms of organization has been the voluntary cooperation of doctors in group practice clinics, but these take a variety of forms which may be described as a spectrum; this is discussed in Chapter 17. In Chapter 18, an analysis is offered of the differential growth of group medical practice in the 50 states in an attempt to identify the conditions that are most fertile for growth of this pattern. Chapter 19 explores the relationship of group financing (or insurance) and group medical practice, with consideration of the impact on costs to the patient.

16

The Growth of Organized Ambulatory Care

Of all components of health service, historically the last to become organized have been the ambulatory services. When hospital care and environmental protection were objects of social planning, the ambulatory services for treatment of the sick were still an individual matter.

In the eighteenth century, steps were taken to provide ambulatory services for the poor in European cities on an organized basis. Since then, a number of kinds of social organization have been developed in connection with hospital out-patient departments, preventive public health services, industrial health services, school and college programs, private group medical practice, and various other governmental and voluntary agency health programs. In aggregate, these separate movements have come to provide a substantial share of the ambulatory health services furnished to the U.S. population. The gradual, incremental nature of these developments has tended to obscure their overall large impact.

AMBULATORY SERVICES ARE, in a social sense, one of the three major components of all health services, the other two being institutional and environmental. By their very nature the institutional services have always required social organization; to develop a facility where patients, away from their homes, could be cared for medically and custodially—from a medieval lazaretto to a 1975 medical center—required group action. Likewise, group or social efforts were required to influence the affects of the environment on health—not only to mobilize manpower and equipment but to impose rules that would control individual behavior.

Not so for ambulatory health services. From the earliest times sick persons sought help from individual healers. It was predominantly a one-to-one, rather than an organized social relationship, whether it was a shaman invoking the supernatural spirits for an ailing patient in a primitive African village or a bewigged and elegant eighteenth-century doctor ordering a concoction for his wealthy European patient in Molière's *Malade Imaginaire*. Even when social rules were enacted, like the ancient Babylonian Code of Hammurabi, to impose controls on the exercise of the healing arts, the provision of services thereby affected remained a personal process between the patient and the doctor (or his equivalent).

A shortened version of Chapter 16 appeared as "From Poor Beginnings: The Growth of Primary Care" in *Hospitals* (the journal of the American Hospital Association), Volume 49, issue 5, March 1, 1975, pp. 38–43, a special issue devoted to ambulatory care, and is reprinted by permission of that journal.

Origins of Organized Ambulatory Service

It was many centuries after the rise of medicine, as a systematic body of knowledge to be taught in schools and applied as a "professional service," before the idea arose that non-institutional care or measures of personal, as distinguished from environmental, intervention might be provided in an organized way. The first "dispensary" was organized in France in 1630 as a place where the poor might come for medical advice and drugs, without entering a hospital bed.[1] It was nearly a half-century later before the same idea was adopted in England, through the initiative of the Royal College of Physicians. In neither country did the hospitals—charitable facilities for the seriously sick poor and destitute—play any part in the innovation. The structures where drugs were dispensed (hence, dispensary) were separate buildings unrelated physically or administratively to hospitals. The motivations of doctors in starting these organized clinics was perhaps a mixture of compassion for the unfortunate with a hostility to the competition from apothecaries—who then, as to some extent now, were the less costly healers of the poor.

A similar story was recapitulated in America, with the first dispensary being organized in Philadelphia in 1786, some 35 years after the founding of the first hospital in the same city in 1751.[2] It was not until the eighteenth century in Europe and the nineteenth in America that hospitals began to consider it reasonable to organize departments for "out-patients" who, like their "in-patients," were expected to be poor. In large part, these clinics were started because of their value for educating medical students about earlier stages of disease. It is worth noting that long after in-patient wards were opened to affluent persons who could pay the costs, out-patient departments remained as they do to this day, essentially for the poor. The reasons, referable to ambulatory service as a matter mainly for private market exchange between doctor and patient, are obvious.

In 1893, the first national "Congress of Hospitals and Dispensaries"—the two types of facilities being considered so different—was held in Chicago. The American Hospital Assoication was founded in 1899 and in 1916 its Committee on Dispensary Work conducted a national survey. It found, by this time, 495 out-patient departments in hospitals, but there were still 185 dispensaries treating general diseases quite separate from any institution. By the end of World War I, practically all the separate dispensaries had become absorbed as part of hospitals, which were now being constructed everywhere.

Separate clinics oriented to halting the spread of communicable diseases, however, became organized, first by voluntary societies and later by official Health Departments, soon after the rise of bacteriology. In 1887 the Victoria Dispensary for Consumption was established in Edinburgh, Scotland, five years after Robert Koch had discovered tubercle bacillus. Voluntary Societies for the

Prevention of Tuberculosis founded similar clinics in the United States in the 1890s.

Charitable clinics for babies, to teach mothers about infant feeding, were started in France in 1890. In New York in 1893, milk stations for impoverished and working mothers were founded by the philanthropist Nathan Strauss, and in 1908 New York City established the first governmental Division of Child Hygiene in its Health Department. As an approach to reducing infant mortality, the idea grew so rapidly that by 1915 there were 538 infant welfare stations under both voluntary and governmental auspices throughout the United States. In 1921, the Sheppard-Towner Act was passed to give federal grants to localities for extending preventive "well-baby clinics" throughout the nation. While terminated because of American Medical Association opposition in 1929, this program was the precedent for Title V of the Social Security Act, on maternal and child health services, in 1935.

Space does not permit review of the somewhat comparable origins of other prevention-oriented clinics for venereal disease, mental hygiene, and other categorical purposes in the early 20th century. Suffice to say that voluntary agency initiative was invariably followed by Health Department organization, to put these clinics on a firmer basis. There was plenty of controversy along the way with the private medical profession—resolved by confining the focus of these clinics to prevention, just as hospitals softened the attacks on their OPDs by confining their services to the poor who were essentially outside the medical marketplace.

Origins of other ambulatory units for specialized population groups may only be mentioned. To thwart the spread of communicable disease and to detect defects which might impair learning, school clinics were organized in America around the turn of the century. A little later, after the first workmen's compensation legislation in this country (it had started in central Europe in the 1880s), industrial clinics were organized in the larger factories. Voluntary societies organized special clinics for crippled children, for cancer, for dental service, for defects of vision or hearing. Special governmental clinic services came later for military veterans, for Indians, for migrant agricultural workers, and others.

One form of organized clinic took shape in America which did not have a precedent in Europe. In the free-wheeling New World society, medical specialization developed more rapidly and without the discipline or requiring memberships (through examinations and other procedures) in royal societies or academies. The specialties were not linked closely to hospital appointments and most of the self-declared specialist's work was done from his private office. In this atmosphere, the coordination of the specialties outside hospital wards or out-patient departments could offer obvious advantages to both doctor and patient. The Mayo brothers saw the benefits of the idea in the small town of Rochester, Minnesota, in the 1880s, and the "group medical practice" concept was born. Like most innovations, the idea was greeted with hostility by private solo-practicing doctors and it grew slowly, taking small spurts from the initiative of younger doctors returning to civilian life after World Wars I and then II. Nevertheless, the share of practicing doctors teaming-up in medical groups slowly grew, to become another stream in the many-faceted movement toward organization of ambulatory care.

This brief historical review would not be complete, however, without mentioning the movement of the 1920s for integrated "health centers," even though it did not succeed in the form advocated. In Great Britain, the Consultative Council on Medical and Allied Services (chaired by Lord Dawson of Penn) had issued in 1920 its report recommending a network of health centers, in which general practitioners, backed up by nurses, social workers, technicians, clerks, etc., would give primary care to everyone. A more modest form of health center was advocated by Herman Biggs, New York State's commissioner of Health, about the same time—the Biggs centers being intended to house all public clinics and offer primary medical care to the poor only. The same concept was proposed by John Pomeroy, Health Officer of Los Angeles County, California. For similar reasons—strong opposition from the private medical profession—none of these ideas got off the ground either in England or America, although they did become implemented in British colonies overseas and in the Soviet Union, which had just had its Revolution in 1917.

In America, some health centers did, in fact, become organized but with a much more restricted purpose. Modeled somewhat after the "settlement house" movement in the first two decades of the 20th century, health facilities were established in the slums of big cities to house under one roof the clinics of the Health Department, the anti-tuberculosis society, the voluntary Visiting Nurse Association, the Milk and Baby Hygiene Association, and so on. They did not offer medical treatment, but they integrated the activities of numerous public and private agencies offering preventive or other ancillary services. In 1920, an American Red Cross survey reported 72 such centers in 49 cities around the nation. Economies in way of shared rentals, common waiting rooms, etc., were achieved, and convenience was an advantage for the poor families who used these centers. In the 1930s, under the New Deal's Public Works Administration, and in the 1940s, through the Hill-Burton Act, further health centers of this type were constructed to house local Health Departments in rural counties or district branches of public health agencies in large cities, with space often provided as well for various voluntary health associations. Not until the 1960s was the comprehensive health center idea reborn, but in another form which we will consider below.

While sketchy, this may be enough of a background to provide perspective on the several currents in the movement toward increasing organization of ambulatory health services in the United States today. It may, at least, serve to show the very different origins of the various currents in the stream, which have in common only their attention to the non-institutionalized patient and the general conceptual theme of furnishing health services to the sick or the well on a teamwork basis.

The Multiple Organized Ambulatory Services Today

With this heterogeneous background, it is easy to see why we can identify some seven or more (depending on how one classifies them) fairly distinct types of organized ambulatory services (OAS) in the United States today. In a sense, of course, all health services are "organized," if we consider that the most isolated medical or dental practitioner is usually assisted by an office nurse or aide, he maintains some sort of record system, he holds informal links with a hospital and with other practitioners, and so on. But if we demand for the definition something more than this—a setting in which several health personnel collaborate, where the decisions are made not by one person but through some team process, or as part of an organizational framework, where the services are usually (though not always) financed in some collectivized or shared manner, then we can categorize OAS units into at least the following types:

- hospital out-patient departments
- public health clinics
- industrial health units
- school health services
- private group medical practice
- special governmental programs
- special voluntary programs

A few words may be said about the current status and trends of each of these.

Hospital Out-Patient Departments

Probably the most ubiquitous type of OAS unit of all is the organized service for out-patients associated with general and special hospitals. Usually subclassified as 1. scheduled clinics, 2. emergency services, and 3. referred services, one or more of these types is found in the great majority of hospitals in the nation. Since more will be said of this crucial form of OAS activity below, we may observe here only that the rate of use of these OPD services has in the last two decades been continually rising, so that today it constitutes some 18 percent of all ambulatory patient-doctor contacts in the nation during a year.

Public Health Clinics

At the local city or county level there are about 1,700 public health agencies in the United States, focussing mainly on organized preventive activities, but probably with no two offering an identical complement of services. In a 1968 survey of all of them, the ten most frequently reported types of personal health service provided were these:[4]

Personal Health Program	*Percentage of Public Health Units*
Tuberculosis	97
Venereal disease	85
Child health	84
Crippled children	72
Dental health	66
Prenatal service	62
Heart disease	57
Mental hygiene	55
Adult health	52
Cancer control	42

The precise content and meaning of each of these categories of programs, of course, differ, but nearly always they included some form of clinic. Based on a comparable survey 20 years earlier, the above figures show a rise in every category, except for a small decline in venereal disease control activities (doubtless as simple penicillin therapy brought these diseases within the easier management of private doctors). In each public health jurisdiction there are typically several clinics or clinic-sessions of each type. In 1970, for example, the U.S. Maternal and Child Health Service reported that about 1,500,000 children made an estimated 5,000,000 visits to the child health clinics, where they receive immunizations, detection of physical or mental disorders, and where their mothers get guidance on diet and child-rearing practices.[5] For definitive diagnosis and treatment the child is typically referred to a private doctor or a pediatric clinic at a hospital OPD or to one of the new-type C. and Y. (children and youth) special clinics in poor districts.

Counting all types of public health program, one cannot offer a firm figure on the number of persons served nor the number of clinic-visits, per year, but there is no doubt that it has been gradually rising. Perhaps more important has been the widening range of categories of clinic sponsored by Health Departments, especially involving general primary care, including treatment of the sick. The days of the narrow categorical public health clinic are probably numbered, in favor of comprehensive primary care units for all people (even low income may cease to be a requirement under conditions of national health insurance) in a district.

Industrial Health Units

While stimulated, as noted above, by the workmen's compensation laws, in-plant health services have gradually widened their horizons. Employers, especially in larger plants, have come to recognize that healthier workers mean greater productivity and that the early detection of disorders can reduce more serious disabilities later.

The number of in-plant or on-site industrial clinics in the United States is not available. A sample survey of the U.S. Department of Labor in 1972 showed, however, that 65 percent of America's nearly 60,000,000 non-farm workers in about 5,000,000 work places were provided with the services of a physician on-the-job, full-time or part-time, or had arrangements with a nearby clinic for the provision of medical care.[6] Only about one-sixth of these were full-time in-plant physicians (thus serving 5,347,000 workers), the rest being part-time, but 21 percent of employees (12,140,000) were in work places staffed by industrial nurses, about 85 percent of whom were full-time.

We know that the adequacy of these OAS industrial units is very much dependent on the size of the plant. Based on another 1972 survey by the National Industrial Conference Board, in establishments of 50,000 or more workers, 100 percent had physicians on the premises, of whom 81 percent were full-time.[7] This staffing declined steadily to 16 percent of plants with under 1,000 employees, and in only about 20 percent of these plants were the doctors full-time. The staffing with nurses is better, so that if we tabulate work places having either physicians or nurses, full-time or part-time, available on the premises, the relationships in 1972 were as follows:

Number of Employees	*Percentage with Physicians or Nurses*
50,000 and over	100
10,000–49,999	90
5,000–9,999	82
2,500–4,999	70
1,000–2,499	59
Under 1,000	33

The range of services varies in much the same way, being broader in the large plants. In the smallest plants, the services may include only first-aid for injuries, while in the largest they tend to include occupational health surveillance, employee examination and placement, general periodic health examination, some non-occupational health care, management of problems like alcoholism and drug abuse, health education, and so on. Since we know that a majority of American workers are employed in establishments of under 1,000 employees, it is likely that less than half are served by systematic in-plant clinics, but the enactment of the Occupational Safety and Health Act (OSHA) of 1970 will doubtless lead to expansion of these services.

Another work-related OAS that should be mentioned is the series of "labor health centers," started by unions, but now usually operated by labor-management trust funds, around the nation. Started by the ILGWU (International Ladies Garment Workers Union) in New York City in 1913, these ambulatory service centers grew noticeably after World War II, with the Sidney Hillman Health Centers of the Amalgamated Clothing Workers of America, the Labor Health Institute (Teamsters Union) of St. Louis, the U.A.W. Health Center in

Detroit, and many others. About 150 such centers now operate, with different scopes of service, but generally stressing diagnostic work-ups, detection of occupational disease, traumatology, primary care, and other services not readily covered by the usual hospital-linked health insurance plans. In California, several such labor centers offer dental care and multiphasic screening examinations.

School Health Services

Originating out of concern for identifying and isolating communicable diseases in school children, as we have noted, organized school clinics have become standard facilities in most of the nation's approximately 90,000 elementary and 32,000 secondary schools. And, as for industrial services, their scopes have gradually broadened from infection control to detection of physical and mental defects, health education, first aid, and special programs to cope with problems of high school youth like drug abuse and teen-age pregnancies.

The great majority of school health clinics and programs are administered by educational authorities. This was so in 80 percent of cities surveyed in 1966,[8] though responsibility is more frequently under Departments of Health in rural school districts. A study back in 1953 found that in 85 percent of city school systems, nurses were employed, and in 63 percent there were school physicians.[9] In the same year over 8,000 doctors in the United States were doing full-time or part-time school health work. In the earlier study of the American Academy of Pediatrics, it was found that 22 percent of all school-age children lived in counties without a regular school medical service; but, put the other way around, 78 percent of children lived in counties with a regular medical or nursing service in the schools.[10] The situation has doubtless improved since then. While it is not feasible to estimate the volume of ambulatory services provided by these programs, it would seem safe to say that the roughly 50,000,000 primary and secondary school children in 1970 were predominantly accessible to first-aid services in school clinics and—if only on the basis of state legislation—had physical examinations at least two or three times during their school years for visual, hearing, or other defects which could impair learning.

As for the approximately 6,000,000 youths in colleges or universities, organized health services are more typically available and comprehensive.[11] Being often away from home, these young adults are usually served by clinics and hospitals or infirmaries offering fairly complete therapeutic and preventive services. The student usually pays a prepaid amount for these services, even in public universities, and the medical personnel are on salaries. While generalization from one institution is obviously not justified, it is of interest that at the University of California-Los Angeles in 1969 there were over 90,000 physician-patient contacts, or more than three per student per year, not counting more than 110,000 laboratory and X-ray procedures, physiotherapy services, immunizations, etc. Even if the rate were half this level at the average college or university in the country, it would constitute a significant volume of organized ambulatory service to young people.

Private Group Practice

In the purely private sector, the grouping of physicians into teams of three or more, with varying patterns of income sharing, took a sharp spurt in the late 1960s and 1970s. The American Medical Association Inventory of Physicians found 6,371 medical groups so defined with 40,093 physicians in 1969.[12] This constituted 19.9 percent of non-federally employed physicians engaged in clinical patient care (excluding interns and residents). While two-thirds of these physicians were in small 3–4 doctor groups, the tendency of small groups has been to grow larger. Looked at another way, about two-thirds of the 40,000 doctors were in multi-specialty groups, and one-third in single-specialty groups.

Unlike other forms of OAS, group practice is found to be more frequent in states of more rural character, lower population density, and more recently developed.[13] One can hardly escape the conclusion that where medical societies are less powerful, where the traditions of private practice are less entrenched, and where the economic rationale for grouping is greater, the hostility to group practice has been weaker and this innovation has grown more successfully. The high failure rate of group practices in the generally hostile professional environment of past years is replaced today by a predominant preference of this form of work among new medical graduates and a steady enlargement in its strength. While today only about 400 or 6 percent of medical groups are linked (over 50 percent of their income) to prepayment plans, it seems likely that such groups are natural seeds for the growth of "health maintenance organizations" of the future.

There has been much discussion of the "productivity" per doctor of physicians in group practice, compared with solo practice. In the estimates offered below, to be on the conservative side, we assume the same productivity for the two modes of practice—that is, an average of 96 office visits per week and 48 working weeks per year, or a total of about 4,600 ambulatory patient-contacts per doctor per year.[14]

Special Governmental Programs

The variety of governmental programs (beyond those reviewed above) for organized ambulatory services to special population groups or for the care of selected diseases is too great to describe fully here. Special public programs for military personnel, for veterans, for Indians, for agricultural migrants, and others operate comprehensive ambulatory care clinics by the hundred. Likewise there are the mental health centers, funded mainly by government, and operated by a variety of local public and voluntary bodies.

Of special interest in recent years are the "neighborhood health centers," initiated by the U.S. Office of Economic Opportunity and then transferred to the supervision of the Department of Health, Education and Welfare, about which a few words should be said. In 1974, there were 103 such neighborhood health centers, plus a further 13 "health care networks" (each containing two or more health centers linked to hospitals), and an additional 33 "family health centers."[15] These 153 clinical entities had a total target population of 5,185,000, and in 1974 actually served about 1,300,000 persons (we do not know the number of patient-visits). Family health centers, the newest type, are intended to be financed by prepaid premiums and are open to self-supporting people who may be above an established poverty line. All these types, however, are constructed only in areas of health care scarcity which, in effect, means localities of very low income, and their services are intended almost exclusively for the poor—although not necessarily recipients of welfare assistance.

The neighborhood health centers are typically well staffed, not only with primary doctors and allied health personnel, but also with specialists and professionals in paramedical fields like optometry, podiatry, or clinical psychology.[16] They are viewed by many as models for organized ambulatory health services that might serve all members of a nearby population some day. Innovative types of health manpower, like nurse practitioners and physician assistants, are being used in many of these health centers, and some are exploring widening their services and financial arrangements to qualify as health maintenance organizations in the future.

Special Voluntary Programs

As with governmental programs, the variety of OAS entities under voluntary auspices, not discussed above, is legion. Special non-governmental clinics for cancer detection, for heart disease, for mental patients, for alcoholism, for family planning, and so on are found in every city. Many of these clinics have been supported by voluntary health agencies for decades. Hundreds have been absorbed into the general out-patient departments of hospitals, but hundreds more remain entirely independent.

Space can be taken here only for noting one new type of voluntary OAS unit that emerged from the problems of alienated youth who organized the so-called free clinics, beginning in 1967. Starting in California, these clinics serve mainly young people separated from their families, who are in need of help for such problems as contraception, abortion of unwanted pregnancies, venereal disease, drug abuse, common respiratory infections, and almost any condition for which treatment can be readily given by a primary care doctor. Organized by the youth themselves, the free clinics are characterized by an easy-going unstructured atmosphere; they are open at night; they operate with a minimum of records or formal procedures; and in general appeal to the anti-Establishment attitudes of their users. Doctors, nurses, and most of the staff give their services without remuneration, so that costs must be faced only for rent, some drugs (many are donated), and often for a clinic-manager. The pattern proved so appropriate to the needs of thousands of young people that by 1970, when a national survey was made, about 170 free clinics were identified in about 30 states.[17]

Many free clinics fail soon after they open, and new ones start. Staffing has been unstable, and equipment has been rudimentary. Yet in some places, such as Los Angeles County, the basic idea has been recognized to be sound enough to lead the county government to subsidize the clinics with drugs and supplies and, moreover, to start a parallel series of "youth clinics" in the official district public health centers, with similar style and objectives. While the whole future of the free clinic movement is quite uncertain, it has clearly taught lessons about consumer initiative in health services and the value of matching clinic procedures to the feelings of its patients.

With this hasty review of the main types of OAS unit today, we may now return to a little closer look at the characteristics of the most numerous of all—the hospital out-patient department.

The Dynamic Hospital OPD

As noted earlier, the rate of use of hospital out-patient departments has been steadily increasing. Especially noteworthy is the fact that, in spite of the availability of Medicare, Medicaid, and other governmental programs to pay for access to private doctors, recourse to hospital clinics—except for a transient slack around 1967—has not declined. Evidently, the demand for ambulatory care exceeds the supply available from individual physicians.

While the several types of hospitals—general short-term, long-term, mental, and other—all tend to offer out-patient services, the most important by far are the OPD services of so-called community hospitals for short-term general illness. Counting all types of hospitals, out-patient visits to the 7,061 facilities in the nation in 1972, according to the American Hospital Association Survey, numbered 219,182,000. Of these the 5,746 community general hospitals provided nearly 163,000,000 patient-visits. The trends in their number and composition over the last 18 years are shown in Table 16-1[18]

It is evident that substantial increases have occurred over this 1954–1972 period, far greater than the growth of U.S. population over these years, in all three categories of OPD service. In 1954, over half of all OPD services were provided in organized clinics (essentially for the poor), the rest divided between emergency and referred services; in 1972, the volume was roughly one-third in each type. The greatest proportionate increase has been in the use of emergency services—about six times—while for referred services the increase was five times and for organized clinics it was about a doubling.

Analyzed by type of hospital sponsorship over the same span of years, the percentage compositions of all OPD services are shown in Table 16-2.

In both years, the voluntary non-profit hospitals gave the lion's share of OPD

Table 16-1
Community Hospital Out-patient Visits, 1954-1972

Type of Visit	*1954*		*1972*	
	Number	*Percent*	*Number*	*Percent*
Emergency	9,419,000	20.2	55,660,000	34.2
Organized Clinic	26,405,000	56.6	53,244,000	32.7
Referred	10,851,000	23.2	53,764,000	33.1
Total	46,675,000	100.0	162,668,000	100.0

services, and this proportion increased from 61 to 67 percent between 1954 and 1972. This has been, however, mainly because of their sheer numbers, which are much greater than the other two sponsorship types. Examining the services in another way, in 1970, when voluntary hospitals had 61.1 percent of the total beds, they provided 53.9 percent of the OPD services, while state and local government hospitals, with 20.9 percent of the beds, provided 31.5 percent of the OPD services. The disparity is more dramatically shown by focusing on the minority of metropolitan counties that have a large public hospital. In 1969, we studied all out-patient services in counties containing a governmental general hospital of 300 beds or more. The OPD services provided by the voluntary hospitals in those counties amounted to 4.5 visits per in-patient admission, compared to 14.0 visits per admission in the public hospitals. Relative to their smaller numbers, in other words, governmental hospitals bear a much heavier share of the OPD load.[19]

We know that the patients attending organized clinics are typically screened for low income eligibility. Numerous studies have shown, however, that a substantial portion of emergency patients—perhaps 30 to 60 percent in different communities—are of incomes higher than would render them eligible for an organized clinic; they come to the hospital simply because they cannot see a private doctor promptly and they have confidence in the hospital's wide range of capabilities. Many studies have shown that the majority of patients coming for these services do not have true emergencies, but rather are seeking non-urgent primary care.[20] Yet the demands continue to rise so steadily, even in hospitals that lack interns and residents who cover so many of the organized clinics in teaching hospitals, that medical staffs have had to adjust with a variety of procedures to offer the emergency services. Most hospitals use a rotational system among their active staff members, but an increasing number are appointing full-time emergency service doctors on salary or other contractual arrangements.

To cope with the rising demands and to make services more convenient for people, an increasing number of hospitals are also developing satellite health centers under their responsibility for ambulatory care. Like the organized home-care movement of the 1950s, this is extending the hospital's services outward into the

Table 16-2
OPD Services, by Hospital Sponsorship, 1954–1972

Hospital Sponsorship	*Percent*	
	1954	*1972*
State & local government	31.7	28.2
Voluntary	60.8	67.1
Proprietary	7.5	4.7
Total	100.0	100.0

community. The use of nurse-practitioners for screening or triage of patients is another way of reducing the load on OPD doctors and permitting more time for care of the serious cases. Establishing "medical arts buildings" for private doctor's offices adjacent to the hospital is still another adjustment. These and other innovations are, in a sense, helping to shape the modern hospital as the community center for medical care, both in-patient and ambulatory. Space does not permit discussion of organizational changes in the equipping, management, and operation of hospital OPDs, but suffice to say that from its second-class status, the out-patient service is coming to occupy an increasingly important place in the overall hospital administrative structure.

General Trends and Issues

Taking an overview of all the forms of organized ambulatory health services, reviewed above as seven principal streams of development, what can be said in conclusion? It is perfectly clear that a rising share of all patient-doctor encounters in the United States are occurring in some sort of organized setting. It is not so easy, however, to quantify this trend or even to measure the proportions today.

To offer a rough order-of-magnitude, however, on the situation in the early 1970s, one may take note that the U.S. National Health survey reports about 5.0 ambulatory doctor-patient contacts per person per year (not counting in-hospital visits). For America's approximately 215,000,000 population in civilian life and outside of institutions, this would amount to a total of about 1,100,000,000 ambulatory medical services per year. Relating this to the few statistical figures we have may permit some such estimates as the following in Table 16-3.

Admittedly the various estimates of ambulatory services and their percentage distributions among various settings are extremely crude. The safest judgment might be that in the early 1970s about half of ambulatory patient-doctor encounters in the United States took place in organized settings, and the other half took place in private doctor's offices. Whatever the accurate figures may be (the determination of which would require more rigorous record and reporting systems

Table 16-3
Ambulatory Services by Type of Setting

Type of Ambulatory Service	*Estimated Number of Visits*	*Percent*
Hospital out-patient departments	200,000,000[a]	18.2
Public health clinics	30,000,000[b]	2.7
Industrial health units	40,000,000[c]	3.6
School and college health services	55,000,000[d]	5.0
Private group practice	185,000,000[e]	16.8
Special government programs	25,000,000[f]	2.3
Special voluntary agencies	20,000,000[g]	1.8
Private medical practice	545,000,000[h]	49.5
All types	1,100,000,000	100.0

a. Count of all institutional OPD services in 1972 by the American Hospital Association (219,000,000), and subtracting those services estimated to be provided to in-patients.
b. Estimate extrapolated from count of child health services tabulated by U.S. Dept. of H.E.W., in consideration of other public health clinics.
c. Estimate based on survey of medically staffed industrial health units by U.S. Dept. of Labor.
d. Estimate based on numbers of elementary, secondary school, and college students with health services, reported by U.S. Office of Education.
e. Estimate based on the American Medical Association 1969 count of 40,093 privately practicing physicians engaged in group practice and assuming the same average number of patients seen per year (4,600) as seen by all doctors (discussed in text above).
f. Estimate extrapolated from count of persons served by "neighborhood health centers," considering numerous other special programs.
g. Estimate extrapolated from approximate "free clinic" attendance, considering numerous other special voluntary programs.
h. This figure is simply the balance derived by subtracting the sum of previous seven figures from the total of 1,100,000,000.

than we now have), there can be no doubt that the proportion of ambulatory services occurring in organized frameworks is gradually rising in the United States.

It may be noted that this estimate does not consider how the doctor is paid, whether by fee-for-service, by salary, or some other method, nor does it consider how the money has been derived—whether from governmental revenues, from voluntary insurance, out-of-pocket, or in some other way. It considers only the manner of delivery of the ambulatory service, preventive or therapeutic.

This question of delivery patterns, however, is perhaps the greatest source of contention in the current national ferment about medical care. Despite the wide consensus that seems to be approaching on some form of national health insurance, acrid controversy continues on the patterns of delivery of care. The degree to which HMOs are to be promoted is hotly debated. The implementation of PSROs (Professional Standard Review Organizations) is fraught with contentious problems. Newly formulated "health system agencies" (or similar bodies with different names) to combine the previous functions of CHP (comprehensive health planning), RMP (regional medical programs for various chronic diseases), and Hill-Burton (hospital construction) programs are the subject of six bills* before the federal Congress.[21] The net effects of all these measures can hardly be predicted, but it seems likely that they will move our overall health care system toward more organized and disciplined patterns.

This judgment is reinforced by the observations in this review of organized ambulatory health services in America indicating that, even without a systematic national plan, they have been moving in that direction. By the very nature of our ever more complex society and our advancing technology, the provision of health services—ambulatory, no less than institutional and environmental—demands increasingly organized systems.[22] Despite the difficulties of bigness and bureaucracy, this movement seems to be the only way to approach the achievement of health care equity in the modern world.

References

1. René Sand, *The Advance to Social Medicine,* London: Staples Press, 1952.
2. Michael M. Davis and Andrew R. Warner, *Dispensaries: Their Management and Development,* New York: Macmillan Company, 1918.
3. Milton I. Roemer, *Evaluation of Community Health Centers,* Geneva: World Health Organization, 1972.
4. Beverlee A. Myers et al., "The Medical Care Activities of Local Health Units," *Public Health Reports,* 83:757–769, September 1968.
5. U.S. Department of Health, Education and Welfare, Maternal and Child Health Service, *Maternal and Child Health Services of State and Local Health Departments, Fiscal Year 1970,* Washington 1971.
6. U.S. Department of Labor, *Occupational Injuries and Illnesses by Industry, 1972,* Washington: Bureau of Labor Statistics Bull. No. 1830, 1974.
7. Seymour Lusterman, *Industry Roles in Health Care,* New York City: The Conference Board, 1973.
8. J. M. Wolf and H. C. Pritham, "Administrative Patterns of School Health Services," *Journal of the American Medical Association,* 193:195–199, 19 July 1966.
9. H. F. Kilander, "Health Services in City Schools—Administrative Aspects," *American Journal of Public Health,* 43:314–321, March 1953.
10. American Academy of Pediatrics, *Child Health Services and Pediatric Education,* New York: Commonwealth Fund, 1949, pp. 115–116.
11. Norman S. Moore and John Summerskill, *Health Services in American Colleges and Universities, 1953,* Ithaca, N.Y.: Cornell University, 1954.
12. "Nearly 20 Percent of Physicians in Group Practice in 1969," *American Medical News,* 15:15, 18 September 1972.
13. Milton I. Roemer, Jorge A. Mera, and William Shonick, "The Ecology of Group Medical Practice in the United States," *Medical Care,* 12:627–637, August 1974.
14. American Medical Association, *The Profile of Medical Practice,* Chicago, 1972.

*The final National Health Planning and Resources Development Act became law in December 1974.

15. Paul B. Batalden (Director, Bureau of Community Health Services, U.S. Dept. of Health, Education & Welfare), personal letter, 27 June 1974.
16. Lisbeth Bamberger Schorr and Joseph T. English, "Background, Context, and Significant Issues in Neighborhood Health Center Programs," *Milbank Memorial Fund Quarterly,* 46:289–296, July 1968.
17. Jerome L. Schwartz, *The National Free Clinic Survey,* Berkeley: University of California Institute of Business and Economic Research, Reprint No. 9, 1971.
18. Derived from the "Annual Survey of Hospitals," American Hospital Association, 1954 and 1972.
19. Milton I. Roemer and Jorge A. Mera, " 'Patient-dumping' and Other Voluntary Agency Contributions to Public Agency Problems," *Medical Care,* 11:30–39, January–February 1973.
20. Paul R. Torrens and Donna Yedvab, "Variations Among Emergency Room Populations: A Comparison of Four Hospitals in New York City," *Medical Care* 8:60–75, January–February, 1970.
21. U.S. House of Representatives, Subcommittee on Public Health and Environment, *Proposals for Health Planning, Development, and Regulation: A Comparison,* Washington: Government Printing Office, 1974.
22. Anne R. Somers, *Health Care in Transition: Directions for the Future,* Chicago: Hospital Research and Educational Trust, 1971.

17

Group Practice: A Medical Care Spectrum

While most organization of ambulatory services has been sponsored by hospitals, health departments, and other agencies, much has been launched by individual doctors voluntarily joining together in groups. This "group practice" movement has taken many forms, varying from simple informal arrangements to complex aggregations of specialists linked with health insurance programs.

Thus, the group organization of private physicians can be conceived as a spectrum of patterns. The movement as a whole has steadily expanded, in response to the complexities of medical technology and the demands for greater efficiency in rendering care to patients.

TO THE RUGGED individualist of American medicine, group practice may still loom as a specter. But a more balanced view shows it to be part of a spectrum—a range of methods of medical service between polar extremes of solo and team performance. As in any spectrum, the lines which separate different bands in the range are not sharp but fuzzy. Moreover, the width and intensity of the bands are changing every day. Group practice is a concept and a trend that has taken many forms in American medicine and, for that matter, in world medicine. An understanding of this can help doctors to evaluate better the bubbling cauldron of medical practice in which they find themselves.

One can see the picture most clearly by historical recollection of the nineteenth century healing art. The doctor—a general practitioner—was not only the keystone of medical care, he was almost the whole arch. He seldom sent a patient to the hospital; there were few specialists for consultation, and not many auxiliary personnel. In 1900 for every 10 physicians there were only 6 other health workers of all types, compared with 90 today.

This lonely, all-encompassing general practitioner is still found in America, but he is rare. Even in rural practice he usually has some access to a hospital and to specialists not very far away. But everywhere, and most strikingly in larger cities, general practice has evolved into other professional forms. These forms constitute an evolution toward increasingly complex teams of doctors and ancillary personnel.

Chapter 17 originally appeared in the *Journal of Medical Education,* 40:1154–1158, December, 1965, and is reprinted by permission of that journal.

Description of Bands

Just as in biological evolution, the earlier forms survive even when the later ones have taken shape. And so we see today the many forms of medical practice operating side by side. As previously noted, they stand as a spectrum in which one can distinguish at least the following 8 bands or stages: solo general practice, specialty practice, single-specialty medical groups, the medical arts building, hospital-based ambulatory medical care, partial coordinated group practice, comprehensive group practice with fee-patients, and comprehensive prepaid group practice.

A closer examination of these bands may shed some light on long-term trends in American medical care.

Solo General Practice

The isolated general practitioner, ancestor of the current race, is the first band in the spectrum. Of course, his isolation is never complete. He renders much of his service with the economic support of health insurance plans or public programs. Even if he has no hospital appointment, he sends patients to specialists and to hospitals. The bulk of his practice, however, is independent home and office care.

Specialty Practice

Most specialists depend on referrals for their practice. Only a small proportion of their patients come to them directly; most are sent by another physician—a general practitioner or another specialist. Whether the arrangement is formalized or not (and it seldom is), there is a certain "social system" to these referrals. The specialist can be represented on a complex community map by a pin to which are radiated paths of patients from many other doctors. The identity of those referring doctors may be largely defined by hospital staff connections. The ease of flow of patients along these paths is influenced by many professional, personal, and economic factors.

Thus, there is a certain "grouping" of medical service even in independent specialty practice. The vitality of medical-staff organization in the general hospital enhances this liaison, both within its walls and outside. The interdependence is fostered, too, by the demands of patients, who increasingly seek specialist attention and request referral or consultation.

Within a given specialty (or within general practice) physicians have also learned the advantages of having close colleagues who will cover for them while they are away. Even telephone answering services facilitate such *locum tenens* arrangements, as does the office nurse.

Single-specialty Medical Groups

An extension of the latter idea is seen in the grouping of 2 or 3 or more specialists of the same field in a common office suite. In 1959 a U.S. Public Health Service survey indicated that there were in this country 392 single-specialty medical groups of 3 or more physicians with some income-sharing plan.[1] There are undoubtedly more, if one considers office-sharing without income-sharing. Waiting rooms, receptionists, telephone service, laboratory, record rooms, and business services are frequently shared by a group of obstetricians or radiologists or internists. A senior man may sometimes invite 1 or more younger colleagues in the same field to join him as partner(s), or even as employee(s).

Such grouping is sometimes associated with a degree of subspecialization within a specialty; internists, for example, may combine gastroenterology with cardiology. In England (less so in America) a group of general practitioners frequently come together with an informal concentration among them in fields like dermatology or minor surgery or pediatrics. Usually, however, the single-specialty medical group contributes more to the convenience of the doctor than to any significant coordination of medical care for the patient.

The Medical Arts Building

European visitors are usually impressed by the sight in many American cities of large buildings which house the private offices of physicians, dentists, and optometrists, along with a drug store, clinical laboratory, and other health-related facilities. The medical arts building, while usually purely commercial in origin, is a step toward coordination of medical care—if only on a geographic level.

A thorough study of the dynamics of medical arts buildings has yet to be made, but certain features are quite evident. They vary greatly in size from small, single-story suburban structures with offices for 3 or 4 practitioners, to large blocks with 100 or more office suites in the downtown section of a city. In the latter a full range of specialists will usually be found, in addition to the laboratory, pharmacy, and other resources. Robert E. Mytinger, in a brief unpublished study of 4 such buildings in Los Angeles, found that the specialists in them tended to refer a large proportion of patients to each other. Acquaintance on a common hospital staff often fostered these relationships. The private clinical laboratory in each building was extensively used, as was the pharmacy. In some of the buildings a conference room which could be used by any of the tenants was provided.

Smaller buildings are often built and owned by physicians themselves, and the suites are rented intentionally to men in a range of specialties. The architectural layouts are often specifically designed to meet the needs of fields like radiology or pediatrics.

While the medical arts building, of course, lacks income-sharing among its occupants and is far from demonstrating full teamwork in patient care, it still encourages a certain level of coordination. Proximity of the many elements of medical care offers great conveniences for the patient as well as the doctor. When 1 of the doctors is away, temporary coverage of his practice is easily arranged. The mere physical association may encourage referrals or, at least, informal consultation.

Within the medical arts building band in the group-practice spectrum, there are various gradations. Some involve professional interplay among their occupants more than others. There is doubtless opportunity for substantial development in this architectural device to bring together the specialties.

Hospital-Based Ambulatory Medical Care

For bed care of the sick, the hospital has long embodied a form of coordinated group practice, but even for ambulatory service this is true. The well-developed out-patient department, especially in a large teaching hospital, presents a symphony of specialties. Sometimes the music is discordant, when the players do not relate effectively to each other, and the poor patient is lost in the clatter. But a growing number of ambulatory service units in hospitals are attempting to offer harmonious "comprehensive medicine."[2]

With the striking increase in the rate of use of hospital emergency rooms (as distinguished from organized out-patient departments) in recent years, medical staffs have been faced with the challenge of proper round-the-clock coverage. A variety of patterns have evolved, from rotation of "on-call" duties among the attending doctors to various forms of full-time salaried appointment.

These patterns of ambulatory service usually involve the part-time groupings of physicians, but at a growing number of hospitals the full professional life of the doctor is based in or adjacent to the institution. A study published in 1960 identified some 268 hospitals where clusters of private medical offices were located in hospitals or in special buildings next to them. While these doctors are typically in private practice, their physical association with a hospital and with each other obviously promotes some interchange and coordination in their professional work.

This is quite aside from the full-fledged group medical practice clinic attached to a hospital, which belongs in another band of the spectrum.

Partial Coordinated Group Practice

A sixth band in the continuum of medical practice may be represented by a number of patterns which bring together diverse specialists in organized working relationships. Here is where the usual definition of group practice begins, that is,

3 or more physicians of different specialties working together at 1 location and sharing income according to some prearranged plan. But the service provided or the dedication of the doctors need not be complete.

There are small medical groups of only 3 or 4 physicians, who obviously cannot provide a comprehensive scope of specialty service. Sometimes these small groups are supplemented by a long panel of specialists "on-call"—a pattern common in southern California, according to a doctoral investigation by Donald M. Dubois. Or the group may be larger, but it may engage the efforts of some or all of its members only part-time, while a good share of professional time is spent in solo practice at another location. (Many of the "labor health centers" fit this model.) Or the group may be large and full-time, but it may limit its services to diagnosis, sending patients back to the referring physician for treatment. Some of the nationally famous clinics built their reputations on such a policy.

These patterns represent partial group practice; and though this type of practice includes the critical feature of income-sharing, it does not stand at the final pole of the spectrum.

Comprehensive Group Practice with Fee-Patients

The classical model of group medical practice, for which praises are sung or epithets hurled, is that involving a full range of medical and surgical specialties, all the necessary supportive services, full-time dedication of the physicians in a well-planned clinic building, sharing of income, and a careful program of self-education and research. To many, the Mayo Clinic is the accepted ideal. This is the pattern responsible for the advantages in terms of sound scientific medicine for the patient and a better life for the doctor. It is also responsible for the alleged disadvantages, in terms of impersonality for the patient and loss of freedom for the doctor.

In the 1959 Public Health Service survey,[1] there were 215 such medical groups with over 10 full-time physicians. Over 5,500 physicians were in these clinics. The patients served by these medical groups are largely private, and for their care they pay fees either individually or through some insurance plan. Only about 10 to 15 percent of all medical groups are associated with a specifically prepaid population for whom the clinic assumes full medical-care responsibility. The latter represent the final band in the spectrum of medical service.

Comprehensive Prepaid Group Practice

The ultimate expression of group medical practice is found in those circumstances where a full panoply of medical resources is combined with an economic arrangement through which a specified population has full access to them.[4] The Kaiser-Permanente Health Plan and the Health Insurance Plan of Greater New

York are the best known models, but there are about 200 others. A comprehensive range of specialty services is provided to a population which prepays for care in the clinic, home, or hospital.

In this pattern of medical care, the responsibility for health maintenance is, in large measure, shifted from the patient to the doctor. Since a fixed annual premium is paid regardless of the individual's rate of illness, there is built-in incentive toward prevention. There are no financial impediments to referral, as in solo practice, nor toward excessive case work-ups or treatment, as may occur in group practice with fee-for-service payment. Liaison among the doctors in the group is fortified by a relationship with patients which is independent of economic considerations. Medical care is shifted from episodic to continuous, from segmental to comprehensive.

Conclusion

This is the spectrum of patterns of medical practice for the ambulatory patient in America today. At what place in the range should one say that "true" group practice begins? Some would say only at band 7, others at band 5 or 4. But the point is that some degree of medical teamwork is operative—at a rising tempo—all along the way.

More important, the trend is clearly toward incresing strength at the coordinated end of the spectrum. A slowly but steadily rising proportion of physicians are practicing in the more coordinated patterns. The growth of "pure" group practices, of the band 7 and 8 types, has not been spectacular; hardly 6 percent of American physicians are now so engaged. The overall movement, however, is clear. And if some quantified account could be taken of the changes at the lower bands in the spectrum, the trend toward medical grouping would doubtless appear more striking.

The basic concept of teamwork among the medical specialties is well established. In our free-wheeling American culture, it is applied in varying degrees and different forms. Experience with the looser forms may pave the path toward greater acceptability of the more structured ones. But all the forms of medical cordination serve as adaptations, partial or complete, to the technical demands of an expanding science.

References

1. Pomrinse, S. D. and Goldstein, M. S. The 1959 Survey of Group Practice. *Amer. J. Public Health,* 51:671–682, May, 1961.
2. Weinerman, E. R. and Edwards, H. R. Changing Patterns in Hospital Emergency Service. *Hospitals* (in press).

3. Rorem, C. R. *Physicians' Private Offices at Hospitals*. Philadelphia: Hospital Council of Philadelphia, September, 1958 (multilithed).
4. Falk, L. A., Mushrush, G. J. and Skrivanek, M. E. *Administrative Aspects of Prepaid Group Practice: An Annotated Bibliography 1950–1962*. Pittsburgh: University of Pittsburgh Press, 1963.

18

The Ecology of Group Medical Practice in the United States

Despite its private professional origins, the group practice idea was opposed by most physicians in its early years. Many social factors influenced its growth or inhibition, so that one finds wide variations in the extent to which clinical physicians of the 50 states are engaged in this organized pattern of health service.

Using multiple regression techniques, colleagues Jorge Mera, William Shonick, and I set out to discover the social and professional factors which were associated with the much greater growth of group practice in some states than in others. The results of this analysis were presented at a conference of the International Epidemiological Association in Sydney, Australia, August, 1973.

OF THE SEVERAL major mechanisms being used to organize the delivery of health services in the world, one of the few to originate in the United States was group medical practice. The hospital, the health insurance program, the public health agency, the visiting nurse association, the rural health center—these and many other social patterns were started by European nations and eventually spread elsewhere. The organization of teams of private physicians, however, for integrated provision of various components of medical care was an American innovation which, in diverse forms, has now been adopted in many other countries. The pioneering demonstration of the idea is usually credited to the Mayo brothers, who started their now famous clinic in a small Minnesota town (Rochester) in 1887.[16]

Group Practice Growth

The social and professional reasons that group practice took root first and then grew in American soil need not be fully explored here. The robust growth of medical and surgical specialization in the freewheeling American culture doubtless was involved.[18] The extensive practice of specialties in private offices, in contrast to their predominant linkage to hospitals in Europe and elsewhere, probably had much to do with it.[14] Also, influences were certainly associated with the

Chapter 18 originally appeared in *Medical Care,* 12:627–637, August, 1974, and is reprinted by permission of that journal.

rapid settlement of the New World, the move across the continent from East to West where, overnight, medical and other resources had to be launched.

The historical development of group medical practice in America has taken place in stages over the last 85 years. Suffice it to say, the process has not been a smooth, continuous one, but rather an irregular flow which moved quite slowly at first, and then took forward leaps after World Wars I and II. It was, in fact, a social struggle encountering much opposition within the medical profession, where it was for years widely condemned as "unethical."[17] It was even inhibited by legal constraints on "corporate practice" in many states. Among the population at large, team service was commonly greeted with suspicion, as rendering medical care mechanistic and impersonal—something acceptable in charity clinics for the poor but not suitable for the private paying patient. Up to 1950, less than 5 percent of all active American physicians were engaged in group practice.

Yet, during the last 20 years or so, group medical practice has gradually come to be accepted as a sound pattern for delivery of high quality medical care in the United States. It has evolved into several forms, the most important categorization probably being the multispecialty and the single-specialty types. The legal forms vary, comprising partnerships, sole proprietorships, nonprofit associations, and corporate entities. Relationships with hospitals may be "open" or "closed." Earnings may be divided among the physicians according to various formulas.[9] Most interesting perhaps is the linkage of a small but increasing proportion of group practices with health insurance or prepayment programs. While the new federal government strategy for promotion of "health maintenance organizations" (HMOs) allows various delivery patterns, the "prepaid group practice plan" has figured prominently.[10] Table 18-1 summarizes the general trend in group practice growth in the United States from 1932 to 1969.

Table 18-1
Growth in Group Medical Practice: Number of Group Practices,* Doctors in Them, and Proportions of Total Active Physicians, United States, 1932-1969

Year	*Number of Groups*	*Number of Physicians in Group Practice*	*Percentage of All Active Physicians*
1932	239	1,466	0.9
1940	335	2,093	1.2
1946	368	3,084	2.6
1950	500	–	–
1959	1,546	12,009	5.2
1965	4,289	28,381	10.2
1969	6,162	38,834	12.8

Source: University of Michigan, School of Public Health, Medical Care Chart Book, 2nd ed. (1964) and 5th ed. (1972).
*For definition, consult the text.

Differentials Among States and "Explanatory" Variables

Despite this story of overall national progress, within the borders of the United States the rate of growth of group practice has been far from uniform among different states and regions. A meaningful measure of these differential growth rates is the *percentage* of all active non-Federal physicians who are engaged in group practice full time in each of the 50 American states. The definition of group practice most widely used is that of the American Medical Association (AMA) (the source of the most recent data) namely:

> three or more physicians formally organized to provide medical care . . . through joint use of equipment and personnel, and with the income from medical practice distributed in accordance with methods previously determined.[15]

Applying this definition (although the AMA definition does not require full-time group practice status), the 50 states ranked by the strength of their group practice development in 1969 are presented in Table 18-2. The above definition, it may be noted, includes both physicians in multispecialty and single-specialty groups, as well as those in a small number of medical groups composed solely of general practitioners. (Separate analyses of the distribution of just the multispecialty groups, by state, are to be made later.) The range of proportions of group practice physicians, expressed as percentages of all active non-Federal physicians (that is, excluding those in employment of the federal government, such as in the military services, Veterans Administration, U.S. Public Health Service, or other federal agencies) extends from 50.1 percent in North Dakota to 4.6 percent in Maryland, or a ratio of about 11 to 1.

The question we set out to answer was: what determines this distribution? What factors in a state's social environment or in its medical setting are associated with a strong, compared with a weak, development of group medical practice? Since group practice is believed to have many valuable attributes, answers to this question might provide clues to social policy decisions which could promote the further extension of this pattern of medical care delivery. In any case, such knowledge could be useful for general social planning.

To answer this question we identified a number of socioenvironmental factors and a number of medical resource factors on which quantitative data were available by states. These factors and acronyms for describing them were as follows:

General Socioenvironmental Factors:

1. Total state population—number from 1970 Census[20] (STATPOP).
2. Aged population—percent 65 years and over[21] (AGED).
3. Youth population—percent under 18 years of age[21] (YOUTH).
4. Income per capita—annual dollars earned per state resident[22] (INCOME).
5. Poverty population—percent of state population in families earning less than governmentally determined threshold, scaled for family size[23] (POOR).
6. Educational level—median years of schooling[20] (EDUC).

7. Population growth—rate of change (usually upward, but in a few states downward) between 1960 and 1970[19] (POPGROW).
8. Density of population—number of persons per square mile[21] (DENSITY).
9. Metropolitan population—percent of population residing in or contiguous to cities of 50,000 or more[21] (METRO).
10. State's year of entry into the United States—the year between 1776 and 1959 when statehood was established[11] (ENTRY).

Table 18-2
Group Practice Strength by States: Numbers and Percentages of All Active Non-Federal Physicians Engaged in Group Medical Practice, in Each State, Ranked by Group Practice Strength (GRPS), United States, 1969

State	*Active Physicians (Non-Federal)*	*Group Practice Physicians*	*Percentage in Group Practice*
North Dakota	579	290	50.1
South Dakota	535	187	35.0
Minnesota	5,671	1,965	34.7
Montana	688	212	31.2
Arkansas	1,629	489	30.8
Wisconsin	5,153	1,494	29.0
Alaska	193	55	28.5
Hawaii	1,106	300	27.1
Oregon	2,925	720	24.6
Nevada	504	122	24.2
Kansas	2,543	588	23.1
Iowa	2,882	663	23.0
North Carolina	5,386	1,087	20.2
Nebraska	1,666	333	20.0
Idaho	646	129	20.0
Louisiana	4,245	824	19.4
Washington	4,827	934	19.3
Mississippi	1,806	329	18.2
Texas	12,566	2,293	18.2
Utah	1,404	253	18.0
California	36,722	6,543	17.8
Virginia	5,388	951	17.7
Oklahoma	2,562	446	17.4
Alabama	3,006	520	17.3
Arizona	2,368	393	16.6
Indiana	5,130	844	16.5
West Virginia	1,822	298	16.4
Colorado	3,717	601	16.2
New Hampshire	1,003	160	16.0
Georgia	4,728	738	15.6
New Mexico	1,042	157	15.1

(continued)

Table 18-2 (Continued)
Group Practice Strength by States: Numbers and Percentages of All Active Non-Federal Physicians Engaged in Group Medical Practice, in Each State, Ranked by Group Practice Strength (GRPS), United States, 1969

State	*Active Physicians (Non-Federal)*	*Group Practice Physicians*	*Percentage in Group Practice*
Tennessee	4,542	673	14.8
Missouri	5,889	874	14.8
Wyoming	313	46	14.7
Kentucky	3,252	460	14.1
Delaware	699	85	12.2
Ohio	13,823	1,646	11.9
South Carolina	2,226	263	11.8
Illinois	15,000	1,726	11.5
Michigan	10,863	1,215	11.2
Florida	9,934	1,103	11.1
Vermont	815	70	8.6
Connecticut	5,625	451	8.0
Pennsylvania	17,584	1,364	7.8
New York	42,290	3,067	7.3
Massachusetts	11,369	701	6.2
Rhode Island	1,398	77	5.5
New Jersey	10,042	540	5.4
Maine	1,058	55	5.2
Maryland	6,790	314	4.6

Sources: Number of non-Federal active physicians from J. N. Haug, and G. A. Roback: Distribution of Physicians, Hospitals, and Beds in the United States, 1969, Vol. 1, Regional State and County. Chicago: American Medical Association, 1970.

Number of group practice physicians from C. Todd, and M. E. McNamara: Medical Groups in the United States, 1969. Chicago: American Medical Association, 1971.

Medical Resource Factors:

1. Office-based physicians—percent of all active (*i.e.*, nonretired) non-Federal physicians with an office-based private practice (thus excluding hospital-based interns, residents, and full time staff as well as physicians engaged full time in teaching, research, or administration)[7] (OFFMD).
2. Active physicians—number of active non-Federally employed physicians in state per 1,000 population[7] (ACTMD).
3. Hospital supply—number of beds in general hospitals per 1,000 population[1] (BEDS).
4. Health insurance coverage—percent of state population under age 65 insured for at least hospitalization[8] (INS).
5. Federal health grants—per capita dollars in federal grants to the state for health purposes[4] (GRANTS).

6. Medical graduates—graduates from all medical schools in the state per 1,000 population[2] (MEDGRADS).
7. Hospital residencies—number of approved residencies at hospitals in the state per 1,000 population[2] (RESIDS).

We analyzed the relationships between these two sets of variables and our measure of the strength of group medical practice development—the percentage of all non-Federal physicians engaged in practice teams of three or more as defined by the AMA—in each state. The analyses were done first through simple correlations, and then through multivariate techniques.

Findings

Since the data used in this study represent the entire population, rather than a sample, we take all our measurements to be actual population parameters (not requiring significance tests). Among the ten socioenvironmental factors examined, the six largest simple correlations with group practice strength (GRPS) are shown in Table 18-3. Among the seven medical resource factors examined, the five largest correlations are shown in Table 18-4. (The complete matrix of simple correlation coefficients among all the variables is available from the authors.)

The simple correlations, of course, indicate the degree of relationship between group practice strength (GRPS) and any one of the independent or "explanatory" variables considered alone. The square of the simple correlation coefficient[2] indicates the proportion of the variation in GRPS from state to state which is due to its correlation with any one of the specified variables considered alone. We see from Table 18-3, for example, that the state's year of entry in the United States

Table 18-3
Socioenvironmental Factors Related to Strength of Group Practice (GRPS): Simple Correlations of Selected Factors with Percentage of Non-Federal Physicians in Group Practice, by 50 States, United States, 1969

Factor	*Coefficient of Correlation (R)*	R^2
State's year of entry into U.S. (ENTRY)	+0.593	0.352
Density of population (DENSITY)	−0.554	0.307
Metropolitan population (percent) METRO)	−0.433	0.187
Youth population (percent) (YOUTH)	+0.351	0.123
Total state population (number) (STATEPOP)	−0.320	0.102
Income per capita (INCOME)	−0.253	0.064

Sources: See references cited in the text.

Table 18-4
Medical Resource Factors Related to Strength of Group Practice (GRPS): Simple Correlations of Selected Factors with Percentage of Non-Federal Physicians in Group Practice, by 50 States, United States, 1969

Factor	*Coefficient of Correlation (R)*	R^2
Office-based physicians (percent) (OFFMD)	+0.598	0.358
Active physicians (per 1,000 population) (ACTMD)	−0.470	0.221
Hospital residencies (per 1,000 population) (RESIDS)	−0.407	0.166
Hospital supply (beds per 1,000 population) (BEDS)	+0.399	0.159
Health insurance coverage (percent) (INS)	−0.238	0.057

Sources: See references cited in the text.

(ENTRY) alone accounts for about 35 percent of the variation in GRPS, as does the percent of office-based physicians (OFFMD), shown in Table 18-4. The individual correlations shown in Tables 18-3 and 18-4 are plausible in the light of the American social scene in general and the medical care scene in particular. These features will be discussed below.

As a totality, however, the differences in group practice strength from state to state are not simply the sum of the influences of each independent variable acting upon the outcome variable. ENTRY and OFFMD cannot merely be added to explain 70 percent of the total variation in GRPS. The several explanatory variables interact with each other. As an illustration of the complexity of these dynamics, we find (in the complete matrix of correlations, not reproduced here) that while ENTRY shows a simple correlation with GRPS of + 0.593, DENSITY in turn shows a correlation of − 0.546 with ENTRY. Thus, the actual "causal" factor underlying the differing values of GRPS from state to state may be due as much or more to DENSITY (that is, low population density) than to ENTRY.

In order to analyze the *simultaneous* effect of the explanatory variables upon GRPS, we used stepwise multiple regression techniques[6,12] principally, with some recourse to factor analytic techniques.[12]* At each step in the regression procedure, the variable entering the equation is the one that yields the most *additional* information about the outcome variable. Thus, it often happens that a

*In the stepwise regression, the dependent variable (GRPS) is expressed as a function (linear) of the explanatory variables. One explanatory variable at a time is introduced into the equation. The first such variable chosen is the one having the highest simple correlation with the dependent variable—in our study, GRPS. The next variable entering the equation is the one having the highest correlation with GRPS after the latter has been "adjusted" for the effects upon it of the first variable. Technically, the next variable chosen is the one having the highest *partial* correlation with GRPS, when the preceding variables are held constant from state to state. This procedure is repeated on the remaining explanatory variables, until the addition of one more such variable to the equation does not yield a statistically significant increment in "explaining" the value of the dependent variable (GRPS). The process then stops.

variable having a high simple correlation with the outcome measure falls out of the equation or enters very late, just because it is also highly correlated with another one already in the equation and therefore adding little *new* information. Conversely, a variable with a low simple correlation with the dependent variable may wind up within the final explanatory equation.

The stepwise procedure applied to our data resulted in an equation which expresses the strength of group practice (GRPS) in a state as a function of six principal explanatory variables, as shown in Table 18-5. In that table, column 3 indicates the proportion of variability in GRPS "explained" by the variables in the equation at each step (R^2). The standardized regression coefficients, shown in column 6, by definition are computed to lie between − 1 and + 1. The rank order of the importance of the explanatory variables is given by the relative size of the *absolute values* of these standardized regression coefficients. Thus, in Table 18-5 the rank of these independent variables in order of their "explanatory importance" is:

Order of Importance	*Variable*	*Order Entered in Equation*
1	OFFMD	1
2	RESIDS	5
3	ENTRY	3
4	BEDS	2
5	EDUC	4
6	POPGROW	6

These six explanatory variables taken together explain 70 percent of the total variation in group practice strength among the states. Inserting the remaining 11 variables into the equation would raise the R^2 to 0.81. We did not use these 11 variables because it did not seem sensible to sacrifice the substantive comprehensibility of the equation to strengthen the explanatory power only from 70 to 81 percent.†

Interpretation and Discussion

Examining first the socioenvironmental factors and their simple correlations with the strength of group practice, one finds that the strongest correlation is with the state's year of entry into the United States—that is, the more recently established states tend to have more group practice. A glance at Table 18-2 shows the mean-

†It must be realized, at the risk of repetition, that the relatively small additional explanatory power of the 11 variables omitted from the final equation is not always due to a low simple correlation with GRPS. For example, DENSITY, not in the final equation, has a relatively strong simple correlation (−0.554) with GRPS. It is much higher, in fact, than the correlation coefficient of EDUC (+0.013, statistically not significant), which is in the equation. The point is that each variable omitted from the equation is well correlated with one or more variables within the equation, which may be regarded as acting as a proxy for it.

Table 18-5

Social and Medical Factors Related to Group Practice Strength: Results of Stepwise Multiple Regression of Group Practice Strength (GRPS) on 17 Original Variables*

Order of Entry into Equation	*Variable*	*Proportion of Variation in GRPS Explained by Each Regression*		*Regression Coefficients*	
		Cumulative	*Additional*	*Regular*	*Standardized*
(1)	*(2)*	*(3)(R^2)*	*(4)*	*(5)*	*(6)*
1	Percent office-based physicians (OFFMD)	0.36	0.36	0.941	0.910
2	General hospital beds per 1,000 (BEDS)	0.47	0.11	4.128	0.391
3	State's year of entry into U.S. (ENTRY)	0.56	0.09	0.083	0.482
4	Median years of schooling (EDUC)	0.61	0.05	–3.120	–0.391
5	Approved residencies per 1,000 (RESIDS)	0.65	0.04	56.161	0.634
6	Rate of population growth (POPGROW)	0.70*	0.06	0.210	0.301

Standard error of estimate = 5.2.

Intercept = –195.139. (Note: Despite this large negative value of the intercept, the average values for GRPS, given by the regression equation, are comfortably positive for each state.)

*Of the original 17 variables, the first six entering the regression equation are presented here. See text for the explanation. If all 17 variables were left in the equation, the R^2 would rise to 0.81. See text for explanation.

ing of this finding; the highest 10 states, in rank order of group practice strength, include newcomers like Alaska and Hawaii (1959) or North and South Dakota (1889), while of the lowest 10, most are among the 13 original British colonies which declared themselves a nation in 1776.

We believe that this measure can be taken as a reflection of traditionalism, in contrast to innovativeness. Group medical practice, as we noted, has been a departure from conventional patterns of medical work. Older communities become encrusted with traditions which inhibit change; in more recently settled places, new ideas can take root more easily. Moreover, such places lack established networks of medical referral among specialists and institutions.

Close behind in the simple social correlations is population density—that is, the less densely populated states tend to have more group practice. Here also, the interpretation would seem to be straightforward. For one thing, newly settled areas are almost by definition thinly settled. We recall the origins of the Mayo Clinic in Minnesota, a state adjacent to the very thinly settled northern prairies of the Dakotas. Perhaps most saliently, the multispecialty clinics, which contain 68 percent of group practice doctors (32 percent being in single-specialty clinics), provide an economically viable form for settlement of specialists in rural regions. In such thinly settled areas, the isolated specialist would have a hard time attracting enough private patients. But a team of specialists (also general practitioners) refer patients to each other and by their greater visibility can attract patients from many miles around. A Federal study of multispecialty group practices by *counties* in 1959, in fact, found the proportions of total private physicians in group practice to be as follows:[24]

Type of County	*Percentage*
Metropolitan	4.6
Adjacent	8.0
Isolated	12.6

Similar interpretations of each of the socioenvironmental factors correlating highly with group practice strength could be presented, but it is perhaps more useful to draw a simplified profile of the setting which appears most favorable for group practice development. It is a state characterized essentially by new settlement and noninhibiting traditions, by a low density population, relatively little concentration in metropolitan cities, relatively large proportions of young people in its small total population, and of relatively low per capita income.

Turning to the medical resource factors, we find that of all physicians (not employed by the Federal Government) in the states with strong group practice, a high proportion are in private office practice, as distinguished from hospital or other agency-related employment. (While at first glance, this might appear to be a tautology, it is not so; one might readily have expected the opposite relationship—more group practice associated with stronger hospital medicine.) These states are characterized by a relatively low overall ratio of doctors to population and a weak development of residency training programs in their hospitals. Yet the hospital bed supply per 1,000 population is high—a factor which we believe is explained plausibly by certain dynamics of the American scene. Because of federal policies in subsidizing hospital construction, highest priorities have been accorded to rural states since 1946; yet it is precisely in those states that the population growth (not to be confused with birth rate) has been slower and, in fact, in some (like the Dakotas) it has actually declined because of large out-migration. The result has been relatively high bed-population ratios in the most thinly settled rural states, especially in the north-central region of the nation. As for the relatively weak insurance coverage, this is doubtless associated with the rurality and low-income levels noted earlier.

The results of the regression analysis shown in Table 18-5, taken together with the simple correlations among the variables, seem to indicate that the strength of group practice (GRPS) is most strongly associated with the percent of office-based physicians (OFFMD). It should be noted that (although the tables are not reproduced here) OFFMD is in turn strongly and negatively correlated with four other variables: ACTMD (−0.790), METRO (−0.612), DENSITY (−0.490), and STATPOP (−0.438) and positively correlated with YOUTH (+0.463). This would seem to indicate that a high level of group practice strength is strongly associated with a complex of variables consisting of high levels of:

- office-based physicians, and
- youthful populations

and low levels of:

- active non-Federal physicians,
- metropolitan concentration,
- population density, and
- overall state population.

Perhaps the high correlation of group practice strength with the percent of office-based physicians (OFFMD) and with weak hospital residency programs means that in such states specialization is only or more readily achieved through group practices in the community.

While the other variables in the equation were of lesser importance, they indicated that high levels of group practice strength are also associated with:

- low per capita incomes,
- high proportions of poverty populations,
- low educational levels, and
- recent entry of the state into the nation.

It may also be noted that the multiple regression analysis drops out two social factors (METRO and STATEPOP) and one medical factor (ACTMD) which figured significantly in the simple correlations. As explained above, this is because these factors are internally correlated with other independent variables which evidently have greater explanatory power. On the other hand, the regression adds in two social factors (EDUC and POPGROW), which were not statistically significant when analyzed by themselves alone.

Conclusion

This analysis of social and medical factors associated with group practice development in the United States supports certain tenable hypotheses about a variety of influences which have evidently been at play. If the confluence of factors in one state could yield eleven times the proportion of doctors in group practice found in another state, it would seem plausible that enlarging those factors in the second state might lead to an increase of group practice. The purpose of this study, after all, was to find clues that could help formulate social policy to promote extension of this pattern of medical care.

Translation of the findings of our study into practical social actions, however, requires that we look beyond their specific circumstances to their more general implications. A pioneering nontraditional atmosphere, a thin population density, a low proportion of hospital-based physicians, a rapid population growth, or poor per capita incomes are hardly conditions to be socially promoted on a deliberate basis, even if this were possible. These were the factors evidently operative in the past, and one might argue that these are the circumstances where most rapid growth of group practice could be expected in the immediate future. Yet it is evident from a glimpse at the recent growth of group practices, some linked to HMOs, that other more general forces are coming into play.

Basically, all the social and medically related factors associated with group practice strength would seem to describe a milieu which creates greater receptivity to innovative patterns of professional teamwork, in contrast to the solo practice of medicine in a free enterprise culture. The question is: can this receptivity be achieved under different influences than operated in the past? Several considerations suggest that it can be. The rising proportion of all physicians engaged in group practice, shown in Table 18-1, suggests that the viability of this pattern in the American environment is increasing. Studies 30 years ago found a high proportion of new group practices organized to decline and disintegrate, presumably due to a combination of internal difficulties and external hostilities;[5] this is manifestly less true today. A recent American study found a majority of new medical graduates to express preference for working in a team setting. A glimpse at Great Britain, where groups of general practitioners have been steadily increasing, points to the effectiveness of governmental subsidies.[3]

The generally changing character of the American medical environment, combined with a program for subsidizing the organization of group medical practices, would probably lead to a further growth of group practice in the future, both in large cities and in the more rural regions where it has grown most successfully in the past. The likely enactment of national health insurance, with more social support for the costs of medical care, will create further pressures for economies which are theoretically more achievable through group practice. Teams of doctors provide a foundation for forming "health maintenance organizations" (HMOs), in which both cost economies and elevated quality have been dramatically demonstrated.[10] Countries with social systems different from the United States achieve the benefits of teamwork medicine, of course, through health centers, polyclinics, and other such facilities.[13] In the more "laissez faire" economies, illustrated by the United States, as well as by several of the countries of Western Europe, Japan, New Zealand, and Australia, the extension of private group medical practice may be expected to play an important part in the evolving health care systems of the future.

References

1. American Hospital Association. Hospitals (Guide Issue), August 1, 1970.
2. American Hospital Association. Medical education in the United States. JAMA 210:1455, 1969.
3. Cameron, J. C.: Group practice in the United Kingdom. *In* New Horizons in Health Care (Proceedings of the First International Congress on Group Medicine). Winnipeg, Canada: Wallingford Press, 1970, pp. 111–15.
4. Dales, S. R.: Federal grants to state and local governments. Soc. Sec. Bull. 33:31, 1969.
5. Dickinson, Frank G., and Bradley, C. E.: Discontinuance of Medical Groups 1940–49. Chicago: American Medical Association, Bureau of Medical Economic Research, Bulletin No. 90, 1952.
6. Dixon, W. J., Ed.: BMD Biomedical Computer Programs. Los Angeles: University of California Press, 1967.
7. Haug, J. N., and Roback, G. A.: Distribution of Physicians, Hospitals, and Beds in the United States, 1969, Vol. 1, Regional, State, and County. Chicago: American Medical Association, 1970.
8. Health Insurance Institute. Source Book of Health Insurance Data 1970. New York, 1971.
9. Jordan, Edwin P.: The Physician and Group Practice. Chicago: Yearbook Publishers, 1958.
10. MacLeod, Gordon K., and Prussin, Jeffrey A.: The continuing evolution of health maintenance organizations. N. Engl. J. Med. 288:439, 1973.
11. Newspaper Enterprise Association: The World Almanac and Book of Facts. 1968 Centennial Edition, New York, 1968, pp. 323–49.
12. Nie, Norman, Bent, Dale H., and Hull, C. Hadlai: SPSS, Statistical Package for the Social Sciences. New York: McGraw-Hill, 1970.
13. Roemer, Milton I.: Evaluation of Community Health Centres. Geneva: World Health Organization, Public Health Paper No. 48, 1972.
14. Roemer, Milton I., and Friedman, Jay W.: Doctors in Hospitals. Baltimore: Johns Hopkins Press, 1971, pp. 49–61.
15. Todd, C., and McNamara, M. E.: Medical Groups in the United States, 1969. Chicago: American Medical Association, 1971.
16. Sigerist, Henry E.: American Medicine. New York: W. W. Norton Co., 1934, pp. 178–80.
17. Stern, Bernhard J.: American Medical Practice in the Perspective of a Century. New York: Commonwealth Fund, 1945.
18. Stevens, Rosemary: American Medicine and the Public Interest. New Haven, Conn.: Yale University Press, 1971.

19. U.S. Bureau of the Census: Current Population Reports. Components of Population Change by County: 1960 to 1970. Washington, 1971.
20. U.S. Bureau of the Census: Statistical Abstract of the United States 1971. Washington: Government Printing Office, 1971.
21. U.S. Bureau of the Census: U.S. Census of Population: 1970. General Population Characteristics, Final Report. Washington, 1971.
22. U.S. Department of Commerce, Office of Business Economics: Survey of Current Business, Vol. 31, No. 4, Washington, April, 1971.
23. U.S. Office of Economic Opportunity: Poverty Facts and Figures, Technical Note No. 1, Washington, January 31, 1971.
24. U.S. Public Health Service: Medical Groups in the United States, 1959. Washington: PHS Pub. No. 1063, July 1963, p. 25.

19

Medical Costs in Relation to the Organization of Ambulatory Care

While some evidence of savings achievable in group compared with solo medical practice is conflicting, most of the evidence suggests that grouping does achieve economies. In other words, the true costs of production of a unit of medical service are lower in a group practice clinic.

These lower costs, however, are seldom passed along to the patient in the form of lower prices; for many historial reasons price competition has not ordinarily been allowed to operate in the medical market. Instead, the lower costs usually yield higher earnings to the doctor, a shorter work week for the same earnings, or both.

It is only when consumers join together in prepayment plans that, in effect, they can "bargain" for lower prices and get the benefit of the cost-savings of this pattern. Comprehensive health care linked to prepaid group practice (later labeled "health maintenance organizations") can also yield substantial savings in lesser use of hospitals and other secondary services. The chapter that follows was co-authored with Donald M. DuBois.

RISING COSTS OF medical care are a worldwide phenomenon, and everywhere they have induced a search for methods of improved economy and efficiency. The rise in costs is real, even after correction for general price inflations. Partly, of course, the rise is due to an increase in the volume of medical services provided or, as it is usually put, the medical-care utilization rate of the population. Since expanding social expectations regard this as desirable (that is, to apply science to human need), the search for economies is seldom expressed in an effort to reduce the rate of ambulatory services provided, beyond elimination of clear abuses. Economies are more often sought through measures to improve the efficiency of production of the services that are offered. On a practical level, this usually means an attempt to achieve the minimum annual expenditure per person served by a medical-care system providing services of satisfactory quality.

The Basic Question

In the United States there is growing evidence that the prevailing pattern of provision of ambulatory care by private individual physicians is relatively extrava-

Chapter 19 originally appeared in the *New England Journal of Medicine*, 280:988–993, May, 1969, and is reprinted by permission of that journal.

gant. Thousands of small, isolated medical offices, furnishing services on an itemized fee basis, constitute a costly method of delivering care. Application of experience in industrial production has long suggested that systematic organization of health personnel and equipment could achieve economies for the usual reasons: specialization; division of labor; and fuller use of time and resources for achieving high capacity in the "production process." In the international context, this has meant the organization of polyclinics, health centers, and a wide variety of related patterns. In America it is usually epitomized as "group medical practice." By this we mean the effective mobilization of a wide range of skilled personnel for both curative and preventive service to the ambulatory patient.

The basic question posed here, then, is whether group practice can reduce the costs of medical care. To avoid confusion, which has been all too common, it is important to clarify the question before the evidence in support of an answer is examined.

First of all, we must consider costs, rather than prices. Prices or charges to consumers, for medical care, are obviously influenced by market conditions of supply and demand. A particular system of organization of ambulatory medical services might yield great reductions in the *cost* of their production, without passing these savings on to the patient in the form of lower medical prices or fees. This can happen under conditions of high demand and limited supply, in which prices are relatively inelastic. There is plenty of evidence that these are precisely the dynamics under which group practice operates in the United States.

Second, we are concerned with total medical care, rather than solely the services of physicians. Thus, the economic effects of group practice must be judged not only by internal production costs, but also by the expenditures generated in the whole complex of medical care, including hospitalization, drugs, and other supporting services.

Third, we must be clear about the unit of measurement of the medical output. Are we thinking of the costs per unit of service provided (such as a physical examination or an injection), costs per illness treated, costs per person served over a given period (for any and all illnesses), or indeed costs per unit of health status achieved—like days of life with unrestricted activity? These are obviously tough and complicated questions, and answers on the comparative economies of different patterns of ambulatory care will depend on which of these output measures we apply.

This paper attempts to state our assumptions on these questions before offering the evidence available to provide answers. We believe that the weight of the evidence suggests that group medical practice *can* yield lower costs per person served, but that the enjoyment of these cost reductions in the form of lower prices and reduced expenditures depends on market conditions in which effective competition is operative. Such market conditions are currently most apparent in the operation of insurance plans, through which the collective voice of consumers can be heard.

The cost effects of group medical practice may be considered under two headings: primary economies, within the group practice operation; and secondary economies, in the provision of total medical care received by the patient.

Primary Economies

General experience in the production of other goods and services certainly suggests that the specialization of labor and larger scale operations of group medical practice should result in lower costs per unit of service rendered. Direct evidence of this is hard to come by, but there is a good deal of indirect evidence.

For years it has been demonstrated that the average net income of doctors in private group medical practice is higher than that in solo practice. This is true specialty by specialty, and also by age group of physicians.[1] It is also relevant that the average hours per week worked by group practice doctors are about the same as among solo doctors, and a few years ago they were even fewer. Hence, the higher group practice incomes cannot be attributed to more hours of work, but rather to higher earnings per man-hour. Since, as discussed below, the fees charged to patients are similar, it follows that the productivity of group practice doctors—that is, their output of services per hour—is higher.

Data on the incomes of doctors in different forms of practice, collected by *Medical Economics* magazine, have been analyzed by Donald Yett.[2] To identify the overhead costs of practice beyond the basic value of the doctor's time, Yett standardized for this value by assuming it to be worth the level of salary paid to doctors of equivalent qualifications in institutional employment (like the Veterans Administration hospitals). On this basis, he found a lower cost of production per patient visit in group practices and partnerships than in either solo practice or expense-sharing medical arrangements.

Richard Bailey,[3] in a study of productivity related to the scale (that is, size or volume) of practice of specialists in internal medicine in northern California, found that the total output of larger clinics exceeded that of smaller units or solo practitioners only because of longer working hours per month; in terms of patient contacts with a doctor per hour, there was no greater productivity with scale. When, however, the *total* medical output of a clinic or private practice was considered, including ancillary X-ray and laboratory services, the larger units or group practices did have higher outputs per hour—measurable in gross income. Our own view is that it is, indeed, reasonable to consider such totals as the aggregate output of medical practice, since the laboratory or X-ray procedure is a type of efficient substitution for or enlargement of physical diagnosis by the doctor. Moreover, one must realize that Bailey's study was confined to nonprepaid arrangements, where, as noted below, pressures for economy in the current market are hardly felt.

In hospital operations, it has also been difficult to analyze costs in relation to scale (usually defined by bed capacity), since larger hospitals (like larger medical practices) offer a richer mixture of services in each day of patient care. Thus, economies of scale may seem to be more than nullified by increases in the quality content of the services. When adjustments are made for this effect, however, and each unit of in-hospital service is separately identified, the cumulative evidence suggests that for sizes up to hospitals of about 600 beds, lower costs per unit of service are generally achieved with increasing scale.[4] This process ought also to apply to out-of-hospital medical services if competition operated to make prices correspond to true costs of production.

Joel Kovner[5] has examined the costs per unit of service among a series of group practices of different size but similar management. He devised ingenious measures of output of specific "identifiable medical procedures" (IMP) and found that the cost of production per procedure was generally lower with increasing scale. Reduction in unit costs was associated with higher numbers of medical specialists, X-ray and laboratory personnel, other auxiliary personnel, and capital.

The difficulty in getting direct hard evidence on this question of primary or internal economies is related to the variation in content of specific services rendered to patients for a given illness in group practice versus solo practice. Bailey's study demonstrates these variations, and it is difficult to adjust for them statistically or to estimate their qualitative effects. In group practice there is typically a higher ratio of low-cost ancillary personnel per doctor than in solo practice. Solo doctors typically employ one or two auxiliaries, whereas in most group practices, three to four and five-tenths ancillary personnel are used in support of each physician.[6] These substitutions of less expensive manpower (for example, blood-pressure measurement done by a nurse) should obviously yield cost reductions. On the other hand, the expenditures per patient seen in group practice may be inflated for the simple reason that more specific services, such as X-ray and laboratory tests, are rendered even though each unit of service is less costly.

The same mechanism presumably applies to the feasibility of using more efficient but expensive equipment under conditions of group practice.[7] A solo practitioner could not ordinarily afford to have a $50,000 "Auto-Analyzer" in his office, even though this machine can perform blood sugar determinations at much lower cost than a laboratory technician working manually. A fair-sized group practice could enjoy this economy, but by the same token its availability probably leads to the performance of more blood sugar tests than would be done otherwise. We urgently need research that can answer these questions on specific unit costs.

Rentals or space costs are part of the cost of medical service, and it appears that waiting rooms, consultation units, and all the other space of ambulatory-care facilities can be used more fully and for more hours per week under group practice arrangements. Thus, capital costs per unit of service rendered would be lower, if the necessary adjustments could be made for the number of units rendered.

Despite these potential internal economies of organized group practice, the prices charged to patients for specific services are not usually lower. The vast majority of group practices in the United States are private, they are not associated with prepayment by a population group, and they charge the fees that have become customary in the general medical market. This has been shown by the study of the American Medical Association Commission on the Cost of Medical Care.[8] In effect, it means that the demand for medical care is high enough and the business relations among doctors are fraternal enough, that competition, which for other goods and services might yield price reductions to attract trade, does not ordinarily operate. It comes into operation only when consumers can bargain effectively on price, such as through certain types of insurance plan, as indicated below.

Secondary Economies

A similar disparity between potentialities and actual demonstrated costs of group practice applies to the secondary economies. The most expensive sector of medical care is hospitalization, whereby the patient must be provided room, board, and other attentions as well as diagnostic and treatment service. If the organized setting of group practice can reduce the use of expensive days of hospital care in a population, therefore, it may be expected to yield important savings. Since many technical procedures, not feasible in the solo medical office, may be done in a group practice clinic without recourse to hospital admission, one would expect economies on this score.

We have no real evidence on the operation of this effect for *private* fee-for-service group practice as compared with solo practice. Under *prepaid* group practice, where price competition is expressible, the evidence is strong. Studies by numerous investigators have shown a much lower rate of hospital utilization—in both admissions and days per 1,000 population per year—among persons served by prepaid group practice than among similar demographic populations served by prepaid solo practice. Most of these studies are based on the membership of the Health Insurance Plan of Greater New York (HIP)[9] and the Kaiser-Permanente Health Plan of the West Coast,[10] compared with that of other health-insurance plans using mainly solo medical practitioners. The findings under the Federal Employees Health Benefits Program, analyzed by George Perrott[11] for 1962–65, indicated this effect to operate, moreover, throughout the nation.

The mechanism of this secondary saving is undoubtedly complex. The saving seems to be only partially due to the elimination of unnecessary admissions for diagnostic work-up. (Indeed, the extensive use of diagnostic tests in group practice may detect more hidden disease, which can mean identification of more cases requiring hospitalization.) More important probably is the influence of fee-for-service incentives on the rate of hospital admissions. Doctors in prepaid group practices are typically on salary, and they do not stand to gain financially by admitting their patients to hospitals. (Indeed, in the Kaiser Plan, the doctors can actually earn more if hospital expenditures are less.) Thus, the rates of tonsillectomy, appendectomy, and other elective surgical procedures are lower under prepaid group practice than under solo practice, either prepaid or not.[12] It is significant that the ratio to population of surgeons, anesthesiologists and ophthalmologists in the United States as a whole is much higher than the ratio of these specialists found for the population of prepaid group practice plans.[13] (Solo surgeons seem to be either not working at full capacity or doing more surgery than is necessary—both of which points are probably true in some degree.)

Group practice may also yield secondary economies to patients in other spheres. Drugs may be prescribed under a judicious formulary that emphasizes lower priced generic products—a policy seldom feasible in solo practice. Moreover, various ancillary services for visual refraction, physiotherapy, or laboratory tests can be provided at lower cost in an organized clinic than in the quarters of private entrepreneurs in these disciplines.

It is these secondary economies on hospital and other expenses that seem principally to account for the lower aggregate costs of medical care provided by the major prepaid group practice plans than by the conventional "Blue" or commercial health insurance plans using mainly private solo practitioners. The comparative study directed by Josephine Williams[14] in 1958 found more ambulatory services provided to prepaid group practice plan (Kaiser) members than to members of either commercial or "Blue" solo practice plans. Yet annual expenditures were lower when out-of-plan expenses were included along with premiums. The California study of state-government employees in 1966 reported the same situation in comparing two prepaid group practice plans (Kaiser and Ross-Loos) with three solo practice plans (Blue Cross-Blue Shield, a commercial carrier, and a medical-society "Foundation").[10]

The recent report of the National Advisory Commission on Health Manpower has summarized the evidence from several sources, from which it may be concluded that the net effect of all the savings operates to make per capita expenditures (including both insurance premiums and out-of-pocket expenses) at least 35 percent lower under the prepaid group practice pattern (Kaiser) than under ordinary solo practice provision of medical care in California.[7] The Commission also found that the trend of rising medical costs from 1960 to 1965 was much lower under the Kaiser plan than that experienced by the total California population—also owing mainly to the secondary economies on hospital utilization.

Ultimate Costs—The Quality Issue

Despite the probability of both primary and secondary economies under organized ambulatory medical care, it may be argued that the savings are false if the quality of care has been sacrificed. Perhaps the greater use of auxiliary personnel may produce primary economies or the reduced rate of hospital days may yield secondary economies, but these might lead to lower rates of recovery from illness. The ultimate goal of any medical care system, of course, is not the rendition of services but the attainment of better health.

Although this tough question cannot be answered definitively, all the evidence so far suggests that health-service systems in which ambulatory care is organized yield greater health benefits than those depending on solo practice. Observations by the AMA Commission on Medical Care Plans concluded that in prepaid group practice clinics, "good medical care is being provided, within the scope of services offered."[15] A study group of the National Advisory Commission on Health Manpower reviewed the nation's largest prepaid group practice program, and found that "the medical care received by Kaiser members was of high quality."[7]

More persuasive was the study of HIP members in 1956, which produced data on the ultimate outcome of services. It found lower perinatal mortality among HIP members than among a demographically comparable sample of New York people served by ordinary solo medical practice.[16] Another New York study of indigent aged persons in 1966 found a lower mortality rate after 65 years of age among those served by HIP group practice clinics than among a comparable sample of people served by private solo doctors.[17]

It has repeatedly been shown that preventive services—health education, immunizations, and periodic examinations—are more readily provided under prepaid group practice.[18] We cannot really prove that prevention always yields cost economies (despite the old saw about the ounce of prevention), but the general medical literature establishes that it can promote health and extend life.

Competition and Incentives

The vexing aspect of the basic question posed here is that the achievement of economies in medical care, in relation to the organization of ambulatory services, depends on many factors beyond the organization itself. Group medical practice in the ordinary private market economy may permit a lower cost-of-production *per unit of service,* but the supply and demand for services is such that the economies usually yield not lower prices but higher medical incomes or reduced hours of work. In terms of expenditures per patient (as distinguished from costs per unit of service), the overall charges to the consumer may actually be higher than in solo practice, because the elaborate facilities of a group practice clinic, combined with the profit motive, may lead to an excessively high volume of specific services per illness or per patient or per person during a year.

It is only when competition on price enters the scene that incentives seem to change and basic economies are passed on to patients by way of lower prices. This observation applies to both the primary economies and the secondary economies, as defined here. Price competition can operate favorably in the American scene when consumers are enabled to bargain in advance of illness and as knowledgeable buyers faced with a choice among alternatives. This is one of the great contributions of the multiplicity of health insurance plans operating in the United States. By permitting the establishment of prices in advance, through insurance premiums, competition among plans has created incentives in some of them not only to achieve economies in producing medical service but also to pass them on to the buyer through wider benefits per premium dollar. When the insurance mechanism is coupled with group practice, the primary and secondary economies of organization can be realized by the population.[19]

In other market situations the lower costs of organized ambulatory services are demonstrated in other ways. Certain social insurance programs for medical care in other countries apply different systems of ambulatory service in different localities, permitting comparison of costs.[20] In the health insurance program of Ecuador, certain localities have organized polyclinics with doctors on good salaries, and other localities permit free choice of private doctor with fee-for-service reimbursement. The per capita costs of the latter method are generally higher, even though the entitlements are the same. Likewise, in India, where 13,000,000 people are covered by a social insurance scheme, roughly half are served by health centers, and the rest by solo doctors. Even though the private doctors here are paid on a capitation, rather than fee-for-service basis, the costs to the system are lower in the health centers. Thus, even when hard bargaining for minimal medical prices is conducted by one insuring agency (rather than multiple plans), the economies of organized ambulatory services, as compared with solo practice, are demonstrable.

Implications for Total Health Service

The implications of organized ambulatory service in the total picture of health care, of course, go much beyond those of costs. Beyond the primary and secondary economies possible when group practice is combined with prepayment, there are relevancies for every aspect of health maintenance. In the whole structure of public health and medical care, the keystone is the physician of initial contact. It is from this point that the patient is referred to all the other elements in the system: the diagnostic procedures, the drugs, the hospital, the nursing home, and so forth. It is at this primary level that prevention and health counseling may be most expeditiously offered, as stressed in the recent Millis Report.[21]

This critical role of the physician of initial contact can hardly be played effectively by the isolated medical practitioner. The complexities of modern health service require the collaboration of many medical and surgical specialists along with a lengthening roster of allied health personnel. Only through organization can all these health workers be effectively used, whether through private group practices, polyclinics, hospital out-patient departments, health centers, or other modes of medical teamwork. The quality advantages of group practice, through the stimulation of colleagues and group discipline, have been appreciated since the Mayo brothers' innovation in the 1880s, but the force of the argument has mounted with the years.

With potential advantages in the sphere of both economy and quality, one may ask why group practice has not grown more rapidly in America. In fact, the growth rate has been impressive since about 1945, if one includes single-specialty along with multispecialty medical groups. The latest survey of the American Medical Association reports that in 1965 there were over 28,000 physicians in nearly 4,300 medical groups.[22] This represented 11 percent of all doctors engaged in patient-care activities, as compared with about 3 percent in 1946—almost a fourfold increase. The growth rate might have been higher except for the individualistic attitudes of most doctors, the administrative difficulties of organizing a medical group, the opposition of the medical community, the obstacles of some state laws, and other factors explored elsewhere.[6] The very rapid growth of office-sharing arrangements—although not meeting the definition of "group practice"—is further indirect evidence of appreciation by doctors of the advantages of some form of grouping over purely isolated practice.

The membership of persons in health insurance plans based on group practice has also not grown as rapidly as one might expect from the fact that in these plans the economies are usually passed on to the consumer in the form of relatively lower premiums in relation to benefit offerings. Enrollment, indeed, had grown in these plans up to about 4,000,000 persons in 1966, but the larger health insurance programs, offering free choice of private doctor, have grown much more rapidly.[23] This is a complex problem, probably related to understandably negative attitudes of most people toward "clinics" (conditioned by experience with crowded hospital outpatient departments for the poor), to the inconvenience of access to a usually distant medical facility as compared with a nearby private doctor, and to the inadequate staffing of some prepaid group practices, which may yield hasty and impersonal care. In the Kaiser-Permanente Health Plan, nevertheless, the rate of growth has actually been more rapid than that in other traditional health insurance plans on the West Coast; the limiting factor has been the ability to recruit physicians who are willing to work in this type of organized setting. In several Kaiser Plan locations, the door to new members has recently been closed, or the growth rate would be still higher.

The extension of the group practice idea in America may depend not so much on its technical and qualitative advantages, which are hard for the average person to appreciate, especially in the face of the impersonalities of most large clinic settings. It may come more because of the cost-reducing potentials that we have tried to review. The conversion of these potentials into achievements, however, seems to depend on intervention of the consumer exercising his right to bargain on price. The cue is becoming gradually more clear to consumers, both through voluntary channels like labor unions and through governmental authorities concerned with paying for care to certain beneficiaries.[24] On a world scale, there is little doubt that isolated medical practice is gradually being replaced by organized ambulatory services.

References

1. Owens, A. Doctors' economic health never better. *Med. Economics* 44:63–67, 1967.
2. Yett, D. Evaluation of methods of estimating physicians' expenses relative to output. *Inquiry* 4:3–27, March, 1967.
3. Bailey, R. M. Appraisals of experience in fee-for-service group practice in San Francisco Bay area. *Bull. New York Acad. Med.* 44:11, 1968.
4. Berry, R. E. Returns to scale in production of hospital services. *Health Serv. Research* 2:123–139, 1967.
5. Kovner, J. *Production Function for Outpatient Medical Facilities.* Ann Arbor, Michigan: University Microfilms, 1968.
6. DuBois, D. M. *Group Medical Practice, an Analytic Study.* Prepared for the National Advisory Commission on Health Manpower, 1967. Pp. 6–18. (Processed.)
7. National Advisory Commission on Health Manpower. *Report.* Vol. 2. Washington, D.C.: Government Printing Office. 1967. Pp.206–228.
8. American Medical Association, *Report of the Commission on the Cost of Medical Care.* Vol. 1. Chicago: The Association, 1964. (General Report.)
9. Densen, P., Balamath, E., and Shapiro, S. *Prepaid Medical Care and Hospital Utilization.* Chicago: American Hospital Association, 1958. (Monograph Series No. 3.)
10. Watts, M. et al. *A Special Report of the Medical and Hospital Advisory Committee to the Board of Administration of the State Employees' Retirement System.* Sacramento, California: The Committee, June, 1964.
11. Perrott, G. S. Federal Employees Health Benefits Program. 3. Utilization of hospital services. *Am. J. Pub. Health* 56:57–64, 1966.
12. Donabedian, A. *A Review of Some Experiences with Prepaid Group Practice.* Ann Arbor, Michigan: University of Michigan School of Public Health, 1965.
13. Dunaye, T. Use of comprehensive medical organization models in physician manpower planning and economic analysis. In DuBois.[6] Appendix A.
14. Williams, J., et al. (Columbia University School of Public Health). *Family Medical Care Under Three Types of Health Insurance.* New York: Foundation on Employee Health, Medical Care, and Welfare, 1962.
15. American Medical Association, Commission on Medical Care Plans. Report: findings, conclusions and recommendation. *J.A.M.A.* 17, January, 1959. (Special Edition.) P. 49.
16. Shapiro, S. End result measurements of quality of medical care. *Milbank Mem. Fund Quart.* 45:7–40, 1967.
17. Shapiro, S., Williams, J., Yerby, A., Densen, P., and Rosner, H. Patterns of medical use by indigent aged under two systems of medical care. *Am. J. Pub. Health* 57:784–790, 1967.
18. Sloss, J. H., Young, W. R., and Weinerman, E. R. Health maintenance in prepaid group practice. I. Planning and early development of project at Community Health Foundation in Cleveland. *M. Care* 6:215–230, 1968.
19. Feldstein, P. J. Proposal for capitation reimbursement to medical groups for total medical care. In *Reimbursement Incentives for Medical Care.* Washington, D.C.: Social Security Administration, 1968. Pp. 87–103.
20. Roemer, M. I. *Medical Care Organization Under Social Security: A study of the experience in eight countries.* Geneva: International Labour Organization, 1969.

21. American Medical Association. Citizens Commission on Graduate Medical Education. *The Graduate Education of Physicians*. Chicago: The Association, 1966.
22. Balfe, B. E., and McNamara, M. E. *Survey of Medical Groups in the U.S., 1965*. Chicago: American Medical Association, 1968.
23. Reed, L. S. Private health insurance: coverage and financial experience, 1940–66. *Social Security Bull.* 30:3–22, November, 1967.
24. United States Public Health Service. *Promoting the Group Practice of Medicine*. Washington, D.C.: Government Printing Office, 1967. (Report of the National Conference on Group Practice, October 19–21, 1967.)

Part Five

Hospital Trends

Perhaps the oldest form of organization of health services has been the hospital, where many health personnel work together to treat many seriously ill patients. Hospital care has become increasingly complex and costly, arousing public concern. Various aspects of hospital organization are explored in this Part.

Chapter 20 reviews the many reasons for rising interest of the general population in the establishment and operation of hospitals, and the social controls evolving in response to this concern. The expanding importance of the hospital has influenced the organizational structure of the whole health care system; Chapter 21 examines this influence, with special focus on its reflection in the engagement by hospitals of salaried and other forms of contractual physician. The patterns by which doctors work in American general hospitals exhibit great variety, and Chapter 22 examines the effects of these varying patterns on overall hospital performance. With the great expansion of hospitals and their use, widespread concern arose in the 1950s that hospitals were being extravagantly overutilized, especially with elimination of financial constraints by insurance; Chapter 23 analyzes the many factors determining the rate of use of hospitals in a community under insurance, especially the bed-population ratio. Chapter 24 explores the increasing social pressures for regulation of hospitals, which need not cause anxiety but must be recognized as an inevitable social development.

20

Hospitals and the Public Interest

Over the centuries, hospitals have increasingly become centers for delivery of the most complicated diagnostic and treatment procedures. As their responsibilities have broadened in scope and number, social concerns have naturally arisen that they should meet certain standards and perform certain functions.

This "public interest" in hospitals became especially prominent in the United States in the early 1960s, as insurance for hospitalization expanded and the utilization of hospital services increased rapidly, along with their costs. The regulatory responses came from both voluntary and governmental sources. Additional aspects of hospital operation were continuously being brought within the orbit of public concern. These trends and issues were analyzed in an article of the same title as this chapter, co-authored with Max Shain. Since 1961, when this article was written, and particularly after the enactment of the Medicare Law of 1965, public controls over hospital structure and function have continued to broaden.

In 1958 the insurance commissioner of Pennsylvania issued a now-famous adjudication on the application of the Philadelphia Blue Cross plan for a premium increase.[1] In explaining his refusal to grant the increase, the commissioner offered a bill of particulars on the operation of both Blue Cross plans and hospitals, suggesting widespread neglect in the control of hospital utilization and costs. In the following months, official investigations were launched in several States on the whole question of hospital management and economics.

The first reaction to these signs of strong governmental intervention into hospital affairs was one of surprise and indignation. What right did an insurance commissioner have to suggest that either a Blue Cross plan or a governmental agency should pry into the operation of institutions that were predominantly under local voluntary auspices? Charges were made of "attacks on the voluntary hospital system" and creeping socialism. At about the same time, Cornell University was called on by the State of New York to help prepare new legal standards for the approval of general hospitals, and we were likewise attacked as accomplices in the crime of governmental interference with free hospital enterprise.[2]

As the dust has settled, it has become clearer to many that hospitals in the United States are, indeed, subject to various forms of supervision by public

Chapter 20 originally appeared in *Public Health Reports* (the official journal of the U.S. Public Health Service), 76:401–410, May, 1961.

agencies. Yet many look at the trends with anxiety. It may help to clarify the changing hospital world if we examine the basis of public interest in hospitals, the voluntary safeguards of this interest, the role of government, and new issues of public concern. Then we may be able to look ahead to future needs for reasonable supervision of hospitals in the American scene.

Basis of the Public Interest

What is the basis of the public interest in hospitals? Fundamentally, it lies in the obligation of the community to protect the health of its members. This responsibility is dispatched through both voluntary and governmental actions. Through a long tradition of political experience and legal precedent, some (though not all) of this theoretical obligation of government is embodied in constitutions. The U.S. Constitution may not spell out "hospitals" or even "health" as subjects of governmental concern, but the "general welfare" clause has been interpreted again and again to include within it the power to safeguard the public health. Except for foreign or interstate activities, however, power in health affairs rests essentially with the State governments. The New York State constitution, for example, states that "the promotion and protection of the health of the inhabitants of the State are matters of public concern."

The States are amply endowed legally to support this public concern. They possess what is called juridically "police power," permitting State governments to protect the health, welfare, safety, and morals of their citizens. The rational foundation of this power may be the need to protect individuals from the harmful acts of others or even from personal imprudence. Hence the State exercises its police power over the sale of drugs or the wages and hours of working people. It may require vaccination against smallpox and quarantine of persons with diphtheria. Likewise it may regulate hospitals since these institutions may intimately affect the life and well-being of the people.

Beyond these philosophical and legal foundations for a public interest in their operation, hospitals derive from the State certain special privileges. At the same time, the State imposes certain obligations on them.

Generally hospitals are incorporated bodies, chartered by the State like other corporations. Directors are substantially relieved of individual responsibility for the wrongdoing of the corporation; instead, the legally created corporate "person" is responsible and liable only to the extent of its collective assets. Considering the possibilities of negligence, harmful acts, and malpractice suits in a hospital, this limited liability is obviously of great importance. As corporations, hospitals have the capacity for perpetual existence, without the necessity of complex transfers of title on the death of individual founders. The responsibilities of corporations are defined by law and are subject to a charter granted usually by the secretary of state in each State.[3]

Because of their usually charitable and nonprofit character, except for the handful of proprietary institutions, hospitals enjoy tax exemptions of many sorts. They are exempt from Federal income taxes and from many excise taxes levied on other enterprises. They are also exempt from local property taxes, and often from local sales taxes on their purchases. Moreover, hospitals may receive gifts from donors who thereby enjoy reductions of their net incomes for tax purposes; hospitals thus receive funds which would otherwise be payable in large part to the government as private income taxes.

Hospitals may receive substantial grants of public money for construction purposes. The extent, of course, differs with the hospital's sponsorship. About one-third of the hospitals in the United States are fully owned by units of government, predominantly State and local, and were built entirely with governmental tax funds. Even excluding special hospitals for tuberculosis and mental disorder, Federal facilities for veterans or merchant seamen, and all long-term facilities, and counting only short-term general hospitals serving local communities, there are more than 1,100 such institutions which have been built substantially from public funds. Beyond this, voluntary hospitals have long received governmental construction grants. Such support has been given since the earliest days of the Republic, when the Pennsylvania Hospital in Philadelphia and the Massachusetts General Hospital in Boston received grants from State legislatures and municipal governments. State governments have in more recent years given such grants to help hospitals in rural communities. Since 1946, of course, the Hill-Burton program has provided substantial Federal money to assist voluntary and public hospital construction on a nationwide scale. Such contributions of public funds have entailed public responsibility for overseeing how the money is spent on the physical plant.

Governmental units purchase services from hospitals on behalf of certain legal beneficiaries. The largest share of these are indigent persons receiving public assistance from State or local governments; that is, recipients of categorical or general assistance. In addition, many States assume responsibility for hospital services to selected persons who are "medically indigent"; that is, unable to pay hospital bills although not on the relief rolls for their general living needs. The new Federal law on medical aid for the aged, enacted in September 1960, may enlarge this group considerably. Then there are a variety of other beneficiaries of governmental programs, such as those for workmen's compensation, vocational rehabilitation, or crippled children, who are ordinarily treated in community hospitals. Finally, there are beneficiaries of the Federal Government, ordinarily served in special Federal hospitals, who may receive care in local general hospitals on occasion; these include veterans, uniformed service dependents, merchant mariners, American Indians, and others. The content of care given to all these beneficiaries is a matter of public concern. In some States, indeed, it is the principal legal foundation for the whole licensure program, with responsibility being assigned to the welfare department because of its authority for overseeing care to the indigent.

Another foundation of public interest in hospitals is their provision of a locale for the work of several licensed health professions. Physicians, nurses, physical therapists, technicians, and others who work in hospitals individually derive their rights to practice from special examinations and licensing procedures. But the very concentration of these personnel under one roof would seem to place a special responsibility on government regarding the technical standards of the environment under that roof. Surveillance over the management of affairs of hospitals provides a channel for some continued assurance of proper performance by these professions, after the initial licensure.

The hospital is also an educational institution, most conspicuously for nurses but also for other occupations. Laboratory technicians, rehabilitation therapists, social workers, dietitians, and pharmacists may receive substantial parts of their basic training in hospitals. Physicians are educated in hospitals throughout their professional lives, not to mention their periods of service as interns and residents and their training years as medical students. Insofar as supervision of education is widely considered a public responsibility in our society, the hospital is partly a school requiring such supervision.

The hospital, furthermore, is an employer of men and women, subject accordingly to the laws of the land controlling the conditions of labor. Exemptions may be made regarding certain wage, hour, and collective-bargaining provisions because of the hospital's usually nonprofit character, but such exemptions are a matter of legislative decision rather than constitutional right. The exemptions could be withdrawn and, as we shall note, there are legislative winds blowing this way. In any event, conditions of work in hospitals are obviously matters of public interest, with about 1,500,000 persons employed in them on a full-time basis.

Finally, there is the question of hospital operating costs, which have obvious importance for the general public. In recent years, public concern about this has become an overriding issue. Not only has there been widespread popular reaction to the sharp rises in hospital costs, but the channel of expression of this reaction has been widened through a separate but closely related social movement: hospital insurance. The Blue Cross plans inevitably reflect hospital costs in their premium charges to subscribers. Being insurance organizations, though nonprofit, they come under the supervision of State insurance commissioners, and these officials must be responsive to public attitudes. Thus, the insurance financing of a major share of hospital costs in recent years—in other words, support by the mass of people rather than solely the sick—has heightened public interest in hospital costs. Obviously, the people have a right to know how their insurance money is being used by hospitals; if there is inefficiency or extravagance, they have a proper concern in eliminating it.

These, then, are the principal reasons for a public interest in hospitals. Perhaps it epitomizes the situation to say that hospitals are essentially public utilities. They are so important to the survival of the community that they have been granted many special immunities and statutory rights. At the same time, their actions may lead to good or poor consequences for the people. For both reasons, citizens and organizations outside the walls of the hospital have assumed a variety of responsibilities for looking in on them and exerting various pressures to assure proper performance.

Voluntary Safeguards

Consciousness of public interest is responsible, at least in part, for the conventional pattern of a board of directors as the top authority of voluntary hospitals. The hospital board is theoretically a kind of built-in protector of the public interest. Its roster is supposed to include persons who represent the community: if not popularly elected, then appointed on the basis of their position as leaders able to judge the interests of the population as a whole.

In practice, we know that the democratic ideal is rarely attained anywhere. Hospital boards may be composed of highly intelligent and responsible persons, but they come predominantly from business and professional groups.[4] Their sensitivity to the needs of humble people may be limited, and their willingness to take particular actions may be strongly influenced by their personal views, which may or may not coincide with maximum protection of the public interest. Moreover, they are often persons who have given substantial donations to the cost of building the institution; hence, they will feel proud and possessive toward it, protecting it against criticism. An attitude of "my hospital, right or wrong" may assure loyalty but not necessarily optimal performance for the general good. These observations should not deprecate the devotion and diligence of most hospital board members, but they do cast doubt on the reliability of the board mechanism for protecting the public interest.

Yet every decision that a hospital board or its administrator makes is laden with public interest. The hospital's handling of funds, its maintenance of the physical plant, its appointment of personnel, its provision of technical services, its policies of staff organization—all affect the adequacy of care given by physicians and others. Not that every decision should be subject to review by a higher authority, but the overall effect of these decisions—or failures to make decisions—is manifestly of great public concern.

There are other boards of citizens at the local level that may examine aspects of hospital operation from time to time. Community chests or councils may look into how funds they have granted are spent. Blue Cross boards may indirectly call for economies. Governmental agencies buying services for various beneficiaries may demand that certain standards be met. But the focus of each of these groups tends to be narrow and their impact is limited.

To provide more general surveillance over hospitals, a number of national nongovernmental associations have taken action. The first such body of wide impact was the American College of Surgeons which, shortly after World War I, developed a nationwide system for approval of hospitals meeting certain standards of organization and practice. Meanwhile the American Hospital Association established limited standards for membership and "listing" in its annual roster. The American Medical Association, through its Council on Education and Hospitals, developed a system of approval of hospitals for internships, residencies, and postgraduate education. Special approvals for such services as tumor clinics, blood banks, and schools for X-ray and laboratory technicians were given by other professional societies or voluntary agencies.

These specialized approvals, on the whole, continue, but in 1952 there was organized an overall system of hospital "accreditation" by a joint commission made up of representatives of the American College of Physicians, American College of Surgeons, American Hospital Association, American Medical Association, and the Canadian Medical Association. This commission undertakes inspections throughout the Nation and has doubtless had a major effect in upgrading hospital performance. The prestige of accreditation has come to be regarded as an essential asset in a hospital's public relations. Withdrawal or the threat of withdrawal of accreditation provides a strong incentive to improve practices. In contrast to the State government licensure systems, the main emphasis of the joint commission's work is on medical staff practices, although a comprehensive review is made.

Despite the notable achievements of these voluntary bodies, their shortcomings must be recognized.[5]

- They are voluntary and no hospital need even apply for their approval; indeed, some of the marginal institutions, in greatest need of improvement, avoid the whole process. Even if an institution seeks approval and fails to get it, there is no penalty except nonapproval. In a one-hospital community, without "competition" for patients, this moral penalty may have little effect.
- The Joint Commission on Accreditation makes a policy of examining only hospitals of 25 beds or more. Yet 800 hospitals in the United States are smaller than this, and these institutions may present the thorniest problems. The Georgia Hospital Association and the Georgia Department of Public Health have been unusual in launching a special accreditation program for these small units.
- These professional societies and commissions are, of course, independent and responsible only to themselves.

While their integrity may be beyond question, they do not unfailingly reflect the public interest. Their viewpoint, indeed, is sometimes parochial; they avoid inspection and accreditation of osteopathic hospitals, for example, despite the fact that these institutions give care to thousands of patients. In the recent contentions between radiologists and hospitals about schemes of organization, these professional societies have stood aloof, not lending their weight toward whatever side they judge to be in the public interest.

In the light of these shortcomings in voluntary mechanisms for protection of the public interest in hospital operations, and in spite of their enormous positive achievements, there remains in a democratic society an overriding need for public supervision of hospitals. Only through governmental authorities, responsible ultimately to the whole people, can this supervision be fully and effectively exercised. The responsibility of government is carried out through the political process. This process in turn, has been increasingly fortified by merit systems for appointment of officials, especially in technical fields. Government agencies may solicit and receive expert advice from many sources, but the final policy decisions must rest with the agencies. They are ultimately accountable to the citizenry, who can vote the top policymakers out of office if dissatisfied. Governments have, in summary, not only the power but also the obligation to protect the public interest.

Role of Government

The principal means by which governmental agencies have come to protect the public interest in the operation of hospitals is through licensing by State authorities. The laws defining this power are relatively new. Before 1945, only 10 States had any form of hospital licensure law, the exercise of public surveillance being confined principally to the State licensure of physicians and other health personnel working in hospitals. The Federal Hospital Survey and Construction Act of 1946, however, was enacted in a period when consciousness of the public interest in hospitals had matured. It contained therefore a stipulation that every State receiving Federal grants for aiding in hospital construction should have a law governing minimum standards of maintenance and operation for at least the subsidized facilities. In time, every State passed such a law, and in all but two States, Delaware and Louisiana, it has come to be applied to all hospitals in the State.[6]

In these State laws, the legislature usually declares that every hospital must have a license granted by a particular State agency, typically the health department. The health department is authorized to issue regulations to carry out the legislative intent, which is usually broadly defined. The Missouri statute, for example, declares it to be the legislative purpose to "provide for the development, establishment, and enforcement of standards (1) for the care and treatment of individuals in hospitals and (2) for the construction, maintenance, and operation of hospitals, which, in the light of advancing knowledge, will promote safe and adequate treatment of such individuals in hospitals," and authorizes the Missouri Department of Public Health and Welfare to adopt, amend, promulgate, and enforce rules to accomplish the purposes of the law.[7]

The adoption of such a statute represents a forceful exercise of the police power of the State. It grants to the public authority the power to determine the precise conditions under which a hospital shall be operated. If anyone sets out to operate a hospital without meeting these standards, he is subject to prosecution.

While these powers are seldom invoked, their existence strengthens the effectiveness of suggestions for improvements made by State agencies.

With such sweeping powers at their disposal, State agencies are faced with many delicate questions about the scope and content of regulations that they adopt. To what precise aspects of hospital operation should the regulations apply? How detailed and specific should they be? Should the regulations tolerate mediocre or second-best practices, so long as they are not proved to be harmful, or should they set more rigorous requirements? Should there be a "grandfather clause" in hospital regulations, permitting more lenient standards for old institutions than for new ones? Should different standards be accepted for large hospitals and small ones, merely because of their size or because of their differing roles in a regional network? In all these questions, the technical considerations must be blended with political judgments. Government officials must decide how far public understanding will support their actions.

The older State hospital regulations tended to construe their authority narrowly. Their attention was concentrated on protection of the safety of patients; they were explicit about details of the physical plant, including such items as fireproof construction, number and location of exits, the maintenance of buildings, and so on. Details of water supply and sewage disposal were also spelled out, in the older public health tradition. Public concern for mothers and babies has also been expressed in special requirements for hospital maternity departments.

The newer State hospital regulations are concerned with much broader aspects of hospital organization. There are requirements on the functions of a governing board and administrator, on the medical staff organization (bylaws, selection of physicians, restrictions, and so on), on detailed clinical records, on the laboratory and X-ray departments, on the nursing service, dietary management, and so on. A few State agencies have ventured into the ticklish problem of requiring admission-discharge control committees. There are also, of course, requirements on physical plant and sanitation. In short, the scope of the hospital licensure regulations in most States today is broad enough to determine whether the hospital is built, organized, equipped, and staffed in a manner adequate to do the job expected in modern society.[8]

The writing, interpretation, and enforcement of hospital licensure regulations, however, are not simple matters. To strike a compromise between the ideal and the practical, it is common for licensure codes to set out certain standards as mandatory while others are simply "recommended." The mere official publication and discussion of the recommended standards serve to encourage higher levels of hospital performance. From time to time a recommended standard will be changed to a mandatory one, so as to promote improvement of hospitals at a realistic pace.

Quite apart from a deliberate objective of the State licensure agency to encourage improvements, standards must be reviewed continually to be certain that they reflect changes in scientific knowledge. Some 10 years ago, for instance, hospital standards stressed the need for ample oxygen for premature infants. The discovery of the danger of producing blindness, retrolental fibroplasia, by providing too much oxygen to premature babies required a quick shift in the licensure standard. The emphasis is now placed on controls to assure a precise concentration of oxygen.

Some might ask, however, whether the licensure standard should not be stated in terms general enough to eliminate the need for frequent amendment. Would it not be easier, for example, to have regulations simply state: "Where premature infants are cared for, a supply of oxygen appropriate to their needs shall be provided"?

The doctrine of generality in licensing regulations unfortunately is deficient on both legal and practical grounds.[9] Primarily, a regulation with the force of law must be specific and clear enough to enable the person or organization being regulated to know what he must do to comply and what he must not do to avoid violation of the law. What guidance is offered to Oklahoma hospitals, for example, by the State regulation that "sufficient registered nurses shall be employed to assure adequate care of patients"? Even if our stage of knowledge does not permit absolute standards on many subjects, certain bare minimum levels may be stipulated. A requirement that "at least one registered nurse for each 20 (or 40 or 50) patients shall be provided by the hospital" can be understood and can be helpful.

The importance of specificity in hospital regulations is heightened by the realities of law enforcement in this field. Even the best-manned State hospital supervising agency, with the most competent staff, could not inspect hospitals frequently enough to assure absolute compliance with the regulations. In a field of service with the high moral purpose of hospitals, moreover, such policing would be repugnant and unnecessary. The issuance of the regulations is ordinarily enough to induce compliance, but only if the standards are clearly stated. If they are open to varying interpretations, not even the best hospital can be certain how to comply, while the poorest may take refuge in their vagueness.

A troublesome aspect of hospital regulation arises from the frequent multiplicity of regulatory agencies in a State and from inconsistencies in the rules issued by each of them. In New York, for instance, general hospital regulations are issued by the State board of social welfare. Specific rules, however, on newborn nurseries, vital statistics, communicable diseases, laboratory and radiology departments, and the handling of cadavers are issued by the State health department for hospitals outside New York City; still other rules on these subjects for hospitals in New York City are issued by the city health department. Educational programs in hospitals are regulated by the State board of regents. State and local fire regulations, multiple dwelling laws, and zoning ordinances affect hospitals through still other jurisdictions.

There are complex historical reasons for this dispersal of authorities for hospital supervision in State governments, not to mention delegations of certain authorities to local governmental units. The intricacies of government are exasperating not only to the population at large but to public officials themselves. Reorganization commissions at the Federal and State levels have attempted to streamline public administration for years, and the task is never ending. There are some, of course, who emphasize the benefits of dispersed governmental authorities as a protection against political czarism. At the same time, in the hospital and health field splintered authorities tend to weaken the effectiveness with which public agencies can protect the public interest.

There are other reasons, however, why many State hospital licensure programs are less effective in practice than they would appear by studying the language of the written regulations. The responsible agency tends to be meagerly financed and staffed. The qualifications of licensure personnel are often modest. Most States seem to rely heavily on registered nurses, whose competence outside the field of nursing care is often limited. At bottom, perhaps, there is a certain hesitation on the part of State governments to pry too closely into the affairs of voluntary institutions associated with so distinguished and ethical a tradition as that of the medical profession and the community hospital.

But the public interest in hospitals, as we have noted, remains wide and is growing wider. The need for effective programs of governmental supervision of hospitals is more pressing than ever, not only because of the greater demands of the public for the highest technical performance in matters of life and death, but because of a number of issues that have become especially prominent in the last few years.

New Issues of Public Concern

Back of the problem of sharply rising hospital costs, mentioned at the outset, are a series of questions demanding action on a broad community basis. The widespread financing of hospital care through insurance has extended the interest in these questions from individual hospital boards to the population as a whole.

One of these new questions concerns the whole level of hospital utilization in a population that is heavily insured. Are hospitals being overused by some patients and some doctors so that the costs rise for everyone? This is a complex question on which there has been a good deal of confused thinking. If there is any improper use of expensive hospital beds, one must be cautious about accusations, since such usage always involves the concurrence of three parties—the patient, the physician, and the hospital. The forces acting on each are manifold.[10] An approach to the problem calls for discipline by physicians on hospital staffs; their judgment on the use of a given bed is decisive. Is there not a place in hospital regulations therefore for some procedure, such as a designated medical staff committee, to assure the proper admission and discharge of patients, so that costly hospital beds are soundly utilized? (The establishment of such a committee in every Blue Cross participating hospital was, in fact, required by the 1958 decision of the Pennsylvania insurance commissioner.)

Closely related to the use of hospital beds is the issue of their supply and location. Strangely enough, no State now exercises control over this basic question. The licensure laws specify that a hospital to be constructed must meet certain standards, and if these standards are met, the hospital must be licensed. The State agency may not examine whether the additional hospital beds are needed, except for the minority, about one-fourth, of hospitals receiving Federal construction funds. Yet studies in the United States and elsewhere have shown that the most fundamental determinant of the expenditures of a Nation or a State for hospital service is the supply of beds provided. The beds that are there tend to be used.[11]

We are not suggesting that too many hospital beds are available and that further construction should be stopped. Far from it; in fact, we believe that a proper meeting of health needs probably demands a higher ratio of beds to population than we now have, especially of beds for the aged. But we are suggesting that any effective public control over expenditures for hospital service by the population as a whole requires a conscious and deliberate control over the supply of beds in a State. This policy has been recommended by some in terms of a "franchise" to be issued by a public agency for hospital construction or extension.[12] Others have called for issuance of approval for all new hospital construction by regional councils set up under State law.[13] However it may be done, the need for some type of governmental control over the supply and location of hospital beds in a State seems to be increasingly accepted.

A third current issue relates to the policies of hospitals on appointment of physicians to their medical staffs. It is well-settled doctrine that the governing board of a voluntary hospital has the authority to permit or deny physicians the right to practice in the institution. There are sound technical reasons for hospital boards to limit the privileges of attending physicians by barring them completely or by defining more narrowly than the State medical licensure laws what they may do within the institution. At the same time the U.S. Supreme Court and other courts have held it illegal, under the antitrust laws, for medical societies to exert pressure on hospital boards to exclude physicians from hospital staff appointments because of their economic patterns of practice. This issue has arisen several times with respect to denial of hospital privileges to technically qualified physicians engaged in prepaid group medical practice—most recently in Staten Island, N.Y.[14,15] Is there not an important question of public policy involved, insofar as the patients of these doctors may need hospital care and the patients are, indeed, contributing to the support of the hospital through insurance payments? Should not a public agency be prepared to protect the public interest in an issue of this sort?

A fourth issue relates to the use of drugs in hospitals. Recent investigations by a U.S. Senate subcommittee into the prices of brand-name drugs have led to a renewed interest in the application of formularies calling for the use of generic-name drugs wherever feasible. Yet, in Pennsylvania, a hospital pharmacist was penalized for filling a prescription with a generic-name form of a drug rather than with the brand-name form of the same drug, as prescribed by a physician. His hospital's official formulary stipulated use of the generic form.[16] The right—or perhaps even the obligation—of hospitals to use drug formularies would seem to be a matter of clear public interest that ought to come within the purview of State licensure regulation.

A fifth issue concerns labor standards. Although employees of voluntary hospitals do not have the protection of the Federal wage-and-hour standards, they may be covered under the State laws. In 1960, the minimum wage law of New York State, for example, was amended to cover the employees of nonprofit corporations, including hospitals. Unless specific exemptions are ordered by the State industrial commissioner, these employees will shortly be paid a minimum wage of $1 an hour [or higher in later years]. In a number of States, furthermore, the right of collective bargaining through hospital unions is protected by law and may be enforced by State labor agencies.[17] The public interest in these fields has been justified on two grounds: first, to assure decent wages for all persons working in the State; and second, to assist hospitals in maintaining a qualified and stable working force in a competitive labor market.

There are doubtless other issues in today's hospital cauldron, but these may be enough to explain the heightened relevance of hospital affairs to the general public interest. All of these questions affect the costs of hospital care, which almost everyone must now finance. They likewise affect the quality of hospital care, which ultimately influences the life or death of patients. There are, indeed, a wide range of professional measures which may be taken to encourage top-quality performance—tissue committees, medical audits, postgraduate education—in certain hospitals. While the administrative task might be complex, would it not be appropriate protection of the public interest to require such measures to be undertaken in all hospitals?

Future Needs

Perhaps to some this sounds like advocacy of an unreasonable extension of governmental authority over voluntary hospital affairs. We can only say that the issues have arisen not from any hunger for authority by public officials, but rather from the experiences and reactions of the general public. Hospitals are becoming more and more important to people, for both their services and their costs. And their conduct acquires therefore the attributes of a public utility, which cannot be left solely to the prerogatives of its managers but requires the increasing surveillance of a public authority. While voluntary discipline can and does reduce the need for governmental controls, an ultimate need for them remains.

Others may regard the delegation of such wide authority to government as unrealistic. What State agency, they may ask, can command the skills necessary to provide the wide scope of supervision called for? Admittedly, there is no State agency now equipped to do the job. It is small wonder that, with their present meager staffs, the State hospital licensure agencies have so often concentrated their attention on the details of physical plant and safety inspection. It is small wonder that, in their present role, hospital licensure authorities have been regarded rather casually by hospital administrators, and the impact of these authorities has been felt to be slight.[18]

A properly staffed and authorized State agency for hospital supervision, however, could be equal to the responsibilities which the times demand. A beginning has certainly been made in a few States which have taken seriously the language of their licensure codes.[19] In one of the Canadian Provinces with a program of hospital insurance encompassing its entire population of about 900,000, there is a division of hospital administration and standards with 23 professional personnel. These include a medical director and consultants in general hospital administration, nursing, dietetics, pharmacy, radiography, laboratory technology, social work, problems of physical plant, accounting, auditing, and health education. In addition there are part-time consultant services provided by other departmental personnel in sanitary engineering, architecture, medical records, and statistics. Records of the Saskatchewan Department of Public Health, Regina, Canada, show that the cost of maintaining this supervisory staff, in relation to the costs of the hospital service itself, is only a drop in the bucket.

In 1957, the American Hospital Association undertook a study to determine an appropriate range and qualifications of staff for State agencies responsible for supervising hospitals. The results do not seem to have been published, but preliminary documents suggested a need for much more comprehensive staffing than prevails anywhere (personal communication from Hilary Fry, January 15, 1958). Not that such staffing would imply a corps of rugged inspectors to crack the whip over hospital administrators. On the contrary, the goal of a State hospital licensure agency must be to upgrade performance and encourage excellence—not to punish or intimidate. To do this, official personnel must play the role essentially of consultants, advising hospitals on how to meet, or surpass, the legal standards and how to continually improve their services within a framework of maximum economy. There is no reason, incidentally, why much of the advice, now purchased at high fees from private hospital counseling firms, could not be given freely by a really sophisticated staff of technical consultants in a governmental agency. This is the custom in Canada and Europe.

To back up the actions of the hospital licensure staff—or perhaps we should call it the supervisory and consultant staff—the official regulations should come to grips with the significant problems of hospital operation in the 20th century.

Here is a list of the 17 chapters in a proposed set of hospital standards which our institute recently drafted at the request of the New York State Department of Social Welfare:

- Administrative organization and services
- Admission and discharge of patients
- General clinical services
- Anesthesia and inhalation therapy
- Laboratory services
- Physical medicine and rehabilitation
- Dental service
- Nursing service and patient accommodation
- Out-patient and preventive services
- Pharmaceutical service
- Medical social service
- Medical records and library
- Educational activities
- Dietary services
- Sanitary functions
- Physical plant
- Special hazard problems

Regulations of this breadth should not be drawn up unilaterally by a State agency. They should be drafted in consultation with representatives of the hospitals. They should obviously be revised at frequent intervals. Their application by the staff, moreover, should be strengthened by the support of an advisory council representing the hospitals, the health professions, and the general public. An important step in the direction of strengthening the overall State programs of hospital licensure was taken by the formulation of "recommended principles" in this field by the American Hospital Association in May 1960.[20]

With proper legal standards and with staffing to apply them, the farflung public interest in hospitals could be adequately protected. Many of the problems that now beset hospital boards and administrators could be reduced. The public would be set at ease in its suspicions about waste or inefficiency in hospital management. The patient would be reassured about the quality of service, not just in those institutions that are manifestly excellent, but in all institutions. The rights of the community to have the best quality hospital service at the lowest feasible cost would be steadily advanced.

References

1. Smith, F. R.: Adjudication in the matter of the filing of the Associated Hospital Service in Philadelphia (Blue Cross). Harrisburg, Insurance Commissioner of the Commonwealth of Pennsylvania, April 15, 1958, p. 8.

2. Royle, C.: Forces at work—the future. Address presented at Annual Blue Cross Member Hospital Meeting, Syracuse, N.Y., Nov. 17, 1959.
3. Hayt, E., and Hayt, L. R.: Legal guide for American hospitals. New York, Hospital Textbook Co., 1940, p. 30.
4. Covert, C.: No "common man" on hospital boards. Syracuse Herald-Journal, October 20, 1959, *See also* Hunter, F.: Community power structure. Chapel Hill, University of North Carolina Press, 1953.
5. Binder, G.: How regulation differs from accreditation. Mod. Hosp. 94:113, May 1960.
6. Abbe, L. M., and Baney, A. M.: The Nation's health facilities; ten years of the Hill-Burton hospital and medical facilities program, 1946–56. PHS Pub. No. 616. Washington, D.C., U.S. Government Printing Office, 1958.
7. Hospital Licensing Law. Missouri, Senate bill No. 422, 67th General Assembly, 1953.
8. Taylor, K. O., and Donald, D. M.: A comparative study of hospital licensure regulations. Berkeley, University of California, 1957.
9. Curran, W. J.: Preparation of State and local health regulations. Am. J. Pub. Health 49:314–321, March 1959.
10. Roemer, M. I., and Shain, M.: Hospital utilization under insurance. American Hospital Association Monogr. No. 6, Chicago, 1959.
11. Shain, M., and Roemer, M. I.: Hospital costs related to the supply of beds. Mod. Hosp. 92:71–73, 168, April 1959.
12. Brown, R. E.: Let the public control utilization through planning. Hospitals 33:34–39, 108–110, Dec. 1, 1959.
13. Columbia University School of Public Health and Administrative Medicine: Prepayment for hospital care in New York State. New York, Insurance Department, 1960, pp. 5–9.
14. Hospitals making peace bid to HIP. New York Times, July 11, 1960, p. 31.
15. HIP disputants charge monopoly. New York Times, July 12, 1960, p. 37.
16. State Board of Pharmacy vs. Joseph V. D'Amtola—adjudication and order. Am. J. Hosp. Pharm. 16:447, September 1959. (Reprint.)
17. Daykin, W. L.: How labor legislation may affect hospitals. Mod. Hosp. 95:65–69, 124–126, July 1960.
18. Roemer, M. I., and McClanahan, M. H.: Impact of governmental programs on voluntary hospitals. Pub. Health Rep. 75:537–544, June 1960.
19. O'Malley, M.: Hospital licensing—its effects and benefits. Indianapolis, Ind., State Department of Health, 1950.
20. American Hospital Association, Board of Trustees: Recommended principles to be followed by licensing programs for hospitals and other medical care institutions. Hospitals: 34:37, 96–97, Sept. 1, 1960.

21

The Hospital as an Organizing Force in American Medical Care

After World War II, the influence of the hospital extended well beyond its walls. Its policies on the organization of medical staffs affected how doctors worked in their private practices in the community. The hospital played an increasing part in the education of physicians and many other types of health personnel. For the care of certain diseases, like serious mental disorders, special governmental hospitals became the main vehicle of public programs, as they did for the care of the poor in municipal or county public hospitals.

During this time, hospitals engaged physicians increasingly on salaries or through other contractual arrangements. A nationwide survey, started in 1959, indicated much more use of "contractual physicians" in hospitals than had been generally realized. Moreover, hospitals of greater technological development showed a greater tendency to engage physicians by contract. Principal findings of this survey, and their significance, were reported in the Fourth Annual Schwitalla Symposium Lecture at St. Louis University in June, 1964.

THE FORCES AFFECTING the shape of medical care in American life derive from many origins; from population changes, from industrialization, from endlessly changing technology, from advancement of education, from the whole democratic process. These forces have been directed along two main channels; those involving modified methods of financing medical care and those involving new patterns for the actual provision of care.[1]

A very great proportion of social energies and political debate in American medicine over the last 30 or 40 years has been concerned with the first of these channels of change. In it we have witnessed the great health insurance movement, with its eddies and currents involving different sponsorships, varied scopes of benefits, diverse population coverages, and so on. In this channel also is the complex of medical care programs supported by general governmental revenues for the care of the needy and other special groups, the treatment of certain diseases, and the purchase of special technical services. Here also must be included the continuing national debates on governmental health insurance for the whole population or part of it (such as the aged), which despite their failure to produce

Chapter 21 originally appeared as "Growth of Salaried Physicians" in *Hospital Progress* (the journal of the Catholic Hospital Association), September, 1964, pp. 79–83, and is reprinted by permission of that journal.

much legislation have had enormous influence on actions taken in the private sector of the medical economy.

In the second channel of medical-social change, that involving new patterns for provision of care, the issues have been somewhat less contentious, though in the long run the developments may well be of much greater importance. It makes one pause perhaps to realize that the issue of dollars and earnings have been more explosive than those involving how doctors work and how people are treated. Perhaps it is because in this second sphere the initiative has been taken less by government and more by voluntary bodies, although even the latter can rock the boat of medical affairs.

The movements affecting patterns of medical care provision might be summarized in four parts: 1. those undertaken by the medical profession itself; 2. those sponsored by public health and related governmental agencies; 3. those initiated by voluntary health agencies, and 4. those launched by hospitals.

The Hospital's Impact

The impact on patterns of medical care in America wrought by the hospital, however, probably exceeds that of all these other social entities. Certainly the average physician and the way he does his work have been more widely influenced by hospital framework. They are salaried members of the hospital team, as is the is felt not only on the doctor's management of his own private patients who are hospitalized, but on the whole fabric of health service organization in the community. A brief examination of the forms taken by these hospital movements will provide a better setting for understanding the role of the salaried hospital physician. We may analyze this hospital movement in terms of four streams of hospital action.

The first stream involves the great number and variety of hospitals devoted to the care of specific diseases. The most important of these, of course, are the mental institutions which contain as many beds as all the general hospitals combined. In addition, there are the tuberculosis hospitals which, while declining in importance with the reduction of this disease, are being steadily replaced by other special hospitals for long-term disorders of any diagnosis. There are some 200 more hospitals in the United States devoted exclusively to the diseases of children, to diseases of the eye or the ear-nose-throat, to orthopedic disorders, to the problems of women, to drug addiction, to alcoholism, or to leprosy.

The point is that in the vast majority of these institutions, the medical supervision of patients is done by physicians who are part and parcel of the organized hospital framework. They are salaried members of the hospital team, as are the nurse and the technician, even though their level of responsibility is higher.In examining overall medical care in America, one must not overlook the vast programs in these special hospitals, just because the patients in them tend to have long-term illness and tend to be somewhat removed from the central stream of community life. Several thousand physicians devote their whole medical lives to this kind of service.

From County to Kaiser

The second stream of the hospital movement affecting American medicine involves those hospitals treating all types of acute or chronic illness in designated population groups for which organized responsibility has been taken by government.[2] Quite aside from the institutions for long-term disorders cited above, the federal government maintains almost 400 general hospitals with more than 100,000 beds for the care of veterans, military personnel, merchant seamen, American Indians, prisoners, and other specific beneficiaries. These institutions, of course, absorb the full-time energies of several thousand physicians on salary.

County and city governments also operate a diverse variety of general hospitals for welfare recipients and other indigent persons. In California and some other western states, the county government is usually responsible, while in the older eastern communities like Philadelphia, New York, or Boston, it is usually the city government; in Louisiana, it is the state government which operates the network of "charity hospitals." Typically, these institutions are staffed by a corps of salaried physicians, often (but not always) affiliated with a medical school faculty. Private attending physicians, on a part-time basis, add to the medical manpower with or without compensation.

Nongovernmental bodies also operate "closed-staff," general hospitals for special beneficiaries, and these constitute a third stream of the hospital movement. Railroads, especially in the West, have maintained such facilities for their workers since the nineteenth century. The Endicott-Johnson Shoe Company and the Hershey Chocolate Company are examples of benevolent managements that have long operated comprehensive medical care programs for their employees plus their families, including maintenance of their own hospitals with organized salaried medical staffs. The Kaiser Corporation on the West Coast developed a medical care program for its workers and dependents during World War II, which included the construction of its own hospitals. The Kaiser Health Plan has now been extended to cover, through insurance payments, over 1,000,000 persons, who receive their hospital care in a network of 15 general hospitals staffed entirely by salaried physicians. (*Note*: By the late 1970s, this comprehensive health insurance plan had grown to some 3 million members with nearly 3,000 physicians, serving in the program's own hospitals and clinics, on full-time salaries.)

In the coal-mining industry, a somewhat similar network of hospitals was developed in the Appalachian region by the union-management sponsored United Mine Workers Welfare and Retirement Fund. Although these 10 general hospitals have now been transferred to other control (the Presbyterian Church Mission), I understand that their basic staffs of salaried physicians are being continued. One must not overlook the several hundred university and college infirmaries, which are essentially small hospitals for a defined population (usually insured) served typically by a staff of salaried physicians.

Other prepaid medical care programs, not tied to a specific company or industry, also operate closed-staff hospitals. Among these are the Farmers Union Hospital Association in Elk City, Okla., and the Group Health Cooperative of Puget Sound in Seattle. The newest and most impressive of these health insurance plans, with its own highly organized general hospital, is operated by a union in Detroit. One should realize, however, that the doctors associated with most health insurance plans, whether sponsored by consumers or providers of service, serve their patients in ordinary community general hospitals, with "open" medical staff policies.

Add Interns and Residents

Finally, within this third stream of the American hospital movement, are those general hospitals—neither governmental nor affiliated with an insurance program—that serve their patients through an organized, salaried, closed medical staff. Some of these have been launched by private philanthropy, like the Henry Ford Hospital in Detroit, the Mary Imogene Bassett Hospital in Cooperstown, N.Y., or in the Hunterdon Medical Center in Flemington, N.J. Others have been developed as in-patient annexes of private group practices, like the hospitals attached to the Crile Clinic in Cleveland, Ohio, the Guthrie Clinic in Sayre, Pa., or the Ochsner Clinic in New Orleans. Most university-sponsored teaching hospitals also must be counted under this heading, since the principal responsibility for patient care in them devolves upon salaried medical school faculty members.

The fourth stream of the American hospital movement affecting medical care is the world of activity involving the modal type of American health facility: the voluntary nonprofit general hospital for short-term illness, with an open staff of private attending physicians. Quite aside from the great impacts on American health service exerted by all types of hospitals so far described, the typical community general hospital is also the scene of a constantly extending pattern of social organization. The growing engagement of salaried physicians in such hospitals is one, but by no means the only, reflection of these important trends.

Between 1931 and 1957, the ratio of physicians in purely private practice in the United States actually declined from 108.2 to 91.1 per 100,000 population. In this period, physicians engaged in full-time hospital service (exclusive of federal government facilities) rose from 7.8 to 21.2 per 100,000. Put another way, this meant that in 1930 one physician in 16 was serving full-time in hospitals, while today it is about one in six. These figures include interns and residents, but there can be no doubt that the same trend applies to full-time hospital physicians who have already completed their training.[3] Moreover, one cannot overlook the vast volume of medical service done for patients in some 800 hospitals (of all sponsorship types) by salaried interns and residents, just because they are simultaneously in training. If these young physicians were not available, their job would probably have to be performed by other contractual physicians, for example, as in VA hospitals.

And Increasing Staff Discipline

We need not explore the historical pressures in the general population and in the health professions themselves in back of these organizing developments, but their current nature may simply be identified. The parliamentary organization of medical staffs, with officers and formal meetings, is one such development. The increasing use of formal procedures for admission of a physician to the medical staff and for definition of his professional privileges and responsibilities is another. The enactment of medical staff bylaws (although not always enforced) defining obligations of the physician on such matters as maintenance of records or procurement of consultations is another widespread fact of hospital life.

The organization of various clinical departments, with further internal structures, tends to bring professional group discipline closer to the decisions of the individual private physician. An extending list of medical staff committees is casting an eye over the actions of doctors in the diagnosis and treatment of their patients (whether private or "public ward" cases). These include committees on pathological tissues, on records, on infections,on drugs, on admissions and discharges, and other professional functions. While these organized measures tend to be more highly developed in larger hospitals, the desire for accredtiation and status is promoting them in hospitals of all sizes.[4]

These essentially bureaucratic measures within the hospital staffs of private attending physicians are being complemented increasingly by organizational decisions requiring engagement of contractual hospital-based physicians inside the essentially open-staff institution. I say "contractual" rather than "salaried" physicians, because the method of payment—while it comes from the hospital rather than the patient—is not always by a flat salary. The various schemes of payment are an intricate story, but they represent essentially a range of compromises between the physician's desire for professional independence and the hospital's need for budgetary planning. The most widely established of these organized elements in community general hospitals are, of course, the departments of radiology and pathology, and surrounding their administration there was widespread controversy a few years ago. Hospitals were accused of the "illegal corporate practice of medicine" simply because they made mutually agreeable contracts with radiologists and pathologists involving payment of salaries for certain services.[5]

Quantitative Findings

In 1959 we set out at the University of California in Los Angeles to determine the extent of engagement of contractual physicians of various specialties by general hospitals throughout the United States, and to examine various correlates of such practices. A mail questionnaire was sent to every general hospital in the country of 50 beds or more and responses were received from 84 percent of this universe. In the final analysis military hospitals were eliminated (although they obviously have many, indeed all, contractual physicians) as well as proprietary hospitals (due to many obvious misinterpretations of our questionnaire). The ultimate tabulation, therefore, was based on 2,434 general hospitals under voluntary nonprofit or governmental (but nonmilitary) sponsorship. While the data did not specifically identify the hospital departments or programs involved, their nature can generally be inferred from the specialties reported. In Table 21-1, the principal findings of this survey are reported, in descending order of frequency for all types of medical contract, either full-time or part-time. The importance of radiology, pathology, and anesthesiology is no surprise, but the 20 percent of general hospitals with contractual physicians in internal medicine may be a bit startling. Most of the hospitals with such appointees, it may be noted, use the internists on a part-time basis and a good proportion of these doctors are probably involved in employee health services, emergency room duties, or possibly EKG readings (though not specifically reported as such). The 15 percent of hospitalswith physical medicine specialists on contract and the 13 percent with doctors devoted to medical education are quite interesting, even though most of these appointments are also part-time.

Without commenting on the implication of each specialty presented in this table, one need only mention a few of the other significant new developments in the way of organized services in community general hospitals. The larger community hospitals are increasingly trying to emulate teaching institutions by appointing directors of medical education, to increase the effectiveness of their training programs for interns and residents, as well as practicing private physicians. A small but growing number of essentially open-staff hospitals are also appointing full-time chiefs of their clinical services, with functions not only in house staff education, but also in the direct supervision of patient care on public wards, in consultations, and in medical research. Some of these appointees are doubtless included under the designations of "medical administration" or "medical research."

Physicians with assigned responsibilities for the hospital emergency room are, as noted earlier, also probably included under other labels in the table. The rapidly increasing utilization of such rooms in recent years is a testimony to the growing public confidence in hospitals and perhaps the declining accessibility of private medical practitioners. Another pattern, still small on the horizon but undoubtedly destined to grow, is the appointment of contractual physicians to supervise organized homecare programs which are now reported to be operating

Table 21-1
General Hospitals with Contractual Physicians: Percentages of General Hospitals (of 50 beds or more) Having Designated Specialists Under Contract, by Time-status, Among 2,434 Institutions in the Continental United States, 1959.

Specialty	*Full-time Only*	*Part-time Only*	*Both Full-Time and Part-time*	*All Types*
Radiology	48.3	39.1	8.4	95.9
Pathology	44.8	39.6	6.5	90.9
Anesthesiology	21.6	8.1	2.5	32.1
Internal medicine	4.9	10.6	4.8	20.3
Physical medicine	6.0	8.0	1.4	15.4
EKG, BMR readings, etc.	1.4	12.2	0.1	13.7
Medical education	4.2	8.7	0.4	13.3
Medical administration	9.9	1.7	0.8	12.4
Surgery	4.1	3.1	4.6	11.8
"Other fields"	2.4	6.0	1.9	10.3
Psychiatry	2.7	3.9	3.0	9.6
Pediatrics	2.5	2.9	1.2	6.7
Obstetrics and gynecology	2.1	3.0	0.6	5.7
Medical research	2.7	1.1	1.2	4.9
Any specialty	—	—	—	98.1

in 7.5 percent of hospitals in the country. The appointment of a hospital-based specialist in preventive or social medicine is still another innovation, rare but significant.

A word is in order about the methods of remuneration under physician-hospital contracts. Looking at all 14 categories of specialty listed in Table 21-1, the commonest scheme of payment is simply by straight salary. While true, this statement is somewhat misleading, however, since radiology, the specialty most frequently found under contract, is remunerated in 70 percent of the hospitals by another method: a share of departmental income (gross or net) by diverse formulas. This is the commonest method also for pathology, that is, in 45 percent of the contracts. Anesthesiology is most frequently (43 percent of the contracts) rewarded on a fee-for-service basis. EKG, BMR readings and the like are also paid for most often by an income-sharing scheme.

The other 10 special fields, while occurring in much smaller proportions of hospitals, are all remunerated most often by salary. The basic data on this question are presented in Table 21-2. The administrative and professional implications of each of these methods of contractual payment are different.

Table 21-2
Remuneration of Contractual Physicians: Percentages of Physician-Hospital Contracts for Designated Specialties, by Method of Remuneration, among 2,434 Institutions in the Continental United States, 1959

Specialty	*Salary*	*Salary Plus Other Method*	*Share of Departmental Income*	*Fee-for-service*	*Two or More Methods*
Radiology	16.7	5.5	69.8	5.0	3.0
Pathology	28.7	8.7	45.0	13.8	3.8
Anesthesiology	31.6	8.4	13.8	43.0	3.2
Internal medicine	54.7	5.7	18.8	16.0	4.8
Physical medicine	60.2	9.9	21.7	6.1	2.1
EKG, BMR readings, etc.	10.2	1.2	49.4	36.8	2.4
Medical education	93.5	6.2	—	0.3	—
Medical administration	94.0	4.7	—	0.3	1.0
Surgery	81.6	6.6	1.7	5.2	4.9
"Other fields"	74.5	5.2	6.8	7.2	6.4
Psychiatry	78.2	8.5	2.1	6.0	5.1
Pediatrics	79.6	10.5	1.2	5.6	3.1
Obstetrics and gynecology	81.3	10.1	0.7	5.8	2.2
Medical research	95.8	2.5	—	0.8	0.8

Implications for Performance

On the qualitative implications of this whole trend toward increasing organization of medical staffs in hospitals, a few final words must be said. A definitive evaluation of its meaning cannot yet be offered, although most leadership in hospital administration would agree that all these movements probably yield improvement in the quality of medical care. This is a subject on which we are trying to get more detailed answers in a current research project at UCLA. In our 1959 study of 2,434 general hospitals, however, we did collect some "circumstantial evidence" on the question. Without taking time to explain the methodology, we gave each hospital a "contractual physician score" to reflect its degree of engagement of such physicians, adjusted for its bed capacity.[6] Our assumption is that this score not only is a barometer of the contractual physicians as such, which it measures directly, but it also gives an indirect reading of the general strictness of organization of the hospital's whole medical staff.

Relationships were then examined with a number of features of each hospital's general program, reflecting its scope and quality of services. This was done by placing all 2,434 hospitals in the order of their "contractual physician scores," which permitted dividing the series into ranked quartile groups. Then, the presence or absence of each of these features of the hospital program (or certain other rates) in each quartile group could be determined. The total series contains both governmental and voluntary hospitals, but the relationships can be more clearly demonstrated by confining the observations to one sponsorship group. This has been done in Table 21-3, which gives the findings for the 1,118 voluntary nonprofit (nonreligious) hospitals in our series.

The data are presented under seven categories which at least indirectly reflect something about the quality of the hospital program: 1. overall performance; 2. amplitude of staffing; 3. diagnostic procedures offered; 4. surgical facilities; 5. other significant therapies; 6. educational functions, and 7. preventive and community service. Of the 26 specific features examined, 20 show a clear and consistent positive relationship by quartile groups to the height of the contractual physician score. Of the remaining six features, for only two (the presence of a premature infant nursery and the presence of a professional nursing school) is the occurrence of the feature in the highest quartile group not at its maximum rate. Whichever may be cause and effect between the medical staff organization in a hospital and the features of its program, it would appear that a high level of staff structuring tends to be associated positively with those services and facilities that connote a higher quality of institutional performance.

Deeper probing of these relationships, of course, would be required to provide practical guidance for hospital administrators, but even these relatively crude findings suggest that the trend toward more contractual physicians in hospitals goes hand-in-hand with a greater likelihood of accreditation, wider diagnostic and treatment functions, more extensive educational activities, and a more positive orientation to preventive and community service.

By the same token, the more disciplined structure of medical staffs in hospitals must inevitably be having an influence on the practice of medicine outside the institutional walls. The operation of a handful of organized homecare programs is perhaps the most direct but the least important way that this extramural influence is now exerted, although its future importance will doubtless increase. The indirect educational influence of the hospital, however, on the doctor's whole mode of practice is continuous and widespread. It brings to bear on community medical practice a sense of teamwork and responsibility that the solo practitioner could rarely acquire in his private office. The absence or weakness of such influence has been a cause for serious concern in European general practice.[7]

Unlike the typical European hospital, the American general hospital holds ties with the great majority of practicing physicians in the locality. These ties are not necessarily and always promotive of excellence, and they may even yield harmful effects for hospitalized patients. Everything depends on the diligence with which doctors help each other, discipline each other, and strengthen each other as a hospital staff. To achieve this esprit de corps most successfully requires at least a skeleton staff of physicians who identify themselves wholly or largely with the

Table 21-3
Contractual Physicians and Selected Features of the Hospital Program: Percentages (and Other Designated Rates) of General Hospitals with Specified Features in Ranked Quartile Groups (According to "Contractual Physician Score") among 1,118 Voluntary Nonprofit, Nonreligious Hospitals in the Continental United States, 1959.

Hospital Feature	*Quartile Groups*			
	Lowest	*Second*	*Third*	*Highest*
Overall Performance				
General accreditation	76.2	89.7	90.4	93.3
Approved cancer program	9.6	16.8	29.6	39.8
Autopsy percentage[a]	23.2	28.7	33.0	43.5
Amplitude of Staffing				
Total personnel[b]	210.0	220.0	230.0	250.0
Professional nurses[b]	34.1	36.3	38.9	39.9
Technical personnel[b]	24.7	27.1	29.3	34.3
Diagnostic Procedures				
Electro-encephalography	10.7	15.7	23.4	38.0
Radioactive isotopes	16.5	31.2	38.3	49.9
Surgical Facilities				
Blood bank	59.7	69.5	71.2	73.2
Post-operative recovery room	60.5	66.8	70.4	71.8
Intensive care unit	4.2	9.6	11.1	15.0
Other Significant Therapies				
Therapeutic X-ray	48.2	58.8	67.0	69.8
Physical therapy	36.8	49.9	57.7	70.8
Dental department	25.2	32.6	48.8	55.2
Premature infant nursery	70.8	73.0	75.0	68.4
Psychiatric beds	2.5	4.5	3.2	7.2
Educational Functions				
Internships	9.8	23.0	37.9	45.5
Residencies	11.5	21.5	34.4	52.6
Medical school affiliation	1.4	1.8	3.8	19.6
Professional nursing school	24.1	29.3	35.4	30.4
Nursing school affiliation	0.7	0.4	1.7	3.2
Preventive and Community Service				
Hospital bed occupany[c]	70.9	73.3	75.3	76.4
Routine chest X-rays	38.3	39.4	47.2	47.0
Outpatient visits[d]	73.4	70.8	98.0	155.1
Long-term beds	1.1	1.5	1.1	3.6
Social service department	6.8	10.4	29.3	46.2

a. Average percentage for each quartile group.
b. Average number of personnel per 100 beds for quartile group.
c. Average percentage for each quartile group.
d. Average visits per bed per year for quartile group.

institution. Their energies must be directed mainly to an institutional ideal, rather than mainly to a private practice, in which the hospital is merely a side issue. This impact on the whole quality of medical care, both inside and outside the walls, it seems, is the chief value to be gained from the increasing engagement of contractual physicians in the hospitals of America.

References

1. Avedis Donabedian and S. J. Axelrod, "Organizing Medical Care Programs to Meet Health Needs," *The Annals* (of the American Academy of Political and Social Science), 337:46–56, September, 1961.
2. James A. Hamilton, *Patterns of Hospital Ownership and Control,* Minneapolis, Univ. of Minnesota Press, 1961.
3. Surgeon General's Consultant Group on Medical Education, *Physicians for a Growing America*, Washington D.C., Public Health Service, Pub. No. 709, 1959, p. 83.
4. "Will the Hospital Soon Be Your Boss?" *Medical Economics,* Vol. 40, No. 12, June 17, 1963.
5. Alanson W. Willcox, et al., *Hospitals and the Corporate Practice of Medicine,* Chicago, American Hospital Association, Monograph No. 1, 1957.
6. Milton I. Roemer, "Medical Staff Organization in General Hospitals: The Influence of Contractual Physicians," *Epidemiology: Reports on Research and Teaching 1962,* London, Oxford Univ. Press, 1963, pp. 307–313.
7. Milton I. Roemer, "The Impact of Hospitals on the Practice of Medicine in Europe and America," *Hospitals,* November 1, 1963, pp. 61–64 ff.

22

The Effect of Staff Organization on Hospital Performance

Our study of medical staff organization in general hospitals in relation to the expected performance of the basic functions was completed in 1969 and published, with the co-authorship of Jay W. Friedman, as Doctors in Hospitals *(Baltimore: The Johns Hopkins Press, 1971). In 1971 the American Hospital Association invited me to present a summary of the study findings at its annual meeting.*

Growth of Salaried Doctors

The increase in appointments of full-time salaried physicians in U.S. general hospitals in the past two or three decades has been too obvious to belabor with statistics. This increase would not be news, of course, on the international scene where the salaried hospital physician nearly everywhere has been the general rule, rather than the exception. The recent American trends, therefore, are simply bringing our hospitals more in line with the patterns that have long prevailed in Europe and elsewhere.

A recent survey of physicians by the American Medical Association showed that between 1963 and 1968 the national supply of physicians increased by 16 percent, while the number of physicians in full-time hospital practice (in nonfederal institutions) rose by 107 percent. Even these figures probably understate the true trend, as they omit physicians in federal hospitals, where full-time appointments predominate, as well as physicians in university positions, administration, and hospital-based research, and all interns and residents. The full-time appointment trend, moreover, cannot be attributed to any special expansion of local and state government hospitals, as distinguished from voluntary ones. Between 1946 and 1967, the beds in local and state government hospitals rose by 44 percent and those in federal hospitals actually declined by 23 percent, while the beds in voluntary hospitals rose by 82 percent. Thus it is evident that the trend toward full-time appointments is referable to voluntary hospitals as much as or more than to public facilities.

Chapter 22 originally appeared in *Hospitals* (the journal of the American Hospital Association), Volume 45, issue 18, September 16, 1971, pp. 70–72, and is reprinted by permission of that journal.

Methods of paying full-time physicians in U.S. hospitals have always been varied, ranging from full-time salaries, to salaries combined with other methods, to sharing of departmental income (gross or net), to an outright concessional contract in which the physician runs a department almost independently, collects all the fees, and pays rent to the hospital. Among these diverse methods, the swing seems to have been toward straight salary remuneration. A nationwide survey that I ran in 1959 showed that salaries were the method of payment among 50 percent of contractual physicians, with another 7 percent combining salaries with some other method and 43 percent following other payment schemes. A similar survey by *Medical Economics* five years later found the salary pattern to have risen to 75 percent and salary plus another method to 11 percent, with only 14 percent using other payment arrangements. While the provisions of the Medicare legislation (that is, considering the services of hospital-based physicians as medical, rather than hospital, insurance benefits) may have altered these trends in the past six years, I suspect that other forces have maintained the straight salary as the most common form of remunerating full-time hospital physicians.

Results of the Trends

The nature of all the technological and social forces responsible for the rising use of full-time physicians in hospitals is well known. They include all the developments of new diagnostic and treatment methods, the expansion of professional education and research in hospitals, the increasing demands for out-patient and emergency services, the expansion of special fields like psychiatry or rehabilitation in hospitals, and the overall pressures for excellence in hospital performance. I think we may expect these forces to continue operating at an increasing tempo, so that the greater part of hospital service in the United States in the future, as in other countries now, may well be provided by full-time physicians. The recent new federal interest in health maintenance organizations under Medicare and Medicaid is perhaps another straw in the wind pointing in this direction.

Health care leaders, as well as the general public, may properly ask what consequences can be expected from these trends in terms of the overall effectiveness of hospitals. In response to this question, the most relevant information that I may be able to contribute here is a report of a study made over the past ten years on medical staff organization and hospital performance.

The main focus in this empirical study was on the medical staff organization in hospitals as a whole, and the salaried physician was analyzed as part of that constellation. Our principal reason for studying the medical staff organization (MSO) was to determine its influence on the hospital's effectiveness in performing the various functions that are increasingly expected in the modern scene.

To tackle this problem, we conducted a number of different studies—historical and international studies, a nationwide statistical survey of 2,400 hospitals, some tangential studies of medical staff bylaws and of hospital death rates as a quality index, and an in-depth investigation of a small sample of hospitals. While each of these studies tended to complement the others, this paper will summarize only the last one—a field examination of the medical staff dynamics and the total program of hospital service in 10 hospitals. These institutions were chosen to illustrate a wide spectrum of MSO patterns, which we conceptualized as ranging from very loosely structured organizations through three midway stages to a very highly structured medical staff organization. The key question was: How is the MSO pattern related to the hospital's performance of five basic functions—in-patient care, out-patient care, professional education, medical research, and functions encompassing prevention, home care, and other wider community roles?

This research problem necessitated development of a quantitative method for scoring the tightness of an MSO pattern. Drawing from general organization theory, we did this by measuring seven basic elements in the MSO structure and operation: 1. staff composition, 2. appointment procedures, 3. commitment, 4. departmentalization, 5. control committees, 6. documentation, and 7. informal dynamics. Under these elements were 19 quantifiable features, the aggregates of which yielded a range of MSO scores from 25 to 84 points on a theoretical 100-point scale.

Improved Hospital Organization

The most predictive among the 19 features, or subelements, of medical staff organization was the calculated strength of "contractual physicians" in the medical staff. We used this broader term to encompass salaried physicians (full-time or part-time) as well as other physicians with contractual ties to the hospital, even though their remuneration was on some basis other than straight time payments. This corollary finding is not merely coincidental, but is causative. The very engagement of contractual physicians by a hospital contributes substantially to the firmness of its overall medical staff organization. The dynamics of this process involve both the supportive role played by these physicians and the reactions they induce in the attending (or voluntary) medical staff. The effect of contractual physicians in hospitals appears to be an elevation of the whole organizational quality of hospitals: strengthening the hand of hospital administration while, at the same time, stimulating firmer group discipline within the medical staff.

Another finding within the MSO dynamics concerned the various control committees for tissue review, medical records, infection, drug use, and so on, which play so large a part in the typical U.S. voluntary hospital. We found that these instruments of group discipline played a relatively lesser role in hospitals at the highly structured end of the MSO scale and a greater role in hospitals at the loosely structured end of the scale. These committees, or equivalent mechanisms, seem to be a type of compensatory mechanism in response to the general permissiveness of the open staff patterns that evolved in U.S. hospitals of the 20th century. Thus, where the general medical staff organization is tighter—the structure usually associated with more use of contractual physicians—less need for these committees is felt, and their operation is actually weaker. This interpretation is supported by both historical and international observations.

Our basic findings on hospital performance were not, of course, all simple and linear, but they pointed in general to the value of the more highly structured MSO patterns in facilitating fulfillment of modern expectations of a general hospital's mission.

The Five Basic Functions

Among the components of in-patient care, the scope and technical development of most clinical department functions in the 10 hospitals of our study were found to be quite similar for the medical needs of "routine" patients or cases of only mild or moderate severity. Differentials were noticeable, however, in the hospital's capacity to serve the difficult or severely ill patients; for these, the range and richness of services were distinctly greater in the hospitals of higher MSO structuring. This generalization applies mainly to medical, surgical, and obstetrical services; for pediatric services, there was a positive association of MSO structuring with performance even for the care of the average patient. As for psychiatric services, the positive correlation is still sharper, for this element of performance was virtually limited to the more highly structured hospitals.

We classified other elements of in-patient hospital care as supportive medical services, and for these our hospital series showed a generally positive relationship to the level of MSO structuring. The differentials were perhaps least marked for anesthesiology, moderate for radiology and pathology, and most marked for physical medicine and rehabilitation. Pharmacy and nursing were classified as supportive paramedical services, and these showed divergent relationships. Pharmacy services were more systematized in the more highly structured hospitals. Nursing services, on the other hand, were most abundant in the less structured hospitals; with relatively larger nursing staffs and fewer technological demands made upon them, these hospitals evidently are capable of giving more "tender loving care" to in-patients.

Ideally, we should like to know the final outcome of any pattern of medical staff organization in terms of patient recovery. This is a thorny research problem, which cannot be discussed in this brief article, except to say that we developed a statistical formula for adjusting hospital death rates to take into account the probable severity of the cases admitted—using the adjusted death rate as an outcome measure on the quality of in-patient care. Application of this formula showed an adjusted mortality rate of 3.41 percent in the most permissive MSO hospitals, 1.51 percent in the moderate MSO hospitals, and 1.88 percent in the most rigorous hospitals. The lack of complete linearity in these figures is due to the inability of our formula to take full account of the greater severity of cases that tend to be served in the more highly structured hospitals. At the poles of the range, nevertheless, the superior performance of the more highly structured hospitals would seem to be clear. In spite of this, we found overall staffing and total expenditures per patient day of care to be somewhat lower in these institutions.

Among the other components of hospital performance, the correlations of scope and development with the level of MSO structuring were found to be more strikingly and consistently positive than for in-patient care. With respect to out-patient services, there were certain reciprocal relationships between the strength of organized clinics and the output of emergency departments, but the tendency was clearly toward greater development in the more highly structured hospitals. For professional education as well as medical research, the correlations with MSO structuring were strongly positive. In the more permissive hospitals these activities were virtually nonexistent; in the medium MSO hospitals they were moderately developed; and in the most rigorous hospitals they were highly developed. Preventive health services were not very well developed in any of the 10 hospitals, but they were somewhat stronger in those with more rigorous MSO patterns. Other community roles of the hospital, such as social services, home care programs, and regionalization functions, were more highly developed and diversified as the level of MSO structuring of the hospital increased.

The significance of the findings in this study, in terms of the impact of the increasing trend to salaried hospital physicians, would seem to be obvious. The reasons for this trend, in terms of the technical and social demands increasingly being made on the modern hospital, have been mentioned. While controversies between the attending staff and hospital authority (both the board and the administration) often are engendered by the appointment of full-time, hospital-based physicians, the net effect is to increase the efficiency of hospital administration. Our empirical study may help to demonstrate the impact of these trends in terms of improving the overall performance of hospitals as key institutions within our general system of medical care.

23

Hospital Utilization under Insurance

The rapidly mounting national expenditures for hospitalization in the 1950s set in motion widespread charges of abuse and a search for culprits. The frenzy of the debate led me, in collaboration with Max Shain, to analyze the accumulated evidence on the determinants of hospital utilization rates and offer a conceptualization of three sets of influences: patient factors, hospital factors, and physician factors. This was published by the American Hospital Association in 1959 as a monograph entitled Hospital Utilization under Insurance.

Among the hospital-related factors, separate studies in Canada and the United States showed the hospital bed supply (beds per 1,000 people) in an area to be a major determinant under conditions of widespread economic support through insurance. In December, 1959, the New York State Joint Legislative Committee on Health Insurance Plans invited testimony on our findings, and the chapter that follows is the text of that testimony. Shortly thereafter, New York enacted the first state "certificate of need" law in the nation, requiring governmental approval of any construction or alteration increasing hospital bed supply (to be based on proof of "public need" for the beds). Soon other states passed similar laws, and in 1974, the National Health Planning and Resources Development Act made such state legislation a condition for receipt of federal planning grants, the policy thereby becoming nationwide.

THE COSTS OF hospital care have been rising steadily in the United States for at least a hundred years, but public concern about it did not become acute until the great extension of hospitalization insurance. When rising costs became reflected not simply in big hospital bills for a small fraction of families, but in climbing insurance premiums for some two-thirds of the population, it was inevitable that public spokesmen should seek evidence of inefficiency or waste in the American general hospital.

Insurance against hospital costs naturally made admission to hospitals easier for both patients and doctors, and some use of a hospital bed for medically indefensible reasons was bound to occur. Although this has provided juicy newspaper copy for muckraking writers, the weight and significance of such abuse dwindles to tiny proportions, when one considers the substantial medical and social reasons for a rising utilization rate of general hospitals under health insurance.

I should like to discuss briefly first the determinants of the hospital utilization

Chapter 23 originally appeared as "Problems of Hospital Utilization under Insurance" in *Hospital Topics*, February, 1960, pp. 24–27, and is reprinted by permission of that journal.

rate; second, the role of the bed supply in a state or region; third, the true meaning and implications of rising hospital costs; and finally, some suggested conclusions for your consideration.

Determinants of the Utilization Rate

Elsewhere, a colleague and I have analyzed in some detail the factors that determine the rate of utilization of hospital beds under insurance.[1] The decision to admit a patient to the hospital, and to keep him there on a given day, depends on the convergence of three sets of factors—conditions involving 1. the patient, 2. the hospital, and 3. the doctor. For a theoretical model, see Table 23-1, p.315.

The patient factors include:

1. *The incidence and prevalence of illness.* While infectious diseases have declined, we know that chronic illnesses associated with aging have greatly increased, and these require long-term hospitalization.
2. *Attitudes toward illness.* With higher educational levels, people tend to seek more medical care. There are also varying levels of anxiety about health.
3. *Costs of medical care to the patient.* When ambulatory service must be privately financed, while hospitalization is insured, the latter will naturally be preferred.
4. *Marital and family status.* Widowhood, divorce, living alone, and mothers at work all render medical care more difficult at home and favor higher use of the protective setting of a hospital.
5. *Housing and social level.* The persistence of poor housing and other concomitants of poverty, combined with insured access to a clean, efficient hospital, will naturally lead the physician to favor the hospital as a locale for medical diagnosis and treatment.

The hospital factors include:

6. *The supply of hospital beds.* Widespread insurance creates a level of medical judgment in which the supply of beds that exists will tend to be more or less fully utilized. More of this later.
7. *The efficiency of bed utilization.* The complexities of hospital administration, staff shortages, hours-of-work, etc., may create bottlenecks and delays in the work-flow and management of cases.
8. *Financing hospital costs.* The prevailing system of hospital reimbursement by insurance plans, through per diem amounts, may create administrative incentives for maximum occupancy of a given bed complement.
9. *Availability of alternative bed facilities.* The utilization of beds in a general hospital will inevitably depend on the supply of beds in nursing homes and homes for the aged, as well as the operation of organized home-care or home-help programs.
10. *Outpatient departments.* The availability of prepaid diagnostic and treatment services in hospital outpatient departments (or other ambulatory care settings) will naturally influence the use of hospital beds.

The physician factors include:

11. *The supply of physicians.* If the supply of physicians is relatively low and if they are extremely busy, doctors will tend to hospitalize more patients to save valuable time.
12. *Method of medical remuneration.* Fee-for-service payment methods have been demonstrated to create incentives for hospital admission, compared to other methods.
13. *The nature of community medical practice.* The feasibility of proper work-ups of patients in private offices or group clinics will influence the tendency to hospitalize.
14. *Medical policies in the hospital.* Early ambulation, medical rehabilitation, prompt consultations, and other policies of a medical staff will affect the length-of-stay of hospital patients.
15. *The level of medical alertness.* The length-of-stay of long-term patients is influenced by the diligence of attending physicians, which may be influenced, in turn, by administrative procedures.
16. *Medical teaching needs.* The needs of clinical teaching may keep selected patients in a hospital for prolonged periods.

Even this hasty summary of factors influencing the hospital utilization rate at any given time and place may be enough to suggest that the forces driving hospital utilization upward in the United States are manifold. On the other hand, "corrective" actions to reduce it, if they are desired in the interests of economy, must come from diverse sources in the community or even in the nation as a whole. Only a small fraction of the problem is soluble by actions that may be taken within an individual hospital or within a Blue Cross insurance plan.

Not that such actions by individual hospitals or insurance plans are useless. Any administrative measure to help assure wise and *proper use* of hospital beds is socially sound. Admission-and-discharge committees on hospital staffs, development of home-care programs, strengthening of out-patient departments, review of questionable cases by an insurance plan, organization of prepayment for home and office care by physicians, are eminently desirable as measures for *improvement and extension* of medical care. They are likely to help assure the use of hospital beds for the cases most needing them, but it is not at all certain that they will reduce the overall utilization rate.

The Question of Bed Supply

The reason for this view is that, under widespread hospitalization insurance, the ultimate determinant of the utilization rate is the supply or ratio of hospital beds. The bed supply sets not only a ceiling on utilization, which is quite obvious, but it more subtly sets a floor as well, since the availability of a bed will inevitably influence the judgment and decisions of busy doctors. This has been the experience in Canada, Great Britain, and throughout the world. We have shown it to be true in large measure also in the United States and in the counties of New York State, where insurance is not yet universal; and I suspect the relationship of utilization to bed supply falls short of a perfect correlation mainly to the extent that important segments of the population are still not insured.[2]

I do not mean to suggest that there is no top limit to the hospital utilization rate, if bed construction were endlessly expanded. There is surely a top limit, but we do not know what it is, nor has any country in the world reached it. In Saskatchewan, Canada, where the general hospital bed supply of 7.5 per 1,000 population is almost double the United States' average, the prevailing attitude of physicians and public in the thirteenth year of a universal hospital insurance plan is that there are not enough hospital beds available.

Despite the many forces contributing to rising utilization of hospitals, the astonishing thing is that the overall rate has actually risen so little. A recent summary of data by the Health Information Foundation shows that in the last twenty-five years, the hospital days used by 1,000 persons in the United States have risen from 712 to 851 days per year, a rise of under 20 percent. Admission rates, of course, have increased more than this, but average length-of-stay has been greatly reduced, so that the net increase in patient-days has been surprisingly small.[3]

The explanation, in my opinion, is that the days of care provided to the population can be no greater than the beds constructed. In the last quarter century, the supply of general and allied beds in the United States has risen from about 3.4 to 4.0 per 1,000 or a rise of hardly 20 percent. Thus, much of the new hospital construction has been necessary just to keep up with the growth in population. Because of the ups-and-downs of illness and other factors affecting hospital occupancy, moreover, the utilization rate is bound to be some 20 or 30 percent below the theoretical maximums of a given bed supply.

The great hue and cry about excessive utilization of hospitals, therefore, simply does not jibe with the facts. Our own studies have shown very little outright abuse. Examination of 1,000 consecutive patient records in three upstate hospitals, by impartial physicians, disclosed only about 4 percent of cases in which the occupancy of a bed did not seem justified by the diagnostic or therapeutic procedures given to the patient, and only about 5 percent in which the duration of stay seemed excessive. Pursuit of the details of these cases with the attending physicians might reduce these figures to even lower levels.[4]

When a hospital bed is used, there are in my opinion nearly always compelling reasons for it. It is rarely due to pure chicanery or extravagance. The reasons may not be explicable solely in terms of pathology. They may involve social causes or causes related to the pattern of medical care organization in the United States. Hospitalization is often a price we pay for poor housing or broken families and it may be, in some cases, a social cost of private, solo fee-for-service medical practice.

But even if we were to undertake the vast social changes required to modify these influences on hospital utilization, the ultimate determinant of the utilization rate—up to a ceiling nowhere reached—would remain in my opinion the supply of beds. I believe this because the reservoir of human need for health service is very large indeed. With tuberculosis reduced, hospital beds are used for other chronic illnesses, for rehabilitation, for better quality psychiatric care. The potentialities of science in surgery, medicine, every specialty, are ever widening. The stresses of life are great, and the survival of people to their 80s and 90s creates an expanding need, now only meagerly met by nursing homes and homes for the aged.

So long as this reservoir of unmet need for hospitalization exists, the elimination of the occasional unnecessary admission will not result in reduced utilization of beds. The bed freed of an "unnecessary" case will simply become filled with another patient. Home care programs and out-patient services have not been shown anywhere to empty hospital beds or reduce utilization; they have instead reserved the available beds for more appropriate patients—which is fine. But we should not be fooled into thinking that the community's expenditure for hospital care has been thereby reduced.

The Meaning of Rising Costs

Indeed, the whole level of hospital utilization has made only a minor contribution to the rising *costs* of hospital care which have preoccupied so many health leaders. While hospital days per 1,000 persons in the last quarter-century have risen about 20 percent, the cost per patient-day has risen from about $5 to over $27, or more than 400 percent.[5] Simple arithmetic will show that the rise in national expenditures for hospital care in this period are, therefore, attributable about 95 percent to the rise in per diem costs and only about 5 percent to the rise in utilization.

The many reasons for this rise in the cost of a day of hospital care are not the subject before us today. Quite aside from inflationary factors, we are all familiar with the steady enrichment in the composition of hospital service that these costs reflect. One need only mention the greater-than-doubling of staff-to-patient ratios in general hospitals in the last twenty years. So far as the impact of utilization per se is concerned, however, there is one point that should be made.

The costs of hospital operation for a given bed complement are mainly fixed. Salaries (67 percent of all costs), fuel, insurance, depreciation, are largely constant costs. Only food and drugs, and possibly some share of laundry costs, are variable—that is, rising or falling with changing occupancy. Therefore, a reduction in hospital utilization of a given bed complement saves very little in hospital expenditures. If—by very rigid policing—hospital days were to be reduced in a given institution by 10 percent, the overall costs would not be reduced by this amount.

The per diem cost of the balance of occupied beds would rise, and the overall reduction in expenditures would be perhaps 2 or 3 percent. As a matter of fact, this whole example is speculative, for the more likely consequence of a program to reduce "unnecessary" days of care, as suggested above, would be to replace them with "necessary" days of care to other patients.

These facts of hospital financing explain why almost all countries with universal insurance or public financing of hospital care have given up the artificial per diem system of hospital reimbursement. They have replaced it with a budget system, by which the hospital is paid for its "readiness-to-serve." It is paid periodic amounts necessary to operate a given bed complement, almost independent of occupancy rate. Under such circumstances, the dependence of the utilization rate on the bed supply becomes crystal clear, and hospitals are financed in accordance with the complement of beds which they hold ready to serve the public—a supply which is determined in some objective way.

Despite all the complaints about the rising costs of hospital care—and hence insurance premiums—let us keep in mind that the nationwide expenditure for all health service, as a percentage of national income, has remained amazingly constant over the years. In 1929, we were spending about 4.1 percent of net national product on health service; in 1957, with all the remarkable developments of medical science, with all the increases in the spectrum of personnel and facilities, it was only about 4.9 percent.[6] It is true that the hospital segment of the "medical care dollar" has increased from about 20 percent to 33 percent nationally (or

Table 23-1
Hospital Utilization under Insurance: Factors Influencing the Utilization Rate of General Hospitals (A Theoretical Model)

	Patient-Factors	*Hospital-Factors*	*Physician-Factors*
Amount	Illness (Age and sex)	Beds (Ratio to population)	Physicians
Attitudes	Education Anxieties	Degree of flexibility	Alertness
Economics	Costs to patient	Reimbursement method	Remuneration method
Technology	Self-care and hygiene	Efficiency of operation	Medical policies (Rehabilitation) Teaching Needs)
Alternatives	Housing Marital status Rural-urban status	Out-patient department Alternative bed facilities Home care	Office practice (Group clinics)

from about 14 percent to 26 percent if one considers only family expenditures), but this is because many services which were formerly rendered in the home and doctor's office, or not at all, are now rendered in the hospital. But the overall impact of total health expenses on our national economic resources remains low. It is still less than expenditures on liquor and tobacco, and enormously less than the outlay for military purposes.

Conclusions

May I conclude with two thoughts for consideration, one on bed supply and the other on financing.

The United States is moving toward a time, in my opinion, when all or almost all the population will be encompassed under some form of hospital insurance protection. Even before that time is reached, however, the development of some form of public control over the *supply* and *location* of all hospital beds would be desirable. Except for the 25 percent of beds built with federal Hill-Burton subsidy, this is now done by no state. Such public authority would provide the ultimate control of hospital utilization—far more effective than the most diligent administrative or professional measures possible within the walls of a given hospital.

But I would emphasize that this should not be interpreted to mean advocacy of a reduced supply of general hospital beds. On the contrary, a serious public determination of the proper bed supply in each state or hospital region—under universal insurance coverage—would, I think, result in a bed-to-population ratio higher than we now have in any area. The ultimate determination of this bed ratio would be "how much hospital care can we afford to provide in order to meet health needs?" And this brings me to my final point.

It is the individual, rather than the social, impact of health costs on economic resources that is so great—especially because these costs strike families unevenly and are disagreeable costs at best. To cope with this, almost every country in the world has underwritten a major share of total medical costs with funds from general *governmental revenues*. In fact, the favorite form of this support is governmental payment of the operating costs of hospitals. Some 80 percent or more of hospitalization costs in Europe are met from public funds and perhaps 90 percent on other continents. Hospitals, in other words, are deemed to be as deserving of solid public support as are schools. Canada has just launched a program of so-called hospital insurance, in which 50 percent of the total costs of general hospital care in the provinces is paid by the federal treasury. The share of governmental support of overall health costs in the United States has, indeed, steadily risen and now stands at about 20 percent of the total, but most of this goes for special categorical programs and the impact of governmental aid on general hospitals remains slight.

Whether utilization continues to rise, levels off, or declines, there is little doubt that hospital costs as a whole will keep on increasing. The long-overdue improvement of hospital wages, hastened by unionization, is bound to cause this, even if technological changes do not. As insurance coverage becomes universal, the desirability of shifting a larger share of hospital financing to the public sector of our economy will become more evident. And—as Canada and Europe demonstrate—this can doubtless be done without loss of motivation or quality in local hospital administration. In fact, all the evidence suggests that the substantial underpinning of hospital operating costs with public funds in other countries has permitted hospital boards and administrators to concentrate on patient care rather than fiscal problems, and has elevated the quality of hospital performance. If this pattern of financing should come to prevail in the United States, the problems of hospital utilization and hospital costs will fall into proper perspective. Instead of attacks and counterattacks on "who is to blame" for the costs of hospital care, attention could be directed to the development of medical and administrative measures which will assure the wisest use of an optimal supply of hospital beds.

References

1. Milton I. Roemer and Max Shain, *Hospital Utilization Under Insurance*. Chicago: American Hospital Association Monograph No. 6, 1959.
2. Max Shain and Milton I. Roemer, "Hospital Costs Relate to the Supply of Beds," *Modern Hospital,* April 1959.
3. Health Information Foundation, "Trends in Use of General Hospitals," *Progress in Health Services,* October 1959.
4. Max Shain, "The Epidemiology of 'Over-Utilization' of Hospitals," publication pending.
5. American Hospital Association, *Hospitals: Guide Issue,* 1 August 1959, p. 384; and E. H. Pennell, J. S. Mountin, and K. Pearson, *Business Census of Hospitals 1935,* Supplement No. 154b *Public Health Reports*. Washington: Government Printing Office, 1939.
6. Derived from the President's Commission on the Health Needs of the Nation, *Building America's Health,* Washington; Government Printing Office, Vol. 4, p. 151; and from recent processed bulletins of the U.S. Department of Health, Education and Welfare, Social Security Administration.

24

The Voluntary Hospital in an Organized Society

The steadily broadening governmental controls over the construction and operation of hospitals, whether public or private, generated many anxieties in the 1960s, and these continue today. Historical review of these trends, however, indicated that these controls led far more to strengthening the general role of hospitals and upgrading their capabilities, than to restricting their freedom.

The concept emerging in the mid-1960s was a creative "partnership" between public and private sectors of the health services. On invitation of the Catholic Hospital Association, I presented the evolution of this concept and these trends in the American hospital scene at the Association's Annual Meeting. Subsequent legislative actions on regionalization, health facility planning, and other matters have confirmed the "prospects" predicted.

THE AVALANCHE OF new legislation on medical care has caused many anxieties for voluntary hospitals. Board members, administrators, and others responsible for the operation of hospitals are apprehensive about future freedom to control their own affairs in the face of increasing financial support from—and therefore economic dependence upon—government. The complex provisions of Medicare are viewed by some as the dramatic prelude to a complete takeover of voluntary institutions by the state.

Historical Background

The concept of the *voluntary* hospital has always been one of degree. Although the medieval hostel for the sick and destitute was a product of charity, developed in close connection with the Christian Church, it depended almost from the beginning on partial support from the sovereign or the state. In thirteenth century England, hospitals were granted the right to levy tolls on local agricultural production. They were supervised jointly by "king and bishop," symbolic of church and state.[1] While charitable donations and the income from property bequeathed to hospitals were the largest sources of support, the local governments of all the main cities of Europe came to contribute increasingly to the upkeep of their major hospitals.

In Latin America today we see the evolution of the voluntary hospital tele-

Chapter 24 originally appeared as "The Voluntary Hospital in an Organized Society: Fears and Prospects" in *Hospital Progress* (the journal of The Catholic Hospital Association), September, 1966, pp. 81–85, and is reprinted by permission of that journal.

scoped into a shorter span of years. Founded by the leadership of the Catholic Church in the eighteenth century, they soon came to be supported by charity or "beneficencia" boards. After a while, the boards were granted by government the right to conduct lotteries, to raise money. Many local governments gave them a specific share of local revenues, such as excises on the sale of wine or beer. In the twentieth century, as the costs of proper hospital care rose, substantial national subsidies were given to the "beneficencia" hospitals. Later in some countries, like Mexico or Chile, the financial support of the hospitals was assumed by government entirely, even though local boards are retained for appointment of staff and other direct responsibilities.[2] In most Latin American countries, the "beneficencia" hospitals remain independent and powerful, despite heavy subsidy from tax sources.

In the United States, the voluntary hospital has been supported mainly by the payments of private patients; unlike other countries, such patients were in the majority. Indigent patients were financed principally by charitable donations or by a surplus from private charges. From colonial times, however, a certain share of voluntary hospital costs has been met by governmental payments on behalf of the poor, usually from city authorities. The New York Hospital, one of the earliest voluntary institutions in British America, was founded in 1771 and received a subsidy from the city government for its first 20 years.[3] As welfare departments were organized in the nineteenth century, such payments became more systematized and provided the first legal rationale for governmental supervision of private hospitals. In New York State, it was only in 1965 that the licensure of hospitals was transferred from the state department of public welfare to the state department of health.

Current Governmental Influences

With the Hospital Survey and Construction (Hill-Burton) Act of 1946, a turning point occurred in the concept of governmental responsibility for hospital affairs.[4] The Depression of the 1930s and the Second World War had led to a much wider conception of health service for the total population—not just the poor—as a proper concern of government. This included a concern that hospital beds be available to the people living at any location in a quantity and quality adequate to meet their health needs. Quantitative adequacy would be fostered by subsidy of construction. Qualitative standards would be assured through a system of state hospital licensure laws.[5]

The actual application of the hospital licensure programs has been much weaker than the theory and the words embodied in the state laws. In a 1959 field study done in upstate New York, we found that most hospital administrators criticized the official inspections not because they were too rigid or demanding, but rather because they were done too casually and infrequently.[6] The fact is that state hospital licensing agencies—now usually part of state health departments—are almost always meagerly staffed, in both numbers and qualifications of personnel. No state reaches even the moderate standards proposed in a study conducted under the auspices of the Hospital Research and Educational Trust of the American Hospital Association, itself.[7]

The impact of the hospital licensure laws, however, has probably been greater from their influence on voluntary self-regulation than through their official execution. It is no accident that the development of the Joint Commission on Accreditation of Hospitals (from the much smaller program originating with the American College of Surgeons in 1918) occurred in 1951, five years after the Hill-Burton Act. The accreditation program has had enormous positive influences on hospital operation in general and medical staff organization in particular.[8] Many governmental programs of medical care, moreover (e.g., the crippled children's services or the vocational rehabilitation programs), specify that participating hospitals must be "accredited"—which means that government has adopted voluntary standards as its own. The new Medicare law does not go quite this far, but it does stipulate that a general hospital which is "accredited" shall be deemed to meet federal standards.

The Hill-Burton Act has also had influences on voluntary self regulation beyond the sphere of licensure. The concept of planned hospital construction, in relation to population needs, could not be long confined just to those new or enlarged facilities built with federal subsidies—only about 25 percent of the construction projects. In the early 1950s, hospital planning councils to exert voluntary "controls" on *all* new hospital construction began to be formed in the major cities.[9] The controls ranged from moral persuasion or indirect influence on capital donors to advising city governments on invocation of zoning ordinances against new construction that was considered unjustified. After about a decade of operation of such voluntary planning councils, a few states—like New York, Pennsylvania, and California—have established such councils under law. In New York, the law has gone furthest, by assigning to the formerly voluntary councils the authority to determine whether a "public need" exists for any new hospital bed construction, without which determination the construction is not permitted.[10]

Governmental influences on voluntary hospitals have been exerted in many other ways as well. The variety of official support programs for specified beneficiaries was great, long before Medicare. Aside from all the public assistance categories (federal, state, and locally defined), there were and are veterans on "home town" service, military dependents, workmen's compensation cases, crippled children's program patients, vocational rehabilitation clients, and other special beneficiaries in selected states. During World War II, there was the federal Emergency Maternity and Infant Care (EMIC) program which paid for services in thousands of hospitals and set up a nationwide hospital cost-accounting procedure.[11] With each of these payment programs, certain technical standards have been stipulated. Moreover, hospital accounting procedures must meet certain requirements of the paying agency. If one considers health insurance, as well as government, to constitute a form of "social financing," we have reached a time when about 65 percent of voluntary hospital costs are being met from social sources.[12]

The Impact Has Widened

Regulatory programs go beyond those tied to specific beneficiaries, as well as general licensure. The use and dispensing of narcotics and alcohol by hospitals have long been subject to direct federal regulation. Federal and state labor legislation affects certain employees, and previous exemptions of nonprofit institutions from the coverage of such laws are being withdrawn.[13] Schools of nursing conducted in hospitals are usually subject to some regulation by state departments of education. Sanitation systems come under the surveillance of local (as distinguished from state) public health authorities, and fireproof construction or fire safety measures are controlled by local fire marshals. The tax-exempt status of nonprofit institutions, of course, is subject to verification by the federal Internal Revenue Service. Indirectly, state insurance departments have influenced the financing of hospitals through their regulation of Blue Cross plans and, to a lesser extent, the indemnity programs of the commercial insurance carriers.[14]

General financial assistance comes from government to voluntary hospitals for purposes unrelated to direct patient care. Aside from construction grants, there is an expanding volume of federal support for research—clinical, laboratory, and even sociological. Schools of nursing get indirect support through grants and loans to nursing students. Institutional food grants by government agencies from agricultural surplus are, of course, a form of support. The strings tied to these gifts have been frail—probably much thinner than those tied to voluntary philanthropic donations. My own experience as a recipient of research grants from both governmental and private sources points to a substantially wider range of investigative freedom in the governmental sector.

It is obvious, then, from this brief account that voluntary hospitals have long come under a variety of influences and controls by government. From their earliest days, but especially over the last 20 years in the United States, they have been recipients of both economic support and technical surveillance from government. The range of these impacts has gradually widened. The authority has extended from the local, to the state, to the federal levels. Yet, and this is most important to realize, this movement has not been accompanied by any perceptible reduction in the initiative and responsibilities of voluntary hospitals. On the contrary, the range of actions of voluntary hospital boards and administrators over the last generation has broadened. The challenges to local hospital leadership today are greater than ever.

If this seems to some like a paradox, it is still not hard to explain. The fact is that over these years the entire community role of the hospital has enlarged tremendously. The cataloguing of this enlargement in the sphere of in-patient care, out-patient service, professional education, research, and prevention has been done too often to repeat here.[15] Thus, the requirements of government have been more than matched by demands and expectations from the total medical and social environment. The opportunities for hospitals to enrich total community health service are almost endless. The role of government has been essentially to set a floor on standards below which no hospital—public or private—would be permitted to fall, and to provide funds which would enable hospitals to stay above that floor. The ceiling, however, remains a matter for each hospital's determination.

The New Legislation

It is against this background that one must view the new health legislation of 1965. The hospital insurance program for the aged under social security doubtless represents a bigger step by government than any in the past, but its direction is not novel. Conceptually, in fact, it may not be so long a step as that taken in the Hill-Burton Act of 1946, which propelled the movements for hospital planning and state licensure. Indeed, it builds upon those movements (and others which followed, like the EMIC or the military dependents "medicare" program) by requiring state agency licensure—or "certification"—as a condition for hospital reimbursement from government funds.

The quantitative impact of Medicare payments on hospital income will, of course, be large, especially if one keeps in mind Title XIX as well as Title XVIII. Persons past 65 years now use about 25 percent of the general hospital days of care provided in the nation, although they are only about 10 percent of the population.[16] With the support of the new law, this share may be expected to rise, perhaps to about 33 percent of the total days (most of which increment can probably be furnished from occupancy of currently unused bed capacity). In addition, there will be the expanded bed days provided for the indigent and medically indigent under age 65, through the benefits of Title XIX. Not all these bed days will be financed by the public program, but the great bulk of them will be (and amendments may reduce the deductibles and cost-sharing features).

Beyond this are the other governmental programs mentioned earlier. One of the unwritten implications of social insurance for health care is the probable integration over the next generation of hospital services for veterans into the mainstream hospital system. (VA facilities will probably be converted into general community institutions, as is now happening to county and municipal hospitals formerly reserved for the indigent.) The same will eventually happen to specialized hospitals for merchant mariners and Indians. Even without substantial further amendments to the Social Security Act, therefore, we may expect that before long 40 to 50 percent of operating costs of all voluntary hospitals will come from governmental sources.

If there are major amendments to the Medicare law, which may reasonably be expected after a few years, the financial impact on hospitals by government will be even greater. The roughly 1.1 million totally disabled persons, and their dependents, now coming under social security (not to be confused with the indigent disabled) will probably soon be added to Medicare enrollment. Perhaps the unemployed, who have usually lost their voluntary health insurance "fringe benefits," tied to jobs, will come next. The political attractions of encompassing health care for children—rich or poor—under a social insurance program may also prove irresistible, especially since, like the aged, they are an economically dependent population. State government programs for temporary disability insurance (in Rhode Island, California, New York, and New Jersey) now cover about 12 million workers, and in California limited hospital benefits are already provided;[17] the step to overall hospital insurance by law for this large population would not be great.

Whatever extension of governmental support for hospital care may occur, however, the important question for voluntary hospitals is not the percentage of impact, but rather the mode of administration. Despite the threatening cliché about the payer of the piper calling the tune, the whole experience of America suggests, as we have seen, that the calling has been reasonable. The command performance for the sovereign has not caused the artist to subvert his art.

The specific provisions of the Medicare law, I believe, demonstrate this very well. The entire administrative structure is built upon the framework of voluntary and local agencies for health service that already exist. The adoption of voluntary "accreditation" as equivalent to meeting governmental standards was mentioned above. The use of "fiscal intermediaries" for direct payment of hospitals under Title XVIII, Part A, is obviously designed to work with and not replace the voluntary health insurance agencies that have developed over the last 35 years. Indeed, the hospitals themselves select the intermediary they prefer to deal with, and the vast majority have chosen the Blue Cross plans. The "certification" of hospitals and other providers of service, moreover, is done not by the federal government directly, but by the state health agencies which have been licensing hospitals for years.[18]

Of course, under a law based on federal tax revenues, federal minimum standards must be stipulated. On a technical level, the principal innovations embodied in these standards have been: 1. the requirement for a satisfactory "utilization review" process in all participating hospitals and extended care facilities and 2. the requirement for satisfactory "transfer agreements" between hospitals and extended care facilities as a condition for participation of the latter. Detailed discussions of these two provisions by professional groups over the months since the law was passed in July, 1965, have only served to confirm their wisdom.[19] Doubts have been expressed about how effectively these administrative measures—designed to promote both equity and quality—will be carried out at the local level, but no responsible leader has questioned their good sense. What is more, medical staffs of thousands of hospitals have been stimulated to introduce measures of self-surveillance on the use of beds and the soundness of patient management which conscientious doctors have long advocated.

The assurance that utilization review and transfer agreements are carried out effectively is a responsibility of both the fiscal intermediaries and the state health agencies. Admittedly there are bound to be some difficulties, especially in small hospitals where serious staff discipline has not been customary. But the attitude of the Secretary of Health, Education and Welfare—who is ultimately responsible to Congress for the whole program—is manifestly flexible, and the future development of the program is looked to in an experimental rather than an authoritarian spirit.[20]

Who Has Been Subsidizing Whom?

On a fiscal level, the key provision of the Medicare law is the requirement that hospital services to beneficiaries will be paid for at "reasonable cost." It has taken many months to hammer out the meaning of this phrase, and the national Health Insurance Benefits Advisory Council (HIBAC)—on which voluntary hospitals and private physicians are well represented—has played a key role in doing so. The past policies and practices of Blue Cross plans, in their reimbursement formulas, have strongly influenced decisions. All the elements of the federal formula cannot be reviewed here, but a few critical components in the cost determination are: 1. the value of services provided by religious sisters may be included; 2. depreciation of buildings and equipment is allowed; 3. the expense of approved educational programs is included; 4. as a growth factor a supplemental two percent of all allowed costs may be added. Excluded from the cost formula are: 1. expenses for research beyond that necessary for patient care, and 2. discounts allowed for charity patients or the courtesy treatment of professional personnel.[21]

It is hard to argue with the rationale of these fiscal policy decisions, although some hospital leaders have quarreled with the accounting basis on which they will be computed. This is to be geared to the cost of services for *aged* beneficiaries only, rather than to the average cost of *all* patients, which has been the Blue Cross method. Since aged patients typically have longer-than-average stays and less use per day of diagnostic and therapeutic services (though probably more use of nursing care), the per diem cost of *their* care is probably lower than the overall hospital average. Strict cost accounting of aged patient care, therefore, will probably place a higher relative burden on prepayment plans financing the care of younger patients, if total hospital costs are to be met. (If so, one can only conclude that older patients in the past—if they paid *average* per diem rates—were actually subsidizing the costs of younger patients.) In any event, the final policy decisions on hospital payment formulas will doubtless evolve through future experience, as they have in the hospital insurance programs of Canada and other countries.

Reverberations of the New Trend

With government support of hospital care for the aged and the poor, and eventually perhaps for nearly everyone, some persons are concerned about the whole humanitarian mission of the voluntary hospital. What is its charitable role, they ask, if government simply pays all the bills? To ask this question, however, displays a narrow view of the function of the voluntary agency in our society. It is surely more than money raising. Unfortunately for hospital development, all too much of the volunteer's energies and talents in the past have been devoted to finding dollars for meeting the deficits of charitable care, rather than to improving the range and quality of hospital service. We may draw a lesson on this point from the National Health Service of Great Britain, where—in spite of the 100 percent government support of hospitals—volunteers are more active than ever. Instead of raising funds for indigent medical care, however, they are supplementing patient services, doing health education, supporting new research, and helping in other positive ways.[22]

Other anxieties have been expressed about medical education and what will happen to the "teaching material" (dreadful phrase) if every patient is insured. In Canada, Europe, and elsewhere, however, this has been no problem. A patient becomes a subject for medical teaching by going to a teaching hospital rather than by being poor. In return for permitting himself to be served by medical students, interns, and residents, the patient in such a hospital is assured of the first-class supervision of professors. There is no dearth of patients in the teaching hospitals of other countries, and none need be expected in the United States even under extended Medicare legislation.

Perhaps the fears of governmental intervention in voluntary hospital affairs would not be so great if the Social Security Act Amendments of July, 1965, had not been followed a few months later by the Public Health Service Act Amendments on "Heart Disease, Cancer, and Stroke." Through the influence of this law, some envisage a gradual domination of all the nation's smaller hospitals by the great urban medical centers. Government, in this context, is seen lurking in the background but encouraging the big hospital fish to eat up the little ones.

In fact, the provisions of the "Heart Disease, Cancer, and Stroke Amendments" embody the height of voluntarism.[23] They simply authorize the U.S. Public Health Service to give grants to "public or nonprofit private universities, medical schools, research institutions, and other public or nonprofit agencies and institutions to assist in establishment and operation of regional medical programs. . . ." These programs would be designed to promote "research and training . . . and related demonstrations of patient care in the fields of heart disease, cancer, and stroke, and related diseases." Regional relationships between a medical center and a peripheral hospital are obviously a two-way matter. Unless both parties agree, there is no "regional cooperative arrangement" in the language of the law. It may be expected that hundreds of such arrangements will be worked out, but only with the willingness of both institutional parties. So far, the emphasis appears to be on programs of professional education, rather than systems of patient referral.

It may be noted that one of the prominent failures of the Hill-Burton Act was in implementation of the functional concept of regionalization. The law has been well applied to decisions on new construction but hardly at all to hospital operations. In spite of a few impressive demonstrations of regionalization (originating prior to 1946) in upstate New York, Maine, Virginia, and elsewhere, the concept of a two-way flow of patients and services in hospital regions had hardly been applied after 20 years of the Hospital Survey and Construction Act.[24] The Hill-Harris Amendments of 1962 gave a further push to this concept by authorizing federal grants specifically for regional projects, but those, too, have been confined essentially to construction planning.

How Willing Are Voluntary Hospitals?

The real meaning of the Heart Disease, Cancer, and Stroke Amendments is to approach the same regionalization objective through the legislative channel of tackling the nation's three top causes of death. No one can tell if this approach will be more successful, but it is certain that it will be no more rapid in implementation than the wishes of the nation's voluntary hospitals themselves.

Another current in the new flood of national health legislation relates to the larger political scene and the advancement of civil rights. Hospitals, of course, cannot be immune from the struggle for racial equity in our democracy, even though this may mean the alteration of many long-established customs. The "separate but equal" doctrine will no longer be applicable in hospitals any more than it is in schools, since the Supreme Court decision of 1954, simply because segregation has usually meant unequal services. As Surgeon General Stewart has said, this does not mean that every hospital room must be shared by patients of two races, but it does mean that hospital facilities—under all the new legislation—must be equally accessible to all patients, in terms of their health needs, without respect to their race or color.[25]

Conclusion

A fair consideration of all these trends, past and current, suggests that the voluntary hospital may look ahead more with excitement than with fear. The expanding force of social organization—both through governmental and voluntary mechanisms—has done far more to enrich than to restrict the performance of voluntary hospitals. Consider the effect of the whole insurance and public medical care movement on the financial support of voluntary hospitals over the last 30 years. Consider the effects of construction, research, and educational subsidies. Consider the influence of standards imposed by licensure and accreditation systems, as well as by the quality requirements of specific medical care programs. American hospital progress has in large measure been built upon these economic and legal foundations.

The prospect of a still greater role for government in the years ahead can properly generate fear only in those hospitals that prefer to stand still. If a hospital aims to adjust its program to the advancing front of medical science, it can expect support and encouragement from an expansion of public responsibility for the public's health. It can face the future with optimism.

The special feature of governmental actions in American culture is that they do not replace private initiative, but rather build upon it. In the health services, as in industrial production, the role of government has been to support and upgrade the performance of the voluntary sector. We are now seeing fewer health programs like the separate Veterans Administration (a *sequela* of the First World War) and more like the integrated system of Medicare for the aged. It has become fashionable to speak of this approach as a "partnership" between public and private entities. It is a useful description, for the goal could not be achieved without the effective participation of both.[26]

Whatever support or social discipline may come from government, the voluntary agency will always have a role that is independent and creative. This role is in the exploration of new ideas before the wide consensus, necessary to launch a public program, is achieved. Such explorations are as needed in the hospital field as in any other. Organized home care, regionalization, systematic rehabilitation, intensive care units, social service departments, "progressive patient care"—

these and other innovations were pioneered by voluntary hospitals. Now they are included in the basic standards and objectives of governmental programs. The same evolution may be expected in the future, so long as we have the vitality and imagination which now characterize both the public and the private sectors of American health service.

References

1. Courtney Dainton, *The Story of England's Hospitals,* Springfield, Ill., Charles C Thomas, 1961, pp. 29–30.
2. A. L. Bravo, "Development of Medical Care Services in Latin America," *American Journal of Public Health,* Vol. 48, April, 1958, pp. 434–447.
3. Henry E. Sigerist, *American Medicine,* New York, W. W. Norton and Company, 1934, p. 204.
4. Leslie Morgan Abbe and Anna Mae Baney, *The Nation's Health Facilities: Ten Years of the Hill-Burton Hospital and Medical Facilities Program 1946–1956,* Washington, U.S. Public Health Service, 1958.
5. Keith O. Taylor and Donna M. Donald, *A Comparative Study of Hospital Licensure Regulations,* Berkeley, University of California, School of Public Health, 1957.
6. Milton I. Roemer and Mary Helen McClanahan, "Impact of Government Programs on Voluntary Hospitals," *Public Health Reports,* Vol. 75, June, 1960, pp. 537–544.
7. Hilary G. Fry, *The Operation of State Hospital Planning and Licensing Programs,* Chicago, American Hospital Association, Monograph Series No. 15, 1965.
8. Robert S. Myers, "Organizing the Medical Staff," *Modern Concepts of Hospital Administration,* J. K. Owen, editor, Philadelphia, W. B. Saunders, 1962, pp. 188–200.
9. American Hospital Association and U.S. Public Health Service, *Areawide Planning for Hospitals and Related Health Facilities,* Washington, Public Health Service, July, 1961.
10. State of New York, Metcalf-McCloskey Law, 1964.
11. Martha M. Eliot and Lillian R. Freedman, "Four Years of the EMIC Program," *Yale Journal of Biology and Medicine,* Vol. 19, March, 1947, pp. 621–635.
12. U.S. Public Health Service, *Medical Care Financing and Utilization,* Washington, Public Health Service, Heath Economics Series No. 1, PHS Pub. 947, 1962, p. 73.
13. W. L. Daykin, "How Labor Legislation May Affect Hospitals," *The Modern Hospital,* Vol. 95, July, 1960, pp. 65–69; 124–126.
14. Max Shain and Milton I. Roemer, "Hospitals and the Public Interest," *Public Health Reports,* Vol. 76, May, 1961, pp. 401–410.
15. John H. Knowles (editor), *Hospitals, Doctors, and the Public Interest,* Cambridge, Harvard University Press, 1965.
16. Derived from data in: University of Michigan, School of Public Health, *Medical Care Chart Book,* Ann Arbor, 1964, pp. 60–61.
17. Alfred M. Skolnik, "Income-Loss Protection Against Short-Term Sickness, 1948–62," *Social Security Bulletin,* January, 1964, pp. 4–12.
18. Margaret Greenfield, *Health Insurance for the Aged: The 1965 Programs for Medicare,* Berkeley, University of California, Institute of Governmental Studies, 1966.
19. American Medical Association, *Utilization Review: A Handbook for the Medical Staff,* Chicago, The Association, 1965.
20. John W. Gardner, "The Creative Partnership for Health," *Medical Tribune,* Vol. 7, No. 75, June 22, 1966, p. 1ff.
21. Ray E. Brown, "The Hospital's Role—The Doctor's Guide to Medicare," *Medical World News,* June 17, 1966, pp. 57–63.
22. Almont Lindsey, *Socialized Medicine in England and Wales: The National Health Service 1948–1961,* Chapel Hill, University of North Carolina Press, 1962, p. 261.

23. The President's Commission on Heart Disease, Cancer, and Stroke, *Report to the President,* Washington, Government Printing Office, December, 1964.
24. Milton I. Roemer and Robert C. Morris, "Hospital Regionalization in Perspective," *Public Health Reports,* Vol. 74, October, 1959, pp. 916–922.
25. William H. Stewart, "Civil Rights and Medicare," *Journal of the American Medical Association,* Vol. 196, June 13, 1966, p. 993.
26. Walter J. McNerney, "The Future of Voluntary Prepayment for Health Services," *New England Journal of Medicine,* Vol. 273, October 21, 1965, pp. 907–914.

Part Six

Quality Evaluation and Regulation

With increasing shares of national income being devoted to health services, and a rising share of these being organized, pressures have mounted for evaluation of programs to determine the level of their accomplishments, or ultimately if they are worth the money spent. In this part, we consider the meaning of the evaluative process, offer examples, and explore social responses in the way of regulation.

Chapter 25 proposes several levels on which health service programs may be evaluated, depending on information available. In Chapter 26, a specific program of medical care is evaluated at the level of final health status outcomes: perinatal mortality rates. Chapter 27 offers a possible strategy for evaluating the quality of hospital performance in terms of another "outcome" measurement–the death rate of patients adjusted for the varying severity of cases admitted to different hospitals. Finally, in Chapter 28, we review the wide scope of governmental regulations that have evolved in the United States to control the quality of health care.

25

Evaluation of Health Service Programs and Levels of Measurement

As more public funds have come to be spent on health care programs, demands have increased not only for greater regulation but also for more evaluation. Is the program worth the costs? How much good is it accomplishing?

In response, social scientists and others have used many methods of evaluation. In this paper, an attempt is made to formulate a sequential ordering of such evaluative methods into six levels. They range from the most ideally desirable (changes in health status attributable to the program) to the most modest or superficial (input of resources). The difficulties associated with evaluative measurements at each level, as well as problems of inference, are also explored.

FOR A HUNDRED years or more clinical medicine has applied, with varying degrees of sophistication and rigor, the method of the controlled clinical trial to test the effectiveness or value of proposed new therapies for individual patients.[1] Only in the last decade or two has serious attention been given to evaluation of the various forms of organization of health services. The problems of this type of evaluation are complicated by an admixture of variables, especially involving differences between the test and control, or comparison, groups with respect to the characteristics of the persons served, the medical technology applied, or other factors outside of the form or pattern of health service organization per se.

Need for Clarification

Because of the complexities of evaluating schemes of health service organization, there has been a great deal of confusion in even deciding what should be evaluated, let alone how to go about doing it.[2] Many different meanings have been attributed to "evaluation," and wide disparity exists in the terminology applied to the goals of a program, its end results, its quality, its effectiveness, its outcomes, and so on.[3] The purpose of this paper is to suggest a framework for analysis of the relative values (evaluation) of various systems or subsystems of health organization (health service programs), to help clear the air and promote

Chapter 25 originally appeared in *HSMHA Health Reports* (Public Health Reports), 86:839–848, September, 1971.

uniformity of terms and concepts so as to facilitate communication among investigators.

Many extensive reviews and annotated bibliographies on the problems of evaluation of health service programs have been issued in recent years. Altman and Anderson, in 1962, prepared an annotated bibliography on the evaluation of medical care.[4] Suchman produced a book in 1967 on evaluative research in the social sciences.[5] In 1966 the Health Services Research Study Section of the Public Health Service commissioned a series of review papers on health services research. Most relevant to the issue posed here are the comprehensive accounts by Donabedian on "Evaluating the Quality of Medical Care"[6] and by Weinerman on "Research into the Organization of Medical Practice."[7] In 1967 Shapiro wrote an excellent summary on "End Result Measurements of Quality of Medical Care."[8] In August 1969 the California Center for Health Services Research issued an annotated bibliography, "Evaluating Outcomes of Health Care."[9] The World Health Organization's selected bibliography, "Methodology in Public Health Studies" (1968), also contains many references on evaluation.[10] In 1969 volume 2 of "A Guide to Medical Care Administration," from the American Public Health Association's program area committee on medical care administration, appeared under the title of "Medical Care Appraisal—Quality and Utilization," prepared by Donabedian.[11] A very useful compilation of readings, "Program Evaluation in the Health Fields" was also assembled in 1969 by Schulberg, Sheldon, and Barker.[12]

With this wealth of reviews on the literature of health program evaluation—and there are more papers and volumes than those noted, MacTavish's bibliography,[13] for example—I do not intend to add another overview, but rather offer a framework that will attempt to integrate the several approaches used into a relatively simple schema.

As organization theorists have pointed out, every system or subsystem has a set of short-term ends, which in turn become means toward more long-term ends.[14] A health service program may have as its immediate end or goal the provision of certain services (for example, prenatal examinations or intensive care of patients with coronary attacks) but the long-term goal is to advance health status. There are several more links in the chain of causation, but the basic point to be recognized is that the system or program can be evaluated on various levels: short term, intermediate, and long term. Several phenomena within each level may be defined and measured.

Donabedian speaks cogently of evaluation or appraisal of the 1. structure, 2. process, and 3. outcome of a medical care program.[11] This entry to the problem is useful, especially his emphasis on the importance of examining process even though the ultimate outcome may be difficult or impossible to measure. My attempt, in a sense, is to refine this typology somewhat further, in order to build a framework into which the whole spectrum of evaluation methodologies may logically be fitted.

If the focus is on evaluation of health service programs (that is, mechanisms of organization of health services in their many aspects) it may be helpful to think of all the consequences as a chain of effects at different levels of depth. Regardless of the immediate short-term ends or goals of a health program, it must ultimately be judged or evaluated by its success in saving lives or reducing disability or advancing health status in some way. Only when the attainment of that ultimate goal becomes difficult to measure or to attribute to a specific programmatic cause, which is frequently true, must we take recourse to evaluation based on less ultimate effects.[15]

Levels of Evaluation

Health Status Outcomes

Ideally, health planners would like to know the effect of any pattern of organization of health services, whether old, new, or projected, in terms of health status changes in the target population. Many studies have used this type of outcome measure with varying degrees of sophistication in ruling out secondary variables.

On the crudest level of a total population, for example, one may compare a large system like the British National Health Service with the U.S. health scene. Observing a higher life expectancy in Great Britain than in the United States, one might conclude that the net outcome of the British National Health Service is superior to that of the pluralistic U.S. system, or "nonsystem."[16] But such a conclusion would be unwarranted without considering the effects of diverse living conditions, genetic factors, and scores of epidemiologic variables that can influence death rates and life expectancy in the two nations, quite aside from their health service systems. Nevertheless, even this crude comparison provides a clue for more searching types of measurement of the effects of the two systems of health service at the deepest level of evaluation; namely, the outcome in health status.

More sophisticated evaluative studies are illustrated by comparisons of the membership of the Health Insurance Plan of Greater New York with the rest of the New York population, matched for sociodemographic characteristics. In the early 1950s an important study showed lower perinatal mortality in a population eligible for this prepaid group practice program,[17] and in the 1960s a study showed a lower death rate among indigent aged (old-age assistance recipients) enrolled in the plan,[18] compared in both instances with matched populations entitled to traditional medical care. The elaborate tasks of sampling, randomization, data analysis, and so on in studies of this type need not be reviewed here.

Health status outcomes have also been applied in comparative studies of populations actually served in varying medical settings, most frequently in hospitals of different types. Lipworth and co-workers found lower disease-specific case fatality rates in British teaching hospitals compared with non-teaching ones.[19] John Thompson and colleagues compared perinatal mortality as an indicator of obstetrical care in two U.S. Air Force hospitals.[20] I found lower postoperative deaths for certain surgical procedures in large, compared with small, hospitals in Saskatchewan.[21]

In all such hospital-based studies, one must make adjustments for the varying severity of cases, and hence risk of death, in different hospitals; and in a 1968 paper two colleagues and I offered a statistical approach to the solution of this problem.[22] If such a statistical adjustment can be perfected, we will have a much firmer basis for judging a hospital's overall effectiveness than the brief inspections of input (hospital resources, policies, practices) on which the Joint Commission on Accreditation of Hospitals or the State hospital licensure authorities now depend.

Beyond mortality data are many other measures of the ultimate outcome of a health service program, in terms of health status, that may be applied, either to total populations eligible or to persons definitely served by the program. Life expectancies, based on modified life table techniques, have been applied to measure the effect of a county public health program. This method corrects for the problem of higher morbidity rates among older persons with chronic disease who are kept alive by active medical care.[23] More sensitive than this are various measures of recovery from illness or days of disability, such as absenteeism from work or school, restricted activity days, or days in bed, of persons eligible for one program as compared with another.[24]

Formulated more positively, health status outcomes may be reflected in measurements of the capacities of persons to function, as applied by Sidney Katz and his colleagues in studies of rehabilitation of the aged sick.[25,26] The effectiveness of family planning programs may be evaluated in terms of subsequent birth rates. There are scores of specific measurements of recovery from certain diseases, improved physical or mental functioning, and other phenomena that may be and have been applied in outcome evaluation of specialized programs.[27] Sanazaro and Williamson have delineated a set of six patient end-results for judging the outcome of cases reaching the attention of specialists in internal medicine.[28]

This type of health status outcome is the usual end point in clinical trials of new drug therapies or new preventive services, like the Salk antipoliomyelitis vaccine or the fluoridation of water supplies to reduce the rate of dental caries. Its application to evaluation of health service programs, however, is complicated by so many variables in the characteristics of the populations eligible or served, the diseases involved, and numerous environmental divergencies that, in practice, it is difficult and costly to apply. To adjust properly for all these confounding influences requires very large or highly selected samples, long periods of observation, and elaborate methodologies. As a practical matter,. therefore, evaluation of health service programs must often resort to measurements of effect that are less ultimate in the chain of influences. Next to health status would be the level that may be described as the estimated quality of service.

Estimated Quality of Service

This level of program evaluation is a component of Donabedian's "process." It can be applied, by definition, only to examination of services actually rendered rather than to the experience of a total population, some members of which may receive no services at all. The measurement rests on the assumption that at any time and place there is a scientific consensus among widely acknowledged experts on what constitutes good or high-quality health service. The consensus typically, though not always, rests on a body of empirical data. The task then is to call upon an expert observer to examine, directly or indirectly, the services actually provided in a program and make judgments on the degree to which the services coincide with these accepted standards of merit. The judgment may be scaled from high to low, may be given a numerical score, or may be subdivided along different dimensions of service.

The most common application of this level of evaluation has been to hospital services through study of patient records. Known generally as the medical audit technique, it has been applied extensively by Lembcke[29] and Rosenfeld[30] as well as others with methodological variations that need not be reviewed here. Numerous investigations have been made of such outcomes as rates of appendectomy (for a physician or for a hospital) associated with nonpathological findings or the proportions of post mortem findings that did not confirm the original diagnosis. The widely publicized study of the quality of medical care received by members of the Teamsters Union under a health insurance plan was based on this audit technique.[31] With somewhat greater difficulty, the study of written records as a basis for evaluation has been applied also to services for ambulatory patients.[32]

Because of the many possible inadequacies of the written record as a reflection of what was actually done (that is, errors of commission or omission in the record), the quality of services may be judged also by visual observation. This technique was used in the well-known studies of general medical practice by Peterson and his colleagues in North Carolina[33] and by Clute in Canada.[34] Visual observations of patients' mouths have likewise been applied in evaluative studies of dental service programs. Prescribing practices of physicians have also been examined as indicators of their quality of performance.[35]

There are endless ramifications to the types of judgmental observations that may be made at this level of evaluation. Instead of applying a standard of excellence, the performance in a particular program may be compared with an average of many such programs, as is the strategy of the Commission on Professional and

Hospital Activities.[36] The old appraisal schedule of local public health programs used by the American Public Health Association was applied largely in this way.[37]

Apart from the fallibilities in judgment of any "expert," this whole level of measuring results is often difficult to apply because of the inaccessibility of records or other objects of observation, because of the expense involved, or for other reasons. Therefore, program evaluation of results must often take recourse to a third level of measurement: the quantity of services provided. This is another facet of Donabedian's concept of process.

Quantity of Services Provided

The basic assumption of this evaluative level is that certain types of health service (not all types) may be regarded as generally beneficial for people, so that a higher rate of providing these services to a population is deemed more favorable than a lower rate. One can immediately think of exceptions to this generalization, but the argument for its usual validity rests on the entire literature and knowledge of the field of scientific clinical medicine. In general, other things being equal, it is assumed that a health service program which yields a high rate of contact between patients and physicians is better than one which yields a lower rate. (This view has been widely held since about 1912; Dr. Reginald Fitz of Boston set that year as the date after which an encounter between a patient and a doctor yielded a better than 50–50 chance of benefit for the patient.) The whole extension of health insurance programs, for example, has been advocated on the basis of the statistical demonstration that insured persons (of given age, sex, and socioeconomic status) get more health services per year than noninsured persons with the same characteristics.[38]

The quantity of health services provided to a population by a program, or the utilization rates if viewed from the standpoint of the recipients, may be of many different categories and subcategories. Most elementary is the determination of the percentage of a stated population reached (that is, provided one or more units of service by the program) during a year. For physician contacts this is often between 50 and 75 percent, even when costs are covered by an insurance or public program.[39]

Beyond this, one may determine the rate of receipt by the eligible population of ambulatory medical services, hospitalizations, prescribed drugs, dental services, and so on. Within ambulatory medical services, one may measure preventively oriented services, like physical examinations or immunizations, or many types of diagnostic or treatment procedures. Dental services may include rates of prophylaxes, fillings, extractions, prostheses, and others. Hospitalization may be measured by cases or admissions, by days of care, by diagnostic category, and so on. All these measurements, of course, depend on minimally adequate medical records and a clear definition of terms.[40]

Such data on the quantity of various types of service received by an eligible population are clearly a program consequence although their appraisal as good, fair, or poor requires further interpretation. When rates of service provided are markedly different from certain well-known experiences, the judgment is easier; for example, we know that the U.S. population as a whole utilizes hospital services at the rate of about 1,100 days per 1,000 persons per year and sees physicians at the rate of about five contacts per person per year. If we then observe that the annual utilization rates in, let us say, the State of West Bengal, India, are 200 hospital days per 1,000 and one physician contact per person, we need not hesitate to conclude that the West Bengal health service system has serious deficiencies. When the differentials are slight, however, we cannot usually make value judgments; yet we can draw simple conclusions on the quantitative effects of a program that can be useful for planning purposes.

When certain medical procedures have been clinically demonstrated to be of dubious benefit (for example, tonsillectomies or uterine suspensions), a high rate of their performance can reflect low programmatic quality. On the other hand, certain procedures may be deemed of generally high value, such as immunizations for the young or proctoscopic examinations of aged persons, and these rates therefore have other meaning. Rates of hospitalization as a whole under different types of insurance plans have been extensively studied as an outcome reflecting possible abuse or overuse of expensive facilities, as well as the compensatory value of out-of-hospital services to the ambulatory patient.[41]

Focusing only on the persons actually receiving services within a program, one may undertake other measurements useful for evaluation. The time spent per patient, or the number of patients seen per physician-hour, is a useful measurement. Within a physician's practice, the proportion of patients given injections or subjected to certain diagnostic tests may be an evaluative index. In a dental program, the ratio of fillings to extractions is widely regarded as reflecting a preventive orientation. The ratio of prescribed to nonprescribed drugs consumed by a population is another index reflecting quality. The rate of noncompliance with medical orders or advice is a special form of program measurement that also has obvious qualitative implications. While interpretations of the meaning of these various quantitative rates, for specified types of health service, must obviously be made with caution, such measurements constitute a level of evaluation that permits interprogram comparisons.[42]

Such relatively simple counts as these may not even be possible, however, if proper records are not kept in a health service program. A common difficulty is the lack of knowledge of the size of the eligible population so that, with no clear denominator, basic rates cannot be calculated at all, and only proportions of patients getting certain services can be measured. Evaluation of a health program may be most feasible, therefore, at still another level: the attitudes of the persons whom the program is intended to serve.

Attitudes of Recipients

Combining quantity and quality, in a sense, is the measurement of a health service outcome that is based on the attitudes of persons entitled to or actually receiving the service. Without knowing the quantitative rates of services provided or their estimated quality (as judged by professional experts), one can ask people how they feel about the program. Many evaluative studies have been based on this type of survey measurement. The impact of diverse types of health insurance plans on persons enrolled has been studied in this way among State government employees in California,[43] among insured persons in New York City,[44] and in other settings. Opinion surveys of the attitudes of British people before and after the National Health Service have been used to evaluate that large program.[45]

Although the judgment of a program member or patient may often be superficial and faulty, this method assumes that such judgment has some validity and will certainly reflect gross problems in a program. For the humanistic and personal aspects of health service, this level of evaluative measure is probably more cogent than any other. Moreover, this type of measurement is probably the best approach to quantification of such frequently espoused criteria for good medical care as accessibility, acceptability, continuity, comprehensiveness, sensitivity, and the like.

Within the population actually receiving services, a quantification of grievances may also be a tool of evaluation. Hospitals and health insurance plans often invite patients to comment in writing on the services they have received, using the rate of specific complaints as a key to program improvement. In more extreme form, a study of the rate of malpractice suits in a series of California hospitals found this measure to reflect the degree of rigor in the organization of the medical staff.[46]

As democratic concepts become more embodied in the provision of health service and as the sophistication of people about medical science broadens, this level of evaluation can become increasingly important. Witness the ferment in the nationwide Medicaid program, associated not only with rising costs but also with documented complaints of poor people about the nature of the services they get.[47] This type of measurement need not require medical records nor the other elaborate forms of data necessary for the three previous levels, but it usually requires population surveys through interviews, questionnaires, or other means, which must be done with care and may be quite costly. On a level still further from the goal of improvement in health status, therefore, one may draw inferences about the operation of a program by measuring the various attributes of the personnel and physical resources made available in it. These are equivalent to Donabedian's concept of structure.

Resources made available

While human and physical resources are ordinarily thought of as inputs rather than outputs of a system, these resources require much effort for production and distribution, so that they may also be viewed as consequences. This concept may be seen clearly in an underdeveloped country, where the results of a national program of rural health improvement may be measured by the simple ratio to population of physicians, nurses, hospital beds, and so on, achieved in rural areas.[48] In the United States an immediate result of the national Hill-Burton program is the number or ratio of hospital beds established in regions formerly undersupplied, and similar measures may be used for personnel trained and working as an achievement of various health manpower development programs.[49] These ratios, it may be noted, apply theoretically to total populations rather than to patients reached.

The assumption, of course, is that personnel and physical resources result in services, just as the services, in turn, are presumed generally to yield benefits for health. Anyone can spot the possible fallacies in these assumptions, and yet they are more likely to be valid than not. For years the local public health promotional program of the Public Health Service reported its progress in terms of the number of counties (among the 3,070 in the nation) served each year by full-time health departments.[50] The assumption was that these structural resources led to certain services which, in turn, reduced communicable diseases, infant mortality, and so on. There was enough independent scientific evidence of the benefits of immunizations, sterilization of baby formulas, early detection of tuberculosis, and so on, to justify these assumptions in a broad sense. More ultimate measures of the results of local health department programs are sought, naturally, but even at this fifth level certain probabilistic conclusions are warranted. In some situations, no more satisfactory evaluative data may be obtainable.

Within this evaluative level of resources made available, measurements may be further refined along qualitative lines. One may count the kinds of physicians available, for example, distinguishing general practitioners and qualified specialists.[51] One may define the range of equipment and the scope of services offered in hospitals and health centers. The whole literature of clinical medicine justifies the assumption, if other data are lacking, that a fully trained surgeon is likely to achieve better surgical results for his patient than a general practitioner. While exceptions may occur, in a complex medical situation it is probable that a professional nurse will be more helpful to a patient than a vocational nurse.

Broadly speaking, a health program may be subjected to an administrative audit in which all its resources are defined and their manner of functioning is described; certain operating procedures imply superior or inferior service.

Beyond this fifth level of evaluation of health service programs, there is still another type of question to be asked: What are the costs of the program? All five levels discussed are measures of benefits but they tell us nothing about the costs and hence of the cost-benefit ratios. Since health service resources are always limited, it is reasonable to attempt to achieve a stated outcome at the lowest possible cost, and the measurement of this cost may therefore be regarded as another type of evaluation.

Costs of the Program

If a stated health objective at any of the five levels can be reached by one method at a lower cost than by another method, there is greater efficiency and higher value in the first method. It means that more money or resources would then be left for meeting other needs or demands.[52]

The costs of a program, while a type of evaluation, are along a dimension different from that of the five levels of benefits discussed. For any quantity of benefits at any of the five levels, there may be a range of costs. The difficulty is to be certain that comparative cost measurements are being applied to health service programs that do, indeed, reach the same results. If not, there must at least be some uniform units of measurement of results, such as days of disability incurred or number of dental services provided, under alternative systems, so that cost-benefit analyses and comparisons can be made.[53] How much should be spent for gaining a stated objective is a matter for social policy decision, and choices must always be made among large sectors like health, military affairs, education, housing, and so on. Within the health sector alone, the choices are difficult enough, but between these large sectors the cost-benefit calculations are so formidable that they are seldom even attempted, and the decisions are usually left to political judgment.

Within the health services, costs can be calculated in several ways. As at the other levels of evaluation, the cost measurement may be applied to the total population eligible or to the population actually served. The first dimension requires calculation of the cost over time per person eligible for service; the second dimension requires only determination of the cost of services actually rendered, such as a physician visit or a hospital day. By either type of measure, comparisons of cost may be made between different methods of seeking to achieve the same goal; for example, water fluoridation versus periodic topical fluoride applications to children's teeth or group medical practice with salaried physicians in contrast to solo practice with fee-for-service remuneration.[54]

These fiscal measurements are complex because hidden costs must not be overlooked. If the cost of an organized home care program is to be compared with equivalent long-term hospital care, one must not ignore the expenses incurred by a family in keeping a sick member at home.[55] One must also not overlook administrative costs in a program's operation; for example, a high rate of personnel turnover in a clinic creates hidden costs for training new employees or reduced efficiency until new personnel learn their tasks. In hospital cost calculations, the shares of professional education and research costs that are properly accountable to patient care are perenially debated. If the laboratory in a hospital is understaffed, a bottleneck may be caused in the flow of patient care, leading to longer durations of stay; this administrative problem might not be reflected in per diem costs but only in cost per hospital case.[56]

In any event, cost figures are a far cry from health status as measurements of the ultimate outcome of a health service program, but they are nevertheless relevant to many larger questions of social policy.

Comment

In this review of five levels of benefit evaluation for health service programs, and a sixth level of cost evaluation, each level is presented along a gradient of depth or ultimacy. In the logic of the means-and-ends chain, this is believed to be generally valid, but as a practical matter there are circumstances in which a less ultimate level of evaluation may actually be more desirable than a more ultimate one. Thus, for example, the secondary variables, outside of the health service program, influencing death rates (level 1) may be so numerous and so difficult to adjust for, that the estimated quality (level 2) or even the simple quantity (level 3) of services provided by the program may be more reliable measures of its effects. For another example, the medical records of services in a program may be so inadequate that an interview with recipients on their attitudes (level 4) toward it, despite all the fallacies of the layman's judgment, may be more reliable than estimates of quality by expert review of written charts.

Because of these difficulties, many efforts to evaluate health service programs properly seek to measure two or more different levels of results at the same time. The studies of old-age assistance clients served by the Health Insurance Plan of Greater New York, compared with the traditional patterns,[18] obtained data on the quantity of different services provided as well as on health status (mortality rates). Our research on diverse health insurance plans in California is determining the quantity of services provided, the attitudes of recipients, and the costs or expenditures under each plan, although we are not getting health status measurements.[57]

The most useful strategy for evaluation would be to determine the effects of health service programs at all five levels plus their costs. Until that can be achieved, we should realize that measurements at any one or more of the six

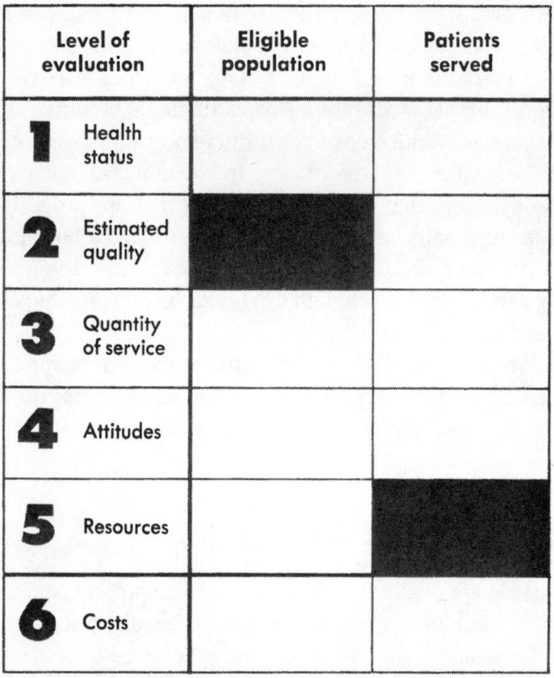

Level of evaluation	Eligible population	Patients served
1 Health status		
2 Estimated quality		
3 Quantity of service		
4 Attitudes		
5 Resources		
6 Costs		

Figure 25-1. Matrix of Evaluation of Health Service Programs

evaluation levels contribute something to our understanding of health service systems and are far more useful than evaluations based on intuition or speculation.

There are endless methodological problems in sampling, data collection, scaling, analysis, and so on not discussed in this paper. It should be pointed out, however, that the health service program to be studied may have varying degrees of complexity, and the problems of evaluation are corresponding. Evaluation may be attempted of an entire national health service system or, for example, of a particular prenatal clinic, or of a large series of program complexities in between. Intermediate complexities might be illustrated by a regional network of hospitals, a health insurance plan, or an air pollution control program.

The more complex the program examined, the more numerous generally are the secondary variables that must be adjusted for. The microsystem questions can usually be answered more rapidly and less expensively than the macrosystem questions. Ease of solution, however, seldom corresponds to the social importance of a question, and we should avoid tackling certain evaluative problems just because they are easily soluble, unless at the same time they are socially salient.

In summary, then, one can conceptualize a matrix of evaluation of health service programs. Along one axis would be the six levels of results that may be measured, and along the other axis the applicability of the measurement to a total eligible population or to only the patients actually served. Within each dimension there would be programs of varying degrees of complexity that may be summarized as macro or micro systems. This matrix could be schematized as shown in Figure 25-1.

Within each of these conceptual cells, evaluation requires the comparison of measurements of at least two entities, defined either across time (before and after) or across space (the model of test and control groups). Studies within any of these conceptual cells can be useful for program evaluation, which can facilitate a rational planning of health services.

References

1. Shryock, R. H.: American medical research past and present. Commonwealth Fund, New York, 1947.
2. B'tesch, S.: International research in the organization of medical care. Med Care 4:41–46, January–March 1966.
3. Kerr, M., and Trantow, D. J.: Defining, measuring, and assessing the quality of health services. Perspectives and a suggested framework. Public Health Rep 84:415–424, May 1969.
4. Altman, I., and Anderson, A. J.: Methodology in evaluating the quality of medical care: An annotated selected bibliography, 1955–61. University of Pittsburgh Press, Pittsburgh, Pa., 1962.
5. Suchman, E.: Evaluative research: Principles and practice in public service and social action programs. Russell Sage Foundation, New York, 1967.
6. Donabedian, A.: Evaluating the quality of medical care. Milbank Mem Fund Q 44:166–206, July 1966.
7. Weinerman, E. R.: Research into the organization of medical practice. Milbank Mem Fund Q 44:104–145, October 1966.
8. Shapiro, S.: End result measurements of quality of medical care. Milbank Mem Fund Q 45:7–30, April 1967.
9. Klein, B.: Evaluating outcomes of health care: An annotated bibliography. California Center for Health Services Research, Los Angeles, August 1969.
10. World Health Organization: Methodology in public health studies: A selected bibliography. OMC/RES/68.5. Geneva, December 1968.
11. Donabedian, A.: Medical care appraisal—quality and utilization: A guide to medical care administration. Vol. 2. American Public Health Association, New York, 1969.
12. Schulberg, H. C., Sheldon, A., and Baker, F., editors: Program evaluation in the health fields. Behavioral Publications, New York, 1969.
13. MacTavish, C. F.: Assessment of the quality of medical care: An annotated bibliography. American Rehabilitation Foundation, Minneapolis, Minn., February 1968.
14. Simon, H. A.: Administrative behavior. Macmillan Co., New York, 1961, pp. 62–66.
15. Hilleboe, H. E., and Schaefer, M.: Evaluation in community health: Relating results to goals. Bull NY Acad Med 44:140–158, February 1968.
16. World Health Organization: Vital statistics and causes of death: World health statistics annual. Vol. 1. Geneva, 1968.
17. Shapiro, S., Jacobziner,. H., Densen, P., and Weiner, L.: Further observations on prematurity

and perinatal mortality in a general population and in the population of a prepaid group practice medical care plan. Am J Public Health 50:1304–1317, September 1960.

18. Shapiro, S., et al.: Patterns of medical use by the indigent aged under two systems of medical care. Am J Public Health 57:784–790, May 1967.
19. Lipworth, L., Lee, H., and Morris, J. N.: Case fatality in teaching and non-teaching hospitals, 1956–1959. Med Care 1:71–76, April 1963.
20. Thompson, J. D., Marquis, D. B., Woodward, R. L., and Yeomans, R. C.: End-result measurements of the quality of obstetrical care in two U.S. Air Force hospitals. Med Care 6:131–143, March–April 1968.
21. Roemer, M. I.: Is surgery safer in larger hospitals? Hosp Manage 87:35–37, 50, 77, 101, (1959).
22. Roemer, M. I., Moustafa. A. T., and Hopkins, C. E.: A proposed hospital quality index: Hospital death rates adjusted for case severity. Health Serv Res 3:96–118, Summer 1968.
23. Sanders, B.: Measuring community health levels. Am J Public Health 54:1063–1070, July 1964.
24. Sullivan, D.: Conceptual problems in developing an index of health: Vital and health statistics. PHS Publication No. 1000, Ser. 2, No. 17, U.S. Government Printing Office, Washington, D.C., May 1966.
25. Katz, S., et al.: Studies of illness in the aged: The index of ADL, a standardized measure of biological and psychosocial function. JAMA 185:914–919, Sept. 21, 1963.
26. Katz, S.: Practical experience in evaluating a health service program. *In* Synopsis of proceedings, outcomes meeting I, California Center for Health Services Research, Los Angeles, May 1969.
27. Hagner, S., LoCicero, V., and Steiger, W.: Patient outcomes in a comprehensive medicine clinic. Med Care 6:144–156, March–April 1968.
28. Sanazaro, P. J., and Williamson, J. W.: End results of patient care: A provisional classification based on reports by internists. Med Care 6:123–130, March–April 1968.
29. Lembcke, P. A.: Evolution of the medical audit. JAMA 199:543–550, Feb. 20, 1967.
30. Rosenfeld, L. S.: Quality of medical care in hospitals. Am J Public Health 47:856–865, July 1957.
31. Ehrlich, J., Morehead, M. A., and Trussell, R. E.: The quantity, quality and costs of medical and hospital care secured by a sample of teamsters families in the New York area. Columbia University, New York, 1962.
32. Kroeger, H. H., et al.: The office practice of internists: The feasibility of evaluating quality of care. JAMA 193:371–376, Aug. 2, 1965.
33. Peterson, O. L., et al.: An analytical study of North Carolina general practice. J Med Educ 31:1–165, December 1965.
34. Clute, K. F.: The general practitioner: A study of medical education and practice in Ontario and Nova Scotia. University of Toronto Press, Toronto, 1963.
35. Furstenberg, F. F., et al.: Prescribing as an index to quality of medical care. Am J Public Health 43:1299–1309, October 1953.
36. Slee, V. N.: Uniform methods of measuring utilization. *In* Utilization review: A handbook for the medical staff: American Medical Association, Chicago, 1965.
37. Hiscock, I. V.: Community health organization. Ed. 4. Commonwealth Fund, New York, 1950, p. 242.
38. Anderson, O. W., and Feldman, J. J.: Family medical costs and voluntary health insurance: A nationwide survey. McGraw-Hill Book Co., New York, 1956.
39. Darksy, B. J., Sinai, N., and Axelrod, S. J.: Comprehensive medical services under voluntary health insurance: A study of Windsor medical services. Harvard University Press, Cambridge, Mass., 1958, p. 62.
40. Densen, P.: Some practical and conceptual problems in appraising the outcome of health care services and programs. Paper presented at Health Services Outcomes Conference, Los Angeles, Dec. 1, 1969.
41. Klarman, H. E.: Controlling hospital use through organization of medical services. *In* Where is hospital use headed? Paper presented at the Fifth Annual Symposium on Hospital Affairs, University of Chicago, 1962, pp. 55–63.
42. Roemer, M. I.: Research in administrative medicine: Comparative analysis of systems of health service organization. *In* Research in social welfare administration. National Association of Social Workers, New York, 1962, pp. 72–81.

43. Watts, M., et al.: A special report of the medical and hospital advisory committee to the board of administration. State Employees Retirement System, Sacramento, Calif., June 1964.
44. Anderson, O. W., and Sheatley, P. B.: Comprehensive medical insurance: A study of costs, use, and attitudes under two plans. Health Information Foundation, Chicago, 1959.
45. Gemmill, P. F.: An American report on the National Health Service. Br Med J (supp.) 5:17–21, July 1958.
46. Blum, R. H.: Hospitals and patient dissatisfaction. Technical Report. California Medical Association, San Francisco, 1958.
47. U.S. Department of Health, Education and Welfare: Recommendations of the task force on Medicaid and related programs. U.S. Government Printing Office, Washington, D.C., November 1969.
48. Roemer, M. I.: The rural health services scheme in Malaysia. World Health Organization, Western Pacific Regional Office, Manila, February 1969.
49. National Commission on Community Health Services: Health manpower: Action to meet community needs. Public Affairs Press, Washington, D.C., 1967.
50. U.S. Public Health Service: Directory of local health units, 1966. PHS Publication No. 118. U.S. Government Printing Office, Washington, D.C., 1966.
51. Mott, F. D., and Roemer, M. I.: Rural health and medical care. McGraw Hill Book Co., New York, 1948.
52. McCaffree, K.: The cost of mental health care under changing treatment methods. Am J Public Health 56:1013–1025, July 1966.
53. Klarman, H.: Present status of cost-benefit analysis in the health field. Am J Public Health 57:1948–1954, November 1967.
54. Williams, J. J., et al.: Family medical care under three types of health insurance. Foundation on Employee Health, Medical Care, and Welfare, New York, 1962.
55. Rogatz, P., et al.: Organized home medical care in New York City. Harvard University Press, Cambridge, Mass., 1956.
56. Lave, J.: A review of the methods used to study hospital costs. Inquiry 3:57–81 (1966).
57. Sasuly, R., and Roemer, M. I.: Health insurance plans: A conceptualization from the California scene. J Health Hum Behav 7:36–44, spring 1966.

26

Comparative Perinatal Mortality under Different Health Care Delivery Models

This chapter presents an empirical study in which the health outcomes of three different models of health care delivery to an indigent population are compared. Particular attention is focused on the "medical care foundation"—a pattern of "health maintenance organization" (HMO) that uses private medical practitioners but provides surveillance over their work. Many claims have been made for the superior performance of this model.

The "outcome" measured was perinatal mortality, as occurring in an indigent Medicaid population in three California counties, one of which had a medical care foundation, while the other two illustrated different delivery patterns. The text reproduced below was co-authored with John Newport.

IN THE NATIONAL debate over health care delivery patterns, the foundations for medical care have figured prominently as an approach to both economy and quality. It has been argued that the achievements claimed for the prepaid group practice (PGP) model, in the way of lower costs and high quality service, could similarly be attained within the framework of traditional individual medical practice if there were 1. insurance for comprehensive physician services (in the office and home, as well as the hospital), and 2. rigorous surveillance over fee-for-service claims.[1] Generally characterized as the medical care foundation (MCF) model, this pattern has been offered as one of the options under the federal government's health maintenance organization (HMO) strategy.

Evaluation of the generally favorable consequences of the PGP model—through measurements of structure and process as well as outcome—have been numerous.[2] It is relevant to note that in regard to outcome investigations of this model, the studies by Shapiro, et al., on the Health Insurance Plan of New York figured prominently.[3] The Shapiro studies, which compared the HIP population with matched non-HIP populations, also focused on perinatal mortality and showed perinatal deaths to be significantly lower among PGP mothers. These differences remained statistically significant even when the comparisons were lim-

Chapter 26 is reprinted, with permission of the Blue Cross Association, from *Inquiry*. Vol. XII, No. 1, pp. 10–17.

ited to childbirths attended by private physicians and when adjustments were made for both age of mother and ethnicity.

The MCF model, on the other hand, has had little quantitative evaluation; evidence of its effects is limited to some suggestive data on cost savings (although some of this is conflicting), and on structural or input appraisal.[4] No evidence has yet been produced on health status outcomes of the MCF model of medical care delivery.

The Study Areas

An opportunity for such evaluative study of outcomes has been presented by research on Medicaid services under different organizational modes in California.[5] Among the modes through which Medicaid families may obtain their medical care, one has been the San Joaquin County Foundation for Medical Care. Other modes have included a prepaid group practice, an OEO neighborhood health center, a county served by a well-developed government hospital out-patient program (as well as a strong health department), and the conventional pattern of private medical practice paid for on a fee-for-service basis.

In the counties demonstrating three of these modes, it was possible to obtain data on childbirths among Medicaid mothers and any associated fetal or infant mortality, which might constitute outcome measurements of the qualitative effects of the several modes. The MCF mode, as noted, was in San Joaquin County; three other small rural counties were also covered by the same foundation. In this area, physician services to Medicaid recipients are covered by a prepaid capitation contract administered by the San Joaquin County Foundation for Medical Care. It is important to note, however, that under this contract Medicaid births occurring in county-operated hospitals are not covered and are not subject to foundation peer review procedures.

The county demonstrating the conventional private practice pattern was chosen by a statistical process aimed at identifying which county, among the 58 in California, was most similar to San Joaquin in terms of both socioeconomic and medical resource variables, but without a medical foundation. Variables examined were:

- total population
- percent employed in agriculture, etc.
- average income per household
- AFDC recipients per 1,000 population
- average monthly Medicaid cost per AFDC recipient
- physicians per 100,000 population
- hospital beds per 1,000 population

By this analysis, Ventura County was selected (Kern County was slightly more closely matched but had to be rejected because it had a medical foundation).

In the area illustrating a well-developed county hospital outpatient department along with a strong health department, it was found, not surprisingly, that Medicaid AFDC (aid to families with dependent children) mothers actually obtained most of their obstetrical services from private physicians and had their deliveries in voluntary hospitals. This was Contra Costa County. Further investigation in this county led to several indications that the local health department had a particularly strong maternal and child health program. The policy for many years has been to encourage, as much as feasible, the early prenatal care of all women, especially the poor, by private physicians. Public health nurses in this county have energetically monitored Medicaid mothers to facilitate their obtaining prompt and continuing prenatal care, expeditious delivery, and effective management of the newborn baby—usually through the private "mainstream" system, but similarly if the mother chose to obtain care at the county hospital (26 percent of the childbirths in 1967 and 1968).[6] It is also noteworthy that in the mid-1960s the Contra Costa County Health Department pioneered the assignment of public health nurses to the clinic of a private medical group—an indication of particularly strong cooperation between the health department and private physicians in that county.[7]

The relative strength of the health department's maternal and child health (MCH) program in Contra Costa County is not meant to imply that in *all* respects this county's public health services are stronger than those in the two other comparison counties. In fact, as measured by money spent per capita in 1968, the Contra Costa County Health Department was not as strong as the one in San Joaquin County, although stronger than the one in Ventura County. Furthermore, the ratio of public health nurses per 100,000 county population was approximately in the same sequence. The salient data are shown in Table 26-1, where it may also be noted that the ratios of public health nurses to the poverty populations (AFDC beneficiaries) in the three comparison counties are roughly equal (although lowest by a small margin in Contra Costa County).

Table 26-1
Health Department Resources in Three Comparison Counties: Selected Indices of Public Health Activity, 1968

	County		
Resource Index	*Ventura*	*San Joaquin*	*Contra Costa*
County population (in thousands)	325	280	539
Health department expenditures per capita	$2.83	$6.61	$4.51
Public health nurses per 100,000 population	6.8	18.0	13.2
Public health nurses per 100,000 AFDC beneficiaries	112	117	110

Practices in the Three Counties

These data must be interpreted, however, in the light of the actual practices in the three counties. In San Joaquin County, a substantial portion of public health nursing time is spent in school health services; by contrast, in Contra Costa County the school nursing program is operated by the Department of Education, so that the health department nurses are able to concentrate their efforts on the community MCH program. As noted, the latter department's policies have emphasized prenatal care by physicians and instructional home visits by nurses to the mothers of newborn babies for many years. Moreover, it happens that in Contra Costa County, the county hospital maintains three satellite MCH clinics, beyond those operated by the health department. Discussions with key personnel in the health departments of the three study counties impressed us that the MCH policies, especially with respect to Medicaid mothers, were decidedly stronger in Contra Costa than in the other two counties.[8]

In summary, in the outcome evaluation study, it was considered reasonable to characterize each of the three comparison areas as follows:

1. A medical care foundation (MCF) area, including San Joaquin County (280,300 population), plus Amador (12,200), Calaveras (11,800), and Tuolomne (20,000) Counties.
2. A conventional private practice (CPP) area—Ventura County (325,000 population).
3. A strong health department (SHD) area—Contra Costa County (539,000 population).

In these three contrasting areas, we set out to examine the end-result experience of Medicaid childbirths.

Method of Data Collection

Broadly speaking, the AFDC mothers in all three study areas are matched populations, since the criteria of eligibility for California's Medicaid program (known as "Medi-Cal") are established at the state level. All three sets of mothers, in other words, are of roughly equal poverty levels. There are differences, however, in their ethnic distribution. Since other studies have shown differences in health behavior among diverse ethnic groups of even the same socioeconomic level, we were fortunate to be able to analyze and adjust the data by ethnic composition.

Moreover, it was important to distinguish in each study area the childbirths occurring in county hospitals (where young house officers in training do most of the deliveries, as well as other obstetrical work) from those occurring in the "mainstream" setting (private physicians and non-governmental hospitals). Reasonable comparisons across areas can only be made within these two subsets. It must be emphasized that the MCF model, on which our evaluation is particularly focused, operates only within the mainstream setting.

The data for analysis were obtained from two principal sources. Identification of Medicaid AFDC childbirths was obtained through the files of fiscal claims from hospitals paid by the Department of Health Care Services, which at the time administered California's Medicaid Program. Corresponding birth and death (either stillbirth or neonatal) data were obtained from the Department of Public Health. The latter department, moreover, has developed a computerized technique for linkage of all births and infant deaths by county throughout the state. The research task, therefore, involved disaggregation of the Medicaid childbirths from the others and tabulation of the data for the three study areas. The total experience reported here applies to the two-year period, 1967 and 1968.[9]

Finally, with respect to methodology, it should be explained that this paper focuses on perinatal mortality rates among Medicaid childbirths partly in the interest of brevity, but mainly in the interest of reliability of the comparisons across geographic areas. Differences in the accuracy of reporting of fetal deaths (stillbirths), as against neonatal deaths (mortality up to 28 days of life), are obviated by use of the perinatal death measurement, since it summates both of these categories. Thus, our definition of the perinatal mortality rate is as follows:

$$\text{Perinatal mortality rate} = \frac{\text{Fetal deaths} + \text{Neonatal deaths}}{\text{Total births (live births} + \text{stillbirths)}} \times 1{,}000$$

A further reason for focusing on perinatal mortality involves the basic objective of the research: evaluation of a model of medical care delivery. Overall infant mortality (deaths during the first year of life, following a live birth) is known to be influenced by environmental conditions and general standards of living, as well as by the provision of medical care. By contrast, deaths occurring shortly before, during, or shortly after childbirth are more exclusively influenced by the level of medical care. Hence, the perinatal mortality rate is believed to be an especially appropriate outcome measure of the quality of service under various models of medical care delivery.

Findings

The basic numbers of Medicaid births and perinatal deaths occurring in the three study areas, classified by ethnic group, are reported in Table 26-2. These figures combine childbirths in both the mainstream setting and in county hospitals. Table 26-3 presents the proportions of all births occurring within these two types of hospital in each study area.

It is evident from these two tables that both the proportions of childbirths in different ethnic groups and the proportions of deliveries occurring in mainstream versus county hospitals differ substantially among the three study areas. From Table 26-2, it may be noted that, contrary to common notions, the greatest proportion of all Medicaid childbirths in all three study areas occur among white "Anglo" families.[10] The proportions of childbirths among the minority ethnic groups, however, vary in the three areas, being subtantially higher for the Spanish surname group in the CPP (conventional private practice) area, moderately higher for this group than for Negroes in the MCF (medical care foundation) area, and substantially higher for Negroes in the SHD (strong health department) area.

From Table 26-3, it is evident that the distribution of childbirths for the total Medicaid population is most mainstream-oriented in the SHD area (74 percent);

Table 26-2
Medicaid Births and Perinatal Deaths: Numbers in Three Types of Health Care Area, by Ethnic Group, 1967 and 1968

	Health Care Delivery Pattern					
	CPP		*MCF*		*SHD*	
Ethnic Group	*Total Births*	*Perinatal Deaths*	*Total Births*	*Perinatal Deaths*	*Total Births*	*Perinatal Deaths*
White "Anglo"	524	22	766	29	1,098	24
Spanish surname	358	8	448	9	193	2
Negro	70	2	315	13	718	13
Other	8	0	45	0	20	0
All groups	960	32	1,574	51	2,029	39

Code: CPP = Conventional private practice (Ventura County)
MCF = Medical care foundation (San Joaquin area)
SHD = Strong health department (Contra Costa County)

Table 26-3
Medicaid Births in Mainstream and in County Hospitals: Percentage Distributions in Three Types of Health Care Area, by Ethnic Group, 1967 and 1968

	Health Care Delivery Pattern					
	CPP		*MCF*		*SHD*	
Ethnic Group	*Mainstream*	*County*	*Mainstream*	*County*	*Mainstream*	*County*
White "Anglo"	40.0	14.6	31.6	17.0	41.7	12.4
Spanish surname	20.5	16.8	10.5	18.0	6.9	2.6
Negro	5.0	2.3	7.1	12.9	25.0	10.4
Other	0.8	0.0	1.0	1.8	0.7	0.2
All groups	66.4	33.6	50.3	49.7	74.3	25.7

Code: CPP = Conventional private practice (Ventura County)
MCF = Medical care foundation (San Joaquin area)
SHD = Strong health department (Contra Costa County)

next so in the CPP area (66 percent); and least so in the MCF area (50 percent). For the different ethnic groups, furthermore, the distribution of obstetrical deliveries between the mainstream hospital setting and county hospitals varies markedly. In all three study areas, white "Anglo" childbirths are more likely to occur in mainstream hospitals than are the childbirths of any of the ethnic minorities. In the SHD area, however, the differentials are small, and 70 percent or more of the childbirths of each of the four ethnic groups, considered separately, occur within mainstream hospitals. By contrast, in the MCF area, unlike the other two, approximately two-thirds of all "Anglo" births occurred in private hospitals, in contrast to only one-third of births among both the Negro and Spanish-surname groups—in spite of the reported influence of the medical care foundation in encouraging private doctor participation in the Medicaid program.[11] That influence, in a word, seems to favor mainly the white "Anglo" mothers.

Perinatal Death Rates

With this background of information to provide perspective, we may consider the perinatal death rates in the three study areas. The basic findings are presented in Table 26-4, tabulated both by ethnic group and by hospital setting. Several observations emerge from these data. First, examining all ethnic groups together, the perinatal mortality rate among childbirths in county hospitals is higher than in mainstream hospitals in all three study areas. (Interpretations of this and other findings will be offered later.) For each ethnic group considered separately, however, there are noticeable exceptions: in the SHD area this relationship is reversed (that is, the mainstream perinatal mortality rate is higher) among Spanish surname childbirths; and in the MCF area it is reversed among Negro childbirths.

Second, it may be observed that (leaving aside the "other" ethnic category, in which the total numbers of childbirths were very low and no deaths occurred) in five of the six study areas and hospital settings, the perinatal mortality rate is lowest among Spanish surname childbirths; the exception is in the mainstream hospitals of the SHD area, where the Negro rate is lowest. As between the white "Anglo" and the Negro perinatal mortality rates, in the county hospital settings, the Negro rates are higher than the "Anglo" rates in the CPP and SHD areas, but lower in the MCF area. In the mainstream hospital settings, the relationships are different, being higher for Negro childbirths in the MCF area and lower in the CPP and SHD areas. In fact, in the SHD mainstream hospital area, the Negro perinatal mortality rate reaches the phenomenally low level (in comparison with national as well as California-wide figures) of 7.9 perinatal deaths per 1,000 total births.

Third, we come to the most crucial findings, from the viewpoint of this study—the differential rates among areas demonstrating different models of medical care delivery. To consider this question, we must focus on the three

Table 26-4
Perinatal Mortality in Three Types of Health Care Area: Rates per 1,000 Total Births* by Ethnic Group and Hospital Setting, 1967 and 1968

Ethnic Group	*Hospital Setting*					
	County			*Mainstream*		
	CPP	*MCF*	*SHD*	*CPP*	*MCF*	*SHD*
White "Anglo"	42.9	56.0	27.9	41.7	28.1	20.1
Spanish surname	31.1	21.2	0.0	15.2	18.2	14.4
Negro	45.5	39.4	42.7	20.8	44.6	7.9
Other	0.0	0.0	0.0	0.0	0.0	0.0
All groups	37.2	37.1	34.6	31.4	27.8	15.3
Total (standardized)	39.7	38.6	24.3	30.1	29.6	15.5

Code: CPP = Conventional private practice (Ventura County)
MCF = Medical care foundation (San Joaquin area)
SHD = Strong health department (Contra Costa County)

*Method of calculation explained in the text.

mainstream columns of Table 26-4. (The three county hospital columns are not so relevant, since the medical care foundation program has no influence on childbirths in these public facilities and the health department influence—according to the Contra Costa County Health Officer—is less marked.) In these mainstream medical care settings, it may be observed that, comparing the MCF area with its essentially matched CPP area, the perinatal mortality rates among white "Anglo" childbirths are substantially lower in the MCF area, among Spanish surname childbirths they are slightly higher, and among Negro childbirths they are substantially higher. Examining the total (but non-standardized) rates for all ethnic groups, the perinatal mortality in the MCF area (27.8 per 1,000) is slightly lower than in the comparison CPP area (31.4 per 1,000); this difference, however, is not statistically significant. Indeed, when the mix of ethnic groups is standardized to California statewide distribution of childbirths in the Medicaid population served by mainstream hospitals (white "Anglo," 53 percent; Spanish surname, 20 percent; Negro, 24 percent; and others, 3 percent), the perinatal mortality rates in the MCF and CPP areas are virtually identical—29.6 and 30.1 respectively.

Finally, the most striking findings to emerge from the data in Table 26-4 are the remarkably low perinatal mortality rates in the SHD area. These rates are lowest in the mainstream sector for each of the three principal ethnic groups examined separately, but especially for the white "Anglo" and the Negro categories. The standardized total mortality rate of 15.5 per 1,000 in the SHD area is almost exactly half of that found in both of the other study areas.

Discussion and Interpretation

From these findings it is possible to draw several inferences with respect to the influence on health status outcome of medical foundations compared with other models of health care delivery, at least as reflected by the impact of these patterns on perinatal mortality in poverty populations in the areas investigated. Before offering these, however, one should consider certain other aspects of the pregnancies of Medicaid mothers that may well have influenced the perinatal mortality rates. Among the many such potential influences, data were available on two that are known to be associated with higher pregnancy risk: illegitimacy and age-of-mother. In general, we know that the risk of perinatal mortality is higher in pregnancies out-of-wedlock (illegitimacy), and in very young mothers (under 20 years of age). General experience also supports the probability of lower pregnancy wastage if prenatal care has been initiated early in the gestational period (during the first trimester).[12]

In Table 26-5, data on these factors affecting pregnancy risk in the three study areas are summarized. Regarding illegitimacy, it may be noted that the rate, and therefore the risk of difficulties, was actually higher in the CPP county than in the MCF county. Regarding percentage of very young mothers, the risk relationship was in the opposite direction, but by a much lesser degree. Most noticeably, however, the highest illegitimacy rate is observed in the SHD county. Regarding very young mothers (under age 20), the risk was slightly greater in the MCF than in the CPP county, but again decidedly higher in the SHD county. Thus, by these two measures, it would appear that the remarkably lower perinatal mortality rates in the SHD than in the other two areas cannot be attributed to any lighter load of pregnancy risks. Indeed, the opposite was true; the lower perinatal mortality rates

Table 26-5
Conditions of Pregnancy in Three Types of Health Care Area: Percentages of Selected Features in Medicaid Mothers, 1967 and 1968

	Health Care Delivery Pattern		
Condition of Pregnancy	*CPP*	*MCF*	*SHD*
Percentage of childbirths that were illegitimate	46.8	41.1	48.5
Percentage of mothers under 20 years of age	33.1	35.3	42.7
Percentage of mothers initiating prenatal care in first trimester	43.0	34.9	49.8

Code: CPP = Conventional private practice (Ventura County)
MCF = Medical care foundation (San Joaquin area)
SHD = Strong health department (Contra Costa County)

in the SHD area occurred in spite of a higher level of pregnancy risk in this county's Medicaid childbirths.

The third row in Table 26-5 tends to support our hypothesis that a decisive influence in the SHD area was the energetic influence of the public health program, especially the work of the public health nurses.[13] In this row, we find that nearly 50 percent of the pregnancies in the SHD area initiated prenatal care in the first gestational trimester, compared with 35 percent in the MCF area and 43 percent in the CPP area. Perhaps one may infer that earlier prenatal care in the SHD area compensated for the greater pregnancy risks in that area. It should be emphasized, however, that in all three areas the study populations were similarly impoverished Medicaid families, so that—aside from the ethnic mixes, which we adjusted for—our comparisons did not require the statistical adjustments for socioeconomic status faced by Shapiro in his HIP studies (cited earlier), or other comparative investigations of perinatal mortality in different population groups.

Conclusions

Returning to the basic question about the influence of medical care delivery models on perinatal mortality outcomes, the following conclusions would seem to be justified by our findings in the California counties studied:

1. The medical care foundation (MCF) model, as represented by the original prototype of this model in the nation (San Joaquin County's), did not yield any significantly better perinatal mortality outcomes in poverty populations than the conventional private practice (CPP) model of health care delivery over the two-year period, 1967–1968. (Although a net decline in perinatal mortality did occur in the MCF area from 1967 to 1968, this decline was almost entirely attributable to births at county hospitals, which are outside the MCF influence.)
2. A county characterized by a strong health department (SHD) with an active maternal and child health program yielded a much lower perinatal death rate than either the prototype MCF or a matched CPP county.
3. In general, perinatal mortality rates were lower for childbirths occurring in the mainstream medical setting than in county government hospitals, regardless of the operations of either a medical care foundation or a strong health department.

The third of these conclusions may be influenced substantially by the risk selection of mothers entering county hospitals for delivery, compared with those served in the mainstream hospitals. How much of the differential is due to these risk factors, as against the circumstances of obstetrical service in the two settings (e.g., poor accessibility, deliveries by young doctors-in-training, etc., in the county hospitals), cannot be assessed from this study.

It appears that in the period covered by this study, the peer review activities of the San Joaquin Foundation for Medical Care were oriented largely toward restraining overutilization of services. In a poverty population, however, a more appropriate emphasis might be encouragement of early prenatal care and the maximum assumption of responsibility by private physicians for minority as well as white "Anglo" ethnic groups.

The superior performance, with respect to perinatal mortality measures, in Contra Costa County may be due to other influences that this study did not identify. It cannot, however, be attributed to the elements reflecting pregnancy risk—illegitimacy and young age of mother—on which data were available. The precise activities of health departments that may be most influential can only be surmised, but our belief is that the activities of public health nurses in bringing expectant Medicaid mothers to relatively prompt and effective medical attention was important.

By way of perspective, it may be noted that the failure of the MCF model to yield a lower perinatal mortality outcome than either a matched CPP model or a SHD model is in contrast to the findings of another study evaluating the San Joaquin County MCF by use of *process* measurements. As part of the same general investigation, it was found that surgical procedures (including obstetrical deliveries) paid for by Medicaid were more likely to be done by a properly qualified physician in San Joaquin than in the matched Ventura County.[14] This is perhaps one more bit of evidence on the crucial importance of outcome, rather than process measurements for evaluating the quality of medical care.

Perinatal mortality, of course, is only one limited type of outcome measurement of health service. For the present, however, it remains to be demonstrated that the individual practice pattern of HMO, implemented in the medical care foundations, has any favorable influence on the qualitative outcome of medical care.

References

1. Egdahl, Richard H. "Foundations for Medical Care," *New England Journal of Medicine* 288:491–498 (8 March 1973).
2. Donabedian, Avedis. "An Evaluation of Prepaid Group Practice," *Inquiry* 6:3–27 (September 1969).
3. See: Shapiro, Sam; Weiner, Louis; and Densen, Paul M. "Comparison of Prematurity and Perinatal Mortality in a General Population and in the Population of a Prepaid Group Medical Care Plan," *American Journal of Public Health* 48:170–187 (February 1958); and Shapiro, Sam; Jacobziner, Harold; Densen, Paul M.; and Weiner, Louis. "Further Observations on Prematurity and Perinatal Mortality in a General Population and in the Population of a Prepaid Group Practice Medical Care Plan," *American Journal of Public Health* 50:1304–1317 (September 1970).
4. Roemer, Milton I. and Shonick, William. "HMO Performance: The Recent Evidence," (A report to the National Academy of Sciences) *Milbank Memorial Fund Quarterly: Health and Society* 51:271–317 (Summer 1973).
5. Gartside, Foline E., *et al. Medicaid Services in California under Different Organizational Modes,* A series of reports, Los Angeles: University of California, School of Public Health, 1970–1973 (processed).

6. Henrik L. Blum, former Health Officer of Contra Costa County, California; personal communication, February 1973.
7. Lindberg, H. G. and Carlson, B. V. "A Public Health Nurse in the Private Physician's Office," *Nursing Outlook* 16:43–45 (April 1968).
8. Field visits to San Joaquin and Ventura Counties yielded discussions with health department personnel in both of these agencies.
9. On a statewide basis, it was found possible to match hospital Medicaid claims with vital record (birth and death) data for 91 percent of the AFDC deliveries in 1967 and 88 percent of them in 1968. In a subsequent study of 1970 experience, however, by detailed investigation of maternity services in a sample of 17 hospitals, it was found possible to account for and achieve matching of over 98 percent of all Medicaid births. (In this year, 1970, the computer technique likewise yielded an approximately 90 percent linkage—or about a 10 percent "fallout.") When comparisons were then made between the perinatal mortality rates calculated from the computerized 90 percent sample with the 98-plus percent sample, the resultant rates were found to be virtually identical. This calculation served to reassure us of the validity of the basic data derived from the computer tapes.
10. This, of course, implies nothing about the birth *rates* among the several ethnic groups, which we know to be generally higher in the minorities.
11. Harrington, Donald C. "San Joaquin Foundation for Medical Care," *Hospitals* 45:67–68 (16 March 1971).
12. U.S. National Center for Health Statistics. *Infant and Perinatal Mortality in the United States* (Washington D.C.: U.S. Public Health Service, Vital and Health Statistics Series 3, No. 4, 1965).
13. The work of these nurses is also reinforced by a reportedly strong peer review program in the local County Medical Society, despite its lack of a medical care foundation.
14. Roemer, Milton I. and Gartside, Foline E. "Peer Review in Medical Foundations: Its Effect on Qualifications of Surgeons," *Health Services Reports* 88:808–813 (November 1973).

27

Hospital Death Rates Adjusted for Case Severity: A Proposed Hospital Quality Index

For decades, the quality of hospital performance has been evaluated mainly by observations, and sometimes measurements, of the "input" of resources and the "process" of work done. In the following paper, an attempt is made to develop an "outcome" measurement of hospital performance, based on the rate of patient deaths adjusted by a proxy indicator of the average severity of the cases admitted to the particular hospital. This indicator (average length-of-stay) is, in turn, corrected for factors other than *the patient's condition which may affect it.*

Based on a sample of 33 general hospitals in one California county, it was found that adjustment of the crude death rate by the method proposed resulted in lower (rather than higher) adjusted death rates for hospitals independently scored as having higher levels of "technological adequacy." The study was done jointly with A. Taher Moustafa and Carl E. Hopkins. Subsequently the evaluative method was tested in other cities (Chicago, Boston, New York, etc.) with varying results, but mainly confirmatory.

HOSPITAL LEADERS HAVE long sought a reliable index of the quality of hospital care in terms of final outcomes. If a hospital does good work, a high proportion of its patients should recover and few should die. In other sectors of health service, the quality of performance is commonly judged by mortality rates: the value of a new therapy for a specific disease is judged by the outcome in recovery or death of patients treated compared with nontreated (or differently treated) patients; the effectiveness of a new public health measure such as the chlorination of the water supply is judged by the outcome in terms of mortality rates for waterborne diseases. A comparable measure of hospital effectiveness might be the hospital death rate, representing the proportion of all patients admitted during a year who die in the hospital.

Chapter 27 is reprinted with permission from *Health Services Research*, Vol. 3, no. 2, Summer 1968, pp. 96–118.

Efforts to Measure Hospital Quality

Outcome measures of the above type have rightly been viewed with much skepticism for evaluating hospital performance. It is pointed out that the types of patients—that is, their diagnoses and severity of illness—coming to different hospitals may be highly variant: Hospital A may have seriously ill patients and difficult cases, while Hospital B may have mainly mild and easy-to-cure cases. Thus, even though Hospital A may offer the most advanced scientific technology, applied with the greatest skill and diligence, its death rate may be higher than that of Hospital B, which may even be poorly staffed, equipped, and operated.[1]

In fact, the crude death rates of large university teaching hospitals are typically higher than those of small nonteaching hospitals. The death rate (number of deaths per number of admissions per year) at a large university teaching hospital in Los Angeles County in 1964 was 9.1 percent, compared with 1.7 percent for a random series of 10 small proprietary hospitals (mainly nonaccredited) in the same county. Hardly anyone would suggest that this means that the quality of care in the teaching hospital is inferior to that in the others. The explanation must be found in the greater proportion of severely ill, high-risk patients coming to highly developed hospitals. A simple statistical adjustment for these diverse mixtures of admissions has not been available.

In the absence of such a statistical device, measurements of a hospital's quality of performance are usually sought along other dimensions. The commonest path taken is simply to examine the *input* side—that is, the staffing, equipment, and services of the hospital—on the presumption that input determines outcome. This is the basis of the whole program of hospital review by the Joint Commission on Accreditation of Hospitals and of the hospital licensing inspection systems of the states.[2] Under these evaluation programs, the structure and function of the hospital are examined in detail: qualifications of staff, organization of medical staff and nonmedical personnel, maintenance of patient records, policies with respect to professional privileges for performing surgery, technical features of the laboratory, X-ray department, operating room, policies with respect to drugs, diligence of the medical staff in reviewing its work through committees or conferences, and so forth. These practices are judged against standards advocated by acknowledged experts and may even be given a numerical score; but none of these scores is a measure of *outcome*. They do not indicate what eventually happens to patients, even though it might be assumed that facilities and practices meeting standards are more likely to lead to a patient's recovery than those that do not.

Within the schedule of data collected by an inspection for hospital accreditation or licensure, certain limited outcome measures may be solicited, but they are always rightfully viewed with great caution.[3] Thus, in the maternity service of a hospital, the rate of infant or fetal deaths, the rate of maternal deaths associated with delivery, or the percentage of obstetrical cases handled by cesarean section may be calculated; in the surgical service, the rate of postoperative or post-anesthetic deaths or of postoperative infections or other complications. It has been customary to set certain figures as the upper limit of tolerance for these measurements.[4] These norms may be useful initial screening devices, but they are obviously crude on several grounds. They take no account of the relative risks of the patients entering the series: a hospital accepting a high proportion of complex surgical cases (for example, cardiac surgery) is bound to have higher post-operative mortality than one accepting few such cases; and a hospital serving mainly low-income patients in poor general health is likely to have higher risk of mortality and morbid complications than one serving mainly high-income patients in good general health. The problem of reporting is also a factor: infections or other complications of surgery may be poorly reported, and deaths may not be attributed to the surgical procedure or anesthesia. These hazards in judging the restricted outcome measures cited are well understood by the Joint Commission and by licensure authorities; they are seldom used as more than faint clues (if the rates appear to be higher than conventional norms) to guide further probing into the operation of certain hospital departments.

One commonly used measure of hospital performance is the "autopsy rate"; years ago it was even heralded by Graham Davis as "the best measure of a hospital's quality." The percentage of autopsies performed, however, is not a measure of the outcome of hospital care. It doubtless indicates something about the diligence and intellectual curiosity of the medical staff—which may, in turn, influence the quality of patient care; but it tells nothing directly about the adequacy with which patients are served while they are alive.

With all these deficiencies in measures of the input side and the very restricted measures of outcome, much reliance has been placed on another approach: the "medical audit," in which a second physician reviews the medical management of specific patients.[5] A medical audit may involve direct visual observation of the work of a physician and ancillary staff, as in the studies of general practice in North Carolina by Peterson and his colleagues.[6] More often, however, the patient's chart is reviewed and judgments are made on the degree to which the recorded diagnostic and therapeutic management of the case coincides with the standards in the mind of the reviewer. Again, the details of case management may strongly influence the outcome in long-term recovery or death, but this is still only a presumption. Moreover, everything depends on the judgment of the reviewer, the accuracy of the written record (which may be faulty both in entries and in omissions), and the presence of other biological or environmental variables, which may not be known to either the reviewer or the original physician.

A variant of the medical audit is the tabulation of procedures carried out for designated diagnoses in a particular hospital or for the patients of a particular physician. For example, how often are liver function tests or gallbladder X-rays done prior to cholecystectomies by Dr. D in Hospital H? How do these rates correspond with the rates for all physicians or all hospitals? Such tabulations have been made for many years on an expanding series of hospitals through the Professional Activities Study (PAS) of the Commission on Professional and Hospital Activities, of Ann Arbor, Michigan. The PAS statistics establish the range of certain practices over a large number of cases; allow determination of means, medians, or modes; and permit identification of deviation from norms by individual hospitals or physicians.[7] Again, however, they do not indicate the outcome of patient care, except insofar as certain crude death rates may be calculated along specific dimensions (with all the hazards noted above).

Another variant of the medical audit is the postoperative tissue examination.[8] If a particular surgeon is found to be removing organs that, in a high proportion of cases, are judged normal by the pathologist's examination, it may be presumed that he is exercising poor surgical judgment. The criterion of "high" varies with the type of operation and the opinion of the observer, although 15 percent nonpathological tissue has been a common benchmark for everyday use. This approach is useful as an evaluation of the clinical judgment of surgeons, but it records essentially only errors of commission, not of omission, and it still tells nothing about the ultimate outcome of the case.

The Approach through Mortality Rates for Selected Diagnoses

With these weaknesses of current and past efforts to measure the quality of hospital performance, the search for hard data on the outcome of hospital care has continued. One approach has been through measures of hospital mortality for selected clinical diagnoses.

Data on selected postoperative death rates in hospitals of different sizes in the province of Saskatchewan, Canada, were examined for the years 1950–53 by one of the authors.[9] Information was available on the universe of five relatively common types of surgical operation performed in all hospitals of this province of about 900,000 population. From the universal hospital insurance plan of the province, data are recorded on every hospital case. For the surgical deaths in 1953, additional information was gathered on the duration of hospital stay before death and on the age of the patient. Institutions were categorized as "small" (under 25 beds), "medium" (25–99 beds), and "large" (100 beds and over); it was presumed that the level of technical services of a hospital increased generally with its bed capacity.

For prostatectomies the case fatality rate was clearly lower in the large hospitals, at 3.8 deaths per 100 operations compared with 8.8 in the medium and 9.8 in the small hospitals. For appendectomies there was no difference by hospital size, the fatality rates being 0.2 per 100 operations in all sizes of hospital (although the average age of the terminal patients was appreciably higher in the large hospitals, suggesting a higher level of surgical risk). For cholecystectomies the lowest case fatality rate was in the medium-sized hospitals, at 1.1 percent, while in the large ones it was 1.6 percent and in the small ones 2.0 percent. (Here again, however, the average age of the deceased patients was higher in the large hospitals—66 years, compared with 49 and 57 years in the other size groups—suggesting a higher level of risk.) For all five surgical diagnoses, the average duration of stay of all patients (not just those who died) was consistently longer in the large hospitals than in the other two size groups, suggesting a greater average severity of case.

In England and Wales, careful case fatality studies were made in teaching hospitals compared with nonteaching hospitals for selected diagnoses in 1951–55.[10] In spite of the possibility that the teaching hospitals were receiving the more complex cases and higher-risk patients, their case fatality rates were lower for all diagnoses examined. These included hyperplasia of the prostate (usually prostatectomy), skull fractures, gallbladder disease (usually cholecystectomy), hernia with intestinal obstruction, appendicitis with peritonitis, peptic ulcer, and ischemic heart disease (usually coronary occlusion). These data suggest higher overall quality of medical care in the teaching hospitals.

A recent analysis of the Professional Activity Study focused on hospital experience in North Carolina with patients admitted for acute coronary occlusion.[11] The overall case fatality rate was 29 percent, ranging from 14 to 80 percent in different institutions. The fatality rates were significantly lower in the larger hospitals, where one might expect more advanced technical services to be offered; they were also lower in hospitals maintaining intensive care units or coronary care units, compared with other hospitals. This, again, suggests higher quality of performance of larger hospitals.

This type of statistical study is difficult and expensive to carry out. Patient records or death certificates or both must be painstakingly collected and carefully analyzed. Moreover, the diagnoses selected for examination represent only a small proportion of all hospital admissions, and they may reflect mainly the skills of a few specialists who handle most of the cases of the given diagnosis in each hospital.

The challenge on a practical level, therefore, is to design a measure that will reflect the outcome of the care of *all* patients coming to the hospital and yet be computable routinely and with relative ease by the average hospital. Within these constraints, can some adjustment be made for the average severity of case treated, so that a hospital's total mortality record will properly reflect the overall quality of the care given rather than the gravity of condition of the patients who enter that hospital's doors?

A Study of General Mortality in 33 Hospitals: The Sample

To tackle this question, a sample of general hospitals in Los Angeles County was chosen for study. From the 166 general hospitals in the county, 20 percent, or 33 hospitals, were selected by stratified sampling methods to represent the main size and control categories. The study hospitals were distributed as shown in Table 27-1. It will be noted that of the 12 conceptual cells in this matrix, 4 are empty, since there are no "very large" proprietary (for profit) hospitals in the county and no governmental general hospitals in the other three size groups. The crude death rates within each size and control category of the series are shown in Table 27-2.

It is evident that the crude death rates tend to be higher in hospitals of larger size and that there is a gradient of rising rates from proprietary to voluntary to governmental control. Yet the more refined studies reported earlier, in which case fatality rates for specific diagnoses are examined, point to the opposite relationship. Certainly, if widely accepted hospital standards have any meaning, one would expect death rates, as an indicator of the quality of hospital care, to be lower in larger hospitals. If accreditation has any meaning as a reflection of the effectiveness of patient care, one would likewise expect voluntary hospitals to have lower death rates than proprietary ones, which have a substantially poorer record of accreditation. In our series of 16 voluntary hospitals, 13 were accredited (81 percent), compared with only 6 of the 15 proprietary hospitals (40 percent). The two governmental hospitals were both accredited. For the entire 21 accredited hospitals of all control categories, the aggregate crude death rate was 3.3 percent, compared with 2.0 percent in the 12 nonaccredited hospitals.

The explanation, as suggested earlier, must lie in the greater severity of cases coming to the larger hospitals and to those under governmental or other nonprofit control compared with the others. If a relatively simple method could be found for *statistical adjustment of crude death rates by a measure of average case severity*, then the adjusted death rates might serve as a useful indicator of the overall quality of a hospital's performance.

Method of Analysis

One can speculate on many possible measures of average case severity, such as the proportion of patients admitted with emergency labels (the "red blanket" cases), the proportion transferred by ambulance from other hospitals, or the proportion referred by nonstaff physicians. Keeping in mind the constraints of simplicity and practicality, however, we set out to find such an indicator or indicators from two official reports already routinely available on hospitals in California. One of these is a one-page Annual Report of Hospital sent by each institution

Table 27-1
Number of Hospitals in Sample, by Size and Type of Control

Size (Number of Beds)	Government	Voluntary (Nongovernmental Nonprofit)	Proprietary (For-profit)	All Types of Control	Total Beds
All sizes	2	16	15	33	–
Small (under 100)	–	7	10	17	1,086
Medium (100–199)	–	3	4	7	1,004
Large (200–499)	–	5	1	6	1,864
Very large (500 and over)	2	1	–	3	2,345
Total beds	1,841	3,098	1,360	—	6,299

Table 27-2
Crude Death Rates* in Sample, by Size and Type of Control

Size (Number of Beds)	Government	Voluntary (Nongovernmental Nonprofit)	Proprietary (For-profit)	All Types of Control
All sizes	7.5	3.0	1.9	3.5
Small (under 100)	–	2.9	1.7	2.2
Medium (100–199)	–	3.1	2.7	2.9
Large (200–499)	–	2.8	2.7	2.8
Very large (500 and over)	7.5	3.8	–	6.0

*All deaths occurring in the hospital except the newborn, as a percentage of all admissions except maternity admissions, during 1964.

to the State Department of Public Health, giving statistics relating to occupancy, admissions, births, deaths, and other items; by law this is public information. The second is the death certificate, on which a wealth of information is available.

Our procedure was as follows: For the 33 general hospitals in our sample, with a total of about 6,300 beds, we secured from the State Department of Public Health copies of the official Annual Report for the years 1963, 1964, and 1965. In the final tabulations we used information only for 1964, because this was the year for which death certificate data were available. From the Los Angeles County Department of Public Health, we obtained official data on all deaths occurring in these 33 hospitals in 1964. This agency codes and enters on punch cards most of the information provided on the death certificate, including the name of the hospital if this was the place of death, so that it was an easy task to identify all the deaths in these hospitals. Of the 70,000 deaths reported in Los Angeles County in 1964, about 8,000 took place in our 33 study hospitals.*

From the Annual Report of Hospital, the total number of admissions and the number of deaths in each institution for 1964 were determined. It was then discovered that several hospitals in our series had no obstetrical (or newborn) service. To render the full series comparable, therefore, it was decided to exclude maternity admissions from the denominators by which hospital crude death rates were calculated. For the same reason, fetal and newborn (under 7 days of age) deaths were excluded from the numerators. Maternal and newborn mortality rates have already been frequently studied[12] and are more readily available than data on the wide spectrum of diagnoses encompassed under the other categories of hospital admission—that is, "medical," "surgical," and "pediatric." Moreover, the distinction between "fetal deaths" and "infant deaths" reported by various hospitals is not always uniformly reliable. For technical reasons maternal deaths were not excluded from the numerators, but they are so rare (less than 3 per 10,000 live births in California, or hardly 1 per 20,000 hospital admissions) that they could be safely ignored in calculating overall hospital death rates.

The crude hospital death rate, then, as defined in this study, is the number of all deaths occurring in the hospital during the year except for the newborn (under 7 days of age), related to the number of all admissions except maternity admissions. Hospital deaths occurring within 24 or 48 hours of admission were not excluded. In past years, the exclusion of such deaths, and also "dead-on-arrival" (DOA) cases, from a hospital death-rate calculation has been justified on the ground that the hospital could not be held "responsible" for the death of a moribund patient. The modern American hospital, however, is expected to have efficient emergency services, which can save the lives of many such patients. An end-result measure of quality, therefore, should include such deaths—at least until more refined measurements can identify cases that are truly hopeless in spite of any medical or surgical procedures.

*Grateful acknowledgment is made to Mr. Martin Donabedian for assemblage of these punch cards.

The final death rate for each hospital, therefore, was calculated by relating the number of deaths, as defined above and reported on death certificates, to the number of admissions recorded on the Annual Report sent to the State Department of Public Health. (The number of deaths indicated on the Annual Report was often slightly lower than the number counted from the death certificates, suggesting that some hospitals might be excluding 24-hour or 48-hour deaths or DOA cases from their reports.)

Possible Indicators of Case Severity

Keeping in mind the constraint of simplicity, it was possible to identify from our two basic data sources several possible indicators of case severity:

Age at death. It is known that after infancy the risk of death increases steadily with age, and the slope of this increase accelerates in the later years. It would follow, therefore, that hospitals admitting a higher proportion of older persons are faced with higher average case severity than other hospitals. By the same logic, a higher average age among the patients who die would probably reflect (although not with absolute certainty) a higher proportion of older persons admitted. Therefore the average age at death might be taken as a rough indicator of the average case severity of patients admitted, older age levels pointing to higher risks.

Socioeconomic status. From many studies, it is known that death rates are generally higher in lower-income populations.[13] Quite apart from the quality of medical and hospital care received after admission, the physiologic state of persons of low socioeconomic status (SES) is likely to result in a lesser chance of survival from a given disease than that for persons of higher SES. This may be caused by poor nutritional status, by previous medical neglect (so that the disease reaches hospital attention only after it is highly advanced), by lower immunization levels (for certain communicable diseases), by higher exposure to serious trauma, and other factors.

By painstaking methodology one could secure a measure of the proportion of indigent or of lower-SES persons served during the year by each hospital. With the constraint of simplicity in mind, however, our approach was confined to examination of the SES of the patients who died. (A crude reflection of the SES mix of admissions might be the proportion of hospital beds reserved for ward, semiprivate, and private patients, but differing hospital policies on this dimension discouraged us from using it.) For the deceased, the death certificates give the last place of residence, and these locations could be assigned to census tracts, which can be classified by their average per capita incomes or average rentals, so that place of residence becomes a fairly reliable proxy measurement of the SES. Another indirect measure of SES might be the last occupation of the deceased or of his or her spouse, which is recorded on death certificates except for children. Tabulations of this sort, however, are laborious and would not meet our constraint of practicality for analysis by the average hospital. Another measure, of simpler application, was therefore sought on the death certificates and was found, to some degree, in the official recording of "color or race." In the current American scene, the nonwhite races certainly tend to be of lower SES than the white race (this being, of course, a social rather than a biologic phenomenon). The proportion of "nonwhite" persons among the deceased may therefore be taken as a rough indicator of the SES among patients served by the hospital and accordingly as a possible reflection of the average case severity.

Diagnoses. Ideally, one would like to examine the exact diagnosis of each patient admitted and classify it according to a scale of gravity, which might be based on case fatality rates derived from the general literature of clinical investigation. A hospital admitting a high proportion of patients with advanced leukemia, for example, would run a higher risk of deaths than a hospital with few such cases. But it is obvious that the task of calculating average case severity by such an analytic process would present formidable problems of data collection.

As an indirect approach to the challenge of using diagnoses as indicators of case severity, it was decided to select from the death certificates two causes of death: cancer and accidents. Cancer was chosen as a disease with a prognosis that is nearly always serious. A hospital receiving a large proportion of patients with cancer—even with the most highly developed medical care—might expect to have a higher death rate than one with few such patients. Selection of a hospital for cancer therapy, moreover, is usually a deliberate medical decision, made with knowledge of the technical resources available in a community or region. Thus the proportion of total deaths that are due to cancer might be expected to influence the hospital death rate.

Admission for serious trauma, on the other hand, is usually an emergency procedure (i.e., not subject to deliberate planning); but such cases would have similar influence on the risk of death in a hospital. A hospital so located as to receive a high proportion of seriously injured patients—such as automobile accident victims—might be expected to have a relatively high death rate. A measure of this diagnosis, moreover, would tend to correct appropriately for inclusion in the death-rate numerator of patients who died within 24 or 48 hours and of DOA cases. Thus the proportion of total deaths that are due to accidents might be causally related to the overall hospital death rate.

Length of stay. Finally, there is a characteristic of hospital cases that might be expected to reflect all the above and perhaps several other factors contributing to case severity: the average length of stay. It is a common observation that older persons have a longer average length of stay as a whole, and even for specific diagnoses. The U.S. National Health Survey shows that the average length of stay rises steadily with age, from 4.6 days per admission in children 1–4 years of age to 14 days for persons 75 years and older.[14] Also, persons of low SES tend to have longer average durations of hospital stay for all diagnoses and for specific diagnoses. The National Health Survey has shown that for appendectomies, for example, persons with low family incomes (under $4,000 per year in 1960–61) have an average hospital stay of 8.7 days, compared with 7.2 days among persons of higher family incomes ($4,000 and over).[15] Furthermore, patients with more serious disorders, regardless of age or income level, obviously have a longer average stay in the hospital than patients with milder conditions. Indeed, the gravity of the case might almost be defined by the relative length of hospital stay. Even for a specific diagnosis, in a person of stated age and SES, the severity of the case (e.g., a severe coronary occlusion versus a light one or a metastasized cancer versus a localized one) would ordinarily be reflected in the duration of hospital stay.

It may be noted that "length of stay" applies to all hospital admissions, rather than solely to decedents, during the year. Since the population at risk consists of all the patients coming to the hospital, this is quite appropriate. Indeed, the variables on decedents only—age, SES, and diagnosis—assume that these measurements would be roughly parallel to the same variables applied to all hospital admissions. A small substudy of five hospitals, with respect to length of stay, showed this to be generally true, although the differences among the hospitals were less for the decedents than for total admissions—which may help to explain the finding, reported below, of greater predictive value for length of stay than for the other variables that define patient characteristics.

A measure of the average duration of stay of all patients in a hospital, then, might be expected to reflect fairly comprehensively several factors, such as age, SES, and diagnoses, contributing to the case severity or level of risk of the overall spectrum of patients coming to that hospital. (This would be an even more reliable index, perhaps, if the DOA and truly moribund cases could be eliminated from the death-rate calculation, which was unfortunately not feasible in this study).

There are several artificial or extraneous influences on length of stay, however, that may keep it from reflecting case severity as such. One of these is the bed supply, or bed/population ratio, in the area: if there is a bed shortage in relation to demand, pressures are created to shorten hospital stays in order to make room for new admissions. A second influence is the time pressure on the attending physician as a practitioner in the community: if he has a heavy load of patients, he is induced to make greater use of the hospital to save himself time,[16] and such pressures may lead him to discharge one patient sooner to make room for another. A third influence is the fluctuation in incidence of disease in the community in relation to a fixed hospital bed supply: when the incidence is high, pressures for hospital admission mount and average hospital stays tend to be shortened; when diseases incidence is low, the opposite occurs.

Occupancy-corrected length of stay. In accordance with the above reasoning, a measurement was sought to correct the average length of stay in a hospital for the operation of those influences extraneous to the patient's morbidity status—in other words, one by which the length of stay would be adjusted upward or downward so as to reflect patient factors such as diagnosis, age, and socio-economic status but not other external factors such as bed supply in the area, pressures on physicians, and community fluctations in illness. Recalling the constraint of simplicity, we concluded that a plausible reflection of these extraneous influences would be found in the hospital's occupancy level.

The level of occupancy of a hospital is, of course, reflected in a simple measurement, the occupancy rate, which records the proportion of the hospital's total bed capacity over a year that is actually occupied by bed patients. As London and Sigmond have noted, this rate reflects the "effective demand of the population served by the medical staff" of the hospital.[17] Correction of the length of stay in a hospital by the degree to which its occupancy rate varies from the average occupancy rate of all hospitals in a series would thus tend to remove the extraneous influences on bed use by patients, so that the corrected length of stay would be a more accurate reflection of the average case severity.†

Data on Patients: Definitions

In summary, then, five measures of case severity could be derived from that data collected on 33 hospitals in Los Angeles County and the deaths occurring in them in 1964. After eliminating deaths of the newborn (under 7 days of age) for the reasons noted, the following measurements were calculated for each hospital:

1. *Crude death rate.* All deaths except for the newborn, including DOAs and other early fatalities, as related to the total number of hospital admissions, except for maternity admissions, during the year.
2. *Average age at death.* The average age, recorded on the death certificate, of all decedents during the year in each hospital. (Deaths of infants between 8 days and one month of age were counted as one month, or one-twelfth of a year, and deaths of infants from 2 to 12 months were counted in twelfths of a year.)
3. *Percentage nonwhite deaths.* Of all the deaths during the year, the percentage for persons of other than the white race.
4. *Percentage deaths due to cancer.* Of all deaths during the year, the percentage due to cancer, as coded on the death certificate (International List rubrics 140–239) for "underlying cause."
5. *Percentage deaths due to accidents.* Of all deaths during the year, the percentage due to accidents, as coded on the death certificate (International List rubrics E800–E999) for "underlying cause."
6. *Average length of stay.* Based on all medical-surgical and pediatric admissions (that

†For certain types of hospital, the occupancy rate could not be expected to introduce an appropriate correction of length of stay as a case severity index. This would apply to university teaching hospitals, where patients may, for their pedagogic value, be kept longer than medically necessary, thereby artificially inflating the occupancy rate. It would also apply to most Veterans Administration hospitals, which operate on a fixed budget geared to high occupancy levels. (Moreover, general VA policy favors comprehensive rehabilitation-oriented care, which leads to long average stays for any given diagnosis.) The effect of this special attribute of VA hospitals on our statistical analysis is discussed later.

is, excluding maternity admissions and the newborn) during one year. This figure for each hospital was drawn from the Annual Reports and not, of course, from the death certificates.

7. *Occupancy rates.* The percentage occupancy during the year of all beds in each hospital except beds reserved for maternity patients. This figure was also drawn from the Annual Reports.
8. *Occupancy-corrected length of stay.* The average length of stay, as defined above, adjusted upward or downward in accordance with the relation of the hospital's average occupancy to the aggregate occupancy of all 33 hospitals in the series. This figure was simply derived from items 6 and 7 above, for each hospital, and from the average of item 7 for all hospitals in the series. Regarding factor 8, it is evident that the *degree* by which extraneous pressures, reflected in the occupancy rate, distort the average length of stay must depend on many factors discussed earlier. Since data on these factors—the bed/population ratio in the area, the practice patterns of doctors, the incidence of disease in the community, and the like—were not available, the correction was made in a simple linear manner: the length of stay for each hospital was simply multiplied by the fraction composed of that hospital's occupancy rate over the average occupancy rate of the full series of 33 hospitals. (A square-root correction, to achieve a more moderate adjustment, was explored, but it yielded less satisfactory correlations than the simple linear route.)

Possible Indicators of Technological Adequacy of Hospitals

Assuming that manipulations of the above data can yield satisfactory measures of average case severity of admissions to a hospital and permit adjustment of the crude death rate accordingly, there are still other questions to be asked. Most important, are there any measurements of the technological adequacy of a hospital that might be expected to have an influence on its death rate?

As already noted, measurements of the various facilities and practices in a hospital are input data that might be expected to influence outcomes. In this research, however, they may also be regarded as an independent check on the validity of our proposed outcome measure. Ultimately, the method of measuring inputs (or technological adequacy) might be subject to modification, if this is necessary to achieve closer correspondence with the evaluations derived from outcome measures, such as the one proposed here on severity-adjusted death rates.

The most commonly used indicator of technological adequacy, in the sense used here, is the accreditation of the hospital. This is indicated, however, only by "Yes" or "No" and permits only crude exploration of statistical relations to mortality measurements. (The Joint Commission on Accreditation of Hospitals tabulates a numerical score for each hospital, but these figures are confidential and not released.) Another indirect reflection of technological adequacy is hospital size; a larger hospital may be expected to have more staffing and equipment conducive to patient recovery. The relevance of the autopsy rate as an indicator of medical staff diligence has already been mentioned. Several other indicators of hospital technological adequacy might be identified for specific aspects of an institution.

It was decided, therefore, to develop for each hospital a score for technological adequacy, which would include several components. Accreditation status could head the list, but the presence or absence of numerous scientific features associated with modern hospital service should also be included. These features were derived from the annual survey of hospitals made by the American Hospital Association and reported in the annual Guide Issue of its journal, *Hospitals*.[18] The final list of features and the scoring system for technological adequacy are shown in Table 27-3, in which it may be noted that commonplace features such as a clinical laboratory or diagnostic X-ray—which would do little to differentiate one hospital from another—were not included. Factors 1. to 3. were assigned heavy weights, since they reflect the net evaluations of independent observers on numerous features of the hospital program. Factors 4. to 9. were included to record the presence of relatively sophisticated elements of modern diagnosis and therapy in the hospital. Factors 10. to 12. were included to reflect a hospital's orientation to extramural medical service and, by implication, a concern for the hospital's role as a community center. Factor 13. was included as an indicator of sensitivity to preventive medicine. The weights assigned to each of these factors correspond to the judgment of the authors on the probable relative influence of these inputs on the outcome of patient care.

By this rating system for technological adequacy, the 33 hospitals in our series scored between 5 and 85 points. Table 27-4 shows the relation of these scores to the crude death rates. It is evident that the hospitals with higher technological adequacy scores (TAS) have consistently higher, rather than lower, crude death rates. The relation of the crude death rates to other indirect measures of technological adequacy is also presented in Table 27-4. For average hospital size and for autopsy rate, the relations follow the same general tendency, but with less consistent fit than the TAS figures.

All in all, the data on a hospital's technological adequacy suggest that greater scientific potential is associated with higher rather than lower crude death rates. Of the various measures of this potential, the TAS would appear to be a relatively comprehensive indicator, with better fit to the crude death rates than other single-factor measures. In the light of other findings about hospital mortality experience, reported above, the relation of the TAS to hospital death rates strongly confirms the general hypothesis that the more highly developed hospitals attract more severely ill patients and more difficult cases. The task, then, is to derive a mathematical function that will adjust the death rates of different hospitals so as to take account of the average severity of illness of patients admitted.

Regression Analysis

Through multiple regression analysis, it was possible to explore the influence exerted on crude hospital death rates by both sets of variables discussed above: the several proxy measurements of case severity and the several measurements of technological adequacy of the institution.

For the 33 hospitals in our sample, a multiple regression was computed among

Table 27-3
Components of Technological Adequacy Score

	Component	*Technological Adequacy Points*
(1)	Accreditation by Joint Commission on Accreditation of Hospitals	20
(2)	Approved residency (or internship)	10
(3)	Approved cancer program	8
(4)	Intensive care unit	7
(5)	Pathology laboratory	5
(6)	Blood bank	5
(7)	Therapeutic X-ray	5
(8)	Postoperative recovery room	5
(9)	Rehabilitation service	5
(10)	Out-patient department	8
(11)	Home care program	8
(12)	Social service department	7
(13)	Chest X-ray on admission	7
	Maximum score for technological adequacy	100

the several variables. The variables can be considered as of four interdependent types:

- *Dependent variable:*
  Crude death rate

- *Hospital features:*
  Type of control
  Capacity (number of beds)
  Autopsy rate (percentage)
  Technological adequacy score (TAS)
  Occupancy rate (percentage)

- *Patient characteristics:*
  Age at death (average, in years)
  Nonwhite deaths (percentage)
  Cancer deaths (percentage)
  Accident deaths (percentage)
  Cancer + accident deaths (percentage)
  Length of stay (average, in days)

- *Modified patient characteristic:*
  Occupancy-corrected length of stay

Table 27-4
Technological Adequacy Scores of 33 Hospitals in Sample, by Crude Death Rate, Hospital Size, and Autopsy Rate

Technological Adequacy Score (TAS)	*Average TAS*	*Average Crude Death Rate, %*	*Average Number of Beds*	*Average Autopsy Rate, %*
5–20 (8 hospitals)	15	1.88	67	21
21–35 (8 hospitals)	28	2.44	59	23
36–59 (9 hospitals)	49	2.95	111	23
60–85 (8 hospitals)	81	3.86	421	47

Through this computation, it was found that the crude death rate in the series of 33 hospitals had its highest correlation with the simple average length of stay, the coefficient being .706 and positive. This meant that, in general, the hospitals with greater average lengths of stay had a higher crude death rate. On the reasoning offered above, this was an important clue for developing a statistical adjustment of the hospital death rate for the severity mix of patients coming to each hospital. The coefficient of correlation with all the other patient characteristics and hospital features was lower.

Examination of the "residual errors" in our series, however, disclosed that one of the 33 hospitals was extremely deviant from the statistical tendencies of the full series. This proved to be the single federal Veterans Administration hospital. As already noted in a footnote, the operational policies of this type of hospital lead to exceptionally long durations of stay, independent of the relative severity of case admitted. It has characteristics, in a sense, of a rehabilitation facility as much as of a general hospital. Therefore a multiple regression of the same variables on the series minus the VA unit was tested.

On this series of 32 general hospitals, then, the multiple regression showed a coefficient of correlation between crude death rate and average length of stay of .794—a stronger correlation than in the series of 33 hospitals. It was reasonable, therefore, to explore the application of a statistical adjustment for case severity derived from the series of 32 general hospitals. The coefficient of correlation with the artificially derived measurement, occupancy-corrected length of stay, was slightly lower, .770. (This is discussed later.)

The coefficient of determination for one variable in "explaining" another is derived by squaring the coefficient of correlation. Thus the coefficient of determination for the crude death rate "explained" by the hospital's average length of stay is .6300 (the square of .7937). In other words, the length of stay alone is found to "explain" 63 percent of the variation among hospitals in their crude death rates. Addition into the regression of the variable, percentage of deaths due to cancer, improved the explanation to 74 percent, while all the other patient characteristics listed above improved it only to 80 percent.

If, then, as discussed earlier, one regards length of stay as an approximate measure of case severity among admissions to a hospital, an equation can be constructed by which the crude death rate may be adjusted for this major disturbing influence. In our series of 32 hospitals, the average length of stay was almost exactly 6 days. To construct an appropriate equation, one must then apply the regression coefficient, which is a measure of the relative *weight* exerted by one variable upon the other. In this instance, the regression coefficient for the influence of length of stay on crude death rate turned out to be 1.00305—or simply 1.0. Thus the crude death rate of a hospital may be adjusted for the impact of its average length of stay (reflecting average case severity) by the equation:

$$\text{LSDR} = \text{DR} - 1\,(\text{ALS} - 6) \tag{1}$$

where LSDR = length-of-stay-adjusted death rate for hospital
DR = crude death rate for hospital
ALS = average length of stay for hospital
1 = regression coefficient
6 = average ALS for series of 32 hospitals

This equation reduces to the simpler form:

$$\begin{aligned}\text{LSDR} &= \text{DR} - (\text{ALS} - 6)\\ &= \text{DR} - \text{ALS} + 6\end{aligned}$$

In words, this equation adjusts the hospital crude death rate upward or downward by 1 death per 100 admissions for each day of average stay above or below the general average stay in all hospitals (6 days, in our series). This manipulation is intended to remove the disturbing influence of average case severity on the hospital's death rate.

Equation (1) provides a series of LSDR figures in which no correction has been made for extraneous pressures on the length of stay unrelated to patient characteristics, as discussed above. Occupancy-corrected length of stay, in the list of variables, incorporates such a correction, based on the occupancy rate as a measure of these extraneous pressures. It must be noted, as mentioned earlier, that the coefficient of correlation for this variable in our series of 32 hospitals (VA institution omitted) was actually slightly lower, at .770, than the coefficient for simple length of stay. The coefficient of determination, moreover, declines slightly from explaining 63 percent to 59 percent of the variation among the crude hospital death rates. It was reasoned, however, that this slightly lower coefficient of correlation between crude death rate and occupancy-corrected length of stay might well be a peculiarity of our small series of 32 hospitals. The importance of taking account of the extraneous distortions of the average length of stay of patients in a hospital justified a second computation, in which the length of stay as corrected by occupancy rate would be forced into the multiple regression as the first variable in the stepwise analysis. In this computation, the occupancy-corrected length of stay for a hospital was derived simply from the formula:

$$\text{OCLS} = \text{ALS} \times \text{OR}/73$$

where OCLS = occupancy-corrected length of stay for hospital
ALS = average length of stay for hospital
OR = occupancy rate for hospital
73 = average OR for series of 32 hospitals

The average occupancy-corrected length of stay for our full series of 32 hospitals proved to be 7.1 days (versus 6 days for the sample ALS). The regression coefficient was no longer a simple 1.0, but 0.94. With this information, a second equation, which may well have greater predictive value in a larger series of hospitals, was derived:

$$\text{SADR} = \text{DR} - 0.94\,(\text{OCLS} - 7.1) \qquad (2)$$

where SADR = severity-adjusted death rate for hospital
DR = crude death rate for hospital
OCLS = occupancy-adjusted length of stay for hospital
7.1 = average OCLS for series of 32 hospitals

The term "severity-adjusted death rate" (SADR) is offered to denote the adjustment of the crude death rate by the occupancy-corrected length of stay rather than the simple average length of stay.

Findings

By these two equations for adjusting the crude death rates, two series of values for the 32 general hospitals in our sample were derived. The principal findings for both series, in relation to the technological adequacy score (TAS), are presented in Table 27-5.

The TAS, it will be recalled, attempts to measure the input side of hospital service. If standards of medical science and hospital administration have validity, one would expect a higher TAS to be associated with a lower death rate adjusted for case severity. In Table 27-5, the 32 hospitals are ranked in quartiles according to their TAS values, and the crude death rates (as shown also in Table 27-4) are directly rather than inversely related to those values. Either of the two forms of statistical adjustment, however, tends to change this relationship substantially.

Table 27-5
Technological Adequacy Scores of 32 Hospitals, by Crude Death Rate and Two Types of Adjusted Death Rate

Technological Adequacy Scores (TAS)	*Crude Death Rate (DR)*	*Length-of-stay-adjusted Death Rates (LSDR)*	*Severity-adjusted Death Rates (SADR)*
5–20 (8 hospitals)	1.88	2.31	3.22
21–35 (8 hospitals)	2.44	2.90	4.19
36–54 (8 hospitals)	2.93	2.96	3.77
55–85 (8 hospitals)	3.64	2.33	2.64

Either adjustment lowers the crude death rate in the highest TAS quartile of hospitals and raises it in the three lower quartiles. The eight hospitals in the highest TAS quartile are mainly (though not entirely) large institutions with a reputation of excellence, which are generally known to attract more difficult medical and surgical cases. Of the two types of death-rate adjustment, it is evident that the SADR approach, which takes account of occupancy pressures, yields a *relatively* lower adjusted death rate for this set of hospitals than does the LSDR approach (without occupancy correction).

By the SADR adjustment, the eight hospitals with highest TAS values are found to have adjusted death rates appreciably lower than those of hospitals in each of the other quartiles. The relationships are almost the exact reverse of those for the series of crude death rates, except for the lowest quartile—eight hospitals, mainly small proprietary institutions in which there is frequently a policy of discharging terminal patients to larger institutions (a tendency that would reduce their crude death rates by a degree that our data could not identify). In any event, the SADR adjustment process appears to achieve a more reasonable fit with TAS values than the LSDR process.

To the extent that this SADR correction does not fully achieve correspondence with the TAS values, it must be recalled that it theoretically explains only 59 percent, and not 100 percent, of the variance. Moreover, there are obviously other factors operating that have not been included in our multiple regression analysis. And it must be realized that the basic data defining death rates on the one hand and technological adequacy on the other are not free from error: the TAS values are drawn largely from hospital reports to the American Hospital Association, which may not always be completely accurate; and the death rates are

Table 27-6
Technological Adequacy Scores of 32 Hospitals, by Quartiles of Crude Death Rates and Quartiles of Severity-adjusted Death Rates (SADR)

	Average Technological Adequacy Score (TAS)	
Mortality Quartile	*For Hospitals Ranked by Crude Death Rate*	*For Hospitals Ranked by Severity-adjusted Death Rates (SADR)*
Lowest	33.2	55.5
II	27.4	40.0
III	54.8	33.1
Highest	48.4	38.8

derived from tabulation of death certificates, which may not always be filled out with one hundred percent diligence.

Examining the relationship of SADR figures to TAS values the other way around gives the results shown in Table 27-6. Here it is seen that if the 32 hospitals are ranked in sequential quartiles from lowest to highest mortality records, the order of TAS values is very different for the crude death rates and for the severity-adjusted death rates. By the crude-death-rate sequence, the low-death-rate hospitals tend to be associated with low TAS values; but by the SADR value sequence, the relationships are reversed—that is, the low-death-rate hospitals are associated with high TAS values. In other words, the SADR values tend to establish an association between high technological adequacy in a hospital and low mortality outcomes.

Another significant relationship is found when the SADR values are related to type of hospital control. If the hospitals in our series are divided between voluntary and proprietary, the following relationships appear:

	Crude Death Rates	*Severity-adjusted Death Rates (SADR)*
Voluntary (16 hospitals)	3.0	3.3
Proprietary (15 hospitals)	1.9	3.5

Thus the crude death rates suggest a higher mortality outcome for the voluntary compared with the proprietary hospitals, while the SADR values reverse this relationship and suggest a slightly lower mortality record for voluntary nonprofit hospitals. In southern California, it should be noted, a number of small hospitals that started out as proprietary institutions have recently been converted to voluntary nonprofit control. Their internal policies and their technological adequacy, however, may not have changed rapidly. An overall comparison of our hospital series according to simple accreditation by the Joint Commission on Hospital

Accreditation may therefore be more meaningful. Applying both forms of death-rate adjustment, the relationships are as follows:

	Crude Death Rates	*LSDR Adjustment*	*SADR Adjustment*
Accredited (20 hospitals)	3.17	2.69	3.41
Nonaccredited (12 hospitals)	1.98	2.52	3.53

By the crude mortality index, the 20 accredited hospitals have a poorer outcome measure than the 12 nonaccredited ones. By the simple LSDR adjustment, the death rate of the accredited series is lowered and that of the nonaccredited series is raised, but the latter still show a lower mortality outcome. By the SADR values, however, the relationship is reversed and the accredited hospitals are found to have a better outcome measure. The massive body of scientific observation and clinical experience behind the hospital accreditation program would seem to justify confidence in this finding as supportive of the validity of the SADR adjustment.

Discussion and Conclusion

This effort to develop an end-point measure of the quality of hospital performance, in terms of death rates adjusted for the severity of cases admitted, is obviously only a crude beginning. It suffers from numerous limitations in our data, and perhaps in our conceptualizations, and should be considered only exploratory.

Our series of 33 hospitals is small. The data from them are not wholly reliable as to characteristics of patients, records of death, or features of the hospitals. The mortality experience examined applies only to one year; a final equation for adjusting the crude death rates would doubtless be better if it were constructed from data for several years. In spite of these weaknesses, our analysis suggests that the average length of stay of patients in a hospital may be taken as a basis for substantial adjustment of crude hospital death rates by average case severity. If the length of stay, moreover, is first corrected by the level of pressure on hospital bed use reflected in the occupancy rate, the severity adjustment is probably more accurate.

The numerical values offered in the equations of this study should not, of course, be regarded as having generalized validity. The data were collected in southern California, where hospital practices are not typical of the nation. The average length of stay of these hospitals, for example, is shorter than in the nation as a whole; and there is an exceptionally high proportion of small proprietary hospitals with relatively low occupancy rates. Our equations, therefore, should be regarded only as paradigms or methods of adjusting death rates, into which numerical figures on average length of stay and occupancy rate should be entered for other geographic regions where they may be applied. It is hoped that other investigators may explore these paradigms in other regions and time periods. They may also discover more refined measures of length of stay or better basic variables by which to adjust the crude death rate as an outcome measure of quality. Moreover, even if length of stay remains the best first approach to adjustment of crude death rates for case severity, better methods of sifting out extraneous influences may be found than linear correction by the occupancy rate. Likewise, better measures of hospital technological adequacy may be designed than that which has been offered here. It should be realized, however, that an outcome measure of hospital quality, in terms of patient mortality, must be kept relatively simple if it is to be widely applied by American hospitals. Almost all our standard biostatistical indices involve an oversimplification of complex phenomena, but it is these shortcuts that enable us to move ahead in day-to-day evaluations and program planning.

With respect to the constraint of simplicity, it will be recalled that the percentage of deaths due to cancer in our series, if entered into the LSDR equation, might have increased its "explanatory" power from 63 to 74 percent. Despite this benefit, it was omitted in the interest of maintaining simplicity. Nevertheless, this additional adjustment—and other patient characteristics such as socioeconomic status or age levels—might be explored in subsequent research. Ideally, these variables should be calculated not just for the decedents but for the whole hospitalized population at risk—that is, for all patients admitted during the year. If hospital record systems were tooled up for such routine data collection, the tabulating task would not be formidable.

A recent report on differential postoperative death rates, incidental to a study of anesthesia deaths, explored the influence of several characteristics of all patients coming to surgery. The authors conclude that "there is evidence that a large part of the variation in institutional death rates is attributable to differences in the age distribution of patients, to differences in the frequency with which high-risk and difficult operations are undertaken, and to the balance between elective and emergency procedures."[19] They found that statistical adjustment for these variables greatly modified the differences among institutions, but that even after taking account of age, sex, physical status, and type of operation, differences remained. These differences, they suggest, may be "real" and therefore reflective of serious problems in institutional performance that warrant corrective action.

Another problem concerns the distinction between *hospital* performance and the performance of *physicians* within the hospital. In this study we have not distinguished between these influences. The hospital is looked upon as a form of social organization that is ultimately responsible for the work of all personnel, including physicians, within it. Insofar as poorly qualified physicians may work in good hospitals, or vice versa, the hospital organization—which includes its scheme of medical staff structure—is still responsible. Every physician working in a particular hospital has been admitted to its staff, and he is influenced (whether effectively or not) by the internal organizational structure when he serves patients.[20]

For the present, an equation is proposed by which the crude death rate in general hospitals may be adjusted for average case severity by the average length of stay, which in turn has been corrected by the occupancy rate (OR). In its generalized form, this equation is:

$$\text{SADR} = \text{DR} - K\,(\text{OCLS} - \text{OCLS}^*)$$

where K refers to the regression coefficient found on statistical analysis; where the other symbols have the meanings explained in the text above; and where the asterisk designates the average value for any given series of hospitals to be studied. As noted earlier, the occupancy-corrected length of stay (OCLS) is derived from a simple linear correction of average length of stay (ALS) as follows:

$$\text{OCLS} = \text{ALS} \times \text{OR}/\text{OR}^*$$

With all its weaknesses, the hospital death rate adjusted for case severity (SADR) derived from this equation is offered as a more objective outcome measure of the overall quality of hospital performance than the currently used measurements based principally on examination of hospital inputs.

References

1. Sheps, M. C. Approaches to the quality of hospital care. *Pub. Health Rep.* 70:877, 1955.
2. Joint Commission on Accreditation of Hospitals. *Model Medical Staff Bylaws, Rules and Regulations.* Chicago: The Joint Commission, 1957.
3. Ponton, T. R. *The Medical Staff in the Hospital* (2d ed.). Chicago: Physicians' Record Co., 1953.
4. MacEachern, M. T. *Hospital Organization and Management* (3d ed.), pp. 204–05. Berwyn, Ill.: Physicians' Record Co., 1962.
5. Lembcke, P. A. A scientific method for medical auditing. *Hospitals, J.A.H.A.* 33:65 June 16, 1959 and 33:65 July 1, 1959.
6. Peterson, O. et al. An analytical study of North Carolina general practice: 1953–54. *J. Med. Educ.,* Vol. 31, Part 2, December 1956.
7. Myers, R. S. and V. N. Slee, Medical statistics tell the story at a glance. *Mod. Hosp.* 93:72 September 1959.
8. Lembcke, P. A. and O. G. Johnson. *A Medical Audit Report.* Los Angeles: University of California School of Public Health, 1963.
9. Roemer, M. I. Is surgery safer in larger hospitals? *Hosp. Mgt.* 87:35 January 1959.
10. Lipworth, L., J. A. H. Lee, and J. N. Morris. Case-fatality in teaching and non-teaching hospitals 1956–59. *Med. Care* (London), 1:71 April–June 1963.
11. Commission on Professional and Hospital Activities. Acute coronary occlusion: Its management in North Carolina. *Record,* Vol. 5, No. 10, Dec. 20, 1967.
12. Rider, R. V., P. A. Harper, H. Knobloch, and S. E. Fetter. An evaluation of standards for the hospital care of premature infants, *J.A.M.A.* 165:1233 Nov. 9, 1957.

13. Stockwell, E. G. A critical examination of the relationship between socioeconomic status and mortality. *Am J. Pub. Health* 53:956 June 1963.
14. U.S. National Center for Health Statistics. *Utilization of Short-stay Hospitals*. Washington: Public Health Service, 1967.
15. U.S. National Center for Health Statistics. *Medical Care, Health Status, and Family Income*. Washington: Public Health Service, 1964.
16. Roemer, M. I. Hospital utilization and the supply of physicians. *J.A.M.A.* 178:989 Dec. 9, 1961.
17. London, M. and R. M. Sigmond. Are we building too many hospital beds? *Mod. Hosp*. 96:59 January 1961.
18. *Hospitals, J.A.H.A.*, Guide Issue, Part 2, Vol. 40, No. 15, Aug. 1, 1966.
19. Moses, L. E. and F. Mosteller. Institutional differences in postoperative death rates. *J.A.M.A.* 203:492 Feb. 12, 1968.
20. American Hospital Association. Statement of general principles of medical staff organization. *Hospitals, J.A.H.A.* 39:77 March 16, 1965.

28

Expanding Governmental Regulation of Health Care Delivery

As noted in previous chapters, the increasing social organization of health services has led to an expanding scope of regulation, both statutory (by government) and voluntary. In this chapter is presented a review of governmental regulations, which tend to be more rigorous than voluntary ones. These are analyzed under four principal categories: (1) resource production (professional licensure, health facility standards, drug controls, etc.); (2) economic support (regulations associated with social financing of health services); (3) physical accessibility (location and regionalization of facilities for health care); and (4) other forms of regulation (prevention, etc.).

The following text was prepared on the invitation of a law journal devoting an entire issue to "Federal Regulation of the Health Care Delivery System."

AS HEALTH CARE has evolved from a purely personal process between patient and healer to an obligation of society, the scope of its regulation by government has steadily expanded. The inclusion of "medical care" as one of the universal human rights, so declared by the United Nations in 1948, was the formal culmination of a long historical evolution witnessed for centuries in countries throughout the world.[1]

As embodied in the Constitution of the World Health Organization in 1948, "Governments have a responsibility for the health of their peoples which can be fulfilled only by the provision of adequate health and social measures."[2] Unlike many other services or commodities, the procurement of which have been left to individual discretion and the operation of the free market, accessibility to health services has been increasingly assumed to be a matter of the entire nation's concern. The legal and moral justification for state intervention to cope with and protect people against the spread of communicable diseases was obvious at an early stage—long before the microbiological causes of infection were understood.[3] As people have come to understand that the well-being of each individual ultimately affects everyone else, equivalent social concern has come to be expressed for all types of disease and trauma.[4]

Assurance that health services will be accessible when needed, or will be

Chapter 28 originally appeared as "The Expanding Scope of Governmental Regulation of Health Care Delivery" and is reprinted by permission of the *University of Toledo Law Review*, Vol. 6, no. 3, Spring 1975, pp. 591–616.

applied to prevent disease from occurring, depends on several prior actions. Especially with the development of a complex technology, it has come to depend on 1. the production of resources to provide the services (manpower, facilities, supplies, etc.); 2. arrangement for their economic support; 3. actions to assure their physical accessibility (geographic location, transportation, etc.); and 4. various degrees of surveillance or control over the performance of health care providers according to reasonable standards of quality and cost. All four of these conditions require social initiative, but the degree and scope of the initiative required can be highly variable among countries. As technology has become more complex and costly, and as social understanding of the concept of health care as a "right" has become more sophisticated, the range and depth of social action to provide for these four conditions has enlarged. In the main, although not exclusively, these social actions have been undertaken increasingly by statute.[5]

To review the evolution of this process throughout human history and in all parts of the world would obviously be beyond the scope of this article. We may, however, examine the highlights of the process, with special focus on the United States and emphasis on the recent period. In so doing we may consider briefly a number of discrete social programs, each of which has in some degree involved governmental initiative toward the goal of assuring health care as a human right.

To better understand these regulatory activities in relation to their ultimate goal, it may be helpful to classify them under the four broad sets of social action for assuring health services noted above. We are presented with a typology of governmental regulation as follows:

- I. Resource Production
  - A. Professional Licensure
  - B. Educational Institutions and Their Control
  - C. Preparation of Medical Specialists
  - D. Health Facilities Production and Standards
  - E. Control of Drugs and Supplies
- II. Economic Support
  - A. Tax-financed Health Programs and Their Control
  - B. Regulation of Private Health Insurance
  - C. Social Insurance and its Control (PSROs)
- III. Physical Accessibility
  - A. Location of Health Facilities
  - B. Organized Ambulatory Health Services
  - C. Regionalization and Distribution of Manpower
- IV. Other Controls of Quality and Costs
  - A. Organized Prevention of Disease
  - B. Encouragement of Self-regulation (HMOs)

As with any classification, there will be some overlap among categories. But the significant governmental action in each sector, particularly in recent years, should be evident.

Resource Production

The manpower, facilities, and material for provision of health services have become increasingly elaborate, and have summoned a complex body of regulation to assure their production according to the best knowledge of the time and place. At least five sets of regulation of resource production can be distinguished.

Professional Licensure

We think today of licensure of any health profession as being the culmination of a specified period of training. For centuries, however, the preparation of doctors or healers was by apprenticeship, through hereditary background or supernatural events. The Code of Hammurabi of ancient Babylonia is usually considered the first social action to regulate the performance of doctors, by prescribing rewards or punishments to surgeons, depending on the outcome of the procedure and the social class of the patient.[6] Ancient Greece and Rome did not regulate physicians, but if they were so identified by the state they were granted certain social privileges. In Baghdad of the tenth century, doctors were examined by an authoritative physician of the Caliph's court. When the guilds were organized in medieval Europe, they were granted legal authority to control the activities of persons doing surgery (barber-surgeons) and compounding drugs (apothecaries).

The first university medical faculty was organized at Salerno, Italy, in the eleventh century. Later, royal decrees were issued calling for examinations of all would-be physicians (not surgeons) by this faculty. In 1140, the Norman King Roger decreed:

> Who, from now on wishes to practice medicine, has to present himself before our officials and examiners, in order to pass their judgment. Should he be bold enough to disregard this, he will be punished by imprisonment and confiscation of his entire property. In this way we are taking care that our subjects are not endangered by the inexperience of the physicians. . . . Nobody dare practice medicine unless he has been found fit by the convention of the Salernitan masters.[7]

In America, in the pioneer setting of the early colonization, there were no medical controls. But after the Revolution, some of the young states enacted licensure laws requiring examinations. They were poorly enforced, however, and so fell into disuse. The American Medical Association was founded in 1847, largely to establish physician eligibility standards and to fight quackery.[8] It was not until after the Civil War that effective medical licensure laws were passed. The first "State Board of Medical Examiners" was established in Texas in 1873, and by 1895 nearly all the states had such laws.

With scores of medical schools, most of them unconnected with universities, state governments, unlike the nations of Europe, could not simply rely on formal educational preparation as a basis for state registration. Neither universities nor independent medical schools were subject to any public supervision. When, after the Flexner Report of 1910,[9] medical schools were drastically reduced in number and improved in quality—through a system of nongovernmental grading—state medical practice laws still continued. Eventually nursing, dentistry, pharmacy, and the other health disciplines modeled their licensure procedures after medicine.

Mobility of health personnel among the states became increasingly frequent, and a common problem was the nonrecognition of licensure in one state by the official state board of another. Gradually reciprocity of licensure recognition developed among many states, but it was by no means complete. Only in 1915, when the National Board of Medical Examiners was established, was a nationwide examination launched. Soon all but a few states recognized this examination as the basis for licensure.[10] However, state boards of medical examiners did not coordinate their efforts until 1968, when they created the FLEX (Federation Licensing Examination) procedure to achieve uniformity.[11] To this day, however, the United States differs from nearly all other countries by requiring passage of a "second examination" beyond having passed the examinations required for earning degrees granted by medical schools from both domestic and foreign medical graduates.[12]

Professional licensure constitutes a very basic form of governmental regulation of entry into the health professions. Economists have, with some persuasiveness, argued that licensure amounts to restraint of trade and creates oligopolies for the health professions.[13] While valid in the sense that the limitation in manpower supply caused by licensure must contribute to heightened prices for health services, this criticism must be weighed against the value of protecting the public interest. The average consumer simply cannot be expected to judge the merit of doctors or others from whom he seeks medical help. Licensure laws, thus, are ultimately intended to protect the people from a lack of technical judgment which they cannot be expected to have.

Educational Institutions and Their Control

As noted above, American schools and colleges for training health personnel are not directly supervised by government. This is very different from most other countries, where institutions of higher education are under the control of a Ministry of Education. This is usually because they are governmental universities in the first place or because they are subject to public supervision by law. This official control of training institutions, of course, makes "registration" of their health graduates a simple pro forma matter.[14]

In the place of government, however, virtually every type of higher educational school in the United States has developed, through an association of such schools, a system of voluntary accreditation.[15] In medicine, for example, the program is conducted jointly by the Association of American Medical Colleges and the American Medical Association. Government, however, does enter the picture in several ways. In its licensure requirements, it specifies often that the candidate must be a graduate of an "accredited" school;[16] similar requirements are imposed for participation of doctors in various governmental programs of medical care.[17] Second, there is, in the Federal Office of Education, the United States Accrediting Commission which approves the various accrediting bodies themselves for all disciplines. Third, one must keep in mind that a major share of professional schools are, in fact, governmental, usually established and sponsored by state governments. About one half of the medical and dental schools in America are in this category. Fourth is the increasing dependence of all professional schools, public and private, on governmental grants for meeting their capital and operating costs.

Regarding the fourth element, governmental subsidy of professional education, governmental influences have been numerous and varied.[18] They have been instrumental, for example, in enlarging the capacity of the nation's institutions to train greater numbers of nurses and doctors. By earmarked grants they have influenced the emphases in research, which may have the effect of strengthening one department or another in a professional school. Special training grants are awarded to institutions which offer education in selected fields, such as subspecialties of psychiatry or public health, or for training new types of personnel, such as nurse-practitioners.[19] Legislation recently enacted by Congress provides funds for establishing programs of "Family Medicine" in medical schools;[20] in 1971, federal grants were given for residency training in family medicine.[21] Thus, governmental perceptions of professional education needs stimulate financial inducements to meet those needs.

Preparation of Medical Specialists

In the early twentieth century, almost all doctors were generalists. Engagement in a specialty was even slightly suspect of charlatanism. The first field to alter this image was ophthalmology, which in 1915 established a nongovernmental board to certify specialized competence in this discipline. Competition from the discipline of optometry seemed to play a large part in this action intended to represent to the general community that certain eye specialists were medical doctors.[22] In any event, with the Depression of the 1930s and with recognition of higher fees being paid to specialists both in the open market and many organized programs, numerous additional specialty boards were established. Today about twenty specialties of medicine and surgery and another fifteen subspecialties designate well-defined regimes of training and require passage of examinations for proper qualification. In British Commonwealth countries, equivalent credentials are offered by the Royal Colleges.

In spite of the nongovernmental sponsorship of this movement, the specialty boards in the United States have acquired a quasi-governmental meaning.

Numerous state and federal public medical programs require certain forms of specialty status for participation, such as the crippled children's services[23] or the vocational rehabilitation program. Other public programs, like workmen's compensation, Medicaid, or Medicare, pay differentially higher fees to specialists than to general practitioners for the same item of service.

In some countries, like Great Britain or Sweden, where the specialties of medicine are tied closely to the hospitals, governmental decisions on hospital staffing largely determine the proportionate numbers among the different specialties. In America, the mix of specialists has been determined essentially by the free market and the independent decision of hundreds of training hospitals offering residencies. This has resulted in what is widely recognized as a relative shortage of general practitioners and pediatricians and a surplus of surgeons. Recognition of this fact is stimulating legislative proposals to control the proportions of specialized residencies approved each year, so as to achieve a better balance for population needs.

In family medicine, the newest "specialty," recertification at five year intervals is a requirement. This is the first medical field to demand such evidence of continuing competence. Other specialties have been discussing the idea to help assure that practitioners keep abreast of advances in medical science. Evidence of the doctor's participation in continuing education is the usual basis considered for such recertification, rather than passage of additional examinations. In several allied health fields—pharmacy, optometry, dietetics, dentistry, and most recently nursing—one or more state governments now require periodic relicensure.[24]

Health Facilities Production and Standards

For centuries the construction of hospitals, along with their staffing and equipment, were entirely matters of local initiative. Originally by the action of churches, and then of city governments, hospitals were built to serve local needs—first for the poor, then for everyone.[25] Some geographic planning was started in European countries at the national level in the early twentieth century, but in America the first national action was taken with the Hospital Survey and Construction Act (Hill-Burton) of 1946.[26]

The principal purpose of this federal law was to provide financial inducements for the construction of general hospitals—and later other types of health facilities—in areas of bed shortage. Each state was required to draw up a "master plan," under which priorities could be established, so that communities of greatest shortage would be helped first.[27] In addition, as a condition for the receipt of any federal grants, the state had to enact a hospital licensure law specifying minimum standards of construction, staffing, and operation.[28]

A few years later, in 1950, the nongovernmental Joint Commission on Accreditation of Hospitals was organized. This was, in fact, a development from an earlier nongovernmental hospital standardization program started by the American College of Surgeons in 1919.[29] The JCAH program places more emphasis on requirements for medical staff organization than do most of the state licensure laws. Moreover, the Commission's stamp of approval has—like the medical specialty qualifications—come to be recognized by government in numerous programs. Under the Medicare law, in fact, JCAH accreditation is accepted as a substitute for certification by a state public health agency.

Regulation of quality standards for both manpower and facilities, it may be noted, has become increasingly a matter of partnership between private and governmental bodies. Essentially, the social status of the health professions has been regarded so highly that the judgment of professional bodies is given official recognition as virtually equivalent to governmental authority. While some have questioned the Constitutional propriety of delegating such public duties to private agencies,[30] this partnership principle seems to be built into American culture and pervades the whole field of health services regulation.

Control of Drugs and Supplies

The production of drugs and medical supplies is done almost entirely through private enterprise in the United States and other capitalist countries. Even in Great Britain and other nations where the costs of health service have been nearly all assumed by governmental bodies, the manufacture and distribution of pharmaceutical products remain in the private sector.

That very fact, together with certain consequences of the private profit motive, has led to a long saga of abuses in the manufacture, advertising, pricing, and distribution of drugs. These abuses have generated, in turn, a series of regulatory reforms.[31] Beginning with the first Food and Drug Act of 1906,[32] controls focused on the honesty of claims on labels and on sanitation in the manufacturing process. Triggered by dramatic tragedies due to harmful drugs, and with matured public understanding, periodic amendments have strengthened this regulatory legislation. The Federal Food, Drug and Cosmetic Act of 1938 demanded prior proof of the safety of a drug—through animal studies—before it could be sold on the market;[33] controls over drug advertising and cosmetics were likewise introduced.[34] In 1962, further regulation was imposed on the scientific reliability of prior drug testing and on the efficacy, as well as the safety, of new products.[35]

Government regulation of the production and distribution of drugs is also exercised in other ways. Programs of government-financed medical care, such as Medicaid in several states, limit the list of drugs which may be prescribed. Since drugs on which there are no patents, or on which the patent has expired, may be sold under a "generic" rather than a "brand" name, at a typically much lower price, the generic form is often mandated.[36] Certain costly drugs, the therapeutic action of which may be achieved by less expensive preparations, may be excluded entirely from an official drug list or formulary.

In recent years, as the problem of drug abuse or dependence has escalated, more stringent regulations have been imposed on certain addictive drugs—barbiturates, amphetamines, tranquilizers, etc.[37] To monitor the use of these drugs, federal laws have come to control them like narcotics, for which a record on the prescribing practices of each doctor is maintained.[38] All these legal measures, of course, impose constraints on the decisions of doctors in the practice of medicine, not to mention the activities and livelihood of pharmacists.

Economic Support

When the procurement of medical care in the open market was a one-to-one transaction, social concern about the process was limited. As economic support for medical service has become increasingly collectivized, regulation of its content has become wider and firmer. This can be observed in several areas.

Tax-financed Health Programs and Their Control

Most directly, the operation of health care programs by government itself is subject to rigorous controls. Medical services for military personnel or veterans, wholly financed by the federal government, are governed by elaborate rules and regulations.[39] Such controls may tend to inhibit innovation; but at the same time they assure a minimum level of quality, which protects the patient.

A more subtle instance of governmental control is the variety of requirements in the numerous government programs that purchase services from private providers on behalf of certain beneficiaries. Federal-state programs for crippled children illustrate well the wide scope of standards required in the way of manpower, facilities, and practices, before services will be paid for.[40] It has been argued that the affluent disabled child, in need of medical care, is not protected by the range of standards applied to a child whose poverty qualified him for such a public program. But this argument really underscores the basic principle involved. In effect, a private individual is free to spend his own money for medical care unwisely, except for the protection offered by the basic licensure laws. Unsound expenditures, however, will not be tolerated for wards of the government; the use of money derived from the whole population must be subject to safeguards. If private individuals are to be similarly protected, new laws must be passed.

Regulation of Private Health Insurance

The same principle of heightened prudence for collectively derived monies ought theoretically apply to insurance of any type—even nongovernmental. To some extent it does. The voluntary health insurance movement has grown to large proportions in the United States, covering now about 25 percent of all personal health expenditures.[41] Some eighteen hundred different insurance carriers are involved and the degree of diligence with which claims from doctors, hospitals, or other providers are reviewed is quite variable. In general, however, it appears that, under our prevailing fee-for-service system of payment, the diligence with which claims (bills) are reviewed—as to the type or duration of the service rendered and in its medical necessity—is relatively loose. Evidence for this is suggested by the differentially higher cost of health services provided under a fee system, compared with the same range of services offered under arrangements in which the doctor is on a fixed salary.[42] It was largely in recognition of this very problem that the "medical foundation" pattern of health insurance was started, emphasizing rigorous review of fee claims as a way to control costs.[43]

More directly included in the sphere of governmental regulation are state insurance laws governing the operation of the health insurance plans. Every state has insurance legislation designed to protect the consumer, but in the 1930s there were enacted a series of state laws granting exceptions for nonprofit hospital insurance plans.[44] These so-called enabling acts recognized the principle of "service benefits," as distinguished from monetary indemnification in the usual commercial insurance, and granted the nonprofit Blue Cross (and later the Blue Shield) plans exemptions from certain statutory requirements on maintenance of reserves, taxes, reporting, etc. In a few states, on the other hand, public hearings were required for approval of premium increases. In defining these exempted insurance programs, the enabling acts often restricted sponsorship, in effect, to medical societies, so that—while facilitating Blue Shield plan organization—they obstructed the founding of prepaid health care plans by consumer groups.[45] One of the issues in the recent promotion of "health maintenance organizations" has been the removal of these restrictive laws in many states.

In any event, both the regulatory laws of the states on health insurance organizations and the surveillance activities of the voluntary plans themselves constitute forms of control over the economic support for health services. These "third parties" place limits on what the doctor or hospital may do and for which payments will be made. While designed mainly to protect the solvency of insurance funds, these controls indirectly affect the freedom of action of the doctor and they influence the content of medical care. Implementation of state insurance laws in Pennsylvania by Commissioner Herbert Denenburg in recent years has illustrated the far-reaching effects of such legislation on the practices of hospitals with respect to surveillance of utilization, charges to patients, and the whole posture of health insurance plans toward protecting the interests of their enrollees.[46]

Social Insurance and Its Control (PSROs)

For many years the only form of social insurance covering medical care in the United States was the workmen's compensation laws, which pay cash benefits and medical costs for work-injuries. From New York State's initial law in 1910[47] to Mississippi's in 1950,[48] the laws of the states imposed an enormous variety of requirements on the medical services to injured workers for which this mandatory insurance would be responsible.[49] Controls over medical fees, limitations on the duration of care for which the insurance would pay, boundaries on the worker's right to freely choose his doctor, and even approval of specific doctors for participation are among the many conditions specified in these laws. In most states, the insurance is carried mainly by private companies, and controversy has been frequent over the administration of these programs. The general trend, however, has been to expand the definition of work-related disorders for which compensation is responsible and the range of medical services to which the worker is entitled.

General disability insurance for short-term disability has been enacted by six states since Rhode Island's pioneering law of 1943. All of these state laws call for physician certification of non-occupational disability, and these doctors are subject to certain regulations in making their decisions.[50] Likewise the federal social insurance for "permanent and total disaiblity," enacted in the 1950s, requires somewhat equivalent certifications from doctors and determination of any potential for the rehabilitation of an applicant.[51]

Most pervasive in its regulatory influence on health service is undoubtedly the Medicare law of 1965, which provides social insurance for most hospital and medical expenses of persons over 65 years of age.[52] The statutory and regulatory influences of this law on hospital and medical practice are wide-ranging. Detailed conditions are laid down on the "conditions for participation" of the various health care providers in the program and on the methods of determination by state agencies whether those conditions have been met.[53] With respect to financial claims for services rendered by hospitals, doctors, and other providers, there are further elaborate regulations intended to be enforced by various "fiscal intermediaries," usually Blue Cross-Blue Shield plans or insurance companies. Important among these are requirements for "utilization review" of all or a sample of cases to determine the "medical necessity" of the service provided, the propriety and length-of-stay of hospital admissions, and other aspects of the care provided.[54]

As costs spiralled in the Medicare and Medicaid programs, there arose a sense of the ineffectiveness of the "utilization review" procedures designed to safeguard against abuse.[55] Scores of fiscal intermediaries were highly variable in the diligence with which they enforced these controls, which were supposed to be implemented on-the-spot by hospitals, nursing homes, and home health agencies.[56] As a result, another approach was taken with the enactment of the Social Security Amendments of 1972 and the requirement of "Professional Standard Review Organizations" (PSROs) to blanket the nation.[57] Some 203 areas have been delineated by the federal government in which PSROs, made up of local doctors, are required to oversee the medical soundness of all hospitalizations under the federal Medicare and Medicaid programs.

The PSRO legislation has generated a storm of controversy among members of the private medical profession who regard it as unwarranted "interference with the doctor-patient relationship," replacing the doctor's individual judgment on a case with "cook-book medicine."[58] There is every expectation that the PSRO surveillance requirements will eventually be extended to out-of-hospital (i.e., private medical office) service and to the care of the general population under a national health insurance law—serving of course to further increase the alarm of many private doctors. Yet, the PSRO legislation is essentially only an extension of the surveillance requirements of the original Medicare law, in response to recognition that the initial controls were not working very well on an individual hospital basis. Numerous questions arise as to the admissibility of PSRO findings as evidence in malpractice actions, and concerning the influence of the whole process on the doctor's sense of freedom to practice medicine according to his own judgment.

Spokesmen for the PSRO concept emphasize that nay standards of "reasonable medical practice" applied will be flexible, that the review of cases is being made by medical colleagues ("peer review"), that the doctor practicing good medicine has nothing to be concerned about, and that in any event there are thorough appeals procedures from decisions of a PSRO on any specific case to protect against bias or faulty judgment.[59] Conceptually the whole PSRO program is simply a further extension of governmental regulation over medical practice, already applied in scores of ways. It would seem that PSRO's impact on a significant proportion of each doctor's work is what causes the anxieties and fears that the concept will be continuously extended in its application.[60]

Yet as stated at the outset, the social financing of medical services would seem inevitably to summon measures of social (governmental) control over how the money is spent. The PSRO approach, indeed, is more lenient than that of most countries in turning controls over to local bodies made up exclusively of practicing doctors themselves. By contrast, in most other countries with social insurance programs for medical care, surveillance is exercised directly by officials of the governmental or quasi-governmental authorities administering the program as a whole.[61]

Physical Accessibility

A variety of governmental measures as well as organized private efforts have been taken to assure geographic accessibility of resources—both health facilities and manpower—to all people. The problem, of course, is particularly serious in rural areas, where the "natural" forces of the free market do not attract the amount and types of health resources required to meet population needs. The corrective influences applied by government may be summarized in terms of health facilities, organized ambulatory health services, and health manpower distribution.

Location of Health Facilities

We noted above the influence of the federal Hill-Burton Act of 1946 on the funding and quality, as well as the location, of health facilities, particularly hospitals.[62] In fact, the effects in improving the distribution of hospitals in the United States have been impressive. Largely because of this subsidy program, the discrepancies between general hospital bed supplies in urban and rural states have been largely eliminated. For example, while in 1942 the six most urbanized states had 4.5 general hospital beds per 1,000 population, compared with 2.2 per 1,000 in the eight most rural states, by 1965 the ratios had been almost equalized; the ten most urbanized states in 1965 had 3.86 beds per 1,000 and the ten most rural had 3.62.[63] Part of this improvement was due to population changes—more rapid urbanization of certain states and slower growth or even decline in the populations of rural states. Still, the equalizing effects on bed availability to rural, as compared with urban, people has been dramatic.

In more recent years the concern of government has shifted from the problem of bed shortages in rural areas to the question of over-building of beds in certain urban as well as rural areas. There is much evidence that the supply of hospital beds is a strong determinant of the rates of bed utilization in an area, and hence the overall community costs.[64] On this theory, New York passed the first legislation requiring approval of all new bed construction—whether or not subsidized by government—in 1964.[65] Within a decade, some twenty-six states passed similar "certificate of need" legislation, requiring proof of the social need for additional hospital beds in an area before construction would be authorized.[66] Other states will doubtless eventually follow suit. Such restrictions obviously further regulate the freedom with which doctors have access to hospital beds for their patients.

Local zoning ordinances, of course, have long influenced the location of hospitals, nursing homes, pharmacies, or other health facilities. At the state level, the location of mental hospitals has typically been based on some sort of state plan in relation to the population to be served. At the federal level, agencies like the Veterans Administration or the Indian Health Service locate their facilities in relation to the distribution of their beneficiaries. The VA, moreover, considers proximity to medical schools as a method for promotion of the quality of service to veterans.

Organized Ambulatory Health Services

The location of physicians' and dentists' offices has long been known to correlate highly with the per capita income of the area. As far back as 1934, it was demonstrated that doctors in Philadelphia were concentrated in the high income neighborhoods, while health needs were greatest in the low income sections.[67] The same disparity is evident in any city, as well as on a state-by-state basis.[68]

These distribution patterns are the foreseeable result of the historical operation of a free market system of health care in the United States.

Recognition and dramatization of the inequities caused by this process have stimulated a number of governmental interventions. The Indian Health Service has built scores of health centers in or near reservations where local doctors were few.[69] The handicaps of migratory agricultural workers led to a special federal network of primary care clinics under the War Food Administration in the World War II years.[70] Manifest shortages in the Appalachian region stimulated a special program of construction of health centers in these impoverished mountain areas.

In the 1960s, several developments led to similar governmental actions to bring organized health centers to the slum areas of larger cities. Serious crowding of city or county hospital clinics pointed clearly to the need for satellite units nearer to the slum neighborhoods.[71] Beginning in 1965, a series of urban "race riots," first in Los Angeles, then in several other cities, dramatized the need for positive actions to improve health care as well as other resources in the urban ghettoes.[72] At about the same time, the medical schools were recognizing the importance of heightening the exposure of students to ambulatory, in contrast to hospitalized, patients. All these forces combined to give birth to the concept of the "neighborhood health center" (NHC)—a facility for comprehensive ambulatory care, both curative and preventive, located in the heart of urban poverty districts.[73] Almost invariably these NHCs were opposed by the local medical societies, and particularly by the handful of doctors who were located in or close to these neighborhoods. Nonetheless, approximately seventy-five NHCs were built with funds from the Federal Office of Economic Opportunity. Soon the United States Department of Health, Education and Welfare established similar health centers and by the 1970s all OEO-funded centers were transferred to the supervision of HEW.

A parallel movement for organized ambulatory care centers was focused on the needs of mothers, children, and youth in poverty areas. Under special authorization of the 1965 Medicare Amendments to the Social Security Act, a series of Maternity and Infant Care (M.I.C.) and Children and Youth (C. and Y.) clinics were established in poverty areas, not to provide the traditional preventive services to these demographic groups, but for comprehensive medical care.[74] Motivated by this trend, many traditional health departments began to widen the scope of their conventional clinics to include generalized primary care. In addition, enactment of the Federal Occupational Safety and Health Administration (OSHA) law in 1970[75] led private industry to strengthen its in-plant health units.[76] School health services widened their horizons from traditional physical examinations for detection of defects and first aid to deliberate programs for coping with drug abuse, teenage pregnancies, and other problems of contemporary youth.[77]

All these and other developments constitute governmental intervention into the central component of medical service—the ambulatory patient-doctor contact. By design, the programs compensate for the shortcomings of the traditional private physician pattern of primary care by setting up organized teams of health personnel in various settings where private medicine could not do the job as well. In addition to the systematized financing involved, they improve the physical accessibility of services for various population groups.

Regionalization and Distribution of Manpower

The regionalization concept embodied in the Hill-Burton legislation of 1946 has been mentioned, but the impact of this legislation did not go beyond the structural aspects of health facilities. The dynamics of a two-way flow of patients and consultant doctors was hardly implemented.[78] The legislation of 1965 on Regional Medical Programs for Heart Disease, Cancer, and Stroke (RMP) was required to make the regional concept operational.[79] Under this nationwide program a variety of activities were launched to transmit the knowledge and practices of teaching medical centers to peripheral hospitals and medical practitioners.[80]

Another closely related governmental strategy was enactment of the Comprehensive Health Planning (CHP) legislation in 1966.[81] Federal subsidies were given to establish health planning agencies at both state and local (or area-wide) levels with consumer majorities on their boards, which would oversee the whole health care system, point up problems, and encourage needed actions.[82] While CHP agencies had few enforcement powers, they provided indirect influences over the construction of health facilities, helped to coordinate various operating programs, and stimulated the initiation of numerous new projects.

With respect to health manpower distribution, for many years actions were taken at local, state, and national levels to attract or direct doctors and others to rural areas of shortage. As far back as the 1920s, New England towns offered subsidies to attract doctors—in the form of rent-free houses or guaranteed minimum annual incomes—and this approach has continued in various forms to the present.[83] In the World War II years and after, several southeastern states set up "rural medical fellowships" through which medical school expenses would be covered with loans, which were "repayable" by an equivalent number of years of practice in a rural area of need designated by the State Health Officer.[84] In 1970, the federal government took action by establishing the National Health Service Corps, through which young doctors and other health personnel could meet military obligations by becoming commissioned in the United States Public Health Service for assignment to clinical practice in areas of need.[85] The boldest approach perhaps is that embodied in the Health Professions Educational Assistance Bill of 1974, which passed the United States Senate but, as of this writing, had not been debated in the House of Representatives.[86] Under this legislation, should it be enacted, all medical schools receiving federal capitation support (which is virtually necessary for the schools to survive) must assure that a certain percent of their graduates locate for two years in areas of need.[87] The method of achieving such assurances is left up to the schools, but such legislation would establish in the United States a type of policy which has long been applied in many other countries to cope with the worldwide problem of maldistribution of medical manpower between urban and rural areas.

Finally, the whole question of physical accessibility of health service is probably heading for its most serious governmental intervention in a series of bills now before Congress on "area health service agencies." Stimulated by the impending termination of authority for both the RMP and the CHP programs, a number of approaches have been proposed which would establish national coverage through a new form of health agency having wide scope and authority for planning as well as regulating all health services in every area of the nation.[88] Undoubtedly to be linked with the financial sanctions possible under national health insurance, these health service agencies would be able to exercise numerous direct and indirect influences not only on location of resources, but also on the mix of specialties, the use of ancillary personnel, the formation of "health maintenance organizations" and the many other means for developing improved accessibility of the population to health service. Obviously, much depends on the final language of this legislation and the general political temper of the times in which it is to be implemented. But the combination of spiralling costs and rising expectations of people generally for adequate health care points to the probability of greater governmental influence through this network of authorities than we have seen in the past.*

Other Controls of Quality and Costs

Throughout all of the previous review of the diverse mechanisms for governmental regulation of or influence on health care delivery, efforts to control the quality and costs of service have been implicit. Anything that brings some health service where there was none before affects the quality as well as the quantity of service. Controls exercised by specialty boards, hospital standards, PSROs, and other devices are obviously directed to quality as well as to cost-monitoring objectives.

Beyond these, there are two other types of governmental action which should be identified to complete the story of regulation.

Organized Prevention of Disease

The role of government in the organized prevention of disease has been so longstanding that it is perhaps taken for granted without realization of its relationship to the regulation of health care delivery. Yet, when a law mandates that children

*Since this article was written the National Health Planning and Resources Development Act of 1974, Pub. L. No. 93-641 (codified at 42 U.S.C.A. § 300k *et seq.* (Supp. 1, 1975)) was enacted.

entering a public school shall have been immunized against diphtheria or smallpox, it is imposing requirements not only upon citizens but also upon doctors; it is, in effect, requiring doctors to immunize their child patients. When a health department conducts a multiphasic screening program that turns up a patient with elevated blood sugar and refers the findings to his physician, it is in effect signalling to the doctor that his patient may have diabetes and needs care. When a well-baby clinic detects inadequate weight-gain in an infant and refers the mother to a pediatrician, he is in effect being advised to search out the cause and give treatment. Similarly, when state laws require silver nitrate drops in the eyes of newborns to prevent infection, they directly influence the practices of obstetricians.[89]

These and many other examples of organized preventive medicine, promoted or enforced by public health agencies, may not fit the ordinary connotation of "regulation," but they have a similar effect. They influence the practice of medicine in countless ways. Even the chlorination of public water supplies to prevent spread of enteric disease indirectly determines the kind of case that the doctor will or will not see, just as water fluoridation changes the incidence of dental caries in a community and thereby alters the mix of patients coming to dentists. Anti-smoking campaigns obviously influence the work of thoracic surgeons who treat cases of lung cancer; and consider the effect on all medical practice that would be caused by discovery of an immunizing agent against cancer—something, incidentally, quite within the realm of possibility.

Encouragement of Self-regulation

The mounting costs of medical care and, indeed, the onerousness of the rising regulation has led to a new governmental strategy for controlling health services in America. Long known by other names, the "health maintenance organization" (HMO) is a mechanism to assure populations a wide range of medical and hospital services for a fixed per capita prepaid sum. It provides inducements to keep people well and to reduce the use of costly hospital care, since doctors may thereby increase (rather than reduce) their earnings. Since 1970, the HMO concept, long considered a dangerous deviance from conventional open-market fee-for-service medicine, has been promoted by the federal government.[90]

In terms of regulation, the HMO approach creates financial incentives for cost-containment and self-regulation in medical practice. In 1973, legislation was enacted authorizing $375,000,000 in federal grants or loans to promote and enlarge HMOs.[91] While correcting the abuse of over-servicing (unnecessary surgery, prolonged hospital stays, etc.) associated with fee-for-service, the HMO opens up the opposite hazard of under-servicing. Aware of this danger, the 1973 legislation required "quality assurance" mechanisms within the structure of governmentally approved HMOs and calls for evaluation of the performance of HMOs by public agencies.[92] It seems altogether likely that the future area health service agencies will have a role in such regulation at the local level. It is obvious that standards must be established to protect the unsophisticated consumer from deficient medical care, beyond the safeguard of his freedom to disenroll from a particular HMO.

From a more far-reaching perspective, the HMO concept is perhaps intended to gradually alter the prevailing pattern of fee-for-service remuneration in American health service. It would encourage a mosaic of mini-systems of health care delivery throughout the nation, which would have numerous incentives to cut costs, while protecting quality simply by making it to the doctor's interest to do so. This, in turn, depends not only on the governmental surveillance noted above, but on the wide dissemination of information on the performance of different HMOs (and also the performance of private medical care) through clearly understandable measurements of the input, the process, and the outcome of the services provided. With full understanding, it may be expected that informed consumers will make reasonable choices about enrollment.

Associated with the HMO movement and, indeed, much else in modern health care delivery, is a rise of so-called consumerism.[93] A larger voice for consumers in policy decisions on the operation of both public and private agencies is expected to offer a countervailing force against potential abuses or greed by the providers of health care. Insofar as laws are increasingly mandating such consumer participation, this constitutes still another form of "self-regulation" in the operation of the health care system.

Conclusion

Given this broad interpretation of the concept of "governmental regulation," it is evident that, in scores of ways, it has been incrementally enhancing its impact on health care delivery. This is seen vividly not only in the United States, but all over the world. As we have noted, it is associated not only with the rising collectivization of the financing of health services, but also with the rising demands of people for assurance that they are getting the best that science can offer. In a word it is the democratization of health services that creates continuing pressures for their regulation.

Conventional wisdom has, for a long time, regarded public controls as objectionable as an invasion of personal freedom. The "police state" has become a cliché in contrast to democracy. Yet it should be clear from consideration of the intricacies of medical science and technology that matters of health and life and death cannot properly be left to the uncertainties of the free market. It is all very well to warn about caveat emptor, but the buyer needs assistance. He cannot possibly be expected to understand and detect the refinements in our increasingly complicated system of medical care delivery. Moreover, the operation of that system in a free capitalist market leads to demonstrated inequities in the distribution of resources (manpower, facilities, etc.) that can be corrected only by governmental intervention.

The challenge that faces all persons concerned with health care delivery is the preservation of personal values—of sensitivities to the feelings and reactions of individuals—in the face of the inexorable expansion of governmental regulation. Small units of organization can usually do this more readily than large ones, whether we consider public entities like the United States Army or private ones like the General Motors Corporation. Within the inevitably large bureaucratic structure of America's health care system of the future, there must be and readily can be sensitivity to such values.

References

1. *See* United Nations, Universal Declaration of Human Rights, art. 25, 1 (1948). Section 1 reads as follows: "Everyone has the right to a standard of living adequate for the health and well-being of himself and of his family, including food, clothing, housing and medical care and necessary social services, and the right to security in the event of unemployment, sickness, disability, widowhood, old age or other lack of livelihood in circumstances beyond his control."
2. U.N. Dep't of Social Affairs, The Impact of the Universal Declaration of Human Rights 3 (1953).
3. *See generally* C.E.A. Winslow, The Conquest of Epidemic Disease (1944).
4. *See* R. Sand, The Advance to Social Medicine (1952).
5. *See generally* F. Grad, American Public Health Association, Public Health Law Manual (1965).
6. H. E. Sigerist, *Primitive and Archaic Medicine,* in 1 History of Medicine 428 (1951).
7. Sigerist, *Henry E. Sigerist on the Sociology of Medicine,* in New York M.D. Publications 312 (M.I. Roemer ed. 1960).
8. *See* O. Garceau, The Political Life of the American Medical Association 14 (1961).
9. A. Flexner, Medical Education in the United States and Canada (1910).
10. *See* H.E. Sigerist, American Medicine 163 (1934).
11. *See* testimony of R. C. Derbyshire, *Hearings on Health Profession Educational Assistance Act of 1974 Before the Senate Comm. on Labor and Public Welfare,* 93d Cong., 2d Sess., at 131 (1974).
12. *See generally* R. Roemer, *Legal Systems Regulating Health Personnel: A Comparative Analysis,* 56 Milbank Memorial Fund Q. 431 (Pt. 1, 1968) (hereinafter cited as *Legal Systems*).
13. *See* M. Friedman & S. Kuznets, Income from Independent Professional Practice (1954).
14. *Legal Systems, supra* note 12, at 434.
15. *See generally* National Commission on Accrediting, Study of Accreditation of Selected Health Educational Programs (1972).
16. *See, e.g.,* Fla. Stat. Ann. § 458.05 (c) (1965), Mich. Comp. Laws Ann. § 338.1806 - 6(d) (Supp. 1975–76).
17. *See, e.g.,* Grants for Maternal and Child Health and Crippled Children's Services, 42 C.F.R. § 51a. 110 (1974) [herinafter cited as Crippled Children's].
18. *See generally* Nat'l Comm. on Health Services, Health Manpower: Action to Meet Community Needs (1967).
19. *See, e.g.,* Nurse Training Act of 1971, Pub. L. No. 92-158, § 3(b), 85 Stat. 469 (codified at 42 U.S.C. § 296d (a) (1974)).
20. 42 U.S.C.A. § 295 *et seq.* (Supp. 2, 1975).
21. Comprehensive Health Manpower Training Act of 1971, Pub. L. No. 92-157, § 107(b), 85 Stat. 457 (codified at 42 U.S.C. § 295e-1 (1974)).
22. *See generally* R. Stevens, American Medicine and the Public Interest (1971).
23. Crippled Children's, *supra* note 17, § 51a. 119.

24. H. Cohen & L. Miike, HEW, Report on Developments in Health Manpower Licensure, at 39–45 (1973).
25. M. MacEachern, Hospital Organization and Management (1957).
26. Hospital Survey and Construction Act, 60 Stat. 1040 (1946), *as amended* 42 U.S.C. § 291 *et seq*. (1974). *See generally* L. Abbe & A. Baney, The Nation's Health Facilities: Ten Years of the Hill-Burton Hospital and Medical Facilities Program 1946–1956 (1958).
27. Hospital Survey and Construction Act of 1946, 60 Stat. 1043.
28. *Id.* at 1044. *See generally* K. Taylor & D. Donald, A Comparative Study of Hospital Licensure Regulations (1957).
29. L. Davis, Fellowship of Surgeons (1960).
30. *See* W. Worthington & L. Silver, *Regulation of Quality of Care in Hospitals: The Need for Change,* 35 Law & Contemp. Prob. 305 (1970).
31. *See generally* O. Anderson, J. Young & W. Janser, *The Government and the Consumer: Evaluation of Food and Drug Laws,* 13 J. Pub. L. 189 (1964).
32. Food and Drug Act of June 30, 1906, ch. 3915, 34 Stat. 768.
33. Federal Food Drug and Cosmetic Act of 1938, Pub. L. No. 717, § 505, 52 Stat. 1052.
34. *Ibid.* § 502, 52 Stat. 1050.
35. Drug Amendments of 1962, Pub. L. No. 87-781, 76 Stat. 780, *as amended* 21 U.S.C. § 321 *et seq*. (1972).
36. *See generally* R. Clapp, HEW, Study of Drug Purchase Problems and Policies (1966).
37. *See* 21 U.S.C. § 353 (b) (1972).
38. *See* 21 U.S.C. § 821 *et seq*. (Supp. 1975). *See generally* Nat'l Comm. on Marijuana and Drug Abuse, Drug Abuse in America, Problem in Perspective (1973).
39. 38 C.F.R. § 17.30 *et seq*. (1974).
40. Crippled Children's, *supra* note 17, § 51a.101 *et seq*. *See generally* American Public Health Association, Services for Handicapped Children (1955).
41. B. Cooper, N. Worthington & P. Piro, *National Health Expenditures, 1929–73*, 37 Social Security Bulletin 3 (Feb. 1974).
42. *See generally* M. I. Roemer *et al.*, Health Insurance Effects: Services, Expenditures, and Attitudes Under Three Types of Health Insurance Plans (1972).
43. *See generally* R. Egdahl, *Foundations for Medical Care,* 288 N. Eng. J. Med. 491 (1973).
44. *See* O. Anderson, State Enabling Legislation for Non-Profit Hospital and Medical Plans (1944).
45. *See generally* H. Hansen, Group Health Association of America, Legal Rights of Group Health Plans (1964).
46. American Medical News, Jan. 10, 1972, at 13. col. 1.
47. Article 14-A of the Labor Law of 1909, c. 674; now, N.Y. Workmen's Comp. Law §§ 1-49 (McKinney 1965).
48. Miss. Code Ann. § 71-3-1 *et seq*. (1972).
49. *See generally* H. Somers & A. Somers, Workmen's Compensation: Prevention, Insurance, and Rehabilitation of Occupational Disability (1954).
50. *See* M. Roemer, *Opportunities for Public Health in Disability Insurance Programs,* 62 Public Health Reports 1657 (1947).
51. Social Security Administration, HEW, Social Security Handbook 92-106 (1966).
52. Social Security Amendments of 1965, Pub. L. No. 89-97, § 102(a), 79 Stat. 291, *as amended* 42 U.S.C. § 1395 *et seq*. (1974).
53. *See, e.g.*, 42 U.S.C. § 1395f *et seq*. (1974).
54. *Ibid*.
55. *See generally* H. Somers & A. Somers, Medicare and the Hospitals Issues and Prospects (1967).
56. *See* U.S. Comptroller-General, Improved Controls Needed Over Extent of Care Provided by Hospitals and Other Facilities to Medicare Patients (1971).
57. Social Security Amendments of 1972, Pub. L. No. 92-603, § 249f (b), 86 Stat. 1429 (codified at 42 U.S.C. § 1320c (1974)). *See generally* L. Henry, Professional Standard Review Organizations—*The Role of the Private Sector,* Viewpoint (July 1973).
58. *See generally 182 PSRO Areas Designated,* American Medical News. Dec., 1973 at 24.
59. *See* R. Covell, *PSROs—Policy and Planning,* in Medical Care Audit 11 (D. Goodman ed. 1974).
60. *See* Institute of Medicine, Nat'l Academy of Sciences, Advancing the Quality of Health Care (1974).

61. M. Roemer, Organization of Medical Care Under Social Security 181 (1969).
62. *See supra* note 29 and accompanying text.
63. Roemer & Anzel, *Health Needs and Services of the Rural Poor,* in Rural Poverty in the United States 311 (1968).
64. Klarman, *Approaches to Moderating the Increases in Medical Care,* 7 Medical Care 175 (1969).
65. N.Y. Pub. Hlth. Law 2802 (McKinney 1971). *See generally* Curran, *Health Planning With "Clout," Certificate of Need Legislation,* 62 Am. J. Pub. Hlth. 1549 (1972).
66. *See* Lewin and Associates, Inc., Nationwide Survey of State Health Regulations, at 164, NTIS Accession No., PB 236660/AS (1974).
67. *See* Bossard, *A Sociologist Looks at the Doctor,* in The Medical Profession and the Public 8 (1934).
68. *See* F. Mott & M. Roemer, Rural Health and Medical Care 169 (1948).
69. *See* U.S. Public Health Services, HEW, Health Services for American Indians (1957).
70. *See* Mott & Roemer, *A Federal Program of Public Health and Medical Services for Migratory Farm Workers,* 60 Pub. Hlth. Rep. 229 (1945).
71. *See* Weinerman, *Changing Patterns in Medical Care: Their Implications for Ambulatory Services,* 39 Hospitals, Dec. 16, 1965, at 67.
72. *See generally* P. Jacobs, Prelude to Riot: A View of Urban America from the Bottom (1966).
73. *See generally* Zwick, *Some Accomplishments and Failings of Neighborhood Health Centers,* 50 Milbank Memorial Fund Q. 387 (Pt. 1, 1972).
74. U.S. Public Health Service, HEW, Promoting the Health of Mothers and Children (1973).
75. Occupational Safety and Health Act of 1970, 29 U.S.C. § 651 *et seq.* (1975).
76. *See* U.S. Dep't. of Labor, The President's Report on Occupational Safety and Health (1973).
77. *See* V. Eisner & L. Callan, Dimensions of School Health (1974).
78. *See* W. McNerney & D. Riedel, Regionalization and Rural Health Care (1962).
79. Heart Disease, Cancer and Stroke Amendments of 1965, Pub. L. No. 89-239, § 2, 79 Stat. 926, *as amended* 42 U.S.C. § 299 *et seq.* (1974).
80. *See generally* Marston, *Regional Medical Programs: A Review,* 43 Bull. N.Y. Acad. Med. 490 (1967).
81. Comprehensive Health Planning and Public Health Service Amendments of 1966, 42 U.S.C. § 246 *et seq.* (1974).
82. *See generally* Stewart, New Dimensions of Health Planning (1967).
83. *See generally* H. Moore, American Medicine and the People's Health 194 (1927).
84. *See* M. Roemer, *Approaches to the Rural Doctor Shortage,* 16 Rural Sociology 137 (1954).
85. *See* 42 U.S.C. § 294 *et seq.* (1974). *See also Health Personnel Will Be Assigned to Critical Manpower-Lacking Areas,* Medical Tribune, June 28, 1972.
86. S. 3585, 93d Cong., 2d Sess. (1974).
87. *Ibid.* § 402. In the final law enacted, this requirement was deleted.
88. *See generally* Staff of the Subcommittee on Public Health and Environment, 93D Cong., 2D Sess., Proposals for Health Planning, Development, and Regulation: A Comparison (1974).
89. *See* M. Rosenau, Preventive Medicine and Public Health (1974).
90. *See* G.K. Macleod & J.A. Prussin, *The Continuing Evolution of Health Maintenance Organizations,* 288 N. Eng. J. Med. 439 (1973).
91. The Health Maintenance Organization Act of 1973, Pub. L. No. 93-222, 87 Stat. 914 (codified at 42 U.S.C. § 300e *et seq.* (1974)).
92. *Ibid.* § 300e(c)(8).
93. *See* Sheps, *The Influence of Consumer Sponsorship on Medical Services,* 50 Milbank Memorial Fund Q. 41 (Pt. II, 1972).

Part Seven

Health Planning

Along with the growing organization of health services all over the world, there has come increasing recognition that deliberate planning of resources and their distribution is required if needs are to be met. The economic mechanisms of the free market are being found inadequate for governing the allocation of services in an equitable or rational way.

In order to understand the dynamics of health care systems in their many subdivisions, social research has been conducted for many years and at an accelerating pace; Chapter 29 reviews the highlights of this research, essential for planning, up to the year 1963. In Chapter 30, we trace the evolution of deliberate comprehensive planning of health services in the United States. As national health planning became more widely accepted in the late 1960s, varying techniques and approaches were taken; in Chapter 31, we examine several of these approaches critically, and offer reasons why it is important for us to focus efforts on the provision of needed health services for communities, rather than become entranced by the refinements of elaborate methodologies. Chapter 32 illustrates this substantive approach by a down-to-earth agenda for comprehensive health planning in rural areas. In the early 1970s, a conservative U.S. government set out to promote a form of cooperative subsystem for health care financing and delivery that had long been tried against much opposition; its virtues as a cost-containment strategy were at last recognized and it received official support and encouragement under a new label: "health maintenance organizations." The HMO also constitutes a type of local subsystem planning, so its effects on costs, on services, and on meeting health needs are examined in Chapter 33.

29

Social Research on Medical Care

The planning of health services depends, first of all, on accurate information about the health needs (diseases and disabilities) of populations, the operation of actual health care systems, and the relative effects of different or alternative methods of organizing health care resources. While the use of such research for deliberate health planning purposes has occurred only in recent years, performance of social studies of disease and health services can be traced back several centuries.

At the 1962 Annual Meeting of the American Sociological Association, I was invited to present an historical overview of the application of sociological research applied to problems of medical care. The paper was prepared jointly with Ray H. Elling (a sociologist). Since then, the tempo of social science research on the causation of disease and the operation and effects of organized health programs has accelerated. Such research aims to serve as a basis for improvement in the effective delivery of health services.

THE FOCUS OF this paper will be on the contribution of social research to the provision of medical care. We will interpret "medical care" to be not coterminous with all health service, but rather to include those health services concerned with the diagnosis, treatment, and rehabilitation of the disabled. Everyone who has studied the field realizes, however, the inseparability of these services from those for prevention of illness or accident, promotion of health, advancement of education and research, and other components of the wide world of health.

Social Change and the Provision of Medical Care

It is now a trite story which begins by declaring the black bag outmoded. As if to underline this, several doctor's bags and their contents have been preserved and are on view in the Smithsonian Institute. But it is well to recognize the implications of the increasing complexity of the medical care system and realize that it is only an extension in the health sphere of a developing complexity in society.

With the development of American society, there has been rapid growth in the population which is expected to continue, coming to 260 million by 1980. The age and sex structure will also continue to change. With greater longevity, the

Chapter 29 originally appeared as "Sociological Research on Medical Care" in the *Journal of Health and Human Behavior,* 4:49–68, Spring 1963, and is reprinted by permission of that journal.

number 65 years and over is expected to rise from the present 16 to 25 million by 1980, while those in the group under 20 years are also expected to increase, from the current 65 to 110 million. These developments will leave a small proportion of active people (perhaps only 48 percent of the population) to produce the resources necessary to support the increased demands for medical care by the elderly and the young.[1] The greater strength and longevity of the "weaker sex" will mean a further increase in the proportion of women.

Other social changes are equally notable. Farming is becoming big business with fewer people producing more food and fibre. The labor force includes more women, fewer farmers and laborers, more sales, services, technical professional, and managerial workers. There has been a general up-grading in the class structure, with evidence for the "professionalization" of labor in several sectors.[2] As one would predict from Ogburn's work, the rate of social change appears to have increased exponentially. The formation of many new occupations has demanded the development of a thick dictionary to keep track of them. This rising specialization of individuals and organizations has resulted in increased interdependence. The person is involved in many contingent relationships. An uneasy "other directedness" pervades the modern scene.[3] As means of adjusting the pieces of this complex society, one out of every five persons changes his residence every year.

There are many apparent consequences of these developments which can be traced out in the medical care system; we mention only the more salient. Technological specialization has brought us the complexity of fifty to one hundred specialized outpatient clinics in a large, urban, medical center; it has meant over 150 different occupations in this center.[4] There are a score of other occupations represented in the hundreds of public and voluntary health agencies in the surrounding community.

East or West, this development in society has entailed ever larger bureaucracies to coordinate the vast range of implements and people needed to accomplish a given health task.[5] With invention in social organization as well as technological invention, a greater potential has been realized; thus, the dimensions of the health tasks themselves have increased. With ministries of health and international agencies to mobilize the technical resources, one can speak with plausibility about eradicating malaria on a worldwide scale. With a vaccine available and several organizations to promote its use, one can speak with reasonable hope for the control of poliomyelitis in this country. With the eventual institution of more adequate mechanisms of payment for and supervision of health care for the elderly, one can look to reduction of much hardship.

But technical competence and complexity have not only brought greater powers and social responsibilities, they have meant greater organizational problems—particularly higher costs. Expenditures for health services in the United States have increased over the last 30 years from about 3.5 to 5.3 percent of the gross national product.[6] They are estimated to have reached 29.0 billion dollars for the 1960–61 fiscal year.[7] The most critical element of our medical care system—the hospital—is increasing in complexity more rapidly than the others; as a consequence, its costs of construction as well as operation have risen precipitously. While the general consumer price index has risen 52 percent since 1945, hospital room rates have gone up 205 percent.[8] The end of this trend is not in sight. These increasing costs have stimulated more broadly based systems of financing. Both governmental and voluntary systems of payment—particularly the insurance mechanism—have moved in to soften the cost burden on the individual and family.

Increased popular desire for the products of a complex medical care system, coupled with concern on the parts of powerful paying agencies (industry, labor, insurance organizations, consumer groups, and government) over meeting the costs of such a system have raised political issues. The patterns of providing care are also under public and professional debate. Medical care has become a focal point of collective bargaining[9] and political action. The current struggle over medicare for the elderly is only the most recent example.

Against this background we may examine past and current development of social research on medical care.

Development of Research on Medical Care

The earliest recognition and study of the social aspects of illness concerned the mode of occurrence of particular disorders. Contagiousness—a social process—was expounded by the Italian Giroloma Francastoro in 1546, based primarily on observations of plague, typhus fever, and other epidemic diseases.[10] Diseases of miners were studied and described by George Agricola in 1556 and a few years later by Paracelsus. Scurvy, a disease due to nutritional deficiency, found especially among seamen, was claimed by Dutch and British physicians to be preventable by drinking lemon juice in the mid-sixteenth century.[11] These were all observations of social phenomena affecting health and they led eventually to practical actions for disease prevention.

One of the earliest applications of research to the overall problem of health and medical care in a population was the work of William Petty, an extremely versatile British physician who lived from 1623 to 1687. He believed in measurements and spoke of data on the diseases, educational level, and other attributes of the population as "political arithmetic." In 1662 John Graunt published the first major work on mortality rates according to cause, season, place of residence, and other variables. Based on this type of social data, Petty proposed in 1676 a state medical service of salaried physicians who would serve everyone. Interestingly, he pointed to the greater stability of the military forces, the church, and the courts because their personnel were on public salaries. He put great stress on the importance of hospitals for both patient-care and professional education, and—much ahead of his time—he advocated "hospitals for the accommodation of sick people, rich as well as poor, so instituted and fitted as to encourage all sick persons to resort to them—every sort of such hospitals to differ only in splendor, but not at all in the sufficiency of the means and remedy for the patient's health."[12]

In the period of the enlightment and the age of revolutions, the social conscience of medicine was expressed in sweeping proposals for health programs. The most important of these was the six-volume comprehensive *System of Medical Policy* (Police), published by the great German physician, Johann Peter Frank, between 1779 and 1817. The emphasis was upon measures of sanitation, protection of mothers and children, accident prevention and—in a later volume—the organization of hospitals and medical care.[13] In England, the early nineteenth century saw the great sanitary awakening, with the issuance in 1842—culminating many years of study and agitation—of the report . . . *On the Inquiry into the Sanitary Conditions of the Laboring Population of Great Britain,* by Edwin Chadwick, a layman, in cooperation with three physicians: Southwood Smith, Neil Arnott and James Philips Kay. While the modern social scientists may not look upon these works as research, they were by no means pure armchair treatises, but were based on abundant field observations and the use of whatever statistical data were available. In America, a comparable study—based on statistical data from in and around Boston—was issued by the Sanitary Commission of Massachusetts in 1850, under the authorship of the energetic and capable bookseller, Lemuel Shattuck.[14] In the early nineteenth century, more than a few important physicians had shown concern for social conditions and their effects on public health.[15]

In the later nineteenth century, building on the collective efforts of trade unions and local friendly societies for many decades before, there arose the social insurance movement, including provisions for the group financing of medical care. The first such national legislation came out of Bismark's Germany in 1883. This was also the period of great discoveries in bacteriology and antisepsis, which changed the whole character of the hospital.[16] The immediate background of these programs of medical care had been the movement for a system of public medical service for the low income groups (not just for paupers, as under the old Elizabethan Poor Laws) led by physicians like Rudolf Virchow and Solomon Neumann in Germany.[17] The research of the later years of the nineteenth century, however, was overwhelmingly concentrated on the discovery of microorganisms and the elucidation of processes in cells which could explain disease. Bacteriology could also provide a scientific grounding for the whole sanitary movement. The practical rewards of such research were so great that it is little surprise that the broad social studies, required for stimulating social action on the improved organization of medical care, had to await the opening decades of the twentieth century.

The major research relating to social action in medical care was bound up with the movement for extension of health insurance in Europe and America. The establishment of the system of Zemstvo medicine in Czarist Russia in 1864—a scheme of public medical care with salaried personnel in rural areas—may not have been ushered in by scientific studies. But the first British health insurance law of 1911 was preceded by a report of the Poor Law Commission in 1909, including the work of figures like Beatrice Webb and William Beveridge.[18] The American Association for Labor Legislation conducted studies which buttressed the movement between 1910 and 1920 for state compulsory health insurance laws.[19] Although none of these passed—under the combined opposition of industry, labor, commercial insurance companies, and medicine—this social research paid dividends in the field of workmen's compensation and in maternal and child health service organization. An occasional physician was deeply conscious of the relations between medicine and society and the need for effective social measures to improve medical care; an example was Dr. James Peter Warbasse, whose collection of essays entitled *Medical Sociology* appeared in 1909.[20]

The halcyon days of the 1920s were not entirely quiet in the field of sociological research, with the Chicago department of sociology under Park, Burgess, and MacKensie in full swing. The theory of social change and cultural lag enunciated by William Ogburn in 1922 had a clear implication for the analysis of problems of medical care.[21] It is of interest that Ogburn himself used a medical care development—workmen's compensation legislation—as his initial case-study for verification of his hypothesis. Studies on the incidence of illness in different socio-economic groups—showing higher rates among the poor—had been made by Edgar Sydenstrycker and other "medical economists" in the U.S. Public Health Service in the early 1920s.[22] Since 1916, Michael M. Davis had studied and written about the organizational problems of clinics and hospitals.[23] In 1927, there appeared a study that brought together most of the American data then available on health needs and medical care in a volume, structured on the theory of cultural lag. It was entitled *American Medicine and the People's Health* with the subtitle "An Outline with Statistical Data on the Organization of Medicine in the United States with Special Reference to the Adjustment of Medical Service to Social and Economic Change." It was written by Harry H. Moore, a "public health economist" of the U.S. Public Health Service who, in our view, deserves greater recognition in the history of this field than he has received.[24]

The year that Moore's book was published was also the year of initiation of the five years of studies that led to the 28-volume report of the Committee on the Costs of Medical Care. Completed in 1932, at the depth of the great economic depression, this sweeping research project, directed by I. S. Falk (a man trained originally in bacteriology), had an enormous influence on both future research and future actions in the field of medical care financing and organization in the United States.[25] Throughout the 1930s and up to the end of World War II, the model for social research on medical care was set by these studies—at least in America. In Europe, the concept of "social medicine" was enunciated by the great Belgian physician René Sand, and much emphasis was put on the dependence of health on social class, with consequent needs for corrective social action.[26] Alfred Grotjahn in Germany, Arthur Newsholme in England, Jacques Parisot in France, Andrija Stampar in Yugoslavia were medical leaders combining administrative actions with field research, education, and writing on the development of systems of medical care which would effectively meet public needs.[27]

Academic sociologists, however, showed relatively little interest in the problems of medical care with a few exceptions. The major exception was Bernhard J. Stern, whose monograph, *Social Factors in Medical Progress,* was published in 1927.[28] This was a study of resistance to medical innovation, primarily historical, and in his later work Stern applied the same historical approach to analysis of other problems of medical care elucidating current forces by examining their origins and trends. Robert Lynd included a chapter on medical care and the medical profession in his classical study of Middletown.[29] James H. S. Bossard, as a part of the prevailing sociological interest in the dynamics of the big city, reported a study on the location of doctors' offices in Philadelphia done in 1933.[30] In 1936 L. J. Henderson—with shades of Talcott Parsons, 25 years later—wrote of "The Patient and Physician as a Social System."[31] Disease and unmet medical needs were regarded as social problems—symptoms or consequences of "social disorganization"[32]—but the social institution of medicine and the problems within it received little attention from formal sociologists. In 1938, Michael Davis made a plea in the *American Journal of Sociology* that sociologists should address themselves to some of the thorny problems of medical care organization and distribution.

More research germane to social action on medical care came from other academic specialties, especially history, economics, and anthropology. Henry E. Sigerist, the great scholar of medical history, showed how historical study could help to explain not only the genesis of medical knowledge and ideas, but also the patterns of medical care of the population.[34] His work both in Europe and America helped to inspire a whole generation of young physicians to recognize the social role of medicine. Richard H. Shryock was another historian whose contributions were primarily to the sociology of medicine.[35] A number of anthropologists, like W. H. R. Rivers, have found the study of medical beliefs and practices a useful channel to understanding whole cultures, and these studies have in turn given perspective to current problems in medical care.[36]

But it was mainly the economists who in the 1920s and 1930s explored and clarified the problems of medical care, from the setting of both the universities and government. As early as 1919, Sumner Slichter wrote about sickness as a major cause of labor turnover.[37] In 1932, Pierce Williams published an important study on the use of insurance as a method of financing medical care, confined at the time largely to industrial groupings.[38] The Committee on the Costs of Medical Care, mentioned earlier, had mobilized young economists like Maurice

Leven and Louis Reed to apply their skills to these problems.[39] Indeed, the whole field of medical care research—even in its strictly sociological aspects—came to be known by the phrase "medical economics." It was the Committee on Research in Medical Economics, for example, which published the interesting empirical study of Gladys Swackhamer on *Choice and Change of Doctors*.[40]

In the latter 1930s, however, there is no question that the major research contribution to action in the field of medical care came from the federal government. At the depth of the depression the U.S. Public Health Service organized the first "national health survey"—providing at the same time work relief by training unemployed workers (under the W.P.A.) as interviewers.[41] This vast field survey provided basic data not only on the extent and types of disease in the American population along with demographic variables; it also demonstrated the relationships of medical care, in all its components, to socio-economic status. It provided the research support for a wide range of social actions on health insurance, chronic disease control, hospital construction, public medical care for the needy, and other problems. The men and women identified with this far-reaching study came from backgrounds in economics, biostatistics, social work, and even chemical engineering (George Perrott). Follow-up of this medical care research in the later 1930s and the early 1940s came principally from the research arm of the Social Security Board, under the able direction of I. S. Falk.

The war years were obviously preoccupied with critical economic and military mobilization, but they were by no means devoid of research toward action in medical care. Indeed, it was the inspiration of post-war planning for a better world that produced major research documents like the Beveridge Report on *Social Insurance and Allied Services*,[42] the Bhore Commission studies in India,[43] or the Hojer studies in Sweden. In the United States, the immediate post-war years included active and vitriolic debate about national medical care insurance, the effect of which was to produce a great deal of social research in tangential but important problems and issues, like voluntary health insurance, hospital planning, rural health needs, and group medical practice.[44]

If we consider the current period of sociological research on medical care to begin about 1950, we can see that it has acquired a very different set of characteristics from that which preceded it. It seems clear that developments in the general socio-political scene of the United States had a strong bearing on the changed approach. As often happens after a war, there was a period of "getting back to normal," when conservative influences became very strong in the United States. With the election of a Republican administration in 1952, the rise of McCarthyism and its inhibiting influence, and the all-pervading influence of the Cold War with Soviet Communism, the direction of social research turned from that geared to broad-scale social-medical reform toward more limited goals. Sociologists, in particular, directed their expanding forces to detailed studies of the internal operation of the whole social institution of medical care.[45]

The convergence of two intellectual developments helps explain the rapid and rich growth of a general field of medical sociology since about 1950. One was the recognition by the medical schools and also the public health agencies and hospitals that social problems required analysis by experts—yet in a manner not identified with the controversial movement toward health insurance and reorganization of medical care. The other was the rapid rise in academic sociology of empirical research methods—an emphasis that favored subjects which were readily quantifiable. Health needs and medical service provided such data, and the centers of medical education and research began to welcome social scientists. The current period since 1950, therefore, has been characterized very largely by contributions to medical care from empirical-theoretical sociologists.[46]

Since 1945, with the publication of such a landmark volume as *The American Soldier*, there has been an effort to interweave theoretical sociology with empirical research on practical problems. With this development sociology has come of age. It has found wide acceptance in the university—the conserver, transmitter, and developer of knowledge. In turn, the broad institutional sectors of our society—family, industry, law, political affairs, health, education, art, leisure, and religion—have increasingly sought the point of view of the quasi-detached student of society,[47] as the complexity and rate of change within each sector have multiplied.

This has resulted in much specialization in sociology itself, including a focus on health and particularly medical care. Several surveys of the general development of medical sociology have appeared in this country and elsewhere,[48] and interest in the field has blossomed overseas, in England and Germany.[49] Two collections of sociological research relevant to medical care have appeared in recent years.[50] A special section of the American Sociological Association has been formed. A text has appeared.[51] Behavioral scientists have joined the medical care section of the American Public Health Association. *The Journal of Health and Human Behavior* has been launched and already a special issue on medical care has come out.[52] Let us now examine some of the principal streams of current research, keeping our focus on medical care (as distinguished from prevention, education, research, or other facets of the health field).

Principal Streams of Current Research in Medical Care

With this background, it is evident why many different streams of study on the problems of health service should be operating side by side. At least five fields of investigation in medical care can be distinguished today.

Health Needs and Medical Care

First is the study of the *health needs of the population and the receipt of medical care*—the heritage of studies starting in the 1930s and providing the foundation for programs of health insurance and other methods of improved financing of medical services. Perhaps the most important current work in this field is the continuing National Health Survey being conducted by the U.S. Public Health Service, as authorized by the Congress in 1957.[53] Based on a nationwide sample of some 38,000 households, this systematic and periodic survey of illness and medical services received by the population provides a wealth of useful data on needs for medical care according to age, sex, income level, and geographic location. It is also providing better data than we have ever had on diagnostic categories of disability, acute and chronic. Important also has been the research of the Health Information Foundation, under the direction of Odin Anderson, in surveying family expenditures for medical care in relation to health insurance coverage in 1953 and again in 1958.[54] Being at a different stage of health insurance planning and operation, the Canadians have done important studies on the utilization of services under various types of insurance program.[55] Studies emanating from Saskatchewan, from the Department of National Health and Welfare (under Dr. Joseph Willard), and from the University of Toronto (especially by Dr. Malcolm Taylor) have provided important lessons for medical care planning in the United States.[56] The long-term study of the Windsor Medical Service by the University of Michigan has provided a model for analysis of the dynamics of prepaid comprehensive medical care.[57]

Studies on rural health needs and utilization of medical care—showing continuing deficiencies in relation to urban experience—have continued to flow from the university departments of rural sociology at Cornell, the University of Missouri, the University of North Carolina, and elsewhere.[58] Major contributions of sociologists in this sphere have been the studies of the attitudes of people toward physicians and the medical care system.[59]

In the urban setting, studies have continued to demonstrate the different patterns of need and care among different segments of the population. Particularly notable is the research done in the Boston area showing that those with the greatest medical care needs, as professionally defined (the elderly and other low-income groups), have the lowest recognition of their needs, the least wherewithall with which to meet their needs once recognized, the longest duration of care once it is received, but the least overall care in spite of great need.[60]

These studies of illness and the receipt of or utilization of medical care—of which those mentioned are only a sketchy sample—are providing data of the greatest usefulness in planning improvements in medical care. They answer questions about the needs for health personnel, hospitals, and other resources for providing service. They permit estimates of costs. They elucidate the differentials in need and demand among different demographic groups, like the aged whose needs are such a pressing socio-political issue today. They help to clear the air of questions and distortions about under-utilization, over-utilization, abuse, and other allegations that seem to inevitably complicate the introduction of medical-care innovations. They even offer by-products in the way of epidemiological data on the occurrence and concomitants of specific disorders. They permit the production of comprehensive, interpretive studies on the distribution of medical care like that published by Herman and Anne Somers in 1961.[61] Note must also be made that theoretical contributions to sociology are as likely in the study of this aspect of human endeavor as in others.

The Organization of Ambulatory Health Services

A second field of investigation discernible in the medical care world today relates to the *pattern of organization of ambulatory health services* in the community. By organization, we mean not only the structure and functions of complex arrangements—like those in clinics or rehabilitation centers, for example—but also the dynamics of the solo office practice.

Relationships among particular role players is a focus of many studies. One of the most researched problems in medical sociology has been the doctor-patient relationship (one might say over-researched considering the range of other problems and resources available to attack them).[62] Much of the relevant theoretical framework for this work was provided by Hughes.[63] Role expectations were regarded as important in themselves in studies by Apple[64] and Reader.[65] But some investigators, notably Hollingshead and Redlich, broadened this interest in patients' expectations to include background variables such as social class.[66] In this view, expectations and conceptions regarding medical care are variables intervening between one's social position and the differential receipt of medical care. It is not only the availability of care but the patient's willingness to participate in it which is important for the final outcome of treatment. Thus, Elling and others examined family disorganization and reflexive self-concepts as independent variables affecting expectations in an illness and participation in a program of treatment.[67] The expectations and practices of patients from different social positions are articulated with different forms of medical care in a study by Freidson.[68] Work currently under way at Harvard Medical School is throwing new light on the long-recognized patterns of low income and "lower class" people seeking care from general practitioners, while the "middle classes" consult specialists.[69] These studies of relations of patients to health professionals are revelant also to hospital dynamics, to be discussed below.

It is one of the disappointing, even if understandable, facts about medical-sociological research that so much of it has been focused on relationships within organized group programs (which have been the minority part of health service in the United States) and so little on the pattern of individualistic office medical care (which predominates in the American scene). One of the few such studies was that carried out by Osler Peterson and his colleagues on the private general practice of medicine in North Carolina.[70] Other work on office practice focuses on the ecological distribution of different types of practices and the relation of practice patterns to medical careers (discussed below).

A number of surveys and analyses of group medical practice in the United States have been made by the U.S. Public Health Service.[71] Studies of the quality of medical care in different group clinics of the Health Insurance Plan of Greater New York were first conducted by Henry Makover,[72] then by others; these have helped to clarify methods of tackling the elusive question of quality measurements.[73] Leonard Rosenfeld and his colleagues applied some of these techniques effectively in their Boston studies on the quality of medical care in hospitals.[74] The whole concept of the "medical audit," developed with the use of hospital records by Paul Lembcke,[75] Robert Myers and Vergil Slee,[76] and others, is now being applied in the evaluation of performance in ambulatory-care clinics. Specialized as this problem may seem to be, it is indicative of the richness of this field that a series of five annual conferences has now been held, under the leadership of Cecil Sheps, on the contributions of research to understanding the problems of ambulatory medical care. To mention only three of the centers tackling this problem, there is the research at Cornell Medical School's comprehensive care and teaching clinic under George Reader,[77] that of Jerry Solon at the Beth Israel Hospital in Boston,[78] and that of the University of North Carolina by Kerr L. White.[79] A small but particularly well-designed study of the benefits of a comprehensive—as against specialized and fragmented—approach to the ambulatory patient was conducted in Chicago by A. J. Simon.[80] A more far-reaching study, the "family health maintenance demonstration," by George Silver and his colleagues has been in process for several years at the Montefiore Hospital and is now available.[81]

British social researchers are also examining the detailed content of ambulatory medical care, under the special conditions of the National Health Service. The studies by Lord Taylor in London,[82] by Gordon Forsyth and Robert Logan in Manchester,[83] and others have helped to clarify the scope and limitations of community general medical practice which has traditionally been rather sharply separated from the hospital and specialty service in Britain (even before the National Health Service). Indeed, comparative international studies of the consequences for patients (and their pocketbooks) of different patterns of medical care organization present invaluable channels for reaching scientific generalizations.[84] Perhaps the ultimate question to be answered—and it has, of course, a thousand subdivisions—is to determine the human consequences of different social organizations of health service. One might hope that these consequences could be defined in terms of health status and survival—as in the perinatal mortality studies of Health Insurance Plan members and non-members in New York City.[85] Even short of this ultimate criterion, a study of results of diverse patterns of care is the soundest foundation for guiding policy decisions.[86]

The Hospital

A third very important sphere of medical care research centers on *the hospital,* both its internal structure and its external relations. As a central link in the medical care chain, considerable work is being done on the hospital, although most of it concerns internal organization.

In a pioneering work, Smith explored the implications of fractionated authority in the hospital.[87] Since that time there have been only a few comprehensive studies of relationships in the general hospital; notable are those by Wessen[88] and by Burling, Lentz, and Wilson.[89] Fox carried through a fascinating study of the system of relationships on a medical research ward.[90] A study by Georgopolis and Mann, to appear soon, has the virtue of comparing several hospitals as to the relations among internal organizational variables, such as cohesiveness, communication, coordination, and effectiveness.[91] Other studies of this more comprehensive character have focused on the mental hospital.[92]

Role relations among hospital personnel is a major category of internal hospital research. Those involving the nurse have perhaps received the most generous attention. Brown has studied the therapeutic effects of nurse-patient relationships.[93] Her work has since dealt with the entire physical and social milieu of the hospital and its probable effects.[94] Only a few of the other works on the nurse's position in the hospital and her relationships to others are cited here.[95]

There are other hospital personnel on whom a little work has been done. Bates, in examining decision-making in the hospital, found the administrator entangled in overlapping spheres of authority involving professional judgments of medical and nursing staffs, on the one hand, and board judgments regarding efficiency and economy, on the other.[96] In a study of the physician as administrator, Goss analyzed his advantages over the lay administrator.[97] Aside from some work on personnel turnover,[98] there is little of relevance to service personnel.[99] With union activity growing in hospitals, this is an important field for further investigation.

Studies of role relations internal to the hospital necessarily involve the patient; however, this concern has usually been secondary. A recent study by Rose Coser focuses primarily on the patient's adaptation to the hospital system. In an insightful summary of the meaning of her work she says, "I found myself analyzing and describing role continuity and discontinuity and those forces that assisted or hindered socialization—the transition from one segment of society to another."[100] She found two main groups of patients: those looking for emotional support and "a home" in the hospital and those looking for technical aid. The support-seekers had much less to look forward to on return to the community, while those seeking technical aid would obviously be "involved" in family and community life upon discharge.

There are few empirical studies of the external relationships of any organization.[101] The hospital is no exception. Various attitude surveys have been conducted.[102] In an important, though unreleased, study of attitudes as related to the quality of care, Blum examined public attitudes toward hospitals with high malpractice-suit rates, as compared with attitudes toward hospitals with low rates. He found public attitudes only weakly related, but there were distinct differences between the high- and low-rate hospitals in medical staff composition and other internal features.[103]

Pattern of medical practice, as related to the hospital, is another topic which has received some attention, following the pioneer work of Hall[104] and Solomon.[105] Ethnic and other background variables in relation to forms of practice have received more recent attention from Lieberson[106] and McElrath.[107] The transmission of drug information and the influence of interns and residents have been studied by Katz and others.[108] In an excellent study, Linn compared mental hospitals making extensive use of tranquilizing drugs with others making little use of them and found that discharge rates had increased equally in both. The author suggested that changes in community and professional attitudes toward mental illness were more important in explaining discharge rates than were techniques in treatment.[109]

Studies of the hospital's place in the community generally and in its health system are relatively rare. Roemer pointed up the extent to which organized overall health services are fractionated even in a semirural county.[110] Babchuck and others report a study of board composition and the position of hospitals relative to other community organizations.[111] Levine and White have examined transfers of resources among health agencies including the hospital.[112] Ivan Belknap is currently completing a study of hospital systems in two Texas communities. A study by the authors on factors related to the hospital's receiving support from its environment is nearly completed.[113] As a part of this work, Elling carried out an intensive study of two well-supported and two poorly supported hospitals in a single urban center and the efforts of these organizations to maintain themselves, in the face of demands made by several citizens' hospital planning committees.[114] But generally speaking, there is little research of a sociological nature relevant to hospital regionalization and planning.[115]

A collection of recent sociological research on the hospital, edited by Freidson, will include chapters on the social history of the hospital; patterns of bureaucracy among medical staff; American and foreign hospitals; goals and authority structure; organizational support; teaching atmosphere of hospitals; negotiation of order in the hospital; alienation of labor; physical environment of the mental hospital ward; ecology of an obstetrical service; and the timetable of treatment.[116]

Programs for Special Groups

A fourth field of work in medical care research may be defined as the study of the *operation of medical care programs for special population groups*. In a sense, these studies cut across the lines of others considered so far, but they are distinguished by the separability of their clientele from the general population. Among these may be mentioned the many studies of the operation of programs of medical care for the indigent, under agencies of government. The Federal Bureau of Public Assistance, the American Public Welfare Association, and the American Medical Association have examined the costs, volume of services, patterns of care, and the administrative difficulties of these state and local public programs. More comprehensive examination of this field is now being made by S. J. Axelrod of the University of Michigan.[117] Likewise, there are studies of the operation of medical services under the Veterans Administration and the more recent "medicare" program for the dependents of military personnel. The medical care needs and services among American Indians have been the subject of a national study.[118] The crippled children's programs in the states are being subjected to repeated critical evaluations, as are the programs of adult restoration under the federal-state program of vocational rehabilitation.

Medical care rendered under the somewhat antiquated workmen's compensation program has also been subjected to fresh scrutiny in recent years.[119] Of special importance also have been the deluge of studies on the needs of and services for the chronically ill, culminating in the four-volume report (already outdated) by the National Commission on Chronic Illness appearing between 1952 and 1959.[120] The care of the mentally ill must also be mentioned under this heading; while most of the studies in this field have been epidemiological or semi-clinical, some have analyzed the receipt of diagnostic and treatment services for mental illness in different social contexts.[121]

These studies of person-specific or disease-specific medical care programs all tend to have a highly practical orientation, and they have usually been stimulated by administrative problems of costs, professional relationships, or obvious qualitative defects. At the same time, they do not lack theoretical interest for the social scientist. They tend to provide data in a well-defined population, in which rates can be readily computed. The questions are usually clear and the answers can be applied in corrective social actions. The situation, in a word, tends to be more subject to deliberate action than is the case for medical care studies involving the larger community or national populations.

Health Personnel

The *development of health personnel* adequate in numbers and quality to the tasks which society expects of them is a fifth sphere of important problems with many facets. Clearly, the planning and provision of medical care involve the recruitment, training, and organization of personnel identified with many occupational groups. The sociology of work is involved.[122] The organization of men and women around their occupational identities has received considerable attention under the rubric of professionalization.[123] Yet it is the flux and flow of individual occupational identities, with which we are faced in this rapidly changing technological society,[124] as much as it is the more corporate action of an occupational group.[125]

Part of this development of one's self-identity as a member of one occupation or another occurs in the course of work. A good example of a study of the division of labor at work is offered by Arnold's study of health department personnel.[126] Working back in sequence, another major facet of this "occupational becoming" occurs as adult socialization in professional schools.[127] There are problems of recruitment to a field which Back, Coker, and others examined for medical students considering public health.[128] There is also the less studied problem of exit from a field. The origin of work group members, in terms of life chances in childhood, has been a concern of several sociologists. Once in an occupation, the organization of members for the establishment of their group is a relatively unstudied aspect of occupational becoming, though Garceau's work on the American Medical Association is notable in this regard.[129] The place of an occupation in society and the changing attitudes of the public toward its members is a further problem of occupational groups. Here one must raise questions of occupational mobility, social status and power, and the mandate of the work group. The person's progress through the world of work is his work career. Stages in the career and their recognition are important aspects of occupational sociology.[130] One of the pressing problems of our time is that, with increasing complexity and the accompanying pace of social change, individuals entering many occupations are no longer able to look forward to nicely laid out career patterns. Professional obsolescence and the need for retraining have become important aspects of most work situations.[131]

Many of these general problems of occupational groups have been studied in the health field. Particular attention has been given to the physician. In many ways, because of the extent of his occupational organization and professional development, the physician has served as a prototype for the study of other occupations. Adams has studied changes in the social positions most likely to produce physicians.[132] With increasing emphasis on technical proficiency, rather than philosophy and bedside manner, and with wider access to medical education, it is suggested that more upward-mobile individuals are to be found in the ranks of physicians today. The physician's development in school has received the attention of several researchers.[133] Hall has studied the stages in the career of the practicing physician.[134] Cohen suggests that the physician's exalted status in U.S. society is due to his having "the best of both worlds," service to humanity and the rewards of entrepreneurship.[135] However, some recent trends suggest that other occupations may have recently developed greater drawing power for the very talented student.[136] Glaser has studied the doctor's particular points d'appui in political action.[137]

The nurse too has come in for considerable attention. Hughes, Hughes, and Deutscher have examined the occupation of nursing in general and its changing character.[138] Devereaux and Weiner trace the origins of nursing in the once clearly defined feminine role of nurturance and care, yet find her cut off from "libidinal replenishment" in present-day scientific medicine and caught in an "ill-defined professional, hierarchical, and social position."[139]

Various studies, as noted under the section on the hospital, have been done on the nurse's position and relationships with others at work. Others by Rohrer,[140]

Goldstein,[141] Habenstein and Christ,[142] Mauksch,[143] and Burkle[144] may be noted here. Various nursing specialties have received some attention. Stewart and Needham report on the operating room nurse.[145] Willie has examined the preferences of public health nurses for patients of "middle" social class backgrounds.[146] Pearsall has examined supervision and nursing.[147] Greenblatt focuses on research and the nurse.[148] Other work relates to the nursing student.[149]

Some studies of other health occupations exist. More and Kohn have examined motives for entering dentistry.[150] Work has appeared on dental students.[151] Kriesberg and Treiman have examined public attitudes toward dentistry[152] and Barthuli has studied dentists' attitudes.[153] The types of careers and training available to medical care and hospital administrators have been explored.[154] Marginal and emerging health occupations have received some attention in the work of New,[155] McCormick,[156] Wardwell,[157] Lortie,[158] and Freidson.[159] An extensive exploration of public health as an occupational complex is currently underway.[160]

Research Needs and Opportunities

With this broad, if not penetrating, review of sociological research relevant to medical care, we are in a position to discuss future needs for research in this field. There is, first of all, a need for grand designs and courageous thinking. Sociological research can be a powerful tool for human betterment, as suggested by the President's Scientific Advisory Committee.[161] In this connection, it seems appropriate to quote from the head of a major foundation:

> There is urgent need of coordination of the many multi-professional, social, economic, welfare and political programs now so conspicuous by their fragmentation, splintering, duplication, ineffectiveness and skyrocketing costs. New patterns for the distribution of health services, better organization and utilization of facilities and personnel, regionalization of activities, new forms of private and governmental cooperation, and a new approach to the joint financing of the essential services suggest some of the challenges. These are acute problems particularly in view of such plans as the medical care for the aged either under the Kerr-Mills Act or the proposed King-Anderson (Kennedy) Bill under the Social Security System.
>
> This is the most demanding era of our history. The future in medical care must be built as daringly and as energetically as were other aspects of our national economy such as industry, transportation, education, agriculture, and housing. The nation is no longer living in a frontier world, nor even in an individualistic world, but in a world demanding cooperation and interdependency. In each phase of the nation's health program the Federal departments, the universities and the professions, the hospitals, industry, labor, and the public must contribute their share of imaginative leadership in the formulation and execution of new patterns of cooperation adapted to the needs and conditions of present day American society.[162]

Consequently, we urge broad, comprehensive but well-designed comparative studies of medical care systems and their consequences at levels of the health organization, the community, the nation. Studies of the scope of that currently under the direction of the National Commission on Community Health Services are important.[163] It is our belief, however, that great benefits are to be derived from the interplay of sociological theory, exacting empirical methods, and concern for practical problems. Work in the field of medical care should be guided by this Elysian mixture.

Starting with the macrocosmic, it is time for systematic comparative studies of relations between health systems and the national societies in which they function. One tires of vitriolic attacks or unlimited praise for this national system or that, based on an individual's fleeting "visit" or disappointing work experience. It is time that such questions were considered scientifically with adequate attention to samples, measures, prior questions, and so on. Comparisons of the functioning of medical care systems themselves, as well as attitudes and relations of the public to them, are needed.

On the intra-nation level, attention to the question of health manpower is needed. What would our knowledge of child development, adolescence, and the maturation of occupational groups suggest to us, if we were to devise a plan for attracting and training 10,000 medical care researchers, planners, and administrators? How can more physicians be developed to work in settings where community and preventive aspects are fully incorporated in their work? What is the optimal number of physicians and nurses? Can a public health nurse be developed to assume the position of family health counsellor, being vacated by the fast-disappearing "family doctor"?

In line with our earlier comments on the need for social as well as technological invention, leaders might be brought together from the fields of sociology, medical care, health and medicine generally, and the general public for the purpose of defining in ideal form the features of an adequate system of medical care for a community. The problems of personnel, financing, facilities, organization, and community conditions should be considered. A system approximating this ideal might be funded and established in an "average" community. A study team could investigate the process of establishment of such a system and devise adequate measures of its effects, to be compared with the same measures taken in a "control" community of like characteristics. Granted it would be impossible to control every variable—for example, the effect of the study process and normal change in the control community. But through such a comprehensive study, we would learn many lessons.

On the intra-community level, there are several questions to be examined: *First,* there is the question of the relationship among health service agencies in a community and the need for a better understanding of the factors that inhibit or facilitate interorganizational cooperation. Some notable work on this has been done in recent months,[164] but far more needs to be known before the much-heralded regionalization and planning of health service can become realities. Particularly those factors which inhibit or facilitate the hospital's functioning as a hub of patient-care need further study. Preventive, diagnostic, treatment, and rehabilitative services are provided by hundreds of voluntary and official agencies. What affects the hospital's ability or the capacity of other health organizations, like the health department, to coordinate this wide range of services?

Second, it is important to understand the relationship between bureaucracy and individual desires, especially emotional needs. With increasing specialization, there is every likelihood that various forms of group practice will be necessary in order that the full armamentarium of medical care can be available to the individual. But availability is only one part of the receipt of care, and enough work has been done to suggest that the very people who need care most are often least likely to involve themselves in the bureaucratized form of organization. The experience in Detroit, where only 5 percent of a labor union chose a group practice as opposed to a solo practice when both were prepaid, is only the most recent bit of evidence on this score.[165] How can the bureaucratized form of care be made human enough to be desirable?[166] If bureaucracy is understood not as "red tape" but as the attempt to organize relationships for the achievement of a goal, then the basic challenge is to rationally organize the technology of modern medical care, while at the same time meeting the infinitely varying needs of individuals. Such organization must find ways of bringing medical care close to where people live, while not sacrificing technical standards.

On the intra-organizational level, there is a desperate need for intensive, comparative studies of clinics and hospitals and their organization as it affects the quality of medical care. Experts in particular medical specialties should be asked to define "good medical care," and organizational forms developed to achieve this—with adequate comparisons of either a before-and-after or a cross-organization nature. Adequate criteria for judging the quality of care will become more and more necessary in the future, so that effective comparisons can be made between different systems of medical care organization—at the agency, the community, the regional, and the national levels.

References

1. Murray Gendell and Hans L. Zetterberg, *A Sociological Almanac for the United States,* New York: The Bedminster Press, 1961.
2. Howard M. Vollmer and Donald L. Mills, "Nuclear Technology and the Professionalization of Labor," *American Journal of Sociology,* 67 (May, 1962), 690–696. See also Nelson N. Foote, "The Professionalization of Labor in Detroit," *American Journal of Sociology,* 58 (January, 1953), 371–380.
3. David Riesman, Nathan Glazer, and Reuel Denney, *The Lonely Crowd,* abridged, New York: Doubleday Anchor, 1950.

4. Arnold A. Rivin, "Your Hospital, a Center for Community Health Services," Chicago: Blue Cross Commission, 1960. See also, George Rosen, *The Specialization of Medicine,* New York: Froben Press, 1944.
5. Alex Inkeles and R. A. Bauer, *The Soviet Citizen: Daily Life in a Totalitarian Society,* Cambridge: Harvard University Press, 1959.
6. Thomas Parran, "Critique of Report" in *Medical Education and Research Needs in Maryland,* Baltimore: Committee on Medical Care, Maryland State Planning Commission, 1962, p. 113.
7. Dorothy Rice, "Public and Private Expenditures for Health and Medical Care, Fiscal Years 1928–29 to 1960–61," *Research and Statistical Note,* No. 22, September 19, 1962, U.S. Department of Health, Education and Welfare, Social Security Administration, Division of Program Research.
8. Charlotte Muller, "Economic Analysis of Medical Care in the United States," *American Journal of Public Health,* 51 (January, 1961), esp. 36–37. *Health, Education and Welfare Trends,* 1961 Edition, Washington: U.S. Department of Health, Education and Welfare, pp. 22 and 61.
9. Joseph W. Garbarino, *Health Plans and Collective Bargaining,* Berkeley: University of California Press, 1960.
10. C. E. A. Winslow, *The Conquest of Epidemic Disease,* Princeton: Princeton University Press, 1955.
11. George Rosen, *A History of Public Health,* New York: MD Publications, 1958.
12. Marquis of Landsdowne, *The Petty Papers,* London, 1927.
13. Johann Peter Frank, "The People's Misery: Mother of Diseases." Translated from the Latin, with an Introduction by Henry E. Sigerist, *Bulletin of the History of Medicine,* 9 (January, 1941), 81–100.
14. Lemuel Shattuck, *Report of the Sanitary Commission of Massachusetts 1850,* reprinted at Cambridge: Harvard University Press, 1948.
15. John Duffy, *Rudolph Matas History of Medicine in Louisiana,* 2 vols., Louisiana State University Press, 1961.
16. Henry E. Sigerist, "From Bismarck to Beveridge: Developments and Trends in Social Security Legislation," *Bulletin of the History of Medicine,* 8 (April, 1943), 365–388.
17. "Dass der groesste Teil der Krankheiten, welche entweder den vollen Lebensgenuss stoeren oder gar einen betraechtlichen Teil der Menschen vor dem natuerlichen Ziel dahinraffen nicht auf natuerlichen, sondern auf gesellschaftlichen Verhaeltnissen beruht, bedarf keines Beweises. Die medizinische Wissenschaft ist in ihbrem innersten Kern und Wesen eine soziale Wissenschaft, und solange ihr diese Bedeutung in der Wirklichkeit nicht vindiziert sein wird, wird man auch ihre Fruechte nicht geniessen, sondern sich mit der Schale und dem Schein begnuegen muessen." Written by Neumann in 1847, as quoted by Alfred Grotjahn. *Soziale Pathologie,* Berlin: August Hirschwald, 1915, p. 3.
18. George Rosen, *op. cit.*
19. Harry A. Millis and Royal E. Montgomery, *Labor's Risks and Social Insurance,* New York: McGraw-Hill, 1938, pp. 321–323.
20. James Peter Warbasse, *Medical Sociology,* New York: D. Appleton & Co., 1909.
21. William F. Ogburn, *Social Change with Respect to Culture and Original Nature,* New York: B. W. Huebsch, 1922.
22. Edgar Sydenstricker, *Health and Environment,* New York: McGraw-Hill, 1933.
23. Michael M. Davis, *Clinics, Hospitals and Health Centers,* New York: Harper and Brothers, 1927.
24. Harry H. Moore, *American Medicine and the People's Health,* New York: D. Appleton & Co., 1927.
25. I. S. Falk, C. Rufus Rorem, and Martha D. Ring, *The Costs of Medical Care,* Committee on the Costs of Medical Care, Publication No. 27 (summary volume), Chicago: University of Chicago Press, 1933.
26. Rene Sand, *Health and Human Progress,* New York: Macmillan, 1936.
27. Arthur Newsholme, *Medicine and the State,* London: George Allen and Unwin, 1932.
28. Bernhard J. Stern, *Social Factors in Medical Progress,* New York: Columbia University Press, 1927.
29. Robert S. and Helen M. Lynd, *Middletown in Transition,* New York: Harcourt, Brace, 1937.
30. James H. S. Bossard, "A Sociologist Looks at the Doctor," pp. 1–10 in *The Medical Profession and the Public,* Philadelphia: Academy of Political and Social Science, 1934.

31. L. J. Henderson, "The Patient and Physician as a Social System," *New England Journal of Medicine,* 212 (May 2, 1935), 819–823.
32. Mabel A. Elliott and Francis E. Merrill, *Social Disorganization,* New York: Harper and Brothers, 1934.
33. Michael M. Davis, "Social Medicine as a Field for Social Research," *American Journal of Sociology,* 44 (September, 1938), 274–279.
34. Milton I. Roemer (ed.), *Henry E. Sigerist on the Sociology of Medicine,* New York: MD Publications, 1960.
35. Richard H. Shryock, *The Development of Modern Medicine,* Philadelphia: University of Pennsylvania Press, 1936.
36. W. H. R. Rivers, *Medicine, Magic, and Religion,* New York: Harcourt, Brace, 1924.
37. Sumner H. Slichter, *The Turnover of Factory Labor,* New York: D. Appleton & Co., 1919.
38. Pierce Williams, *The Purchase of Medical Care Through Fixed Periodic Payment,* New York: National Bureau of Economic Research, 1932.
39. Louis S. Reed, *The Healing Cults: A Study of Sectarian Medical Practice,* Committee on the Costs of Medical Care, Publication No. 16, Chicago: University of Chicago Press, 1932. That these studies had primarily an economic focus, rather than an emphasis on social organization, was brought out by Michael Davis in a session commemorating his work at the last annual meeting of the American Sociological Association, Washington, D.C., August 29, 1962.
40. Gladys V. Swackhamer, *Choice and Change of Doctors,* New York: Committee on Research in Medical Economics, 1939.
41. U.S. Public Health Service, *Illness and Medical Care Among 2,500,000 Persons in 83 Cities, with Special Reference to Socio-Economic Factors* (a collection of 27 reprints), Washington: U.S. Government Printing Office, 1945.
42. William Beveridge, *Social Insurance and Allied Services* (American Edition, reproduced from the English Edition by arrangement with His Majesty's Stationery Office), New York: Macmillan Co., 1942.
43. Health Survey and Development Committee, *Report,* (4 vols.), Delhi, India: Government of India Press, 1946.
44. Michael M. Davis, *Medical Care for Tomorrow,* New York: Harper & Brothers, 1955. Also Franz Goldmann, "Medicine as a Social Instrument: Organization of Medical Care," *New England Journal of Medicine,* 244 (March 8, 1951), 363–370.
45. Robert Straus, "The Nature and Status of Medical Sociology," *American Sociological Review,* 22 (April, 1957), 200–204.
46. Hugh R. Leavell, "Contributions of the Social Sciences to the Solution of Health Problems," *New England Journal of Medicine,* 247 (December 4, 1952), 885–897.
47. For a classic presentation of what one might term the sociologist's code, see Robert and Helen Lynd, *op. cit.,* "Preface."
48. William Caudill, "Applied Anthropology in Medicine," pp. 771–806 in A. L. Kroeber (ed.), *Anthropology Today,* Chicago: University of Chicago Press, 1953. Oswald Hall, "Sociological Research in the Field of Medicine: Progress and Prospects," *American Sociological Review,* 16 (October, 1951), 639–645. Hugh Leavell, *op. cit.* H. E. Freeman and L. G. Reeder, "Medical Sociology: A Review of the Literature," *American Sociological Review,* 22 (February, 1957), 73–81. Ray Elling, "Die Medizinische Soziologie in den Vereinigten Staaten: Ihre Rollen and Interessen," pp. 273–293 in Rene Koenig and Margaret Toennesmann (eds.), *Probleme der Medizin-Soziologie,* Koelner Zeitschrift fuer Soziologie und Sozialpsychologie, Sonderheft 3, Koeln/Opladen: Westdeutscher Verlag, 1958. George Rosen and Edward Wellin, "A Bookshelf on the Social Sciences and Public Health," *American Journal of Public Health,* 49 (April, 1959), 441–461. George Reader and Mary Goss, "The Sociology of Medicine," pp. 229–246 in Robert K. Merton, Leonard Broom, and Leonard S. Cottrell, Jr. (eds.), *Sociology Today,* New York: Basic Books, Inc., 1959. Steven Polgar, "Health and Human Behavior: Areas of Interest Common to the Social and Medical Sciences," *Current Anthropology,* (December, 1961), 122–162.
49. Rene Koenig and Margaret Toennesmann, *op. cit.;* also Manfred Pflanz, *Sozialer Wandel und Krankheit,* Stuttgart: Ferdinand Enke Verlag, 1962. Also: R. M. Titmuss, *Essays on the "Welfare State,"* London: Allen and Unwin, 1958.
50. E. Gartly Jaco (ed.), *Patients, Physicians and Illness,* New York: The Free Press of Glencoe, Inc., 1958. Dorrian Apple, *Sociological Studies of Health and Sickness,* New York: McGraw-Hill, 1960.

51. Norman G. Hawkins, *Medical Sociology,* Springfield, Ill.: Charles Thomas, 1958.
52. *Journal of Health and Human Behavior,* Special Issue on Medical Care, 3 (Spring, 1962), George G. Reader, Special Editor.
53. U.S. Public Health Service, *Health Statistics from the U.S. National Health Survey,* a series of reports from 1957 onward, Washington: U.S. Government Printing Office.
54. Odin W. Anderson and Jacob J. Feldman, *Family Medical Costs and Voluntary Health Insurance: A Nationwide Survey,* New York: McGraw-Hill, 1956.
55. For example, Research Division, Department of National Health and Welfare, *Voluntary Medical Care Insurance: A Study of Non-Profit Plans in Canada,* Ottawa, 1954.
56. Of particular interest is a paper which points out the stronger linkage between "lower" classes and a governmental system of care even under a generally available system. Robin F. Badgley and Robert W. Hetherington, "Social Class and Patterns of Utilization of Health Services in Wheatville," paper presented to the Eighth Annual Meeting of the Canadian Public Health Association (Saskatchewan Branch), Regina, Saskatchewan, April 25, 1962.
57. B. J. Darsky, N. Sinai, and S. J. Axelrod, *Comprehensive Medical Services under Voluntary Health Insurance,* Cambridge: Harvard University Press, 1958.
58. Robert L. McNamara and Edward W. Hassinger, *Extent of Illness and Use of Health Servicies in a South Missouri County,* Columbia, Missouri: Agricultural Experiment Station, Research Bulletin 647, 1958.
59. Earl L. Koos, *The Health of Regionville,* New York: Columbia University Press, 1954.
60. L. S. Rosenfeld and A. Donabedian, "Prenatal Care in Metropolitan Boston," *American Journal of Public Health,* 48 (September, 1958), 1115–1124.
61. H. M. and A. R. Somers, *Doctors, Patients, and Health Insurance,* Washington: The Brookings Institution, 1961.
62. M. I. Roemer, "Social Science and Organized Health Services," *Human Organization,* 18 (October, 1959), 75–77.
63. Everett C. Hughes, "Dilemmas and Contradictions of Status," *American Journal of Sociology,* 50 (March, 1945), 353–359.
64. Dorrian Apple, "How Laymen Define Illness," *Journal of Health and Human Behavior,* 1 (Fall, 1960), 219–225.
65. George Reader, Lois Pratt, and M. C. Mudd, "What Patients Expect From Their Doctors," *The Modern Hospital,* 89 (July, 1957), 88–94.
66. A. B. Hollingshead and F. C. Redlich, *Social Class and Mental Illness,* New York: Wiley, 1958. See also L. Schafer and J. K. Myers, "Psychotherapy and Social Stratification: An Empirical Study of Practice in a Psychiatric Outpatient Clinic," *Psychiatry,* 17 (February, 1954), 83–93.
67. Ray Elling, Ruth Whittemore, and Morris Green, "Patient Participation in a Pediatric Program," *Journal of Health and Human Behavior,* 1 (Fall, 1960), 183–191. See further, Donald K. Ryan, *et. al.,* "Participation in a Longitudinal Study of Negro-Infants and Children," *Public Health Reports,* 75 (November, 1960), 1085–1090.
68. Eliot Freidson, *Patient's Views of Medical Practice,* New York: Russell Sage Foundation, 1961.
69. H. Jack Geiger, "Patterns of Choice and Use of Physicians by Families," paper presented at the Annual Meeting of the American Sociological Association, Washington, D. C., August 29, 1962.
70. O. L. Peterson, R. G. Spain, L. P. Andrews, and B. G. Greenberg, "An Analytical Study of North Carolina General Practice, 1953–1954," *Journal of Medical Education,* 31 (December, 1956), part 2.
71. David Pomrinse and Marcus Goldstein, "The 1959 Survey of Group Practice," *American Journal of Public Health,* 51 (May, 1961), 671–682.
72. Henry Makover, "The Quality of Medical Care: Methodology of a Survey of the Medical Groups Associated with the Health Insurance Plan of Greater New York," *American Journal of Public Health,* 41 (July, 1961), 824–832.
73. E. F. Daily and M. A. Morehead, "A Method of Evaluating and Improving the Quality of Medical Care," *American Journal of Public Health,* 46 (July, 1956), 848–854. Also E. R. Weinerman, "An Appraisal of Medical Care in Group Health Centers," *American Journal of Public Health,* 46 (March, 1956), 300–309.
74. Leonard S. Rosenfeld, "The Quality of Medical Care in Hospitals," *American Journal of Public Health,* 47 (July, 1957), 856–865.

75. Paul A. Lembcke, "Medical Auditing by Scientific Methods," *Journal of the American Medical Association,* 162 (October 13, 1956), 646–655.
76. R. S. Myers and V. N. Slee, "Medical Statistics Tell the Story at a Glance," *The Modern Hospital,* 93:3 (September, 1959), 72–75.
77. R. K. Merton, G. G. Reader, and P. L. Kendall (eds.), *The Student Physician,* Cambridge: Harvard University Press, 1957, pp. 3–79.
78. J. N. Solon, C. G. Sheps, and S. S. Lee, "Delineating Patterns of Medical Care," *American Journal of Public Health,* 50 (August, 1960), 1105–1113.
79. K. L. White, T. F. Williams, and B. G. Greenberg, "The Ecology of Medical Care," *New England Journal of Medicine,* 265 (November 2, 1961), 885–892.
80. A. J. Simon, "Social Structure of Clinics and Patient Improvement," *Administrative Science Quarterly,* 4 (September, 1959), 197–206.
81. George A. Silver, "Objectives of the Family Health Maintenance Demonstration" in *The Family Health Maintenance Demonstration,* New York: Milbank Memorial Fund, 1954. See also, George A. Silver, *et al., The Family Health Team,* Cambridge: Harvard University Press, 1962.
82. S. Taylor, *Good General Practice,* London: Oxford University Press, 1954.
83. Gordon Forsyth and R. F. L. Logan, "Studies in Medical Care: An Assessment of Some Methods" in *Towards a Measure of Medical Care,* London: Oxford University Press, 1962.
84. A comparative study of this sort was presented recently. While it suggests that patterns of medical care organization explain the apparent greater efficiency of Swedish and British health care systems, as compared with that of the United States, it does not have other variables such as cultural homogeneity of the population controlled. Nevertheless, the contribution of the study is great. See Osler L. Peterson, "Quantity and Quality of Medical Care and Health," paper presented at the Annual Meetings of the American Sociological Association, Washington, D.C., August 29, 1962.
85. Committee for the Special Research Project in the Health Insurance Plan of Greater New York, *Health and Medical Care in New York City,* Cambridge: Harvard University Press, 1957.
86. Mindel C. Sheps, "Approaches to the Quality of Hospital Care," *Public Health Reports,* 70 (September, 1955), 877–886.
87. Harvey L. Smith, "Sociological Study of Hospitals," unpublished Ph.D. dissertation, University of Chicago, 1949.
88. Albert F. Wessen, "The Social Structure of a Modern Hospital," unpublished Ph.D. dissertation, Yale University, 1950.
89. Temple Burling, Edith M. Lentz, and Robert N. Wilson, *The Give and Take in Hospitals,* New York: G. P. Putnam's Sons, 1956.
90. Renee C. Fox, *Experiment Perilous: Physicians and Patients Facing the Unknown,* Glencoe, Ill.: The Free Press, 1959.
91. Basil S. Georgopoulos and Floyd C. Mann, *The Community General Hospital,* New York: Macmillan, 1962. This study is being followed up at the Survey Research Center, University of Michigan by Jack Kirscht.
92. Ivan Belknap, *Human Problems of a State Mental Hospital,* New York: McGraw-Hill, 1956. M. Greenblatt, D. J. Levinson, and R. Williams (eds.), *The Patient and the Mental Hospital,* Glencoe, Ill.: Free Press, 1957. William Caudill, *The Psychiatric Hospital as a Small Society,* Cambridge: Harvard University Press, 1957. Erving Goffman, "The Characteristics of Total Institutions," pp. 43–93 in *Symposium on Preventive and Social Psychiatry*. Washington: Walter Reed Army Institute of Research, 1958.
93. Esther Lucile Brown, *Studies in Interpersonal Relationships in a Therapeutic Setting,* New York: Russell Sage Foundation, 1951.
94. Esther Lucile Brown, *Newer Dimensions of Patient Care:* Part I—"The Use of the Physical and Social Environment of the General Hospital for Therapeutic Purposes," New York: Russell Sage Foundation, 1961. Part II—"Improving Staff Motivation and Competence in the General Hospital," 1962.
95. Ivar E. Bery, "Role, Personality and Social Structures: A Study of Nursing in a General Hospital," unpublished Ph.D. dissertation, Harvard University, 1960. Ronald G. Corwin, "The Professional Employee: A Study of Conflicts in Nursing Roles," *American Journal of Sociology,* 66 (May, 1961), 604–615. Norman H. Berkowitz and Warren G. Bennis, "Interaction Patterns in Formal Service-Oriented Organizations," *Administrative Science Quarterly,* 6 (June, 1961),

25–30. Joan S. Dodge, "Nurses' Sense of Adequacy and Attitudes Toward Keeping Patients Informed," *Journal of Health and Human Behavior,* 2 (Fall, 1961), 213–216.

96. Frederick L. Bates, "Authority and Decision-making in Voluntary Hospitals," Ithaca, New York: Sloan Institute of Hospital Administration, Graduate School of Business and Public Administration, Cornell University, 1959 (processed). On another administrative concern, see Seymour Warkov, "Certain Aspects of Organizational Effectiveness: The Problem of Irregular Discharge from the Tuberculosis Service of Veterans Administration Hospitals," unpublished Ph.D. dissertation, Yale University, 1958.

97. Mary E. Goss, "Physicians in Bureaucracy: A Case Study of Professional Pressures on Organizational Roles," unpublished Ph.D. dissertation, Columbia University, 1959. For other analyses, see Oswald Hall, "Half Medical Man, Half Administrator: An Occupational Dilemma," *Canadian Public Administration,* 2 (December, 1959), 185–194. Robert N. Wilson, "The Physician's Changing Hospital Role," *Human Organization,* 18 (Winter, 1959–60), 177–183.

98. Edward Levine and Samuel Wright, "New Ways to Measure Personnel Turnover in Hospitals," *Hospitals,* 30 (October, 1957), 53. On nurse-turnover, see Joan S. Dodge, "Why Nurses Leave and What To Do About It," *The Modern Hospital,* 94 (May, 1960), 116–120. For a study of other aspects of a special category of persons, see John R. Pope, "Psychological Testing of Dietary Personnel," *Hospital Progress,* 41 (April, 1960), 106–114.

99. Of some relevance here is Irving Babow, "Minority Group Integration in Hospitals: A Sample Survey," *Hospitals,* 35 (February, 1961), 47–48 ff.

100. Rose L. Coser, *Life in the Ward,* East Lansing, Michigan: Michigan State University Press, 1962, p. 147.

101. Amitai Etzioni, "New Directions in the Study of Organizations and Society," *Social Research,* 27 (Summer, 1960), 223–228.

102. Eliot Freidson and Jacob J. Feldman, "The Public Looks at Hospitals," New York: Health Information Foundation, 1958. United Hospital Fund of New York, "Public's Attitudes Toward Hospitals in New York City and Their Financing, May, 1958," New York: *The Fund,* 1958. Milton I. Roemer and Rodney F. White, "Community Attitudes Towards Hospitals," *Hospital Management,* 89 (January and February, 1960), two parts.

103. Richard Blum, *Hospitals and Patient Dissatisfaction, a Study of Factors Associated with Malpractice Rates in Hospitals,* California Medical Association, Medical Review and Advisory Board, 1958.

104. Oswald Hall, "Types of Medical Careers," *American Journal of Sociology,* 55 (November, 1949), 243–253.

105. David N. Solomon, "Career Contingencies of Chicago Physicians," unpublished Ph.D. dissertation, University of Chicago, 1952.

106. Stan Lieberson, "Ethnic Groups and the Practice of Medicine," *American Sociological Review,* 23 (October, 1958), 542–549.

107. Dennis C. McElrath, "Perspective and Participation of Physicians in Prepaid Group Practice," *American Sociological Review,* 26 (August, 1961), 596–607.

108. James Coleman, Elihu Katz, and Herbert Menzel, "The Diffusion of an Innovation among Physicians," *Sociometry,* 20 (December, 1957), 253–270.

109. Erwin L. Linn, "Drug Therapy, Milieu Change, and Release from a Mental Hospital," *AMA Archives of Neurology and Psychiatry,* 81 (June, 1959), 785–796.

110. M. I. Roemer and E. A. Wilson, *Organized Health Services in a County of the United States,* Washington: U.S. Public Health Service, Publication 197, 1952.

111. Nicholus Babchuk, *et al.,* "Men and Women in Community Agencies: A Note on Power and Prestige," *American Sociological Review,* 25 (June, 1960), 399–403.

112. Sol Levine and Paul White, "Exchange as a Framework for Interorganizational Relationships," *Administrative Science Quarterly,* 5 (March, 1961), 583–601.

113. A preliminary analysis of internal factors related to support is given in Ray Elling and Milton Roemer, "Determinants of Community Support," *Hospital Administration,* 6 (Summer, 1961), 17–34. A more complete presentation of the theory and method of the study and a comparison of support received by voluntary non-denominational and local governmental hospitals is given in Ray Elling and Sandor Halebsky, "Organizational Differentiation and Support," *Administrative Science Quarterly,* 6 (September, 1961), 185–209.

114. Ray Elling, "The Hospital Support Game in Urban Center," to appear in Eliot Freidson (ed.),

The Hospital in Modern Society, New York: Macmillan (Free Press), 1963. See also L. Vaughn Blankenship, "Organizational Support and Community Leadership in Two New York State Communities," unpublished Ph.D. dissertation, Cornell University, 1962.

115. An important study has just appeared, on behaviors and attitudes of professionals and others in several rural hospitals with regard to "regionalization." Walter J. McNerney and Donald C. Riedel, *Regionalization and Rural Health Care, an Experiment in Three Communities,* Ann Arbor: The University of Michigan, Graduate School of Business Administration, Bureau of Hospital Administration, 1962. See also Leonard S. Rosenfeld and Henry B. Makover, *The Rochester Regional Hospital Council,* Cambridge: Harvard University Press, 1956.
116. See note 114.
117. Pearl Bierman, "Meeting the Health Needs of Low-Income Families," *The Annals of the American Academy of Political and Social Science,* 337 (September, 1961), 103–113.
118. U.S. Public Health Service, *Health Services for American Indians,* Washington: U.S. Government Printing Office, U.S. Public Health Service, Publication 531, 1957.
119. Louis S. Reed, "Medical Care and Rehabilitation under the New York Workmen's Compensation Program," *American Journal of Public Health,* 50 (September, 1960), 1264–1273.
120. Commission on Chronic Illness, *Chronic Illness in the United States* (4 vols.), Cambridge: Harvard University Press, 1952–1959.
121. Joint Commission on Mental Illness and Health, *Action for Mental Health,* New York: Basic Books, 1961. The already cited work by Hollingshead and Redlich is a landmark in the field of medical care for mental illness. Also of interest here is the review by John Clausen, *Sociology and the Field of Mental Health,* New York: Russell Sage Foundation, 1956.
122. Everett C. Hughes, *Men and Their Work,* Glencoe, Ill.: Free Press, 1958. Edward Gross, *Work and Society,* New York: Thomas Y. Crowell, 1958.
123. A. M. Carr-Saunders, "Professions" in E. B. A. Seligman and A. Johnson (eds.), *Encyclopedia of Social Sciences,* New York: Macmillan, 1951, V. 11–12, 476–480.
124. Rue Bucher and Anselm Strauss, "Professions in Process," *American Journal of Sociology,* 66 (January, 1961), 325–334.
125. This view is presented in William J. Goode, "Community Within a Community: The Professions," *American Sociological Review,* 22 (April, 1957), 194–200.
126. Mary F. Arnold, "Perception of Professional Role Activities in the Local Health Department," *Public Health Reports,* 77 (January, 1962), 80–88.
127. Morris Rosenberg, with the assistance of Edward A. Suchman and Rose K. Goldsen, *Occupations and Values,* Glencoe, Ill.: The Free Press, 1957. R. K. Merton, G. Reader, and P. L. Kendall (eds.), *op. cit.* Howard S. Becker, *et al., Boys in White: Student Culture in Medical School,* Chicago: University of Chicago Press, 1961. E. L. Quarantelli, "The Career Choice Patterns of Dental Students," *Journal of Health and Human Behavior,* 2 (Summer, 1961), 124–132.
128. R. Coker, *et al.,* "Public Health as Viewed by the Medical Student," *American Journal of Public Health,* 49 (May, 1959), 601–609. Also, R. Coker, *et al.,* "Patterns of Influence: Medical School Faculty Members and the Values and Specialty Interests of Medical Students," *The Journal of Medical Education,* 35 (June, 1960), 518–527.
129. Oliver Garceau, *The Political Life of the American Medical Association,* Cambridge: Harvard University Press, 1941. See also D. R. Hyde and P. Wolff, "The American Medical Association: Power, Purpose, and Politics in Organized Medicine," *Yale Law Journal,* 63 (May, 1954), 951–976. One humorous but very important article compares the organizing behavior of different occupational groups: Melvin Levine, "Professors, Physicians, and Unionism," *AAUP Bulletin,* 48 (September, 1962), 272–276.
130. Many of these problems are dealt with in Sigmund Nosow and William H. Form (eds.), *Man, Work and Society, A Reader in the Sociology of Occupations,* New York: Basic Books, 1962.
131. The recent passage of the Manpower Training Act underlines the problem of technological employment and obsolescence.
132. Stuart Adams, "Trends in Occupational Origins of Physicians," *American Sociological Review,* 18 (August, 1953), 404–409.
133. See note 127. Perhaps of special relevance to the topic of this paper is a study that examined differences in orientation toward questions of medical care organization among senior and freshman medical students. In the particular school under study, Seniors were more "liberal" in

orientation than Freshmen. To the extent that this represented change while in school and not a long term trend in entrants, it appeared to come about through a process of faculty, peer-group influence. The value climate of this school was such that the liberal faculty were the most preferred by the students; the liberal students (as measured by a conservatism-liberalism scale) were most chosen as hypothetical representatives of the school and these same students received the best grades and the most academic honors. R. H. Elling, "Outlook on Medical Organization Among First and Fourth Year Medical Students," unpublished M.A. thesis, University of Chicago, 1955.

134. Oswald Hall, "The Stages of a Medical Career," *American Journal of Sociology,* 53 (March, 1948), 327–336.
135. Werner Cohn, "Social Status and the Ambivalence Hypothesis," *American Sociological Review,* 25 (August, 1960), 508–513.
136. Editorial, "Applicants for Medical Training," *Journal of Medical Education,* 35 (October, 1960), 949–950.
137. William A. Glaser, "Doctors and Politics," *American Journal of Sociology,* 66 (November, 1960), 230–245.
138. E. C. Hughes, H. M. Hughes and I. Deutscher, *Twenty Thousand Nurses Tell Their Story,* Philadelphia: J. B. Lippincott, 1958.
139. George Devereaux and F. R. Weiner, "Occupational Status of Nurses," *American Sociological Review,* 15 (October, 1950), 628–634.
140. John H. Rohrer, *et al., Nursing Services in a Premature Infant Center,* New Orleans: Tulane University Press, 1953.
141. Rhoda Goldstein, "The Professional Nurse in the Hospital Bureaucracy," unpublished Ph.D. dissertation, University of Chicago, 1954.
142. R. W. Habenstein and E. A. Christ, *Professionalizer, Traditionalizer, Utilizer,* Columbia, Mo.: University of Missouri Press, 1955.
143. Hans O. Mauksch, "Nursing Dilemmas in the Organization of Patient Care," *Nursing Outlook,* 5 (January, 1957), 31–33.
144. Jack V. Buerkle, "Patterns of Socialization, Role Conflict, and Leadership among Nurses," *Sociology and Social Research,* 44 (Nov.–Dec., 1959), 100–105.
145. D. D. Stewart and C. H. Needham, *The Operating Room Nurse,* Fayetteville: University of Arkansas, 1955.
146. Charles V. Willie, "The Social Class of Patients that Public Health Nurses Prefer to Serve," *American Journal of Public Health,* 50 (August, 1960), 1126–1136.
147. Marion Pearsall, "Supervision—A Nursing Dilemma," *Nursing Outlook,* 9 (September, 1961), 91–92.
148. Milton Greenblatt, "The Nurse in Research," *Nursing Research,* 1 (February, 1953), 36–40.
149. I. Deutscher, *et al., Formal Education and the Process of Professionalization: A Study of Student Nurses,* Kansas City, Mo.: Community Studies, Inc., 1958. H. W. Martin and F. E. Katz, "The Professional School as a Molder of Motivations," *Journal of Health and Human Behavior,* 2 (Summer, 1961), 106–112.
150. D. M. More and Nathan Kohn, Jr., "Some Motives for Entering Dentistry," *American Journal of Sociology,* 66 (July, 1960), 48–53.
151. E. L. Quarantelli, "Attitudes of Dental Students Toward Specialization and Research," *Journal of the American College of Dentists,* 27 (June, 1960), 101–107.
152. Louis Kreisberg and B. R. Treiman, "Factors Affecting the Public Attitudes and Beliefs about Dentists," Paper presented at the Annual Meeting of the American Sociological Association, New York, 1960.
153. E. F. Barthuli, "Occupational Attitudes of Dentists," *Sociology and Social Research,* 20 (July–August, 1936), 548–551.
154. M. I. Roemer, "Medical Care Administration in the United States: Personnel, Needs and Goals," *American Journal of Public Health,* 52 (January, 1962), 8–19. Robert J. Mowitz, "Training Health Administrators," *Public Health Reports,* 75 (November, 1960), 1062–1066. Editorial, "Hospital Administration as a Career," *The Hospital,* London (February, 1961), 93–94. Frederic C. LeRocker, "How Good Are Master's Degree Programs," *The Modern Hospital,* 97 (December, 1961), 87 ff. G. Hartman and S. Levey, "Doctoral Study in an Emerging Profession," *Journal of Medical Education,* 4 (March, 1962), 296–301.

155. Peter K. New, "The Osteopathic Students: A Study in Dilemma," pp. 413–421 in E. G. Jaco (ed.), *Patients, Physicians and Illness,* Glencoe, Ill.: Free Press, 1958.
156. Thelma A. McCormick, "The Druggists' Dilemma: Problems of a Marginal Occupation," *American Journal of Sociology,* (January, 1956), 308–315.
157. Walter I. Wardwell, "A Marginal Professional Role: The Chiropractor," *Social Forces,* 30 (March, 1952), 339–348.
158. Dan C. Lortie, "Anesthesia: From Nurse's Work to Medical Specialty," pp. 405–412 in E. G. Jaco (ed.), *Patients, Physicians and Illness,* Glencoe, Ill.: Free Press, 1958.
159. Eliot Freidson, "Specialties Without Roots: The Utilization of New Services," *Human Organization,* 19 (Fall, 1959), 112–116.
160. Thomas Parran, "Committee on Professional Education," *American Journal of Public Health,* 51 (March, 1961), 471–473. The research is entitled, "The Joint Committee Study of Education for Public Health." It is sponsored by the American Public Health Association, the Association of Schools of Public Health, and the State and Territorial Health Officers Association, with representation from the United States Public Health Service and the Department of Health and Welfare in Canada. The staff of the study are William P. Shepard, Director, Ray H. Elling, Field Director, and Walter F. Grimes, Research Associate.
161. "Strengthening the Behavioral Sciences," The White House, Washington, D.C., April 20, 1962, U.S. Government Printing Office, 1962 (pamphlet).
162. Willard C. Rappleye, M.D., President, Josiah Macy, Jr., Foundation, "Labor, Management, and Medicine," presented at a meeting of the Section on Occupational Medicine, New York Academy of Medicine, April 5, 1962.
163. American Public Health Association, *This is the News,* (May, 1962), 1–2. Consult National Commission on Community Health Services, 1790 Broadway, New York 19, New York, Dean W. Roberts, Executive Director.
164. Eugene Litwak and Lydia F. Hylton, "Interorganizational Analysis," *Administrative Science Quarterly,* 6 (March, 1962), 395–420. R. H. Elling, "The Hospital Support Game," *op. cit.* Sol Levine and Paul White, *op. cit.* Walter J. McNerney and Donald C. Riedel, *op. cit.*
165. However, in the few companies where union members had chosen the group practice pattern, the selection of this pattern in the second year rose strikingly.
166. An associated problem is how to make publicly controlled bureaucracies more attractive as places of work for health personnel so that second-rate individuals are not giving the care through these organizations. An empirical study of the problem is given by Jack Elinson, "Physician's Dilemma in Puerto Rico," *Journal of Health and Human Behavior,* Special Issue on Medical Care, 3 (Spring, 1962), pp. 14–20.

30

Evolution of Health Planning

Systematic planning of health services to better meet the needs of the American population became formalized and deliberate on the eve of the Great Depression of 1929. Since the landmark work of the Committee on the Costs of Medical Care (1928–32), several other broad overview studies have been done, but most health planning has been focused on specific sectors of the health field.

A review of the development of these more focused planning efforts was prepared in 1974, categorized with respect to the planning of health facilities, health care financing, public health preventive services, health manpower, and health care regulation. The concept of "comprehensive health planning" in 1966 was a culmination of this movement, which has since 1974 been carried still further through federal and state legislation. The text that follows was the opening presentation in a "Colloquium on Health Service Planning and Administration," sponsored by the Yale University School of Medicine and several Connecticut health agencies.

TO TRACE THE background of our current scene in comprehensive health planning, it is worth recalling that until barely a decade ago planning outside of very narrow or local sectors had a dangerous socialistic flavor. The Soviet Union had launched the first 5-year plan for its total social and economic development in 1928, and this—along with a persistent laissez faire economic philosophy—was enough to scare other nations away from the concept for nearly 20 years. It was only after World War II that most countries, and expecially the developing ones, found it reasonable to design broad step-by-step plans for their general socio-economic development.

Health Planning Background

Perhaps it is more than coincidence that 1928 also marks the date when the first broad-scale planning of health services was started in the United States. This was the year when several foundations joined forces to launch a 5-year study of the total problems of health services in America. The name of the Committee on the Costs of Medical Care was much more restricted than the scope of its work

Chapter 30 was issued previously only as a processed document, in the *Proceedings of the Colloquium on Health Service Planning and Administration* (New Haven, 1975). It is published here for the first time.

(perhaps intentionally), since it encompassed not only medical care costs, but also problems of health manpower, facilities, public health, modes of organization or delivery, and just about every type of health issue that occupies the attention of comprehensive health planning (CHP) agencies today. The CCMC's final report, *Medical Care for the American People,* was issued in October 1932, and happily was reprinted a generation later, in 1970, by the federal Department of Health, Education and Welfare.[1]

It was after World War II, in 1948, that the Federal Security Administrator, Oscar Ewing, reported to President Truman on *The Nation's Health—A Ten Year Program.*[2] In 1952, on a more thorough basis, the President's Commission on the Health Needs of the Nation produced its 5-volume report on *Building America's Health.*[3] The next effort of comparable scope was that of the National Commission on Community Health Services, which between 1962 and 1966 issued some 10 volumes making planning recommendations on every aspect of health needs and services in America.[4]

All these may be considered comprehensive health planning efforts in the United States prior to the enactment of P.L. 89-749 in November 1966. They all served as catalytic agents toward some social action in the public or the private sector of health or both. These actions, however, have tended to be in circumscribed categories of the health field, and I think we will get a better appreciation of the developments leading up to our current scene if we consider the background as consisting of several more or less concurrent paths of health action. To oversimplify a bit we can classify these paths under five main headings: health facilities, health financing, public health programs, health manpower, and social controls.

Health Facility Planning

Perhaps it is because buildings are such permanent things and they affect health affairs for many years after that the earliest planning efforts seem to have been made in health facility planning. Just after World War I, the New York Academy of Medicine made a study of hospital bed needs in the nation's largest city. Basing their calculations on available morbidity data, they estimated that for every four persons sick on an average day, one should be occupying a hospital bed. On this basis, they reported in 1920 that about 5.0 beds per 1,000 population were needed—and, indeed, this was about the number that New York had. For the time being, it was concluded that no more construction was needed, although as we know, additional hospitals were built as transportation improved and people came to New York from miles around for their care.

It is of interest that, as part of the CCMC studies, one was devoted to an estimate of the population's need for hospital beds. As in the New York Academy of Medicine study, they started with the volume of morbidity, based on a nationwide household survey. Then, a committee of doctors estimated the number of days of hospitalization, according to 1930 policies, that would be required for this sickness load. Assuming a 90 percent hospital occupancy, they concluded that 4.62 beds per 1,000 would be adequate. Fifteen years later, despite the changes in both medical science and the rates of morbidity, the standard of 4.5 to 5.0 beds per 1,000 was written into national hospital legislation.

With the Depression striking in 1929, hospital construction stopped, but was resumed as part of the Public Works Administration of the New Deal in the 1934–40 period. This required some planning, and PWA funds, intended primarily to provide jobs, added to the supply of municipal, county, and state government hospitals throughout the land. Then with World War II, hospital construction again stopped, but a recognition of the need for "post-war planning" gave birth to the National Commission on Hospital Care.[5] From these distinct planning efforts there emerged the information background that led to enactment of the Hill-Burton National Hospital Survey and Construction Act in 1946. It is notable that the phrase "hospital survey" was written into the very name of the law; studies of each state's hospital supply, its unmet needs according to stipulated standards, and its priorities were required as a condition for federal construction grants.

This was clearly planning legislation in the hospital sector. Amendments to the law over the years have reflected the perception of changing needs for health facilities, including "diagnostic and treatment centers" in 1954, and grants for hospital planning in regional or local areas in 1964.[6] The latter amendment clearly paved the way to the CHP Law of 1966 and, indeed, the funds allotted under this provision were converted to support of CHP activities in December, 1967. Also at the state level, after New York State broke the ice with the Metcalf-McCloskie Law of 1964 requiring state approval for all new hospital construction, based on proof of social need for beds, similar "certificate of need" laws were passed in about 25 other states, putting some teeth in the control of hospital construction, whether government-subsidized or not.

Health Care Financing Planning

The state workmen's compensation legislation starting in 1910 and reaching all the states by 1950 constituted planning in the sector of paying for the costs—in earnings lost and medical care—of work-related injuries. As early as 1915, similar bills were introduced in several state legislatures to provide insurance to workers for general medical care, although in the atmosphere of World War I, none of them passed.

The 1920s were silent in the health care financing sector, but with the birth of the New Deal, the Federal Emergency Relief Administration (FERA) put the first federal money into medical care for the poor and paved the way to the public assistance provisions of the Social Security Act of 1935. Those provisions certainly involved planning for more adequate health care of the poor, with amendments successively over the years up to the Title XIX Medicaid program of 1965.

For the self-supporting population, the original planning of the Social Security Act had contemplated a title on health care insurance, but in the interest of avoiding a battle (that might jeopardize the whole Act) it was not included. Instead Titles V and VI provided for federal grants to the states for general public health and for maternal and child health services. Only four years later, however, Senator Wagner introduced in Congress the first National Health Insurance Bill, which would have offered grants to the states to help them develop state health insurance plans. Hardly was this introduced in 1939, when Hitler marched on Poland, World War II began, and social legislation took a back seat for several years.

The Second Front was not yet opened at Normandy Beach in 1944, when as noted earlier, "post-war planning" began in many sectors of American life. Among these was health insurance, and in 1943, the first version of a new National Health Insurance and Public Health Act was again put forward by Senator Wagner, along with Senator Murray and Congressman Dingell. This was an omnibus bill with provisions for subsidizing hospital construction, medical education, strengthening public health services, and other health programs. It also provided social insurance for general medical care. Over the next six or eight years, modified versions of the Wagner-Murray-Dingell Bill were proposed, and in 1946, it was one section on hospital construction that was separately enacted as the Hill-Burton Law.

Hearings on these bills brought forth a storm of opposition, especially from the American Medical Association and the insurance industry. Though no bill was ever reported out of Committee and brought to a Congressional vote, there is no doubt that the debate itself accomplished a great deal of good; by serving as a "threat" of government action, it furnished a powerful goad for the expansion of voluntary health insurance. The Blue Cross plans, sponsored by hospitals, the Blue Shield plans, sponsored by medical societies, and the commercial insurance companies pushed the sale of their insurance products like never before. It was a race against time, and by 1961, the number of Americans covered with at least hospitalization insurance had spiralled up to 135,000,000 from 24,000,000 in 1943.[7] This was really voluntary planning for the social financing of hospital-based medical care on a grand scale.

By the late 1950s, however, it became obvious that the weakest health insurance coverage applied to a sector of the population with the highest volume of sickness and usually meager financial resources: the aged. Since most voluntary health insurance was tied to employment, those who were retired usually lost their protection, quite aside from the fact that many insurance carriers specifically barred coverage of persons after age 65. And so there began another seven or eight years of controversy on health insurance—first limited to hospital care and then extended to a wide range of benefits—for the aged alone. Despite the revival by the private medical profession of the awesome spectre of "socialized medicine," in July, 1965, Title XVIII was added to the Social Security Act, providing for a broad scope of medical, institutional, and home care services for the aged. In my view, despite various deficiencies, this law, soon dubbed "Medicare" by the newspapers, constituted a major breakthrough in planned public financing of medical services for the 10 percent of our population with the heaviest illness burden.

It was only to be expected that this action would lead to pressures for extending social insurance protection to the rest of the population. With Medicare and Medicaid injecting billions of new dollars into the medical market place, without a commensurate increase in health manpower resources, prices were bound to rise. Even if they hadn't—at about twice the rate of the general cost-of-living index—the renewed introduction of bills for national health insurance would probably have occurred. Within five years, Senator Kennedy introduced the "Health Security Act of 1970" and by 1973, at least a dozen proposals for national health insurance, stemming from all points on the political spectrum, were in the Congressional hopper. While the debate continues to this moment, it seems generally agreed that within the next year or two, the United States will cease to be alone among the world's industrialized countries without a system of social insurance for general medical care. That dubious distinction was shared with Australia until just last August, when a law was passed to replace that country's program of subsidized voluntary insurance with a universal scheme providing broad benefits.

It is surely no accident that the CHP Law was enacted barely a year after Medicare, but before discussing this we should take a glimpse at the third path of development leading to the current health planning scene.

Public Health Services Planning

In a sense all public health activity, from the earliest medieval efforts to quarantine towns against the plague, represents planning. On a national scale in the United States, however, we may look upon the Chamberlain-Kahn Act of 1918, authorizing federal grants to the states for venereal disease control, as the first national planning action to tackle a specific disease. The appropriations for this purpose soon ended, as did those for maternal and child health services under the Sheppard-Towner Act of 1921, under the conservative federal philosophy of the 1920s. It took the Depression and the Social Security Act of 1935, as we have seen, to reinstate federal grants for various public health purposes. Although these included medical care for crippled children, the emphasis was clearly on disease control through prevention.

In most of these grant programs, it is significant that the State Health Departments were required to submit a "state plan" on how the money would be spent. Over the years, additional categorical grants were added—for industrial hygiene, for tuberculosis, for cancer control, for mental hygiene, for "services to the chronically ill,'' and other purposes. The very multiplicity of these grants, each with its own requirements and standards, was one of the stimuli for the CHP Law of 1966.

In the non-official sector, a major national planning effort took place under the auspices of the American Public Health Association, culminating in Haven Emerson's *Local Health Units for the Nation* in 1945.[8] This was a master plan, if there ever was one, to blanket the nation with local health departments of adequate strength to offer the ''basic six'' community health services—communicable disease control, environmental sanitation, maternal and child health, vital statistics, health education, and laboratory services. By combining counties of small population, it was considered feasible to cover 3,100 counties with 1,200 health jurisdictions. While there were plenty of criticisms of the restricted scope of public health services proposed, the concept of multi-county health units had a real impact on subsequent developments. Another integrative planning movement that gained momentum after World War II was the organization of hundreds of local ''health and welfare councils'' in cities and counties, not only for voluntary fund-raising but also for coordination of countless categorical agencies and programs.

Still another component of the public health planning path was the movement for an integrated physical locale for public health activities. In 1920, the British Consultative Council on Medical and Allied Services, chaired by Lord Dawson of Penn, issued its report recommending a network of ''primary health centres'' as the places from which all organized preventive service, as well as primary care from general practitioners, would be offered.[9] A similar idea almost became law in New York State under Health Commissioner Biggs a few years later and was propounded also in California by Los Angeles Health Officer Pomeroy. Not until the 1930s did health centers take shape on any broad scale, and then only for preventively oriented Health Department services. It took the urban riots of the 1960s to produce the ''neighborhood health centers,'' with comprehensive medical care for the poor, in the United States, and other developments to yield several hundred integrated treatment and prevention centers in Britain. These surely constitute a kind of physical planning for delivery of comprehensive ambulatory services, which we see spreading throughout the nation and the world every day.

Health Manpower Planning

National or even statewide planning of the output of health manpower came somewhat later than planning in other sectors of the health field. The Flexner Report of 1910 did, indeed, have an effect on the output of doctors, but this was incidental to its objectives of improving quality of medical schools, which we can examine later. The education of doctors, nurses, pharmacists, or other health personnel, however, was long regarded as a matter to be settled by the free market. As long as nurses were needed, for example, hospitals would train them, and similarly for colleges or other training institutions for all the classes of health professionals.

The first national overview of the social need for doctors in the United States was taken by Joseph W. Mountin and his colleagues in the U.S. Public Health Service in 1949. By using the simple planning technique of expecting the level of physician-supply actually achieved by the upper half of the states to be reached everywhere, he estimated a shortage of 17,400 doctors by 1960; if the best fourth of the states set the standard, the deficiency would be 45,000.[10] It is noteworthy, however, that the first federal legislative action to assist in the planned training of health personnel applied principally to manpower outside the open marketplace of private medical care. The Health Amendments Act of 1956 was principally for the training of professional public health personnel.[11] A whole series of federal grant programs for strengthening the training of nurses and other health workers soon followed, but the world of medical school subsidies was not entered until 1963. Gradually, governmental support for the education of doctors and dentists increased on both federal and state levels, as consensus was achieved between government and the American Medical Association that the nation did, indeed, face a shortage of physicians. The Bane Report on *Physicians for a Growing America,* appearing in 1959, was a crucial planning document demonstrating the need for further governmental support of medical education.[12]

Beyond the question of numbers, the better adaptation of medical educational content to the needs of society was explored in the early 1960s by the Association of American Medical Colleges, and in 1965 *Planning for Medical Progress through Education* by Lowell T. Coggeshall appeared.[13] While covering scores of topics, the thrust of this planning document was to increase AAMC influence in modernizing both the substance and methods of training doctors. Another broad-scale planning effort in this field was the report of the *National Advisory Commission on Health Manpower* in 1967.[14] Among its many recommendations was an emphasis on the need for new types of allied health worker and the importance of better organization of health services as essential to the optimal use of all types of health manpower. About the same time came the Millis Report, with its emphasis on the great need for more general practitioners or family doctors.[15]

Numerous other planning efforts have been undertaken regarding nursing, dentistry, pharmacy, and almost every class of health manpower which time does not permit us to review. It is quite evident now, however, that the great ferment in the health manpower field throughout the nation today, in training nurse practitioners and physician assistants, in promoting a new specialty of Family Medicine, in modifying and shortening educaton for the specialties, comes as a result of these planning efforts. The Health Manpower Act that passed the U.S. Senate recently contains provisions that would not have been dreamed of in the previous decade—such as those requiring many medical graduates to serve in areas of doctor shortage or limiting the numbers of specialists trained in various fields.

Planning for Greater Controls of Health Service

Finally we may look at the health planning path which, in a sense, has been more complicated by obstacles and traps than any other—the movement to improve or protect the quality of health care and to control its costs. The founding of the American Medical Association in 1847 was a planning effort to upgrade the quality of medical practice, although the first effective state medical licensure laws were not enacted until after the Civil War 20 years later.[16] Certification of the specialties came much later, starting with ophthalmology in 1916 which, as Rosemary Stevens has so well shown, grew mainly out of competition from the optometrists.[17] In time, specialty certification undoubtedly represented social planning on a national, though nongovernmental, level for quality assurance in medical care.

Equivalent efforts in planning for improved hospital standards, under the sponsorship of the American College of Surgeons in 1918, met great resistance at first; not until 1952, after state hospital licensure laws had been virtually mandated by the Hill-Burton Act, did the Joint Commission on Accreditation of Hospitals take shape.[18] The hospital accreditation movement, also nongovernmental, has had great influence in upgrading the standards of medical work in American hospitals which, by comparison with European, were rather free and easy.

Most of the planned controls over the quality and costs of health service have probably come as an appendage to categorical programs paying for medical care. The crippled children's programs administered originally by the Children's Bureau set rigorous standards for participating doctors and hospitals, as did this Bureau's later Emergency Maternity and Infant Care (EMIC) program for servicemen's families during World War II. Some, but not all, voluntary health insurance plans scrutinize claims for the propriety of the service rendered, in addition to the charges, as do governmental welfare medical assistance programs (Medicaid) and the fiscal intermediaries under Medicare. In the insurance field the "medical foundation" model of "health maintenance organization" (HMO) counts heavily on careful scrutiny of doctor's bills as the way to control costs of comprehensive care under individual practice fee-for-service patterns. The most recent chapter in this story is the PSRO (professional standard review organization) amendment to Medicare and Medicaid which, despite the current controversy, will eventually establish peer review of medical care quality and costs as a routine feature of our health care system.

The HMO idea itself, formalized in a Presidential "Health Strategy Message" of February, 1971, was another approach to cost containment. "Prepaid group practice" and "comprehensive health cooperatives" had been operating under consumer and other sponsorships for half a century or more. Since they modified customary patterns of both medical service and financing they were generally regarded as social deviants; compared with the "Blue" and commercial insurance plans their aggregate enrollment was small. But the spiralling of medical costs in the late 1960s and the flexibility of the HMO concept, with an attractive new label, suddenly converted it to fashionable respectability.[19] Health maintenance organizations, under both individual fee-practice and salaried group practice models, were promoted by the federal government several years before the HMO Act of December 1973 authorized funds and defined standards. From a planning perspective, HMOs may be regarded as mini-systems of comprehensive health service in which local initiative and profit incentives induce local planning with minimal government intervention.

The whole hospital regionalization movement may also be regarded as a planned effort to promote quality services.[20] The objective was to assure patients living anywhere of the quality of service that their illness required, either by arranging referrals from peripheral to central facilities, consultations in the opposite direction, or the upgrading of service quality in the smaller hospitals. From the pioneering of the Bingham Associates program in Maine in the 1930s and the Commonwealth Fund program around Rochester, New York, in the 1940s up to the Regional Medical Program for Heart Disease, Cancer, and Stroke (RMP) in the 1960s, regionalization has constituted geographic planning of technology on an efficient and rational basis. The enactment of the RMP law just a few months after Medicare surely meant that Congress wished to see some planning actions for quality of care of the three major diseases killing older people, as well as a planned system for paying their medical and hospital bills.

This sketchy review of the background of health planning in America is far from complete. National surveys of illness, starting with the first official one in 1935 and becoming regularized as the Continuing National Health Survey in 1957, are surely instruments for planning. So are the periodic inventories of the nation's hospitals by the American Hospital Association and of physicians by the American Medical Association. Comparable surveys of psychiatric clinics by the National Institute for Mental Health, of occupational health units by the National Industrial Conference Board, of HMOs by the Group Health Association of America, and others provide essential data for planning.

Is there anything new and different, then, about the comprehensive health planning movement which got its legislative start in 1966, and which this conference is exploring in depth? I think the answer is "Yes—in several respects."

Comprehensive Health Planning Today

First, I would say, is the concept of comprehensiveness. As our review of the last 50 years or so has illustrated, the vast majority of planning efforts have been within distinct sectors of the health field. Progress has surely come from these efforts, but there are obvious interdependencies which require a total system approach—easier said than done—if health problems are to be solved. To provide a solid opportunity for learning how to do this, the CHP Law gives the State Councils the task of allocating funds from a block Public Health Service grant for seven or eight categorical health purposes which had previously been subject to separate rules from Washington.

Second, the 1966 law and subsequent appropriations have established comprehensive health planning as a function to be carried out by every state and local area in the nation. As of early 1974, there were 56 state and territorial CHP agencies—34 of them in State Health Departments or umbrella Health and Welfare Agencies, with the balance in other state offices. At the local or "area-wide" level within states were 198 CHP agencies, of which 150 are nonprofit private corporations, the balance under other sponsorships, though none—I regret to say—lodged in local health departments.[21] The solution of many health problems is inherently beyond the power of the most competent and affluent local jurisdictions, but it is equally true that other problems cannot be solved without local effort.

Third is the strong role mandated for health consumers or ordinary citizens, as distinguished from health professionals, in the planning process. This may be little more than "window-dressing" if consumers do not become educated about the intricacies of health issues. But the potential of developing a sophisticated consumer voice in health policy determination is an ultimate safeguard in protection of the public interest.

It has perhaps become a cliché to point out that CHP agencies are usually not very effective in achieving rational planning because their authority has no teeth in back of it; they lack sanctions to enforce their decisions. But if we take the long view, I believe we can look upon these last eight years as a tooling-up period for more effective planning in the future. It has been a period when the several thousand people—professional and lay—involved in CHP councils have become educated about the problems of developing a better, more equitable health service system. The opportunity to use that knowledge will, in my opinion, become greatest when this nation develops a national health insurance program, which is not very far off. Such a program will provide, at least potentially, economic sanctions for achieving various ends in the distribution of health resources in proportion to population needs and the setting of priorities when resources are not sufficient—which are after all the purposes and meaning of comprehensive health planning.

This is certainly not to imply that solid achievements cannot be chalked up to CHP agencies over the past years. In Connecticut, for example, the five areawide agencies can point to numerous achievements in promoting screening programs for chronic disease detection, getting new district Health Departments established, inducing cooperative activities of agencies in the mental health field, and so on.[22] But I am convinced that much greater opportunities lie ahead, in association with national health insurance.

References

1. Committee on the Costs of Medical Care, *Medical Care for the American People* (First Printing: University of Chicago Press, 1932), Reprinted by U.S. Dept. of Health, Education and Welfare, Washington, 1970.
2. Oscar R. Ewing, *The Nation's Health:* A Ten Year Program, Washington: Federal Security Agency, September 1948.
3. President's Commission on the Health Needs of the Nation, *Building America's Health,* Vols. I–V, Washington: Government Printing Office, 1952.
4. National Commission on Community Health Services, *Health is a Community Affair,* Cambridge, Mass: Harvard Univ. Press, 1966.
5. Commission on Hospital Care, *Hospital Care in the United States,* Chicago: American Hospital Association, October 1946.
6. U.S. Health Services and Mental Health Administration, *Hill-Burton Progress Report 1947–1970,* Washington (HEW Pub. No. HSM-73-4001), 1972.
7. Health Insurance Council, *The Extent of Voluntary Health Insurance Coverage,* New York, 1962, p. 10.
8. Haven Emerson and Martha Luginbuhl, *Local Health Units for the Nation,* New York: Commonwealth Fund, 1945.
9. England & Wales, Ministry of Health, Consultative Council on Medical and Allied Services, *Interim Report on the Future of Medical and Allied Services,* London: H. M. Stationery Office, 1920.
10. Joseph W. Mountin, E. H. Pennell, and A. G. Berger, *Health Service Areas: Estimates of Future Physician Requirements,* Public Health Bull. No. 305, Washington: Government Printing Office, 1949.
11. National Commission on Community Health Services, *Health Manpower: Action to Meet Community Needs,* Washington: Public Affairs Press, 1967, pp. 144 ff.
12. Report of the Surgeon General's Consultant Group on Medical Education (F. Bane, Chairman), *Physician's for a Growing America,* Washington: U.S. Dept. of Health, Education and Welfare, 1959.
13. Lowell T. Coggeshall, *Planning for Medical Progress Through Education,* Evanston, Ill.: Association of American Medical Colleges, 1965.
14. *Report of the National Advisory Commission on Health Manpower,* Vol. I and II, Washington: Government Printing Office, 1967.
15. Citizen's Commission on Graduate Medical Education (John S. Millis, Chairman), *The Graduate Education of Physicians,* Chicago: American Medical Association, 1966.
16. Richard H. Shryock, *Medical Licensing in America, 1650–1965,* Baltimore: Johns Hopkins Press, 1967.
17. Rosemary Stevens, *American Medicine and the Public Interest,* New Haven: Yale University Press, 1971, pp. 111 ff.
18. Milton I. Roemer and Jay W. Friedman, *Doctors in Hospitals: Medical Staff Organization and Hospital Performance,* Baltimore: Johns Hopkins Press, 1971, pp. 21 ff.
19. William R. Roy, *Health Maintenance Organization Act of 1972,* Washington: Science and Health Communications Group, 1972.
20. Leonard S. Rosenfeld and Henry B. Makover, *The Rochester Regional Hospital Council,* Cambridge, Mass: Harvard University Press, 1956, pp. 3–13.
21. Comptroller General of the United States, *Comprehensive Health Planning as Carried Out by State and Areawide Agencies in Three States,* Washington: General Accounting Office, April 1974.
22. Marcus R. McCraven, "Paper to the Democratic and Republican Platform Committees," New Haven: South Central Connecticut Comprehensive Health Planning, Inc., processed, 1974.

31

Planning Health Services: Substance versus Form

When the Comprehensive Health Planning Law was enacted by the U.S. Congress in October, 1966, nationwide interest in the health planning process naturally expanded rapidly. New training courses were organized, engineering and administrative personnel from other disciplines entered the field, and a variety of health planning methods were formulated.

Unfortunately, much of this work was done by technicians with little or no knowledge of the health services, the information available about health conditions, or the sociopolitical realities of the American health care system. As a result, much of the methodology applied–for example, that drawn from the methodology used in planning military operations–was poorly adapted to the requirements of the "open system" of pluralistic programs constituting American health services. There emerged a great preoccupation with so-called sophisticated and quantified techniques, which proved to be of little value in the practical achievement of improved health care for communities. In the following paper, a critique of these developments is offered, and suggestions are made about more down-to-earth ways of analyzing community health problems and possible paths to their solution. The paper was presented at the 1968 Annual Meeting of the Canadian Public Association.

In the last few years, "planning" has become a very respectable word in the North American health vocabulary. It wasn't always so; for many years, the word and the concept were strictly avoided because they smacked of socialism. It was the Soviet Union that launched its initial Five-year Plan in 1928—ten years after its revolution—embarking on a course, incidentally, that had not been envisaged by Marx and Engels. Planning came to mean the examination of a total economic and social scene, with a deliberate outline of phased steps over prescribed time periods to solve certain problems and then move on to the next ones.

Background of Health Planning

Planning requires a classification of problems and disciplines to solve them, among which are the tasks of providing health service. It was after World War II that the planning of health services became a prominent national issue—mainly

Chapter 31 originally appeared in the *Canadian Journal of Public Health,* 59:431–437, November, 1968, and is reprinted by permission of that journal.

in the underdeveloped countries. The post-war period of reconstruction gave a fresh opportunity to new governments, like that of India, to build their health systems according to some sort of ideal model in a step-by-step process.[1] It was probably no accident that the Bhore Commission invited consultation from Dr. Henry E. Sigerist in 1944, a few years after his studies of the Soviet health system. In the same year, Dr. Sigerist came to Saskatchewan to advise the newly elected government of that province on what was probably the first comprehensive planning approach to health services on this continent.[2] There were similar bold approaches in Israel, the Union of South Africa, Indonesia, and elsewhere.[3] During the War, the Beveridge Report gave a new purpose to the fight for "Freedom from Want," and outlined plans for the British National Health Service which was launched in 1948. In 1952, Chile—inspired by the British model—started its Servicio Nacional de Salud.

In the more affluent countries, not so devastated by the War, like Canada and the United States, progress in organization of health services has been substantial but on a more piecemeal basis. In both our countries, the chief movement has been in the sphere of improved and collectivized methods of financing, mainly through the insurance device. Voluntary insurance for hospitalization expanded rapidly. In Canada its success, along with the even greater impact of the social insurance model in Saskatchewan after 1947, led to the nationwide federal-provincial hospital insurance program in 1957. With the much firmer base for financing of hospital operating costs throughout Canada, great improvements were possible in hospital staffing and technology, the supply of health personnel was expanded, and methods of administration were advanced.[4] Progress in public health work, medical education, scientific research, and other sectors of health activity went along with this.

In the United States, serious discussion of overall health planning could not be expected until the first round was won in the fight for national health insurance. For the basic requirement of planning, when one cuts through the platitudes, is control over the allocation of resources and the use of those resources, and this is very difficult without control over the flow of money. It was only after enactment in July 1965 of health insurance for the aged—our modest Medicare law—that discussion could begin in earnest on "comprehensive health planning." It is true that 20 years earlier the Hill-Burton Act had called for construction of hospitals according to a "master plan," but this significantly could be implemented only for those facilities receiving federal subsidy—about 25 percent of all construction projects and a much smaller proportion of total hospitals. A few months after Medicare, Public Law 89-239 for "regional medical programs for heart disease, cancer, and stroke" (now generally called RMP) was enacted, focusing on the quality, rather than simply the financing, of health services. Then, a year later, in October 1966 the Comprehensive Health Planning Law (P.L. 89-749) was passed, offering grants to the states for general planning of health manpower, facilities, and services—along with other provisions.[5]

In Canada, with nationwide hospitalization financing coming in 1957, attention to overall planning came earlier. The Royal Commission on Health Services was appointed in 1961 and its report was issued in 1964.[6] Many bold measures were called for, but the most important was doubtless the proposal for nationwide insurance for physician's services. After the usual debate, legislation to carry this out was passed last year and, although there are some unsettled problems in provincial-federal relations, the program is to be implemented later this year. With organized financial support for the bulk of hospital and physician services—constituting about two-thirds of all national health expenditures—Canada will soon be in a position to move ahead even more rapidly in systematic planning of its total health services.

Approaches to Planning

This economic foundation for delivering health services has greatly accelerated the interest of health leaders in the whole planning process. Since most medical people have been identified with one or another specific sector of the health field, rather than the total panorama, few have been familiar with planning strategies. Our organized health services in North America are characterized by fragmentation. One man is familiar with communicable disease control, another with medical care of the poor, another with hospital operation, and another with professional education. All of these are segments of health planning, but the very essence of planning is an overview of all the parts in combination. Handicapped by the blinders of specialization, we health workers have had to turn elsewhere for assistance in gaining a broad overview of our own field.

I am not so sure about Canada, but in the United States health leaders have turned for this assistance to the economists and public administrators. By reason of their responsibilities in other public programs, that is, programs clearly financed by public funds and controlled by governmental authorities, these social scientists have developed some very useful tools for analysis of complex organized activities. The most highly developed techniques were hammered out where the money was big, in the military systems, especially that of the Air Force. The task was to figure out how all the thousands of steps in the production and distribution of weapons, training of personnel, and countless specific actions along the way could articulate so that a bomb could be dropped from an airplane at a specific time and place. The methodology was called "systems analysis."[7] Vast new organizations of scientists were formed to make these analyses, such as the RAND (Research and Development) Corporation or the Systems Development Corporation, to name only two of them.

In calculating the wisest course of action for a military program, there are always alternative paths possible. The choice among several paths ought to depend on a weighing of the relative benefits to be gained, in relation to the costs, of various decisions. This often involves intricate construction of theoretical models (defining the alternative paths) and measurements of the numerous inputs and outputs. This is known as "cost-benefit" or "cost effectiveness" analysis.[8] It depends on "model-building" and "simulation techniques." The data on different combinations of factors (variables) are fed into electronic computers, and through multiple regression and other techniques, quantitative answers are derived. When this whole process is done in a governmental agency, in order to plan the spending of the taxpayers' money wisely, it is called "planning, programming, and budgeting" or PPB. The elegance with which this was done in the U.S. Department of Defense (under Secretary Robert McNamara) was so highly regarded that in 1965, President Johnson directed all departments of the federal government to start to apply similar analytical techniques to all their activities.[9]

In Great Britain, during World War II, a somewhat similar analytical process was applied to military operations, and it was called "operations research." Soon after the War it was applied to studies of the operations of the health services, with determination of the quantity of services being delivered under various circumstances and at various costs.[10] More recently, the public administrators have spoken of the "program evaluation and review technique" or PERT.[11]

Sketchy as this review is, it may be enough to clarify the point that various techniques of measurement and evaluation of organized social actions have been applied, with great sophistication, to military and other extremely costly governmental operations. Through this effort, techniques have been developed in what is essentially "planning," and these techniques are now believed to be useful in planning other complex sets of actions, such as the health services. To oversimplify a bit, the techniques for estimating the most economical and effective method of delivering a bomb are now being applied to the delivery of a shot of penicillin.

One can immediately detect differences between the tasks of military logistics and those of medical care. Aside from the moral value of humanism versus violence, the principal difference is probably that the military (or other governmental) function is essentially a "closed system" under a single central authority, while health service—in North America, at least—involves an infinitely complex set of relationships between public and private sectors. On further probing, however, this difference turns out to be not so basic as it might seem, for the military process also involves numerous articulations with the private economy (manufacture and delivery of weapons, induction of soldiers, etc.). And the health services, on the other hand, involve enormous influences of central authority on the operations of private local entities (hospitals, physicians, etc.), as in the Medicare programs of both Canada and the United States.

The problem lies not in a confusion between nuclear bombs and the cobalt type, or between khaki uniforms and the nurse's type. It lies rather in a confusion of means and ends, of form and substance.

The point is that the various tools of planning developed by the economists and public administrators are useful, and doubtless have broad generic value. But still they are only tools. They become relevant for planning of the health services only if they are applied to the appropriate substantive problems. The right questions must be asked, or the instruments cannot give useful answers. This leads to an examination of the questions that health leaders are posing to the experts in planning methodology.

The Nature of Health Planning Problems

The questions on planning, posed by public health or medical leaders, are bound to be derived from their past experience. Because of the great fragmentation of organized health services noted earlier, these experiences usually fall along certain dimensions (and to subcategories within them), which tend to shape one's view of the health world. These experiences are bound to determine the questions posed for planning, which have been oriented along the following lines.

Disease Categories

Physicians naturally see the health world in terms of disease entities. They have been educated this way. There is tuberculosis, which has its etiology and pathology, its diagnosis and treatment, its prevention, its rehabilitation, its ups and downs, its mysteries and challenges. One can engage in fascinating planning exercises along the path of this one disease or, indeed, any other single disease, like cancer or poliomyelitis or kwashiorkor. Each disease has its special biological and social concomitants which give the clues to both its prevention and treatment.

The trouble is that, useful as the disease concept may be for clinical management of the individual patient, or even for special public health campaigns, it is not necessarily the soundest approach to overall planning. There are hundreds of diseases, which take thousands of forms. Organized programs may be focused on one disease to the exclusion of all others, as has indeed been the practice. Success may be achieved in a campaign against malaria without any impact on all the rest of morbidity. Other categorical programs attack other diseases, leading to endless duplication and complication in the health services. It is this very complexity that has highlighted the current urgent concerns for planning. One of the principal planning efforts in Latin America has taken the disease-specific approach and, aside from providing some interesting teaching exercises, it has proved to be of little practical value in the actual process of national health planning.[12]

Categories of Person

Another approach to the health world is through certain classes of person. There are children who have special health problems, as well as industrial workers and military veterans and poor people and Indians and pensioners and agricultural migrants and government employees and many others. Special health service programs are organized for these demographic groups largely because of distinctive social or political pressures. With limited resources, one group is accorded priorities ahead of another.[13] Some good may be accomplished for the favored group, but often at the expense of other groups and always at a price of duplicated and complex administration. Planning along this dimension involves a jungle of processes which fragment families, neighborhoods, and cities with separate programs. Even a single individual may be fragmented when his status as a factory worker, a veteran, and fraternal lodge member entitles him to use three separate medical care channels for the same disease problem—let alone other channels for special diseases.

The Defined Agency

Still another approach to the health services is through specific organized agencies that have evolved inside or outside government for various purposes.[14] There are the health departments, with their focus principally on prevention, the welfare departments serving the poor, the cancer societies, the visiting nurse associations, the voluntary health insurance plans (hundreds of these), the hospital associations, the Red Cross, and countless others.[15] There is a nationwide voluntary agency in the United States whose mission is totally devoted to hemophilia—a disease so rare that most physicians never see a case of it. Passionate loyalty to the specific program of the agency develops in its most dedicated members. Planning is attempted within the bailiwick of each of these programs, quite separately from all the others and sometimes even in competition with them.

To coordinate these diverse efforts, community "health councils" are sometimes formed, bringing together representatives of many public and private agencies. There may be a special council, moreover, for agencies in one disease-related field, like mental health or nutrition. The task then becomes to coordinate the planners or to plan the planning, so that the total health needs of a total population in a community can be reasonably met.

None of these three approaches, in my view, meets the requirements of comprehensive health planning. For the very essence of planning is to analyze the total landscape of health needs in populations, and this cannot be done along the parochial channels of paricular diseases, particular persons, or particular agencies. Planning requires rather the viewpoint of "community"—that is a geographic area where people live. "Community" may be defined as a neighborhood, a town, a county, a district, a region, a province, or a nation. Within it, at any of these levels, are many different kinds of people who are afflicted by many different sorts of diseases. The past has endowed us with many different formal agencies to cope with these problems, but the boundaries of these agencies—whether legally or voluntarily defined—are often obstructive rather than conducive to comprehensive health planning today.[16]

The Community Approach: Health Services

The community approach, in the sense used here, poses a different sort of question for the methodologists of planning. It asks: how can the needed health services be best delivered, for control (prevention or treatment) of any disease in any person? To answer this question, one must think in terms of *health services*—not in terms of diagnoses, demographic traits, or agencies.

The health services are technical processes definable along other lines. They involve the skills of trained personnel applied to people living at home—the ambulatory services. They involve attention to persons needing removal from their homes—the institutional services. Within either of these settings, the services must be both preventive (that is, directed to the nonsymptomatic person) and curative (to the person who has signs of illness). The health services must be provided by appropriately trained personnel and rendered in properly constructed and equipped facilities. Coordination among the full range of personnel and facilities is necessary, especially at their point of impact on the patient. To support these resources, there must be an adequate flow of money, and there must be standards of performance and review to assure quality.

Consideration of these several basic categories of health service, of course, requires more refined breakdowns in the final planning process. The ambulatory services include, for example, the activities of scores of types of personnel: general physicians, diverse specialists, professional nurses, auxiliary nurses, pharmacists, laboratory technicians, physical therapists, dentists, dental aides, optometrists, social workers, and many others. The preventive services require most of these personnel, plus certain others, like sanitary engineers, sanitarians, health educators, nutritionists, public health nurses, etc. The institutional services involve the construction, staffing, and operation of general hospitals, but also of mental hospitals, chronic disease facilities, rehabilitation centers, etc.

The coordination of this wide range of personnel and facilities presents many alternatives for organization. Different mixes of personnel, and different channels of communication and supervision may be explored. The outcomes of these several patterns can be quantified in terms of volume of services provided, reduction of disability, unit-costs, and other measures. Likewise, the mechanisms for raising money are of several types, and the implications of alternative methods can be explored. Regarding the review of quality, there are many subdivisions along which performance may be analyzed; standards can be stipulated for each of the medical, nursing, laboratory, dental, hospital, pharmaceutical, and other services. All of these rubrics of analysis, it may be noted, relate to the delivery of services to total populations in communities, and are not categorized by disease entities, personal pedigree, or agency lines.

The effective and efficient provision of these several types of service in communities, in my view, constitutes the substance of planning. The articulation of different communities and the transfer of services or patients across community borders constitutes regionalization.[17] Transportation is necessary because of the complexities of scientific technology and the practical limitations of time and place; brain surgery cannot currently be offered at every crossroads, so that patients or skilled services must be transferable from one place to another. The training and distribution of the necessary personnel (or "health manpower" in 1968 parlance) and facilities, the achievement of the necessary financial support, and the maintenance of appropriate quality controls in geographic areas—these are the substance of planning the delivery of health services.

In its ultimate implications, this substantive picture is not difficult to draw. The subdivisions of disease categories, population classes and agency jurisdictions are terribly complex, but the basic requirements of delivering health service to the people in communities are conceptually simple. For the ambulatory services, health centers are needed, with a spectrum of personnel for medical, dental, psychiatric, and related services both curative and preventive. For the institutional services networks of hospitals and related facilities are necessary. The financial support must be on some social basis—by insurance or taxation—if everyone is to get the care he needs. The quality promotion must be systematized through some form of teamwork with smooth communication and discipline, if uniform standards are to be maintained.

Substance versus Form

We all know, of course, the political and social obstacles to the implementation of this health service picture. The path to rationality in any social system must often follow a tortuous route through a labyrinth of traditions, vested interests, and power alignment.[18] Yet this is the substantive goal that must be seen if planning is to move us ahead. With this overview, all the tools of systems analysis, cost-benefit calculations, operations research, and all the rest can be useful. We can study the rate of utilization of ambulatory or institutional services by populations, the costs and achievements under different organizational designs, the gaps in resources that need to be filled. The planning measurements can help us get from here to there—from the current confused reality to a more rational future. Without a substantive goal before us, without this overview, we can become lost in the methodologies.

To observe some of the efforts at so-called comprehensive health planning in the United States today, one might get the impression that concentration on the tools and techniques is regarded as a protection against any unpleasant confrontation with the controversial realities. The realities of current health service organization are beset with issues.[19] There are arguments about the sources of money, as between the private and the public sectors. There are issues of power and who shall exercise it. There are numerous questions about the patterns of medical service—both ambulatory and institutional—and how coordination may be achieved.[20] When state or community health planning councils contain members from special groups, with different and often conflicting interests in the status quo, there is naturally reluctance to face these issues squarely. Refuge is taken in the study of methodologies or the focus on some specific disease, which avoids the necessity of taking the comprehensive community view of health services.

On a worldwide scale, however, the perspective becomes more clear.[21] The substance of planning in most countries has come to mean the organization of total health services in defined geographic areas. It is often epitomized simply as "regionalization," with authority for preventive, ambulatory, and institutional services integrated in local areas. Implementation is largely dependent on the flow of funds through the public sector. By definition, planning means an overview at a central level, where all parts of the landscape can be seen. Usually this means national governments, but certain planning responsibilities may be delegated to provincial levels. At the local level, many public and nongovernmental entities may be involved in the final delivery of health services, but their financial support and their minimum standards of operation usually come from authorities at a higher echelon.

This is also the direction in which we are moving in North America. In the United States, about 60 percent of the $45,000,000,000 spent annually on health services is now flowing through organized channels—governmental and voluntary.[22] In Canada, the proportion is probably higher. This visibility of expenditures heightens social concern for both economies and quality. Far more concern than ever before is being shown about the patterns of medical care through which this money is spent. The keystone role of day-to-day physicians' service is being probed, and various forms of teamwork are being promoted.[23] There is increasing recognition of the decisive role of the primary physician, and his influence on disease-prevention, on the one hand, and hospital utilization on the other.[24] Group practice, neighborhood health centers, expanded hospital out-patient departments, and organized home care programs are all around us. There is deliberate planning of expanded health manpower.[25] Hospitals and related facilities are being studied in area-wide constellations, whether or not they have received federal construction grants.[26] Environmental control of the water and air is transcending the usual political jurisdictions.[27]

These are the substantive issues of planning, and the primary task is to understand their nature before we sharpen the tools for their study. Planning techniques can be well taught in graduate schools of business or public administration, but the responsibility for training "health planners" must remain with schools of public health, where the substantive knowledge is found. While analytical tools are needed, we must avoid the fallacy of Pythagoras, who thought that because the world could be described quantitatively, the ultimate reality was to be found in numbers. We must avoid the sterile cul-de-sac of the medieval scholastics who became so obsessed with form that they failed to examine the substance of the world around them. We must keep our eye on the ball of health services for the population in the communities where they live. We must work toward a goal of comprehensive preventive and curative service for everyone, as a right of citizenship. This is the substance of health planning.

References

1. Government of India: Health Survey and Development Committee, Report (4 volumes). New Delhi, 1946.
2. Sigerist, Henry E.: "Saskatchewan Health Services Survey Commission" in *Henry E. Sigerist on the Sociology of Medicine,* Milton I. Roemer, Editor. MD Publications, New York, 1960, pp. 209–228.
3. Roemer, Milton I.: *Medical Care in Relation to Public Health: A Study of the Relationships between Preventive and Curative Medicine throughout the World.* World Health Organization, Geneva, 1956.
4. Roth, F. Burns: "How a Plan Administrator Sees Hospital Insurance." The Canadian Hospital, 1957, *34:*34.
5. Forgotson, Edward H.: "1965: The Turning Point in Health Law—1966 Reflections." Amer. J. Public Health, 1967, *57:*934.
6. Royal Commission on Health Services. Report, Volume I. Queen's Printer, Ottawa, 1964.
7. McKean, Roland N.: *The Economics of Defense in the Nuclear Age.* Harvard University Press, Cambridge, 1963.
8. U.S. Vocational Rehabilitation Administration: *An Exploratory Cost-Benefits Analysis of Vocational Rehabilitation.* Washington, D.C., August 1967.
9. Executive Office of the President: "Planning-Programing-Budgeting" (Bulletin No. 66-3) October 12, 1965. See also: Kissick, William L.: "Planning, Programming, and Budgeting in Health." Medical Care, 1967, *5:*201.
10. Davies, J. O. F.: "Problems for Operational Research in the National Health Service" in *Towards a Measure of Medical Care: Operational Research in the Health Service.* Oxford University Press, London, 1962, pp. 1–17.
11. American Public Health Association: *Health Program Implementation through P.E.R.T.,* 1966.
12. Pan American Health Organization: "Health Planning: Problems of Concept and Method." Scientific Pub. No. 111, Washington, D.C., 1965.
13. Roemer, Milton I.: "A Co-ordinated Health Service and the Problem of Priorities." Israel Journal of Medical Sciences, 1965. *1:*643.
14. Morris, Robert, Binstock, Robert H., and Rein, Martin: *Feasible Planning for Social Change.* Columbia University Press, New York, 1966.
15. Wasserman, Clara S. and Paul: *Health Organizations of the United States and Canada: National, Regional and State.* Cornell University, Ithaca, 1961.
16. Sigmond, Robert M.: "Health Planning." Medical Care, 1967, *5:*117.

17. Lembcke, Paul A.: "Regional Organization of Hospitals." Annals of the American Academy of Political and Social Science. January 1951, pp. 53–61.
18. Stern, Bernhard J.: *Society and Medical Progress*. Princeton University Press. Princeton, 1941.
19. Greenberg, Selig: *The Troubled Calling: Crisis in the Medical Establishment*. Macmillan Company, New York, 1965.
20. Stewart, William H.: *New Dimensions of Health Planning*. University of Chicago, Chicago, 1967.
21. World Health Organization: "Planning of Public Health Services." Fourth Report of the Expert Committee on Public Health Administration. Technical Report Series No. 215, Geneva 1961.
22. Rice, Dorothy P. and Cooper, B. S.: "National Health Expenditures, 1950–66." Research and Statistics Note. U.S. Social Security Administration, Note No. 3, February 1, 1968.
23. U.S. Public Health Service: "Promoting the Group Practice of Medicine." Report of the National Conference on Group Practice. October 19–21, 1967. P.H.S. Pub. No. 1750, Washington, D.C. 1967.
24. Citizens' Committee on Graduate Education (John S. Millis, Chairman): *The Graduate Education of Physicians*. American Medical Association, 1966.
25. Report of the National Advisory Commission on Health Manpower, Vol. I. Office of Science and Technology, Washington, D.C., 1967.
26. National Commission on Community Health Services: *Health Care Facilities*. Public Affairs Press, Washington, D.C., 1967.
27. National Commission on Community Health Services: *Changing Environmental Hazards*. Public Affairs Press, Washington, D.C., 1967.

32

Comprehensive Health Planning for Rural Areas

Because of their deficiencies in health care resources (personnel and facilities), rural regions have been the object of deliberate planning efforts for many years. In 1948, Dr. Frederick D. Mott and I published the first national overview of this field in a book entitled Rural Health and Medical Care *(New York: McGraw-Hill).*

With the national comprehensive health planning movement in the late 1960s, the interest of rural organizations was reactivated. A seminar on "Health Problems in the Great Plains with Special Attention to the Implementation of Comprehensive Health Plans" was held at Lincoln, Nebraska, in May, 1969. The paper presented at this seminar is reproduced in the following pages. It illustrates the down-to-earth approach to health planning discussed in the previous chapter, and stresses the dependence of rural health care improvements on actions required at the national level of government.

Earlier Rural Health Planning

During World War II, leaders here in the Great Plains and elsewhere in rural America were tussling with the problems of "post-war planning," as it was called. Among the many sectors was health service, and the community representatives who participated in the planning efforts included farmers, teachers, doctors, nurses, shopkeepers, accountants, and many others. As the U.S. Public Health Service officer assigned to this duty, with the War Food Administration, I had the opportunity to work with many of these dedicated community people.

Our approach to health planning in this period was along five lines. While the terminology and the popular phrases were a little different a quarter-century ago, the substance of health discussions were strikingly similar to the analytical framework of "comprehensive health planning" in 1969, and the language of the relevant federal legislation of 1966 and 1967. In 1944, we spoke of the problems and the solutions required for rural health improvement under these five categories:

1. health personnel—greater numbers and better distribution;
2. health facilities—hospitals and other facilities in the numbers and places needed, tied together in regional networks;

Chapter 32 was issued previously only as a processed document, in the *Proceedings of the Great Plains Agricultural Council* (Lincoln, Nebr., 1969). It is published here for the first time.

3. economic support for health care—a system which would be based on the principle of charges according to ability to pay and would eliminate financial obstacles to all needed services;
4. maximum disease prevention—through organized community programs of many types; and
5. quality promotion—through measures of education, surveillance, and technical organization of medical and related services.

In today's Comprehensive Health Planning legislation, we speak of "health manpower" instead of "personnel"; "health facilities" are still "facilities"; and "services" is the current planning shortcut word for earlier specification of "economic support," "disease prevention," and "quality promotion."

I do not mean to imply that there is nothing new under the sun, or that no progress has been made in the last generation, but rather that health planning has actually been going on for some years. Since the end of World War II, we have been doing a great deal of planning—some of it through legislation, like the Hill-Burton Hospital Survey and Construction Act of 1946 or the Medicare Law of 1965, and some of it through voluntary efforts, like the Blue Cross hospital insurance movement or the extension of private group medical clinics. The "new look" in planning of the last four years has been much more in the sphere of methods and tools, I would say, than of the substance and goals of health service.

I hope, therefore, it will not be deemed old-fashioned if I approach the subject of "comprehensive health planning in rural areas" along the same five paths that we mapped out 25 years ago. In this way, we can also take note of progress that has been made over these years and estimate the direction in which we are moving.

The Great Plains Setting

First, however, a word about the Great Plains region as a setting for health planning. From the viewpoint of conventional modern planning concepts—concepts dealing with resource allocations, distance, time, and communication—the Great Plains present the quintessence of the planning challenge. The ecology of people, the tasks of transportation, the organization of technology—these are the main issues. It is to be noted that stickier problems in the sphere of economic support are, in my opinion, not prominent issues. This is not a poor region today, like the southeastern states, although there are, of course, some pockets of poverty. This is not a region of massive illiteracy, as in the rural stretches of many other nations.

The health planning challenges of the Great Plains are mainly in the sphere of *organization,* rather than of financing. In some obvious ways, this makes the task easier, but in other ways it becomes harder, because the rockiest roads to innovation in the health services are in this sector.

Moreover, many of the problems of rural health service organization in the Great Plains cannot possibly be solved within the boundaries of the plains themselves. They require decisions and actions elsewhere in the nation. This is doubtless true of any specific region one would consider. It should be recognized, no matter how deep our commitment may be to the American traditions of self-help and local initiative. For the particular problems which I refer to, local community leaders can probably make their greatest contribution by articulating statements of rural needs, so that they can be heard throughout the land. In the remarks that follow, I should like to call attention to planning tasks that demand such nationwide action, as distinguished from those that can yield reasonable prospects of accomplishment at the local community or the state level.

Health Manpower Planning

For a long time the shortages of doctors and other health personnel in the rural areas of America have been recognized, but until recently this was spoken of mainly as a "maldistribution." The assumption of this concept was that, altogether, we had enough physicians, dentists, nurses, etc., in the nation, but they were too heavily concentrated in certain places—mainly the big cities. The task, therefore, was to induce a better geographic distribution of the existent manpower supply.

This was attempted by offering various attractions to encourage settlement of doctors and others in small towns and rural areas. The programs of the American Medical Association, the Sears Roebuck Foundation, the rural medical fellowships of several states, the rural health center program of the University of Kansas Medical School, the Tennessee Medical Foundation program—these were some of the better known efforts along this line. Highly important also has been the Hill-Burton hospital construction program, which favors the rural states and has doubtless had secondary effects in attracting doctors to rural regions by providing them with good facilities in which to work.

The net effect of all these efforts to attract doctors to rural regions, however, has not been very impressive. Statistical data for 1963, comparing doctor-population ratios in rural or semi-rural counties with those in metropolitan counties, show about the same degree of disparity as that found in 1940. If there has been any improvement in the access of rural people to physicians and dentists, it has been not by reason of the choices of professional office location, but rather by improvements in roads and transportation, enabling rural people to travel more readily to the cities. A recent study of doctors in Iowa, moreover, reported the distressing finding that 41 percent of the rural practitioners would like to change their locations, compared with 19 percent of the urban doctors.

If planning is to be effective in this health manpower sector, therefore, it would seem necessary to take action that would increase the total national supply of doctors and dentists. Only when the total reservoir is greater can we expect the under-served rural regions to acquire a larger share. Medical and dental educations are expensive, and enlargement of the universities, for greater outputs in these professions, demands support by state and federal governments. This has been the trend, of course, in the last twenty years, but the subsidy provided has barely enabled the university schools to keep pace with the growth of population. (In fact, if it were not for our importation of several thousand foreign-trained doctors each year, our doctor-population ratio in the United States would have steadily declined.) If the medical manpower supply is to be substantially improved, much greater governmental support will be necessary.

In the face of rising demands for health service, among both rural and urban people, we have managed to get along with our static ratio of doctors, only because of a substantial improvement in the supply of nurses and other paramedical personnel. But still greater numbers of these health workers are also needed to meet the demands. Planners also must explore innovations in the more effective *use* of health personnel. The scarce and valuable time of the physician or dentist can be made more productive, it has been well demonstrated, by the organization of group practice clinics and other forms of sensible medical teamwork. Such teamwork can also spare the doctor from workdays, as found in the Iowa study, of 11 or 12 hours—which pave the way for early heart attacks, not to mention the effect of exhaustion on the quality of a doctor's work.

Health Facilities

The planning tasks for improvement of health facilities in rural regions are less formidable. In this sector, we have made a good deal of progress. The ratio of hospital beds to population in the predominantly rural states of the nation is now as good as or better than it is in the heavily urbanized states, while in 1940 it was far worse. Here in the Great Plains States, in fact, are found the highest bed-population ratios in the country. This is partly due to the vigorous hospital construction efforts of the last 20 years and partly to the relatively slower rate of population growth in these states, compared with the national average.

In the hospital sector, the planning needs—unlike the manpower requirements—are not so much quantitative as organizational. If we study the occupancy levels of hospitals in the thinly settled Plains states, we find that the small hospitals in the small towns have low occupancy rates, while the larger hospitals in the urban centers of rural regions—like those in Lincoln or in Omaha or Des Moines or Kansas City or Tulsa—have high rates. The small hospitals, in other words, are half-empty while the large ones are overcrowded.

A few years ago I made a study of this phenomenon and found that the degree of discrepancy between occupancy levels of differently sized hospitals was almost inversely proportional to the population density of the state. It was much greater, for example, in a thinly settled rural state like Nebraska than a more heavily and more evenly settled state like Ohio. This suggests that for hospital care, rural people are tending to bypass the nearby small-town hospital, in favor of the more distant big-city institution, where specialists and other technical resources are concentrated.

For health planners, this would seem to call for either one of two courses of action: 1. greater expansion of the larger urban hospitals to accommodate the heavier demands being made upon them, thereby allowing the smaller rural hospitals almost to wither on the vine; or 2. upgrading the quality of the small rural hospitals, so that people close by will use them. I would hope that the latter course of action would be chosen, even though it is the more difficult option. It would mean, however, attraction of qualified medical specialists to the small towns—involving the whole manpower challenge discussed earlier—and also the development of regional ties between rural hospitals and urban medical centers.

This concept of professional ties between hospitals in a region is one that has been discussed for several decades, but only recently—with the national legislation on Regional Medical Programs for Heart Disease, Cancer and Stroke—have we seen progress in implementing it, beyond a few pilot areas. There is certainly great potential in the RMP movement, which has hardly yet been exploited. In most states, the activities are now heavily focused on programs of continuing education for doctors—a good enough way to begin—but much more could be done to develop a genuine two-way flow of patients and services among the different hospitals of a regional network. In no type of geography would this vitalized concept of regionalization be more applicable than in the Great Plains States. To achieve it would require statesmanship, not only among hospital boards, but also among the medical staffs of hospitals throughout a region. This initiative can indeed be taken locally, without any exercise of authority at the national level. The necessary statesmanship may be more likely to develop, however, if some of the remaining *economic* problems in medical service are solved.

Economic Support for Health Care

Earlier I suggested that the main health problems of the Great Plains States were organizational, rather than economic, but this is not to imply that all problems of health economics have been solved. The voluntary health insurance movement has made great progress and many contributions over the last thirty years, and has eased the financial access to hospital care, for the great majority of families. The weakest level of insurance protection, however, is found among rural families, such as those in the Plains States. It is weakest both in extent of population coverage and in the degree of financial protection enjoyed by those families who have any insurance. The situation is probably somewhat better now than it was in 1963, when a study was reported on this question, but in that year, 36 percent of rural nonfarm people and 49 percent of rural farm people in the United States had no insurance at all for hospitalization. Protection against the costs of out-of-hospital medical services, for both rural and urban people, is considerably less.

The Medicare Amendments to the Social Security Act of 1965 were a great step forward—despite the great opposition against this important and helpful law. This program has been a boon for aged people, both rural and urban, and both doctors and hospitals have learned from the program that social insurance does *not* strike the death knoll on their freedom. Most of the difficulties of the program have come from the escalation of medical and hospital prices under it, but the containment of this trend would involve greater social controls, which our government has hesitated to apply.

The success of the Medicare program has led Governor Rockefeller of New York to propose that, now, the rest of the national population should be provided the same health insurance protection as the aged. Senator Yarborough of Texas, the new Chairman of the U.S. Senate Committee on Labor and Public Welfare (which covers health legislation), proposed the same action last week! Thus, national health insurance is no longer a left-wing slogan, but is advocated by highly placed spokesmen of our two national parties. This should provide a clue, it would seem, for health planning groups at all levels.

If universal population coverage for comprehensive health care benefits should be achieved in the United States—as I think it will be—it would be of special value for rural people. For, more than urban people, who are tied to salaried employment in industry or business—with fringe benefit health and welfare provisions—rural people tend to be self-employed or working in small establishments, in which voluntary insurance has always been harder to organize. This has also been the experience in the Scandinavian countries and elsewhere, where, after a century of voluntary insurance, social insurance had to be enacted to reach the nonurban population adequately.

The planning of "services"—as defined in the Comprehensive Health Planning legislation—would be far more effective with an underpinning of national health insurance. When proper economic support for medical care—in the office and home, as well as in the hospital—is assured, then many other positive consequences can follow. A much stronger foundation would be laid for attracting doctors to rural areas. Opportunities would be presented for encouraging teamwork in delivery of medical service, and in applying peer review to assure maintenance of quality. Most important, the access of every person, rich or poor, to the benefits of science would become equalized. Any priority decisions, necessary in the face of resource scarcities, would depend on medical judgment of the patient's health needs, rather than his pocketbook.

Action in *this* sphere of rural planning is probably dependent on initiative at the national level. Conceivably a wealthy urban state might enact social insurance legislation on its own—as four urban states have done, for example, to provide short-term disability insurance. But rural states, like those in the Great Plains, could not be expected to take such action by themselves. They would be the greatest beneficiaries, however, of national action.

Quality Promotion

Several of the planning actions already discussed have implications for the promotion of a continually improved quality of health service, but still other efforts are called for.

The former Chairman of the Council on Rural Health of the American Medical Association, Dr. Ben N. Saltzman, stated only a few weeks ago: "There are communities so isolated that present modes of health care do not apply. These are communities whose inhabitants actually know little about good health care. . . . Their care would be on a par with that provided by native witch doctors."

The key word in Dr. Saltzman's indictment is "isolated"—for it is continuous contact with, and stimulation from, colleagues that is essential to maintain the quality of medical care. Such contacts are possible in well organized hospitals, and they can also be attained in the provision of day-to-day ambulatory care through group practice clinics. Similar medical teamwork can be achieved in the new type of "neighborhood health centers" launched by the U.S. Office of Economic Opportunity, and it can be achieved in hospital out-patient departments, which need not be restricted to the poor.

Continuing education, such as the RMP movement is providing, is also important for quality maintenance. Beyond this, there are two basic approaches to quality control. One is retrospective and the other is prospective. In the retrospective approach, there are systems of surveillance of previous medical performance—medical audits, claims reviews, etc.—and one hopes that exposure of past mistakes will encourage greater diligence in the future. For the prospective approach, the delivery pattern is so organized that colleague review, consultation, and assistance are built into the health care system in advance. This is the approach in the university hospital, where doctors are trained, and I think there is little doubt of its superiority. Planning of medical care programs for such prospective quality promotion takes both imagination and courage. It involves innovation, and the planners must have a clear sense of direction to see it through.

Disease Prevention

Finally, we come to planning challenges in the sphere of disease prevention and health promotion. This I have left for the last, not because prevention is least important, but rather because the modern approach calls for incorporation of preventive health services into the basic program of personal medical care. The public health agencies, which in the past have been identified with specialized preventive programs, have another role for the future.

The historical reasons for separate programs of communicable disease control, through immunizations and other measures, of maternal and child health services, of health education, of multiphasic screening for chronic diseases—the reasons for these programs being separated from the curative services were never technical, but social and political. It was believed that therapy was a private matter, and only prevention could be undertaken by the health agencies of government. We realize now, however, that this separation of preventive and curative services has caused technological inefficiencies for both, not to mention the personal difficulties caused for the patient. In the health patterns to be planned for the future, all these preventive services for individuals—with the obvious exception of environmental sanitation—should be given by the same personnel and in the same facilities as personal medical care.

The Health Department, however, has another and larger task. To assure that the whole complex system of health services works properly, there is need for a center of coordination. To protect both patients and providers of service, some sort of guiding authority is needed in every community or region. An agency is required to see to it that quality standards are met, that people are served according to their needs, that grievances are redressed. Gaps in service must be identified and wasteful duplications eliminated. All of this is "health planning," which must be a continuous process. There must be responsiveness to changing needs, whether they are due to changes in the population and its diseases or to advances in scientific potential.

This is the future role of the public health agency, in my opinion—along with the maintenance of environmental health protections. In fulfilling such a role, it would obviously behoove the Health Department to engage the participation of all sorts of interested citizens, as do the comprehensive planning agencies today. In a region like the Great Plains, health departments in the past have not been characterized by enormous power and impact, but this coordinating and planning role for total health services would greatly widen their mission for the benefit of everyone.

The Great Plains States, like the rest of America, are undergoing urbanization. A rising proportion of the total population is living in cities, while a relatively smaller rural population is able, with mechanization, to produce more agricultural commodities than ever before.

This urbanization process cannot be resisted, for—while there are short-term difficulties—the long-term effect is to enrich the lives of everyone. The family that stays on the farm, or in the small town or village, still benefits from the goods and services produced in or emanating from the expanding metropolitan centers. To be assured of those benefits, however, there must be social planning and organization. In the health services, this is as true as or truer than it is for education, housing, clothing, or other essentials of life.

I have tried to review some of the features of this planning and organizing process, as it relates to rural health services. The challenges to those now invested with the responsibilities for comprehensive health planning in this great rural territory are tough but exciting.

33

Health Maintenance Organizations— Strategy for Planning

Many ways were sought to control the spiraling of health care expenditures in the 1960s and 1970s. Among these was official national support for a pattern of health care organization, long operating as a minority current in American health services and known by such terms as "health cooperatives" or "prepaid group practice." The basic concept, with some modifications, was given a new label: "health maintenance organization" (HMO), and promoted with federal subsidies.

In addition to their cost-control effects, HMOs also constituted a form of health planning by relatively small local and voluntary subsystems for comprehensive health services offered to defined populations for fixed prepaid amounts. The concept continued to generate controversy, and in 1972 the Institute of Medicine of the National Academy of Sciences commissioned the preparation of a general review of the new evidence on HMO performance, accumulated since the last such review appearing in 1969. The following chapter, co-authored with William Shonick, is the text of that general review, indicating the apparent strengths, weaknesses, potentialities, and planning implications of the idea.

Introduction

In a "health strategy" message of February, 1971, the President gave new prominence to an idea which had been evolving in the United States for half a century or more. Basically, the idea involves the assumption of responsibility for the health of a population by an organized entity, in consideration of a fixed, prepaid amount of money. Incentives to increase medical earnings through maximizing services are theoretically replaced by incentives to maximize earnings by prudent use of costly services. Initially a contentious deviance from the

Chapter 33 originally appeared as "HMO Performance: The Recent Evidence" in *Health and Society* (Milbank Memorial Fund Quarterly), Summer 1973, pp. 271–317, and is reprinted by permission of that journal.

conventional open-market, fee-for-service concept of medical care, the idea gradually gained social acceptance in the 1950s and 1960s, as experience demonstrated that it could yield medical care of good quality at lower than prevailing average costs. By the 1970s, the spiraling of medical costs had become so alarming that a conservative federal administration decided to push the idea and to give it a glamorous new label: the "Health Maintenance Organization," or HMO.

Clearcut evidence of the effects of HMOs has not been abundant but it has gradually mounted. Avedis Donabedian (1969) published a comprehensive evaluation of the principal model of HMO—that based on group practice organization—and since that time additional evaluative evidence has accumulated. Most of this evidence compares the prepaid group practice (PGP) model with other patterns of health care delivery, but some of it concerns the model of the "medical care foundations," in which the key principles of HMOs are implemented under a pattern of physician's service offered through individual rather than group practices. This paper will review this recent evidence and offer interpretations of its meaning, with respect to social policy decisions on HMO strategy.

The definition of HMO applied here is an organization which:

1. makes a contract with consumers (or employers on their behalf) to assure the delivery of stated health services of measurable quality;
2. has an enrolled population;
3. offers a stated broad range of personal health service benefits, including at least physician services and hospital care;
4. is paid on an advance capitation basis.

Regarding element 3. in this definition, the investigations reviewed here have been applied to HMOs with rather widely varying scopes of benefits, not all of which offer protection for *all* physician and hospital services used or needed by a population. At this point, however, we believe there are lessons to be learned from study of some HMOs which may not fit perfectly under an ideal definition.

Since 1969, there have been published a number of other general review papers which examine the whole question of HMOs and their consequences: for health, economy, and other values. In offering this review we have naturally made use of these papers, in particular those by Herbert Klarman (1971), John Glasgow (1972), Merwyn Greenlick (1972), and Ira Greenberg and Michael Rodburg (1971) in the *Harvard Law Review*. We shall, of course, in addition review the main findings of several other studies reported separately.

The recent material has not only provided additional empirical evidence but has also extended and deepened our understanding of the various dimensions along which analysis must proceed if we are to infer, from the accumulated evidence, generalizations useful for social policy decisions.

Previous Studies

Research on comparative performance under alternative forms of organization of medical care delivery had been going on with ever increasing frequency since the issuance of the final report of the Committee on the Costs of Medical Care (1932). Particular interest centered around the performance of prepaid group practice (PGP) as compared with other modalities for delivery of care. In attempting to design research which would provide information about these effects, the investigators were faced with evaluating a phenomenon whose input consisted of a number of different and perhaps separable factors and whose output similarly consisted of a number of separately identifiable elements.

On the *input side* have been included the factors of 1. prepayment by the subscriber, 2. practice in a group setting, 3. paying the physician by salary, and, in some cases, 4. owning or at least controlling the operation of the associated hospitals. Although each of these components was often present in the operation of a PGP, not all of them existed in "pure" form in every PGP studied. The degree to which each of these factors was present varied among the PGPs studied; attributing an appropriate aliquot part of the observed effect to these several input factors was often the aim of later research, using ever more refined designs.

Similarly, on the *output side,* the criteria to be applied in judging the effects produced by the PGP, as compared with alternative practice modalities, were increasingly broken down by researchers into more particular elements, such as patient satisfaction, effects on hospital use, and the like.

As the number of such studies proliferated, publications reporting their results began to be interspersed periodically with review articles summarizing and analyzing the current state of the findings on various facets of the question. In attempting to draw generalizations about the performance of PGP from the published results, the several reviewers formulated various typologies for analysis.

The earlier reviews did not discuss in great detail the various components of PGP (noted above), in general considering all such organizations to be members of one generic group. These earlier evaluation articles each focused on some particular aspect of the performance results of PGP, as compared with alternative forms of organization of practice. Klarman's initial review (1963) addressed itself to the effects of the PGP and other practice modalities upon hospital utilization; Weinerman (1964) dealt mainly with patients' perception of the medical care provided in prepaid group practice.

Donabedian's 1969 review constituted a landmark in its attempt to analyze the research results according to a broad series of criteria, considering the entire spectrum as the necessary basis for evaluating medical care system performance. He grouped these criteria, and the parameters for measuring them, as follows:

1. Patient satisfaction:
    - frequency with which consumers choose PGP, when this choice is available

- expressed opinions of subscribers
- frequency of out-of-plan use by PGP members

2. Opinions of participating physicians:
   - concerning conditions of medical practice
   - concerning the nature and behavior of subscribers
3. Health service utilization rates:
   - from hospital and insurance records
   - from survey questionnaires to subscribers
4. Costs to patients:
   - premiums paid (from insurance records and surveys)
   - out-of-plan expenditures from surveys
5. Economic productivity:
   - theoretical analysis of expectations
   - economic analysis of empirical data
6. Quality of medical care:
   - influence of pattern on ways of using medical services (through survey questionnaires)
   - qualifications of physicians and hospitals used (from records and surveys)
   - physician performance (from direct observation and "audits" of medical records)
7. Ultimate health outcomes:
   - mortality rates on matched samples

Format of the Present Study

While this Donabedian analysis, in its multifaceted approach to PGP performance, was the most comprehensive up to 1969, it was based entirely on the author's study of previous individual investigations which he had identified and considered relevant. Indeed, Donabedian specifically states that his "review was made without reference to Klarman's 1963 and Weinerman's 1964 reviews . . ." referred to earlier in this paper.

The present review will consider the evidence on HMO performance that has been newly accumulated since the Donabedian paper, along with material that he did not include, especially from the Klarman (1963) and the Weinerman (1964) papers. In the light of present-day perspectives on HMOs, our analysis will be classified along somewhat different evaluative categories, as follows:

1. Subscriber composition
2. Participation of physicians
3. Utilization rates
4. Quality assessments
5. Costs and productivity
6. Health status outcomes
7. Patient attitudes

With respect to each of these features, we will attempt to report empirical findings under both the PGP and the "medical care foundation" (MCF) models of HMO. Finally, we will offer a few interpretive comments about the apparent need for surveillance of HMOs, the implications for comprehensive health planning, and the indications for further required research.

Subscriber Composition

The performance of HMOs will naturally be influenced by the composition of their memberships. Rates of utilization, costs, health status outcomes, and other measures for evaluation are inevitably influenced by the demographic composition of HMO members, their pre-existing medical conditions, and related factors.

A. T. Moustafa et al. (1971) reported on the characteristics of persons choosing among a series of five health insurance plans, two of which represented the PGP model (Kaiser-Permanente Health Plan or Ross-Loos Medical Group Plan). They found that married persons with children, in contrast to single persons, were more likely to choose the more comprehensive HMO-type plans, but that, otherwise, educational or income levels showed no significant relationship to plan choice. When, for some reason, persons changed their plan affiliation (at an annual open-enrollment period), those in comprehensive benefit plans—whether HMO-type or commercial insurance with wide benefits—were most likely to shift to another plan of comprehensive benefit scope.

The social acceptance of the idea of group medical practice, in contrast to the traditional pattern of individual practice, was investigated over several years in three cities (Detroit, Cleveland, and Cincinnati) by C. A. Metzner et al. (1972). A substantial majority of persons surveyed expressed preference for the idea of getting their care through group practice arrangements, even though many had no actual experience with such arrangements. The preference tended to prevail for all demographic breakdowns but was somewhat stronger in persons of higher educational and middle income levels. While this study did not explore *prepaid* group practice, the findings would seem to have implications for the HMO model as well.

Virtually all the investigations cited in the review by E. R. Weinerman (1964) were included by Donabedian (1969), and we shall not repeat them here. However, Weinerman's own analytic contribution is worth noting. He drew these inferences on the initial choices, among different patterns of delivery, made by subscribers to health insurance plans (Weinerman, 1964:882):

> The fee-for-service plans still attract a majority of workers in a dual choice situation, especially when their benefits are broad in scope. The advantages of initial enrollment have been indicated. Certainly, the organizational effort preceding the election date is of enormous impact. . . . The group practice method is still new and unfamiliar to most patients and to most doctors. . . . The comparative advantages of group practice health plan benefits are often complex and difficult for the

> average worker to decipher. Most significant is the repeated observation that enrollees respond primarily to the prospect of comprehensive benefits, and seem less concerned with the alternative of group versus solo practice.

It would seem to follow that greater familiarity with the PGP pattern is likely to increase the tendency of persons to like it, in spite of some of the impersonal "public clinic" connotations of *large* group practices.

In 1973, there were reported, for the first time, the actual characteristics of random samples of *total memberships* enrolled in various types of insurance organization, including HMO models. Studying health insurance plans in southern California in 1968, Roemer et al. (1973) found that significantly higher proportions of persons with generally greater risk of sickness were members of PGP organizations than were in commercial insurance or provider-sponsored (Blue Cross and Blue Shield) plans. This was reflected by slightly higher proportions of plan members aged 41 years and over, substantially higher proportions of families with a history of one or more chronic illnesses (60.6 percent in PGP plans, in contrast to 46.6 percent and 37.4 percent in the two open-market plan-types), and somewhat greater proportions of persons scoring high on a "symptom sensitivity" test. They also found a slightly greater proportion of foreign-born and nonwhite persons in the HMO-type plans, although the average family incomes in those plans, paradoxically, was slightly higher ($11,309 compared with $10,987 and $10,398 in the other two plan-types).

These studies suggest that any advantages that may be found for HMO-type plans, in terms of lower costs or better health status outcomes (as reflected in the pre-1969 research reports), cannot be attributed to their containing a smaller membership of high-risk persons, but would seem to be associated with the opposite.

With respect to the medical care foundation model of HMO, we have found, unfortunately, no documentation on the nature of its subscriber composition. We can only point out that the MCFs operate predominantly in relatively small counties of low urbanization. Moreover, as Richard H. Egdahl (1973) notes, a major share of member composition in many foundations has been derived from Medicare and Medicaid beneficiaries in recent years.

Participation of Physicians

The performance of HMOs is bound to be influenced by the qualifications of physicians as well as of other personnel entering this pattern of health service. It is also likely to be influenced by the satisfaction of professional personnel with their general conditions of work (including earnings) in this setting.

Prepaid Group Practice

Careful investigation of the qualifications of doctors in PGP (compared with others) has not been made, except for what may be inferred from the espoused policies of PGP organizations. The policies of large HMO models, like the Health Insurance Plan of Greater New York (HIP) and the Kaiser-Permanente Plan, are believed to result in careful selection of properly qualified specialists for all positions requiring specialty status (Greenberg and Rodburg, 1971). Insofar as general practitioners are selected for primary care, qualifications under the new specialty board in family medicine are encouraged. Similarly rigorous criteria for appointment, however, evidently do not apply to all HMOs, such as some of the new ones with small group practice units organized mainly to serve Medicaid beneficiaries in California (Nelson, 1973).

Empirical studies have recently been made regarding the satisfaction of physicians with the conditions of work in PGP. The earlier literature on group medical practice gave the impression that, with or without prepayment, difficulties and dissatisfactions were rampant (Dickinson and Bradley, 1952). D. M. Du Bois (1970) studied in 1966 a small series of private group practices that failed and disintegrated, comparing them with a series of private group practices that grew and prospered; he concluded that organizational failure was mainly associated with "policies in conflict with the professional role"—in a word, commercialization. Other relevant factors were a hostile professional environment and poor administrative management.

Based on a national survey in 1970 of private multispecialty medical group practices, Laurence D. Prybil (1971) found that the annual turnover rate—a long-used index of job dissatisfaction—was less than 5 percent. The respondents were from institutional members of the American Association of Medical Clinics ($N = 237$), a series that might admittedly be expected to have especially high stability. Even this low rate of turnover, however, seemed to be declining; it involved physicians mainly under 45 years of age, and most of those who left went to other positions in organized settings rather than into solo practice. Low turnover was also confirmed by the study of Austin Ross (1969), who found problems of remuneration in group practices to be the major cause of departure. David Mechanic (1972) in a recent national survey also found high rates of satisfaction in group practice—95 percent were either "very" or "fairly" satisfied (over 50 percent were "very satisfied")—with no differences evident in comparison to satisfaction with solo practice. Of course, one may infer that only those physicians who like the concept enter group practice in the first place.

Focusing more specifically on *prepaid* group practice, Mechanic found these doctors most satisfied of all subgroups with opportunities for professional contacts, total time of work required, and leisure opportunities; they were least satisfied with respect to time available per patient, income level, office facilities, and community status. Nevertheless, in aggregate "general satisfaction with one's practice," the PGP physicians reported "very satisfied" in 52 percent of the cases, which was precisely the same percentage as reported by fee-for-service solo practitioners. A turnover study in the Northern California Kaiser-Permanente PGP over the period 1966–1970 by Wallace H. Cook (1971) reported under 10 percent departures per year for employed doctors and less than 2 percent for Permanente Group partners.

Considering the socially marginal character of prepaid group practice in American medical culture, the remarkable point would seem to be how little dissatisfaction is evident among physicians who have "bucked the tide" and engaged in this pattern of work. One can readily speculate that, with the steady growth of open-market private group practice (now up to about 20 percent of clinical physicians, according to the AMA Survey reported in 1972) and the general national promotion of the HMO idea, participation in PGPs will become regarded as less and less "deviant," will attract more doctors, and will become associated with greater stability.

Medical Care Foundations

In regard to the medical care foundation HMO pattern, participation of physicians is, of course, open to all members of local medical societies. Except for young physicians-in-training, doctors in full-time research, education, or administration, and some physicians in full-time salaried hospital employment, one may assume that local medical societies (not necessarily the American Medical Association or the black physicians' National Medical Association) contain in their memberships virtually all private clinical practitioners in their areas. In the Physicians' Association of Clackamas County, Oregon, for example, it is reported (Bechtol, 1972) that all but two members of the County Medical Association participate in the foundation. Such widespread participation, of course, implies wide free choice for patients, but says nothing about the specialty or other technical qualifications of the physicians, beyond the licensure and "ethical" requirements for medical society membership.

Studies of the San Joaquin County Foundation for Medical Care by the UCLA School of Public Health cast some light on the participation of these physicians in the care of Medicaid beneficiaries. One study (Gartside and Proctor, 1970) found a higher proportion (85 percent versus 78 percent) of all physicians and particularly of certain qualified specialists (strikingly so in pediatrics and obstetrics) from the foundation area to be serving Medicaid patients than in a closely matched comparison county (Ventura) without a medical foundation. Another UCLA study (Roemer and Gartside, 1973) found that, in the performance of surgical operations, the work was more often done by properly qualified surgeons in the San Joaquin Foundation area than in the comparison county. These findings would suggest that, in the nonmetropolitan type of county where medical foundations have tended to develop, they exert a positive influence on the qualifications of doctors serving the poor; similar disciplinary influence might possibly apply to the care of all patients in foundation-type HMOs.

Utilization Rates

The data on differential utilization rates for health services under HMOs, compared with other medical care arrangements, have continued to accumulate. One of the principal advantages long claimed for the HMO model, of course, has been its association with relatively lower use of expensive hospital days, resulting in substantial cost savings. Before reviewing the recently produced data on this (and other) utilization features, we should consider some of the earlier interpretations of them not included in the benchmark Donabedian paper of 1969.

Hospital Utilization

The Klarman review (1963) was one of the earlier assessments of the general influence of health insurance on hospital utilization. Some of his interpretations, not reported in the Donabedian review (1969), should be cited. Drawing upon the studies of Osler Peterson in the United States and of G. Forsythe and R. Logan in Great Britain, Klarman noted that the concern of the 1930s about underutilization of hospitals shifted, in the 1960s, to concern about overutilization. Which concern is "correct," he notes, cannot be determined, since no objective standards for "proper" utilization exist. This implies that lower hospital utilization rates cannot appropriately be used as evidence of good performance without reference to what type of utilization is being reduced—"necessary" or "excess." Donabedian (1969) attempted to address this question by pointing to studies which analyzed certain aspects of hospital utilization between different practice modalities, in particular the diagnostic composition of this differential. Although the final verdict is far from being rendered, the prevailing pattern in the various studies of admission rates for the Health Insurance Plan of New York (HIP), as compared with other types of practice organization in New York City, was substantially lower in precisely those diagnostic categories most often suspected to comprise unnecessary admissions—tonsillectomies and upper respiratory infections.

There are two additional analytic points covered by Klarman (1963) which were either omitted or skimmed over by Donabedian. One concerns the early findings of 1940–1946 that Blue Cross-insured persons had higher hospital admission rates and lower average lengths of stay than did the general United States population. The other was the finding that, although HIP subscribers experienced lower hospitalization rates than persons under Blue Shield-Blue Cross, they showed the same rates as persons who used a union self-insured plan for ambulatory care. In the latter comparison, both the HIP subscribers and the self-insured union members used a self-insured hospital plan, leading to a hypothesis that control, specifically, of hospital use is a deciding factor. This is an important point, since it represents an attempt at identifying which structural variables in PGP affected which output results.

M. I. Roemer and M. Shain (1959) had reviewed the available evidence up to that time on hospital utilization under insurance. They conceptualized the determinants both of rates of hospital admission and hospital days in an area as derived from three sets of influences operative under conditions of economic support through insurance: patient, hospital, and physician factors. Roemer and Shain speculated that, while all these factors must theoretically exert an influence under the cost-easing operation of insurance (and there was support from empirical data for the influence of most of these factors), the most pragmatically effective mechanism of *control* was probably through constraints on the supply of hospital beds, that is, the bed-population ratio in an area. As we shall see, the subsequent findings on hospital utilization under the HMO models have continued to point to the bed supply as an important explanatory variable. The enactment of "certificate of need" laws on hospital construction in some 20 states, moreover, seems to reflect a growing consensus on the importance of the influence of bed supply on bed demand, with obvious implications for community costs (American Hospital Association, 1972).

Subsequent to the Donabedian review, additional publications dealing with hospital utilization levels of HMOs continued to accumulate. These consisted both of additional reports of empirical results and newer evaluative and analytic works.

Another Klarman paper (1970) concentrates its analysis upon "expected savings in health services expenditures" from the PGP pattern, thus again exploring the general criterion of his 1963 paper. Reviewing again the HIP studies summarized in the Donabedian review, Klarman clarifies certain aspects of the unavoidable confounding of the many causative (independent or input) variables in those studies that resulted from the special circumstances of the HIP structure and the New York City location. Included in these variables are group practice organization; prepayment by the subscriber; capitation payments to the 30-odd medical groups, accompanied by the diverse methods of payment by the groups to the physicians; the use of part-time as well as full-time physicians; the unique nature of the New York municipal hospital system; and the limited access which HIP physicians had to community hospital beds. From these studies, as well as others involving Kaiser-Permanente, Klarman concludes that the evidence indicates that limiting physicians' access to hospital beds has been an important factor in keeping the utilization of hospitals low under the PGP pattern.

Hill and Veney (1970) offer new empirical evidence from a Kansas Blue Cross-Blue Shield experiment on insured outpatient benefits. This experiment confirmed earlier evidence supporting the proposition that increased ambulatory insurance benefits per se for patients led to no reduction in hospital use and, in fact, result in at least a temporary increase of such use. These findings, Klarman argues, effectively rule out the availability of ambulatory care benefits as an explanatory cause for the reduced hospital utilization generally experienced by PGP organizations.

Besides limiting access to beds, Klarman notes that the salary or capitation forms of paying the physician may reasonably be expected to contribute to decreased hospital utilization on theoretical economic grounds. He cites the work of Monsma (1970), who showed that fee-for-service physicians derive a marginal increment in earnings for the performance of additional service (surgery, for example) while capitation payments (and salary) do not offer such an increment. This theory fits the findings noted in Donabedian's review that the excess hospitalization of the fee-for-service arrangement over that of PGP care modalities is centered in surgical diagnoses, particularly in tonsillectomies, cholecystectomies, "female surgery," and appendectomies. It is also supported by Bunker's findings (1970) that surgery rates are much lower in England (where there are relatively fewer surgeons, most of whom are on salary) than in the United States.

Klarman's most recent review (1971) broadened the field surveyed from PGP to the generalized HMO concept. Thus, besides reporting on some additional research and giving further analysis of PGP experience, he considered the data on medical care foundations reported in the literature and analyzed the factors in the MCF form of organization which might affect performance. Dealing with savings on hospital utilization under PGP, Klarman has summarized some of these results in the following generalizations: 1. It has been widely held, based on the implications of two HIP studies conducted in the 1950s, that there is a saving of about 20 percent in patient days and admission rates under PGP plans, compared to other health insurance plans; and 2. These results have been "subsequently reinforced in several ways."

Most of the "reinforcing" studies discussed by Klarman were cited and described by Donabedian in 1969, but there have since been additional ones. Moreover, Shapiro (1971) estimated a 25 percent lower rate of hospital utilization for HIP compared with other matched subscribers.

The Social Security Administration (1971) reported that per capita Medicare *expenditures* for hospital use were, respectively, 18 percent and 11 percent lower in northern and in southern California for Kaiser-Permanente, compared with care under other auspices. While these differentials are for expenditures rather than for use, it is probably safe to assume that they reflect patient-days utilized as well as possible differences in per diem costs. In any case, Klarman discusses this finding under his "utilization" category. A surprising datum in this same report is that HIP per capita Medicare expenditures did not differ from those for care under other auspices. Klarman speculates that this may be due to unreported utilization by the over-65 age group in the New York City municipal hospital system. He also notes that the differential in hospital utilization between HIP subscribers and other persons, reported in the past, was always quite small in the over-65 age group. If the zero difference currently reported by the Social Security Administration (SSA) is not due to an easing of HIP physician accessibility to beds, then the possibility exists that the difference in under-65 hospital utilization has been considerably greater than 20 percent.

A newly issued and more complete report by George St. J. Perrott (1971), describing the experience of the Federal Employee Health Program for the years 1961 through 1968, focuses mainly on hospital utilization among 8,000,000 federal employees insured under different types of plans throughout the country. Over these years, the rates for both hospital admissions and aggregate patient-days in the prepaid group practice plans have consistently remained the lowest, compared with the open-market "Blue" or commercial indemnity plans. These variations have prevailed for each age-sex level examined separately; they are especially striking for elective surgical admissions (such as tonsillectomy, appendectomy, and gynecological surgery).

Klarman (1971:29) notes, as a conclusion of his overall studies, that increasingly he has "come to single out the control exercised through bed supply" as a potent determinant of hospital use in the observed experience of PGP models, compared with that of other modes of health care organization.

"Foundations" and Hospital Use

Turning to the medical care foundation form of HMO, Klarman in his 1971 review notes that savings from reduced hospital utilization should not be expected from this form of organization on both theoretical and empirical grounds, although thus far evidence for the latter is slim. Since the prevailing method of payment to the physician under the MCF type of HMO is fee-for-service, there remains the incentive for the physician of higher income for additional services, according to Monsma's type of analysis. While the MCF type of HMO does not alter the method of paying the physician, it does broaden the ambulatory service benefits available to the subscriber. Empirical results have failed to indicate that such a broadening lowers hospital utilization rates. In addition to the Kansas findings of the Hill and Veney study (1970), Klarman also reminds us of the Avnet study (1967) for Group Health Insurance (GHI) in New York and of the reported results from extended out-of-hospital Blue Shield benefits offered in Maryland and described by Kelly (1965). All of these substantiated the theoretical expectations of no decrease (and, indeed, an increase) in hospital utilization when "physician services are broadened in a solo practice fee-for-service setting." In the Saskatchewan setting, Roemer (1958) had reported the same finding—increased hospital use associated with prepaid comprehensive doctor's care, compared with no insurance for ambulatory care—as far back as the late 1950s.

In recent years, further data on hospital utilization continued to be reported. Another study of government employees (state, rather than federal) insured under different types of health plan was reported from California (Medical Advisory Council to the California Public Employees Retirement System, 1971). Hospital utilization findings in this PERS (Public Employees Retirement System) study corresponded generally with those found for federal employees, with aggregate days per 1,000 per year being much lower than in PGP plans. Unlike the federal study, the California one also reported utilization under the medical care foundation plans, which are relatively numerous in this state. Interestingly, the utilization rates for both hospital days and ambulatory doctor visits were *higher* under the foundation-type plans than for any of the other plan-types. The experience applied to a 12-month period in 1962–1963.

Still another comparison of hospital utilization under the PGP type of HMO with other types of health insurance plan in California is given by Roemer et al. (1973). This study examined the experience of random samples of the total memberships of the three main types of plan, selecting two examples of each type. In contrast to some others, this study found the differential for hospital admission rates to be relatively small; but, because of a very short length of hospital stay under the PGP plans, the differential in aggregate hospital days was great—526 days per 1,000 per year in the PGP plans, compared to 864 and 1,109 days in the commercial and provider-sponsored plans, respectively. In this investigation, out-of-plan hospital use (determined through study of a subsample) was found to involve 7.2 percent of the admissions, many of them for maternity care (short-stay cases). These cases, like those in the earlier Densen studies of HIP experience, are included within the group practice hospitalization rates reported above.

Roemer et al. (1973) also analyzed hospital utilization according to several demographic breakdowns. It became evident that the low use rate (in days per 1,000 per year) of the group practice or HMO-type plans was largely referable to the experience of families with dependents and families of other than Protestant faith. With respect to social class (as measured by educational attainment and occupation), hospital day rates in all plan-types were consistently higher in the lower-class group, but the markedly lower rate under the HMO-type plans prevailed for both social classes. The same was true of families with and without a history of chronic illness—much greater hospital use in the "chronically ill" families, but markedly fewer days in the HMO-type plans for both types of families.

Interpretations of Hospital Experience

The total complex of causes contributing to the lower use rates of hospital days in the PGP type of HMO remains a matter for discussion and research. As noted earlier, the absence of fee incentives, especially for elective surgical operations, has been credited by much of the data (and theoretically justified by Monsma).

Easier financial (if not geographic) accessibility to ambulatory care under these plans has also been considered causative, but both the findings of the California PERS study (Medical Advisory Council, 1971) and the numerous studies of ambulatory care insurance for private doctor's care in Kansas, Saskatchewan, Maryland, and elsewhere, reported above, would not seem to support this contention. The constraint exercised by a limited hospital bed-population ratio, however, in the PGP plans would seem to be clear. The less-than-average supply of hospital beds in the Kaiser-Permanente Health Plan (below 2.0 per 1,000 members) obviously places an upper limit on the number of hospital days of care that can be provided. Striking evidence of this influence of bed supply is furnished by the differentials noted earlier in this paper on hospital expenditures for Medicare beneficiaries in the Kaiser-Permanente Health Plan in 1971, compared with other California Medicare beneficiaries; on the other hand, in HIP of New York, where the Medicare members use ordinary community hospitals, their hospital use expenditures were just the same as those of non-HIP Medicare beneficiaries (Social Security Administration, 1971). The degree to which this latter finding is due to the "opening up" of HIP physician accessibility to community hospital beds in New York, or to the other factors which Klarman postulates, cannot be determined on the basis of available data.

The point is that PGP doctors can evidently "live with" a constrained bed supply; they adjust by being prudent on hospital admissions, doing the maximum diagnostic workups on an outpatient basis, and keeping patients hospitalized for relatively short stays. Whether this results in better or poorer health for the patient is a serious question yet to be answered (refer to the section on Health Outcomes). That it results in cost savings (refer to the section on Costs and Productivity) is beyond doubt.

Aside from the PERS study reviewed above, meaningful data on hospitalization under the medical care foundation model of HMO are sparse. The Physicians' Association of Clackamas County, Oregon (Haley, 1971), reported that for 1969–1970 the average length of stay of Clackamas County patients at one Portland hospital was 5.18 days, compared to 6.82 days for patients from metropolitan Portland. No other data about the characteristics of these patients or the rate of admissions are given; since Clackamas County is essentially suburban to Portland and since its population characteristics doubtless differ from those of the central city, it is difficult to interpret these figures.

A still unpublished study of the Clackamas County Foundation by the UCLA Survey Research Center (Berkanovic, 1973) gives other data on hospital utilization under this pattern. Based on 1971 experience of Medicaid beneficiaries enrolled in the Clackamas County foundation, the preliminary findings suggest a *higher* hospital utilization rate (by a factor of 1.5 to 2.0), in days per 1,000 persons covered per year compared with a Medicaid population in a neighboring county using open-market patterns without a foundation.

Ambulatory Care Utilization

Donabedian (1969) noted that the sparsely reported data on ambulatory care utilization tended to indicate that, in general, such utilization increased under plans which insured for out-of-hospital benefits. The increase, however, was no different under PGP than under fee-for-service private practice. Also, there seemed to be no evidence of flagrant or obvious overutilization of ambulatory services.

Klarman (1971) attempted to assess the import of various published reports on physician-population ratios, in an effort to arrive at generalizations about respective ambulatory care utilization rates in PGP and in other delivery forms. Physician-population ratios presumably give indirect evidence of patient-doctor contact rates—if productivity levels are assumed constant. Based on the reported evidence of physician-population ratios, Klarman noted the often contradictory results of published studies, beginning as far back as 1940. In some cases the savings, in terms of per capita expenditures for physician care, were found to be greater than the proportionately lower physician-population ratio, presumably because of lower rates of reimbursement of physicians in PGP plans.

The actual rate of physician visits per capita is estimated by Klarman to be 4.50 per year for Kaiser-Permanente, compared to 4.42 for the general California population, after adjustment for out-of-plan utilization as well as for telephone and other nonphysician contacts reported as visits in the California-wide data. These estimates are based on the report of the National Advisory Commission on Health Manpower (1967) and on the Columbia University survey of three plan-types in 1962. The greater number of visits and the generally lower physician-population ratio in Kaiser-Permanente implies a higher level of production for the latter's physicians, but Klarman believes the Manpower Commission's report overstates the general California physician-population ratio. Data (Social Security Administration, 1971) on ambulatory care from the Medicare program could be used without the dubious intervention of "adjustments," except that only expenditures, not medical visits, are reported. Per capita expenditures for physician's care were 7 percent less for Kaiser-Permanente, Northern California, the same as other sources for Southern California, and 35 percent higher for HIP, as reported by SSA in 1971. Expenditures may, indeed, reflect utilization differences, but the relationship can be confounded by different levels of earnings and different productivity rates of physicians. Thus, the picture presented by Klarman (1971) provides very little information on differentials in utilization rates for ambulatory services between PGP and other forms of medical care delivery.

The Roemer et al. study (1973) does provide some comparative data on ambulatory services. Basically, the findings showed much lesser differentials among the plan-types than for hospital days; the PGP-type plans had doctor-contacts at the rate of 3,324 per 1,000 persons per year, compared with 3,108 in the commercial and 3,984 in the "Blue" plans. A revealing categorization in which these relationships, however, did not prevail was by educational level of the family head. Among persons with college education, ambulatory care use was higher under the PGP plans than under either of the other two plan-types. It would appear that better educated and probably more sophisticated persons are able to make greater use of ambulatory care in the relatively complex framework of the large prepaid group practice plans found in California; this is less true under conventional conditions of private medical practice.

Another study in California (Kovner et al., 1969) examined the effect of family income on ambulatory care utilization under two HMO patterns: both the prepaid group practice (the Ross-Loos Medical Clinic Plan) and the medical care foundation (San Joaquin County) patterns. The study found that, in both these HMO patterns, the effect of income was virtually nil—eliminating the usual correlation between poverty and low utilization of outpatient services.

It has been shown both theoretically and empirically that merely extending insured ambulatory service benefits will not reduce hospital utilization under fee-for-service practice; the same economic theory indicates that there is reason to believe that paying the physician either by capitation or salary should lead to decreased hospital utilization. If one adds to this the influence of substantial ambulatory diagnostic and treatment facilities found in a group practice setting, as well as a restriction on available beds, one may expect a *relatively* higher level of ambulatory, compared with hospital, utilization under the PGP type of HMO.

A revealing demonstration of these dynamics is given in the ratios between doctor visits and hospital days reported by Roemer et al. (1973) in the three plan-types. These are shown in Table 33-1.

It is apparent that the PGP-type plan gives almost double the *relative* emphasis on ambulatory compared with hospital bed service, of either of the open-market plan-types.

Further evidence of the influence of the PGP model of HMO on the ratio between ambulatory and hospital services came from the Columbia (Maryland) Plan in 1969–1970. Malcolm Peterson (1971) reported that physicians' office visits were occurring at a rate of about 8.0 per person per year (of which 40 percent were for well-person care), compared with 4.6 nationally; hospital days, by con-

Table 33-1
Ratio between Doctor Visits and Hospital Days in 3 Plan-types

Plan-type	*Doctor Visits per 1,000/Year (a)*	*Hospital Days per 1,000/Year (b)*	*Ratio (a):(b)*
Commercial	3,104	864	3.6
"Blues"	3,984	1,109	3.6
Group practice	3,324	526	6.3

trast, were at a rate of 335 per 1,000 per year, compared with about 1,100 days nationally. Although these rough figures were not adjusted for age, socioeconomic status, etc., they are still striking.

Quality Assessments

Regarding the persistently difficult question of quality evaluations, an excellent review of all the methodologies was produced by Robert H. Brook (1972) as a doctoral dissertation at the Johns Hopkins School of Hygiene. Although the evaluation of HMOs, in comparison with other patterns of medical care, figures only tangentially in this work, Brook concludes that both "process" and "outcome" measures should ideally be used in combination. Among outcome measures, he advocates greater application of the so-called tracer technique, in which the incidence of morbid sequelae of specified pathological conditions (e.g., middle ear infection leading to deafness or hypertension leading to stroke) is traced under varying subsystems of medical care.

In the last several years, investigators do not seem to have devoted much effort to quality assessments of HMOs based simply on "structure" or the input of resources (personnel, equipment, etc.). The unitary medical record and the greater convenience of interspecialty consultations were emphasized as structural avenues to quality care in the *Harvard Law Review* paper by Greenberg and Rodburg (1971), but these factors in the PGP model have not been subjected to quantified comparisons with ordinary medical practice. Williamson (1971) has demonstrated the discrepancies between "input" measures of the qualifications of doctors, and "output" measures of the quality of their work, pointing further to the importance of using process and outcome measures in combination as a basis for quality evaluation.

With regard to "process" evaluations, the recent years also do not seem to have produced medical audit studies comparing HMO services with traditional patterns of medical care delivery. The belief continues to be widely held, nevertheless, that peer review—whether on a day-to-day basis or on the post-hoc basis of claims surveillance in medical foundation plans—helps to assure the quality of the doctor's work. Yet Weinerman (1969), commenting on group practice (whether prepaid or not), noted: "Group conferences, medical audits, and informal office consultations . . . are common in the descriptive literature but infrequent in daily practice."

The Roemer et al. study in California (1973), from its examination of samples of actual medical records in doctors' offices or clinics, developed a "rationality index" as an approach to quality evaluation. This index was based on such documentable criteria as completeness of the medical history, extent of physical examination, frequency of consultations, and other elements of service. With the use of "factor analysis" technique, the value of this index for the HMO model plans turned out to be 0.527, compared with 0.515 in the "Blue" plans and 0.503 in the commercial plans. The fallacies of medical record analysis as a reflection of the actual medical care process have long been recognized, yet there is no reason to expect less complete records in private medical offices than in prepaid group clinics, and it is the comparative values that the above indices reflect. In fact, one might suspect that in private offices, where fees are paid for each unit of service, records would be more nearly complete than in prepaid clinics where the doctors are on salary; if so, the differentials on "rationality" indicated above may understate the relative performance level under the HMO pattern.

Another dimension of the quality of medical care is often considered to be the degree to which preventive services are provided and used. Under HMOs, there has long been discussion of the effect of incentives to preventive service, aside from the influence of early, rather than late, attention to overt symptoms. Roemer et al. (1973) have produced some of the first hard data on this question through the examination of medical records (and hospital records) under the PGP versus open-market patterns. Indicators of prevention, identifiable in patient charts, were such items as "checkup" examinations of adults, well-child examinations, vaginal cytology tests, routine rectal examinations, chest X-rays, serological tests for syphilis, and immunizations. Summating these, by "factor analysis," a "preventive service index" was derived for the three types of health plan. It was computed as 0.452 in the HMO-type plan, compared to 0.404 in the "Blue" and 0.384 in the commercial insurance plans.

Another reflection of prevention in HMOs is given in data reported by Lester Breslow (1972), derived from 1965 studies in Alameda County, California. In the sample of the "Human Population Laboratory" in that county, those persons who were insured under the Kaiser-Permanente Health Plan had a "health maintenance examination" within the past year more frequently than those covered by open-market plans; the comparisons were, respectively, 58 percent versus 43–46 percent for men and 63 percent versus 49–57 percent for women.

A study of schoolchildren in whom physical defects had been detected was reported by Cauffman and Roemer (1967), with information on utilization under the different types of health insurance plans that covered the various children's families. They found that any type of health insurance coverage, compared with noninsurance, was more likely to be associated with treatment of the child's defect, but that children in families covered by PGP health insurance plans were more likely to have received a general "checkup" examination than children in families covered by open-market plans.

Costs and Productivity

The economic dimension of HMOs, compared with other modes of medical care delivery, must distinguish between the overall expenditures by the patient or the community, on the one hand, and the "costs of production" or the productivity

Table 33-2
Annual Family Expenditures for Medical and Hospital Services in 3 Plan-types.

Plan-type	*Average Premium*	*Out-of-pocket Expenditures*	*Total Costs*
Commercial	$208	$156	$364
"Blues"	257	190	447
Group practice	271	52	323

of the subsystem, on the other, whether or not any productive efficiencies are "passed along" to the consumer in the form of lower prices. Each of these questions will be considered separately.

Expenditures by the Consumer

With regard to expenditures by consumers or costs to patients, the Roemer et al. California study (1973) produced data on the PGP model of HMO, as compared with conventional patterns. It analyzed annual expenditures by family units for physician and hospital services in terms of 1. insurance premiums (whether or not paid partly or wholly by employers) and 2. out-of-pocket expenditures. The basic findings for families of all sizes in the three plan-types are shown in Table 33-2.

Thus, it is evident that the average family premiums of the PGP-type plans are higher, but that the out-of-pocket expenditures for medical and hospital services are so much lower than in the other two plan-types that the aggregate costs are the lowest among the three types of plan. When family size is held constant, the same general findings prevail. There are, however, different relationships by other demographic breakdowns. In families of three to four members defined as "lower income" (under $11,000 per year), the lowest aggregate expenditures occur in the commercial plans; they are $391 in the latter plans, compared with $417 in the PGP-type plans. These findings may reflect the lower illness risk composition in the enrollment of commercial plans (reported earlier) as well as the lower available family incomes (even in the "under $11,000" category), also reported earlier.

For the medical care foundation model of HMO, the available data are, again, confined largely to the experience of Medicaid beneficiaries on the California scene. In a comparison (Gartside, 1971) of the four-county area covered by the San Joaquin County foundation with a similar county lacking a foundation, the monthly costs per eligible person average $5.81 for physician services in the MCF area and $6.66 in the comparison traditional area; the state-wide average, adjusted for the mix of Medicaid categories, was $7.33. The overall average costs for all types of health service were actually higher in the MCF than in the comparison area ($10.43 versus $10.13), although this was due almost entirely to a higher expenditure for nursing-home services in the San Joaquin area.

The MCF of Clackamas County, Oregon (Haley, 1971), reported that "generally costs in Clackamas County are 23 percent under the cost of service outside the county," but clear data in support of this statement have not been issued.

Production Efficiencies

In considering the crucial question of production efficiencies under the HMO model, studies on economies of scale within prepaid group practice have figured prominently. Herbert Klarman, (1970; 1971) goes into this subject at some length. He notes at the outset that empirical results represent experience drawn entirely from fee-for-service practice since "little, if anything, has been published on variation in productivity among medical groups in the same prepayment plan" (Klarman, 1971:30). By implication at least, he minimizes the dangers of extrapolating conclusions, reached on the basis of findings from the fee-for-service group practice milieu, to the PGP model, asserting that the caveats of Roemer and Du Bois (1969) about the noncomparabilities of the two practice media "pertain to who gets the benefits of any savings, but do not appear to bear on the issue of variation in physician productivity by the size of the medical firm" (Klarman, 1971:30). Although this particular point is well taken, it would still seem that such extrapolation should be made with extreme caution.

First, much of the fee-for-service practice data have been obtained in single-specialty settings, and PGP is typically carried on in a multi-specialty setting. Second, in view of the important influence on other performance criteria believed to be associated with different methods of paying physicians, one would hesitate to assume that there is no impact on productivity just because one cannot at present make a clear-cut case for it. After all, until Monsma's work (1970) articulated the issue, there was no commonly accepted theoretical explanation for the method of physician payment influencing HIP versus non-HIP hospitalization differentials in New York City. It may very well be, for example, that the management option of "pacing" physician visits, by control over the appointment system when the physician is on salary, can be more strongly asserted in large PGPs than in smaller ones. It may also be that substitution of lower-paid personnel for part of the physician's time is more feasible in the PGP model.

Many of the research findings cited by Klarman appeared in Donabedian (1969), but Klarman noted some additional works and further refined the economic analysis. The major studies again concern the work of Boan (1966), Bailey (1968), and Yett (1967). The study by Yankauer et al. (1970) is new. Klarman notes that theoretical considerations have led economists to expect returns to scale in medical care output on a priori grounds, and that Boan's and Yett's work seems to support this hypothesis. Bailey (1968), however, draws opposite conclusions. His findings (focused on specialists in internal medicine) lead him to infer that physicians in larger group practices earn more because of the profits earned on a proportionately higher rate of ancillary services performed in their establishments. The output, in terms of clinical visits per physician per unit time, was found to hold constant with increasing size of medical group. Bailey interpreted this to mean that the proportionately greater use of ancillary services by the larger groups of internists apparently did not represent a substitution of the time of allied health personnel for that of physicians, but could be viewed as merely incremental services delivered by larger groups.

Yankauer et al. (1970) reported a similar finding based on a nationwide survey of pediatric practices. This study also found the number of physician visits per unit time to be virtually constant with increase of size of the group practice. Delegation of tasks by the physician was generally in the administrative, technical, and clerical functions, but not in patient care functions. Where the latter type of delegation was found to occur, it was in response to relative local shortages of pediatricians, rather than in relation to the size of the medical group.

Klarman notes that the conflicting interpretations placed on these findings cannot be resolved by further analysis of existing data, but require additional research on medical care production, designed to answer the open questions. For the present, he concludes (1971:31) that "economies of scale have not yet been demonstrated empirically."

It should be noted that arguments which postulate a possibly greater willingness to delegate patient care tasks to ancillary personnel are related to the circumstances found more widely under large PGP conditions. These include the feasibility of close supervision of such tasks by the physician, a relative lack of concern by him that his income position may be eroded, and, in the case of large, self-sufficient PGPs, lessened fear of retaliation by competitors. Moreover, it is difficult to see why one could expect any increase in productivity, as measured solely by physician visits, under conditions which closely prescribe the tasks reserved for physician performance. In particular, in a PGP situation the number of visits to be handled by a physician per hour would largely be determined by the scheduling mechanism, and could resemble the moving assembly line in industry.

It is also necessary to note that defining physician productivity solely in terms of office visits, in fee-for-service private practice, can be illusory. Since, in the American scheme of things, physicians typically prescribe treatment for the same patient in the office and in the hospital, it is not unreasonable to postulate that solo practitioners and small private groups run up physician visit "scores" by hospitalizing freely. In that case, as Roemer and Shain (1959) have pointed out, the private physician can ostensibly increase his efficiency of practice by hospitalizing patients, passing along the heavy diagnostic work to the hospital and the expense to insurance plans. The larger, better equipped group practices may reasonably be expected to handle more of these cases in the office—spending more time with the patients, doing more tests, and hospitalizing less. Bailey's (1968) data tend to support this hypothesis, at least for solo as compared with group practice.

The important missing data in Bailey's study are the total utilization by and cost to the patients per year, per illness, etc. Lacking a defined subscriber population, these data are virtually impossible of meaningful interpretation. (If one wished to dramatize the deficiencies of these data, one could argue that all the data on visits to a particular physician might pertain to two or three patients with chronic illness making repeated visits, with astronomical cost to themselves or their insurance carriers.)

Boan (1966) stated the conclusions from his research in Canada straightforwardly. He found that physicians in group practice, compared to solo practice, had higher ratios of allied health personnel per physician, lower costs per physician for such personnel, and lower costs of investment per physician. However, these results are not strictly proof of economies of scale, since only the dichotomy between solo and group practice is examined. Furthermore, the applicability of nationwide Canadian results to the United States scene remains open to question. Direct inferences on returns to scale can be made only if one assumes that Boan's conclusions follow from observation on two discrete points along the size-of-firm scale—solo and larger than solo—and if one is further willing to assume that his upward slope of the returns-to-scale line would hold if the group practices were categorized along an increasing size scale.

Yett (1967) measured total tax-deductible expenses per physician as related to output (of computed patient visits) per physician, and found definite economies of scale. The result would suggest that practices in which the physicians were more productive, in terms of visits produced, exhibited a smaller overhead cost per physician visit. It would seem that a cost function analysis of this type does not directly address the question of economies of scale in terms of larger versus smaller group practices, and, a fortiori, does not shed light on what one might expect in an HMO situation. Furthermore, it does not directly address the problem of physician output as a function of size of practice (measured by number of physicians involved), which was Bailey's concern.

However, subsequent work by Reinhardt and Yett (1972), at the University of Southern California, has produced insight on this crucial subject. The published work concentrates on fitting production functions to national data reported to the magazine *Medical Economics* (MEDEC). These investigators are now tackling the question of the output of physicians (measured in patient visits per physician per week and, separately, by annual gross patient billings per physician) as a function of inputs. The latter consist of the services of medical auxiliary personnel, cost of plant and medical equipment, medical supplies used up in the conduct of practice, and the amount of physician's time (hours per week) occupied "strictly on practice-related activities." Physicians' visits are totaled over three sites: office, home, and hospital. The Reinhardt-Yett study defined "returns to scale" as the relative increase in number of visits per physician associated with the same percentage increase applied to all input factors.

Without reference to mode of practice, their results were that the output (visits per week) of the individual physician showed the expected increasing returns to scale, if inputs were to be increased in relatively small private practices. Comparing solo practices to single-specialty group practices, they found that the latter produce "between 4 and 13 percent more patient visits than do solo practitioners at any given level of factor input." The report cautions that these results may be flawed because of the lack of data on total medical group output, instead of output of individual physicians. So few data were available on mixed-specialty groups that they decided to exclude all multi-specialty group data from the group-solo comparisons in this study. Furthermore, the preponderance of the single-specialty groups studied was very small, consisting of three to six physicians.

Included among the USC (1972) findings were these points: 1. "Solo practitioners tend to work fewer hours and employ fewer aides per physician than do their colleagues in groups or partnerships"; 2. quite apart from the longer hours worked, group practice physicians produced more visits per hour than those in solo practice—4.5 percent more for general practitioners, 6.2 percent for pediatricians, 13.8 percent for obstetricians-gynecologists, and 4.0 percent more for internists; 3. up to about four or five aides per physician, the total number of patient visits per week per physician increases with additional aides; and 4. adding more physician time as an input will increase patient units by a greater factor than an increase of proportionate size in any other input.

Another USC study by Kimbell and Lorant (c. 1970) used the responses to the Seventh Periodic Survey of Physicians by the American Medical Association as its data for analyzing production functions of solo physicians, and the data of the AMA's Survey of Medical Groups for analyzing group practice relationships. Economies of scale were measured in terms of *office* visits as a function of the inputs: physician time, number of allied personnel employed, and number of examining rooms (representing capital investment). Among their findings on solo practice were these: 1. an increase in physician time increases the number of office visits by a greater factor than an identical percentage increase of any of the other inputs—in fact, more than the increase in allied personnel and capital (examining rooms) combined (a given percentage increase in allied personnel will have a greater effect on office visits than the same percentage increase in examining rooms, although increases in the latter will also increase the output); 2. physicians who charge higher initial fees have a lower output of office visits; and 3. the total R^2 (the proportion of the total variation due to the "explanatory" variables) is only 0.13, so that other factors not in the analysis explain much more of the production than those included.

Regarding group practices, Kimbell and Lorant found that: 1. the most important factor in increasing office (as well as total) patient visits by far is still physician time input; 2. there are decreasing returns to scale in office visits (and total visits) for an increasing size of output (i.e., an increase of about 10 percent in input factors will increase output by only about 8 percent, although, for gross revenues, the return to scale is almost constant, tending to agree with Bailey's findings); and 3. practices using an incentive plan for income distribution "had 10 percent greater apparent efficiency" than practices applying completely equal sharing or salaries. "Efficiency" was measured by the degree to which the group practices produce above or below the output predicted by the model. The R^2 achieved by this analysis of group practices was about 0.80, so that the explanation of output by the input variables was much better than for solo physicians.

Another recently reported study on medical care productivity is that of Newhouse (1973). This paper addresses the question of costs per physician visit in different practice patterns, and a principal determinant was found to be whether or not the practice shared income equally or divided it among the members of the practice in proportion to the number of visits each doctor produced. It followed that solo, fee-for-service practice was found to yield the lowest overhead costs per visit, since this form of organization represents the most direct relationship between the income received by the physician and the visits produced by him. The sample studied comprised 20 practices, varying from 11 solo practices to two 5-physician groups, and three outpatient clinics of hospitals. Newhouse states "there is the obvious qualification that the sample is extremely small," and much of the paper is devoted to showing that equal income-sharing should theoretically lead to increased unit costs per visit.

Effects of Size

In concluding this section on the literature dealing with economies of scale, a number of points must be noted. In using production functions in private fee-for-service practice, investigators have often considered patient visits as the key output measure. It would seem to be a questionable assumption, however, that more visits per hour are uniformly desirable. Clearly, the desirable number depends on patient care considerations, and flatly to equate an increasing number of visits per hour with greater efficiency cannot be excused by appealing to the assumption of "other things being equal." Studies of productivity which do not include some simultaneous observations on the content or quality of care are of doubtful usefulness at best, and may even be misleading.

Similar considerations hold in studying *economies of scale* in private fee-for-service practice. Assuming that physicians will keep unit (per visit) overhead costs down, if their income is directly tied to the net earnings of the visits they produce, might also imply that doctors would do almost anything they can "get away with" to maximize their net incomes. In a period of physician shortage, and in consideration of legal restrictions on competition entering the field, it would again seem to be questionable whether this type of motivation is widely operative.

Finally, with the preceding two points in mind, it might be germane to restate

Klarman's 1972 summary on the research to date in the following manner: General economic theory, as outlined by Boan, Fein, and others, indicates that group practice should be more efficient than solo practice, all other things being equal, in terms of productivity. Monsma's theoretic formulation indicates that *prepaid* practice is expected to be more efficient than fee-for-service practice, in terms of avoidance of unnecessary utilization of expensive procedures. Research to date has not effectively proven these reasonable hypotheses false. In any event, the entire question of production efficiencies touches only one aspect of the HMO concept; other aspects of incentives to economy, when a fixed annual premium is paid for a broad scope of services, will be considered in the following sections.

Health Outcomes

PGP and Health Outcomes

The ultimate measure of HMO performance, as suggested earlier, is how healthy these organizations keep their members, compared with other patterns of medical care delivery. The sparsity of data on this crucial question, up to 1969, was evident in the review by Donabedian. It had been largely confined to the experience of the Health Insurance Plan of Greater New York and focused on mortality in the very young and the very old.

Since then, some few additional outcome data have been produced on this key question, but not always with conclusive results. A study by William I. Barton (1972), though based on a nationwide mortality study in 1964–1966, provides the first such nationwide data on infant mortality in relation to health insurance coverage. After adjustment for race, region, parental education, and live-birth order, the mothers with some health insurance coverage had significantly lower infant mortality rates than those not insured; when adjustment was made for family income, the infant mortality rate was still slightly lower for the insured childbirth cases (23.3 per 1,000 live births compared with 24.5), but the difference was not statistically significant. This study, unfortunately, does not come to grips with the HMO question. In fact, it was found, paradoxically, that mothers with more comprehensive health insurance coverage actually had *higher* infant mortality rates than those with more limited coverage; the author, however, speculates that this unexpected finding reflected characteristics of the mothers, rather than being attributable to the extent of insurance protection. He postulates that women with more complete insurance coverage were probably higher-risk mothers in the first place—in other words, a previous pregnancy complication had induced them to secure broader insurance protection.

The first American report applying sickness absenteeism as an outcome measure for comparing prepaid group practice with other patterns appeared in 1971.

Robert L. Robertson (1971) studied work loss in 1966–1967 among schoolteachers covered under a PGP-type of HMO, compared with teachers covered under a "Blue" plan. Although in this, as in other comparative studies, the effects of self-selection could not be completely eliminated (since membership in either type of insurance plan is the individual's own decision), the findings suggest a slightly lower rate of "work-loss from sickness or injury" for both men and women teachers covered by the HMO-type plan. The size of the differences varied with age level, and the greatest difference characterized younger females. The overall age-standardized mean days of work loss were 3.88 days per year in the HMO-type plan for males compared with 4.01 days in the "Blue" plan; the parallel figures for females were 5.93 days compared to 6.41 days.

"Foundations" and Health Outcomes

With respect to the medical care foundation pattern of HMO, an as yet unpublished study from the UCLA School of Public Health (Newport and Roemer, 1973) examined perinatal mortality among mothers covered by Medicaid through the San Joaquin Foundation for Medical Care, compared with a closely matched county (Ventura) lacking a foundation and using traditional methods. Newport and Roemer found that, excluding county hospital births, which are not influenced by MCF procedures, the perinatal death rates were lower in the foundation area for "white Anglo" childbirths, but higher for childbirths in black and Spanish-surname families. When ethnically standardized for the mix of these groups in the state-wide Medicaid population, the perinatal death rates in the foundation and matched comparison areas were virtually identical: 29.6 deaths per 1,000 total births in the former group and 30.1 in the latter. More interesting, perhaps, was the finding that in a third area, admittedly not matched to the foundation county, but lacking a foundation and having a strong county health department (with an active maternal and child health program), the perinatal death rate was *half* of that in either of the study counties, at 15.5 deaths per 1,000 births.

While these were the only recent health outcome studies with a direct bearing on evaluation of HMO performance, other investigations have been providing new approaches to the use of adjusted mortality data for evaluating the performance of complex organizations. Moses and Mosteller (1968) revealed large differences in the death rates for specified surgical operations made in large teaching hospitals throughout the country, even after adjustments for various patient characteristics. Roemer et al. (1968) developed a formula by which crude hospital death rates could be adjusted for average case-severity, so that adjusted death rates could serve as a basis for evaluating the overall quality of hospital performance. These methodologic studies may provide clues for evaluation of HMO performance on the basis of mortality outcomes.

Patient Attitudes

While more substantial data on health status outcomes is awaited, some idea of the quality of service in a medical care program may be validly inferred from the attitudes expressed by consumers or patients. Although consumer attitudes may be influenced by many factors in health service delivery unrelated to technical excellence, it is reasonable to consider that the speed and degree with which the service helps a person to recover from illness or to maintain his health is an important determinant of attitudes. This becomes more plausible as patients become better educated about health care requirements.

Since the Donabedian review, additional studies have reported relatively high degrees of satisfaction with health services associated with HMO patterns. The favorable population attitudes toward group practice in general, even when experience with such clinics was lacking, were noted earlier from the study by Metzner et al. (1972). Weinerman's paper (1964) on patient attitudes toward prepaid group practice plans showed a high degree of overall satisfaction in spite of many complaints about the impersonality of the doctor-patient relationship in a "clinic setting." His general summary of numerous studies up to 1964 is worth quoting (Weinerman, 1964:886):

> In general, the various investigations of attitudes of group health members suggest much appreciation for the technical standards of group health care, but less satisfaction with the doctor-patient relationship itself. In one way or another patients report disappointment with the degree of personal interest shown by the doctor and with the availability of his services when requested. Much more rarely is there criticism of the quality or the economics of group health care.

The dynamics of a sort of psychological trade-off—that is, tolerance of unsatisfactory doctor-patient relationships in return for judgment of good technical service and a "good buy" financially—in patient acceptance of the PGP pattern are reflected in the findings of Roemer et al. (reported in 1973, although based on a 1968 investigation). This study solicited the attitudes of health plan members along two dimensions: satisfaction with financial protection and with medical care received. Regarding financial protection, the preference for the PGP pattern, compared with open market plans, was overwhelming, prevailing in all types of family (large and small), in all religious categories, in all social classes, in families of either high or low geographic mobility, and whether or not the family had a history of chronic illness.

With respect to satisfaction of plan members with "the medical care received," the positive attributes of the PGP plans were not so impressive, although the occurrence of frank dissatisfaction was substantially *lower* in those plans, compared with private medical practice patterns. Definite dissatisfaction was reported by 8.6 percent of PGP plan families, compared to 17.4 and 20.3 percent in the commercial and "Blue" plan-types.

When these responses are analyzed by social groupings, some interesting differentials become evident. The low level of frank dissatisfaction with the PGP-type patterns, compared with the others, prevails in all social subgroups. For certain subgroups, however, the HMO-type plans also show the highest level of "very satisfied" members: these include 1. single-person family units (compared with larger units), 2. Protestants (compared with other faiths), 3. families with no history of chronic illness (compared with sicklier families), 4. adult men alone (compared with adult women), and 5. geographically mobile families (compared with relatively stable ones).

Similar general findings were reported by Greenlick (1972) regarding the Kaiser-Permanente Health Plan in Portland, Oregon. While his respondents indicated substantial general satisfaction with the plan, that satisfaction was most often attributed to the financial advantages ("reasonable premiums" for the benefits offered) and to the actual care received after the doctor was reached, but over 50 percent of the respondents complained about the time it took before they got an appointment—in other words, access to the doctor.

Another study of patient satisfaction (Leyhe and Procter, 1971) was focused on Medicaid recipients enrolled in a PGP plan in California, compared with other such persons getting care through traditional private doctor mechanisms. The investigators in that study concluded (Leyhe and Procter, 1971:II) that:

> No appreciable differences were found between responses of . . . [the PGP] enrollees and of those who used individual practitioners. . . . Medi-Cal enrollees of this private group practice apparently appraised their medical care as equivalent in almost all respects to that received from individual practitioners. This private (prepaid) group practice was not seen by the majority of the enrollees as having the objectionable features often attributed to public clinics.

Of the 51 questions used in this patient attitude survey, only four yielded significant differences between PGP and non-PGP respondents. In three of these questions, OAS (old-age security) Medicaid patients expressed the familiar objection that they had difficulty reaching a physician by telephone, could not see the same physician continuously, and did not get house call service. In the remaining question of these four, the *non-PGP* sample of AFDC (aid to families with dependent children) clients complained that they had difficulty obtaining ambulatory care because of problems with transportation—a service the PGP plan provided for its members.

One other conclusion of this study worth citing is that ". . . it became evident that patient education pertaining to the current source of care is extremely important." Since about 20 percent of the respondents reported that they had had no identifiable source for medical care before being accepted into the Medicaid program, this conclusion seems to suggest that a pattern of delivery with a clearly identified, physically accessible source for primary care is likely to be more successful in reaching previously underserviced populations with medical service.

Meaning of Attitudes

Several comments are in order about patient attitudes toward prepaid group practice, typically associated with HMOs, as compared with traditional patterns. First, the policy of "dual" or "multiple choice" among plan types, always followed by the Kaiser-Permanente Plan and increasingly followed by other HMO-type plans, helps to assure that only persons willing to accept the "clinic pattern" of service will join such plans in the first place. Second, on the other hand, the clinic pattern clearly departs from traditional custom and experience among self-supporting families, and it is small wonder if the inevitable impersonalities, especially if the clinic is a large one, cause irritations or, at least, require psychological adjustment. Third, it must be realized that some of the dissatisfactions with PGP patterns are basically a result of the insufficient numbers of doctors in those programs—a situation which, in turn, relates to nationwide shortages; in light of the high incomes attainable in private practice, the PGP plans have understandably had difficulties in recruiting qualified physicians to fill all their posts.

Finally, it must be recognized that managerial problems are far from solved in most large-scale medical care organizations, whether for ambulatory or for inpatient service. The hospital literature is full of reports about the "insensitivities" of patient care in large hospitals, whether or not prepayment is in the picture. There are obviously improvements needed in the efficiency of managing patient flow in organized medical care systems. In a sense, the most remarkable fact is the increasing degree of satisfaction that seems to be characterizing clinic services in spite of their departure from traditional patterns.

In regard to patient attitudes toward the medical care foundation pattern of HMO, compared with conventional private practice, there is little reason to expect much difference since conventional patterns of medical care are indeed applied by the foundations. The California PERS study (Medical Advisory Council, 1971) did, however, solicit three levels of satisfaction ("satisfied," "not entirely satisfied," or "dissatisfied") toward different aspects of the four plan-types used by these state government employees. The responses showed overwhelmingly high "satisfaction" in all plan-types across the three dimensions: plan administration, doctor's care, and hospitalization.

The differences were all very small, by these measures; but for the foundation plans, compared with the PGP model of HMOs, satisfaction levels appeared to be slightly higher for doctor's and hospital care, and slightly lower for plan administration. It is doubtful if these figures have any statistical significance. More important, they are bound to be strongly influenced by the general social settings, since, in California, the medical foundations operate in the smaller and more rural counties, while the PGP plans are largely concentrated in metropolitan counties.

Out-of-plan Use

A reflection of patient attitudes toward the PGP pattern of HMO is bound to be given by the extent of out-of-plan use. Since the Donabedian review, the new data seem to suggest that this use is somewhat lower than reported in the earlier studies. Greenlick's report (1972) on the Portland branch of the Kaiser-Permanente Plan found that about 10 percent of persons had some out-of-plan use during the previous 12 months, but since this might have ranged from little to much service for these persons, he estimates that it would amount to under 10 percent of the total services.

Roemer et al. (1973) analyzed out-of-plan use separately for ambulatory doctor and hospital services. They found, through examination of medical records, that 12 percent of the ambulatory doctor contacts of PGP plan members during one year occurred with private doctors outside the plan; for hospitalizations, the out-of-plan admissions were 7.2 percent of the total. The relative lowness of these figures suggests that, in spite of some dissatisfactions, a decision of PGP plan members to seek care elsewhere (and pay privately—which may not be such a hardship, when premiums have been paid by employers, as is commonly true) is made relatively rarely. Moreover, even these low figures may be an overstatement, since the questionnaire used did not distinguish between outside care sought because of dissatisfaction (impatience for an appointment or the like) and such care sought in an emergency occurring outside the plan's geographic area—a type of care financially covered by "out-of-area" indemnity benefits.

In the previous section, it was noted that out-of-pocket outlays for doctor's and hospital services by PGP plan members were strikingly low, even though these figures included certain small in-plan copayments that are levied on certain membership groups in the HMO-type plans of the UCLA study (Roemer et al., 1973). The general extent of out-of-plan use in PGP plans, by various measures of services or expenditures, would seem to be lower than in the earlier studies summarized by Donabedian (1969). It would seem reasonable to conclude that, as people have become more accustomed to the PGP model of medical care, they have been more inclined to stay with it, in spite of some difficulties; perhaps over the years there has also been improved efficiency in PGP operations. There still remain, nevertheless, obvious problems to solve in the sphere of plan-patient relationships within the HMO model.

HMOs and Planning

The whole HMO strategy has important implications for planning. In a sense, it shifts planning responsibilities from central governmental authorities to local voluntary bodies, within certain ground rules. It says that for a fixed monetary sum, the HMO must keep its customers happy, or at least sufficiently satisfied to stay with that HMO and not to leave it for the open market or to join another one. Within the constraints of money and membership expectations, the HMO would have wide leeway to provide health services in a variety of ways. The evidence so far suggests that, given a promotional boost by government "seed" grants, the potentials of HMOs, based on the PGP model, to provide good health service at relatively lower costs than the traditional open-market private medicine model are substantial. Reasonable interpretation, however, of the evaluative data on HMO performance, summarized above, requires certain "caveats."

Nearly all of the studies on effects, whether based on structure, process, or outcome, have been made on relatively large, stable, and well-established HMO models. It is altogether possible—and some of the recent California experience mentioned (Nelson, 1973) underscores the hazards—that some HMOs, especially the newer ones, may yield a very different performance record. As the American Public Health Association (1971) pointed out in an official policy statement, there are two principal hazards in the HMO concept: inequitable "risk" selection among enrollees and poor-quality care through underservicing.

Safeguards against both of these hazards are feasible through a process of public surveillance. Regarding risk selection or, more accurately, membership composition, standards with respect to age, sex, socioeconomic status, and past illness history could be set and applied to the actual enrollees of each HMO. Recurrent "open enrollment periods" are another device to help assure that every HMO is serving its fair share of high- and low-risk persons. Without such procedures, one or another HMO could offer competitively wider benefits or particularly low premiums simply by excluding or reducing its load of high-risk members.

Regarding the hazard of underservicing or other strategies for cutting HMO costs at the expense of quality, the surveillance procedures are more difficult and complex. There seems to be an increasing consensus that monitoring would be required along all principal channels of evaluation: input, process, and health outcomes. In January, 1972, a conference was sponsored by InterStudy and headed by Paul M. Ellwood (1973), who has done so much to promote the HMO concept, in order to grapple specifically with the problems of quality assurance under HMOs. The report of this conference suggests that the main emphasis was on the importance of developing sharpened measures of "clinical outcomes," as essential tools of a "Health Outcomes Commission" (in government) to promote quality assurance.

The general question of quality assurance has, of course, acquired greater national importance as collective financing of medical care (through both government and voluntary insurance) has increased—quite aside from the issue of HMOs. In January of 1973, still another major national conference was held on this question (U.S. Department of Health, Education and Welfare, 1973), again stressing the importance of developing reliable measurements of both medical care process and outcome. The enactment of P.L. 92-603, the 1972 amendments to Medicare and Medicaid, adds further impetus to the need for quality criteria, with the new legal requirement of "professional standard review organizations" (PSROs) to blanket the nation. More research on formulating readily applicable measurements of both medical care process and outcome is obviously needed.

With several bills pending in the U.S. Congress for promotion of HMOs, including versions backed by both major political parties, it is a fair guess that the future holds expansion of HMO patterns of both major types—the PGP and the medical care foundation models. In the light of both continuously rising health care costs and the agreed-upon persistent need for comprehensive health planning (one item in the 1973–1974 Presidential budget contemplated for expansion, in contrast to the cutbacks in so many other sectors of the health field), one may reasonably look upon the HMO strategy as a peculiarly American approach to planning, in which responsibilities are delegated to numerous local mini-systems, in contrast to the usual European strategy of centralized controls. The private sector, through HMO development, would be vested with responsibilities and incentives to regulate itself and to meet the health needs of the population. As we have seen from the accumulated evidence, there is much reason to have confidence in the soundness of this strategy. Yet, as we have also seen, when and if HMOs become more a "mainstream" than a "vanguard" phenomenon, there will be enormous needs for continuing vigilance to protect the interests of consumers both inside and outside of health maintenance organizations.

References

American Hospital Association. Review of 1971 Certificate-of-Need Legislation. Survey report. Chicago: American Hospital Association. 1972.

American Public Health Association. "Health maintenance organizations: a policy paper." American Journal of Public Health 61 (December):2528–2536, 1971.

Avnet, Helen H. Physician Service Patterns and Illness Rates. New York: Group Health Insurance, 1967.

Bailey, Richard M. "A comparison of internists in solo and fee-for-service group practice in the San Francisco Bay area." Bulletin of the New York Academy of Medicine 44 (November):1293–1303, 1968.

Barton, William I. "Infant mortality and health insurance coverage for maternity care." Inquiry 9 (September):16–29, 1972.

Bechtol, Thomas A. (General manager of the Physicians' Association of Clackamas County, Oregon) Personal communication, July 10, 1972.
Berkanovic, Emil. Prepayment vs. Fee-for-Service for Medicaid Recipients. Unpublished data, University of California Survey Research Center, 1973.
Boan, J. A. Group Practice. Ottawa: Royal Commission on Health Services, Queen's Printer, 1966.
Breslow, Lester. "Health maintenance services in health maintenance organizations." Association of Teachers of Preventive Medicine Newsletter 19 (Winter):2, 1972.
Brook, Robert H. A Study of Methodologic Problems Associated with Assessment of Quality of Care. Doctoral dissertation, Johns Hopkins School of Hygiene (May, processed), 1972.
Bunker, John P. "Surgical manpower: a comparison of operations and surgeons in the United States and in England and Wales." New England Journal of Medicine 282 (January 15): 135–144, 1970.
Cauffman, Joy G., and Milton I. Roemer. "The impact of health insurance coverage on health care of school children." Public Health Reports 82 (April): 323–328, 1967.
Committee on the Costs of Medical Care. Medical Care for the American People. Chicago: University of Chicago Press, 1932.
Cook, Wallace H. "Profile of the Permanente physician." P. 104 in Somers, Anne R. (ed.), The Kaiser-Permanente Medical Care Program. New York: Commonwealth Fund, 1971.
Dickinson, Frank G., and C. E. Bradley. Discontinuance of Medical Groups 1940–49, Bulletin No. 90. Chicago: American Medical Association, Bureau of Economic Research, 1952.
Donabedian, Avedis. "An evaluation of prepaid group practice." Inquiry 6 (September): 3–27, 1969.
Du Bois, Donald M. "Organizational viability of group practice." Pp. 378–414 in Roemer, Milton I., Donald M. Du Bois, and Shirley W. Rich (eds.), Health Insurance Plans: Studies in Organizational Diversity. Los Angeles: University of California School of Public Health, 1970.
Egdahl, Richard E. "Foundations for medical care." New England Journal of Medicine 288 (March 8): 491–498, 1973.
Ellwood, Paul M., et al. Assuring the Quality of Health Care. Minneapolis: InterStudy, 1973.
Gartside, Foline E. The Utilization and Costs of Services in the San Joaquin Prepayment Project. Los Angeles: University of California School of Public Health (January, processed), 1971.
———, and Donald M. Procter. Medicaid Services in California under Different Organizational Modes: Physician Participation in the San Joaquin Prepayment Project. Los Angeles: University of California School of Public Health (January, processed), 1970.
Glasgow, John M. "Prepaid group practice as a national health policy: problems and perspectives." Inquiry 9 (March): 3–15, 1972.
Greenberg, Ira G., and Michael L. Rodburg. "The role of prepaid group practice in relieving the medical care crisis." Harvard Law Review 84 (February): 887–1001, 1971.
Greenlick, Merwyn. "The impact of prepaid group practice on American medical care: a critical evaluation." The Annals of the American Academy of Political and Social Science 399 (January): 100–113, 1972.
Haley, Thomas W. "Physicians' Association of Clackamas County." Hospitals 45 (March): 8, 1971.
Hill, Daniel B., and James E. Veney. "Kansas Blue Cross-Blue Shield out-patient benefits experiment." Medical Care 8 (March–April): 143–158, 1970.
Kelly, Denwood N. "Experience with a program of coverage for diagnostic procedures provided in physicians' offices and hospital out-patient departments—Maryland Blue Cross and Blue Shield plans (1957–1964)." Inquiry 2 (November): 28–44, 1965.
Kimbell, Larry J., and John H. Lorant. Production Functions for Physician Services. Los Angeles: University of Southern California. Human Resources Research Center (undated, processed), c. 1970.
Klarman, Herbert E. "The effect of prepaid group practice on hospital use." Public Health Reports 78 (November): 955–965, 1963.
———. "Economic research in group medicine." Pp. 178–193 in Beamish, R. E. (ed.), New Horizons in Health Care. Winnipeg, Canada: First International Congress on Group Medicine, 1970.
———. "Analysis of the HMO proposal—its assumptions, implications, and prospects." Pp. 24–38 in Health Maintenance Organizations: A Reconfiguration of the Health Services System. Chicago: University of Chicago Center for Health Administration Studies, 1971.

Kovner, Joel W., L. Brian Browne, and Arnold I. Kisch. "Income and use of outpatient medical care by the insured." Inquiry 6 (June): 27–34, 1969.

Leyhe, Dixie L., and D. M. Procter. Medi-Cal Patient Satisfaction under a Prepaid Group Practice and Individual Fee-for-Service Practice. Los Angeles: University of California School of Public Health (June, processed), 1971.

Mechanic, David. Physician Satisfaction in Varying Settings. University of Wisconsin (mimeographed, undated), c. 1972.

Medical Advisory Council to the California Public Employees Retirement System. Final Report on the Survey of Consumer Experience under the State of California Employees Hospital and Medical Care Act. Sacramento: Medical Advisory Council, California Public Employees Retirement System, 1971.

Metzner, Charles A., Rashid L. Bashshur, and Gary W. Shannon. "Differential public acceptance of group medical practice." Medical Care 10 (July–August): 279–287, 1972.

Monsma, George N. "Marginal revenue and demand for physicians' services." Pp. 145–160 in Klarman, Herbert E. (ed.), Empirical Studies in Health Economics. Baltimore: Johns Hopkins Press, 1970.

Moses, Lincoln E., and Frederick Mosteller. "Institutional differences in post-operative death rates: commentary on some findings of the National Halothane Study." Journal of the American Medical Association 203 (February 12): 7, 1968.

Moustafa, A. Taher, Carl E. Hopkins, and Bonnie Klein. "Determinants of choice and change of health insurance plan." Medical Care 9 (January–February): 32–41, 1971.

National Advisory Commission on Health Manpower. Report. Vol. II:197–228. Washington: Government Printing Office, 1967.

Nelson, Harry. "Investigation of prepaid health programs asked: possible fraud in some cases hinted by L.A. County unit." Los Angeles Times, February 24:1, 1973.

Newhouse, Joseph P. "The economics of group practice." The Journal of Human Resources 8 (Winter): 37–56, 1973.

Newport, John, and Milton I. Roemer. "Health service outcome under medical care foundations: perinatal mortality in Medicaid childbirths covered by a county medical foundation compared to other delivery models." Publication pending, 1973.

Perrott, George St. J. Federal Employees Health Benefit Program: Enrollment and Utilization of Health Services 1961–1968. Washington: Department of Health, Education and Welfare, Public Health Service, 1971.

Peterson, Malcolm L. "The first year in Columbia: assessments of low hospitalization and high office use." Johns Hopkins Medical Journal 128 (January): 15–23, 1971.

Prybil, Lawrence D. "Physician terminations in large multi-specialty groups." Medical Group Management 18 (September): 4–6, 23–25, 1971.

Reinhardt, Uwe E., and Donald E. Yett. Physician Production Functions under Varying Practice Arrangements. Technical Paper Series No. 1. Washington: U.S. Department of Health, Education and Welfare, Community Health Service, 1972.

Robertson, Robert L. "Economic effects of personal health services: work loss in a public school teacher population." American Journal of Public Health 61 (January): 30–45, 1971.

Roemer, Milton I. "The influence of prepaid physician's service on hospital utilization." Hospitals 16 (October): 48–52, 1958.

———, and Donald M. Du Bois. "Medical costs in relation to the organization of ambulatory care." New England Journal of Medicine 280 (May): 988–993, 1969.

———, and Foline E. Gartside. "Peer review in medical foundations: its effect on qualifications of surgeons." Health Services Reports 88 (December): 808–813, 1973.
cember), 1973.

———, Robert W. Hetherington, Carl E. Hopkins, Arthur E. Gerst, Eleanor Parsons, and Donald M. Long. Health Insurance Effects: Services, Expenditures, and Attitudes under Three Types of Plan. Ann Arbor: University of Michigan School of Public Health, 1973.

———, A. Taher Moustafa, and Carl E. Hopkins. "A proposed hospital quality index: hospital death rates adjusted for case severity." Health Services Research 3 (Summer): 96–118, 1968.

———, and Max Shain. Hospital Utilization under Insurance, Monograph Series No. 6. Chicago: American Hospital Association, 1959.

Ross, Austin, Jr. "A report on physician terminations in group practice." Medical Group Management 16: 15–21, 1969.

Shapiro, Sam. "Role of hospitals in the changing health insurance plan of Greater New York." Bulletin of the New York Academy of Medicine 74 (April): 374–381, 1971.

Social Security Administration. Medicare Experience with Prepaid Group Practice Enrollees. Washington: Social Security Administration Office of Research and Statistics (March, processed), 1971.

U.S. Department of Health, Education and Welfare. Quality Assurance of Medical Care. Monograph. Washington: Regional Medical Programs Service (February, processed), 1973.

Weinerman, E. Richard. "Patients' perceptions of group medical care." American Journal of Public Health 54 (June): 880–889, 1964.

———. "Problems and perspectives in group practice." Group Practice 18 (April): 30, 1969.

Williamson, John W. "Evaluating quality of patient care." Journal of the American Medical Association 218 (October 25): 4, 1971.

Yankauer, Alfred, John P. Connelly, and Jacob J. Feldman. "Physician productivity and delivery of ambulatory care: some findings from a survey of pediatricians." Medical Care 8 (January–February): 35–46, 1970.

Yett, Donald E. "An evaluation of alternative methods of estimating physicians' expenses relative to output." Inquiry 4 (March): 3–27, 1967.

Part Eight

Prospects Ahead

If past trends continue, it seems highly likely that the future will bring further organization of health services in a variety of ways. Collective or social actions are being increasingly applied to the financing of health services, and systematic organization is coming to characterize more and more features of health care delivery.

In Chapter 34, we take an overview of past trends and probable future developments in the entire health care system, which is analyzed according to six major components. Chapter 35 also surveys the health care system as a whole, emphasizing interdependence of changes occurring on the financing side and the service delivery side of the complex. The process of social change in most countries has started with the collectivization of financing (usually through health insurance), and this has led to forces promoting the more systematic delivery of services; Chapter 36 reviews these worldwide developments. For some years, the enactment of a law for national insurance of the major components of health care has been promoted in the United States, but some–impatient with the slow progress–have come to oppose this in favor of a "national health service" to be financed directly by general revenues; the implications of this political issue are explored in Chapter 37. Finally in Chapter 38, a blueprint for an ideal future U.S. health care system is drawn.

34

The Future of Social Medicine in the United States

Forecasting the future may reasonably be based on observing the direction of trends from the past. In this chapter, trends in various components of social medicine in America are examined with respect to health insurance, hospitals, medical practice, public health services, health personnel, quality surveillance, and certain categorical health programs, and increasing social organization is predicted. The principal forecasts are an increasing collectivization of medical care financing, a heightened organization of the delivery of services, and a widening scope of social controls.

In the decade or more since this text was presented at the 1966 Annual Meeting of the American Sociological Association, the changes predicted have, indeed, been occurring.

The Background of Social Forces

Estimates about the future are bound to be based on trends of the past, and so it may be appropriate to start these remarks with a quotation from a generation ago:

> The present trend . . . gives strong evidence for expecting increasing governmental assumption of responsibility for medical care, growing private and professional organization for more rational medical payment, and finally state and eventually federal programs of compulsory health insurance. . . . The price of more efficient and effective medical service may well be the complete loss of the "human touch" which medicine has prized for so long. . . . Whatever may be the details of the future picture, however, one conclusion may be drawn with certainty: that the institution of the private family doctor with all its individualistic and sentimental attachments is passing and in its place is developing a system of medical service more highly organized, more efficient, and . . . more generally available to the American people.

The relative accuracy of this forecast from 27 years ago is less attributable to the perspicacity of its author—for these were the closing lines of my M.A. thesis in sociology submitted in 1939—than to the conspicuous clarity of the trends in

Chapter 34 is reprinted from *The Pharos* of Alpha Omega Alpha, April, 1967, *33*, pp. 42–50, with permission of the Editor.

social medicine in America for the quarter-century (i.e., 1914–1939) before these lines were written. In the subsequent quarter-century, the trends have been no less clear. It does not require prophetic wisdom, therefore, to hazard some predictions about the future of social medicine in the United States.

In the usual academic style of the day, my 1939 approach to the trends in American medicine analyzed them in terms of biological, historical, economic, technological, sociological, political, and professional influences determining the direction of change. Our view today perhaps may be sharper. It is quite evident that the forces shaping the health services come from many sources, but they can probably be put under three broad headings.

First, there are the scientific and technological developments. Knowledge and its technical applications seem to grow exponentially. The management of scientific techniques requires increasing specialization. For a meaningful final output in the way of service, this demands organization and administration. Examples in all sectors of health care—in hospitalization, ambulatory service, public health—are too well known to repeat.

Second, there are developments which are fundamentally biological. Past achievements have affected the nature of disease. In place of acute infections, the predominant place is taken by the chronic disorders, both physical and mental, which are far more complex to treat. Along with this the composition of the population has changed, yielding a higher proportion of the very old and the very young, in relation to those in middle adult years. These biological ratios have profound economic implications for health service, since they mean that the productive working population has an increasing load of dependent age groups to sustain, and these are the very age groups that biologically have a higher incidence and prevalence of disease. To carry this load, of course, requires social organization.

Finally, there are the social developments, which include many features. Industrialization and urbanization are basic. Religion plays a lesser role and mass education a greater one. Family structure and function change, while larger social entities, especially government, play a greater part in the daily lives of people. Communication and transportation change the relation of people to each other. Democratization leads to rising expectations in health service as in other processes to serve human need.

All three of these sets of forces—technical, biological, and social—influence the shape of American medicine. The direction is clearly the same as it was in 1939, toward greater organization. Every push, of course, induces a reaction, and there are many resistances to change. But change in the social structure and function of medicine nevertheless continues. That is the definition, I believe, we may give to the much-debated phrase: "social medicine." It is the social structure and mode of operation of the social institution of medicine. The latter is meant to include, of course, more than the actions of medical doctors. As an academic discipline, "social medicine" has also included—especially in

Europe—study of the social factors influencing health and disease, a subject we usually define as epidemiology. But in the American context, and certainly in the context of this conference of sociologists, we are speaking of the social structure and function of the wide range of health services.

Trends in the Components of Social Medicine

To forecast the future of social medicine in the United States, we must examine it in smaller pieces. I should like to use a classification for this that is not pure, in the sense of following a single axis or dimension. It is a series of components in the social structure of medicine that are prominent and salient in the American scene: 1. health insurance, 2. hospitals and other health facilities, 3. medical practice, 4. public health services, 5. health personnel and quality surveillance, 6. categorical health care programs. This is by no means a comprehensive coverage of every facet of social medicine, but it may be enough to clarify the general character of important past trends and, therefore, the probable shape of the future.

Health Insurance

From the viewpoint of the general population, one of the most prominent features of medical scientific advances has been the rising cost of their application. To cope with these costs, for centuries one response of social groupings of people has been through insurance. As in other collective welfare measures, American responses came many decades after European, but since about 1930 insurance for meeting the costs of medical care has become an increasingly prominent feature of social medicine in this country.

The growth of this social device in the last 35 years has been phenomenal. From less than 5 percent of the population, the coverage has extended to over 75 percent. The benefits, however, have been limited largely to payment of the costs of hospitalized illness—that is, hospital bills and physician fees for in-hospital care. Of the total costs of medical care of all types, insurance supports only about 24 percent of the burden, since benefits for out-of-hospital care, including physicians' services in the home and office, dental care, drugs, and other items, are only meagerly financed through this device.

While the earliest health insurance plans in America were initiated and sponsored by consumers or their employers, the real growth of this mechanism has been through the entry of other sponsoring entities. The providers of service (hospitals and physicians) themselves launched the Blue Cross and Blue Shield plans. Then, with actuarial feasibility demonstrated, the commercial insurance carriers—which had sold other forms of group insurance to industrial populations earlier—began to underwrite hospital and medical benefits. Labor-management negotiations for "fringe benefits" gave enrollment a great push. This coincided with the stimulus to both provider-sponsored and commercially sponsored plans presented by the "threat" of national governmental health insurance proposed in a series of bills between 1943 and 1952.

The pattern of benefits and sponsorship of health insurance in America was quite different from the European model. Since hospital care was largely offered in public institutions anyway, health insurance benefits applied mainly to out-of-hospital physician's care. Sponsorship was largely by labor or other consumer groups themselves. In one important respect, however, the American development parallels the European and permits us, I think, to make some projections to the future. This is the observation that voluntary insurance leads to mandatory or social insurance for medical care in the long run.

It appears to be both the successes and failures of voluntary health insurance that account for this development. The successes demonstrate the economic and administrative feasibility of medical care insurance, as far as it goes. The failures relate to its not going far enough—that is, substantial sectors of health need, for many reasons, being left unprotected by the voluntary insurance approach. The most glaring such gap perceived in the last decade has been insurance of the aged—a sector of the population with greatest medical needs, generally low economic resources, and growing in proportionate size. This accounts, of course, for the "Medicare" legislation on health insurance of the aged enacted in 1965.

There can be little doubt that the future holds further expansion of governmental health insurance. The totally disabled (with or without indigency status) are a likely next group to be covered; then, perhaps the unemployed who now have wage-loss insurance but face termination of their job-connected health insurance. Perhaps children—about 25 percent of whom nationally are in impoverished families—will be next encompassed under this protective umbrella. Then, what about military veterans (and also their families), to whom the nation has long paid political tribute by way of a separate medical care system, but who could be readily served in ordinary community facilities under insurance protection? Before long, the non-covered sector of the population may be so small—perhaps 5 or 10 percent—that the political attractiveness of 100 percent coverage would be too obvious to resist.

Insurance extension will also doubtless occur for benefits as well. The medical foolishness of protecting only against the costs of severe illness requiring hospitalization, while ignoring earlier stages when the disease might be arrested, is getting increasingly recognized. We have only to look to Canada and the report of its recent Royal Commission on Health Services to see the probable path in this country as well.

Extension of health insurance protection in both coverage and benefits will not mean that the existing private organizations in the field will disappear from the scene—any more than they did in Europe. On the contrary, they were integrated into the European systems with essential instrumental roles. This is seen clearly enough in the provision for "fiscal intermediaries" of the new Medicare law, as it was developed in the earlier so-called medicare program for military dependents since 1956. The precise form of this integration, of course, differs in the American and European settings, and it will doubtless differ in the future here from its pattern in the Social Security Amendments of 1965. But one may surely expect that social entities as viable as the large insurance agencies—nonprofit and proprietary alike—will continue to play an administrative role in any broader social insurance that America evolves.

This much discussion of health insurance in a forecast of trends in social medicine would hardly be warranted if this were solely a financial device. In the polemics of the field it has, indeed, been argued that insurance is "only a payment mechanism" that does not affect the substance of medical care. But, in fact, this is true only in the short run, when insurance simply pays for the same pattern of medical care that prevailed before. In the long run, however, the collectivization of medical costs makes their volume socially visible; it provides the public who pay these costs an opportunity to exercise controls—through appropriate technical agencies—over the quality and economy of the services that the money is spent on. This has many meanings for the operational patterns of medical and hospital care, some of which will be examined below.

Hospitals and Other Health Facilities

With or without the enormous expansion of economic support for hospitals, the role of these facilities in the overall health care system was bound to change. Hospitalization insurance accelerated that change, as did expanded governmental support for hospital construction and operations over the last 20 years. The technological rationale for centers of elaborate equipment and staffing, required by scientific advances, was matched by an economic base to support these expanded resources.

In the total spectrum of medical care, hospital-centered services have obviously become steadily more important. The proportion of the personal medical care dollar devoted to hospital costs rose from about 20 cents to 30 cents between 1930 and 1960, but this is only a faint reflection of the trends. The rate of admissions to hospitals has steadily increased, approximately doubling over the last generation. Our supply of hospital beds has coped with these demands by a sharp reduction in the average length-of-stay per case. This means an intensification of diagnostic and treatment services rendered per day—a fact reflected by a steady rise in the ratio of hospital personnel to patients over the years.

The greater place of the hospital in service to the patient is paralleled, of course, by its greater significance in the professional life of the doctor. This trend has been quite different between America and Europe, where ambulatory or "community" medical practice is generally quite separate from hospital practice. In the United States, however, the vast majority of clinical physicians have hospital appointments, and the organized processes in the hospital have come to play an increasing part in their professional lives. This means that the sovereignty of the private practitioner is subjected to the increasingly collective discipline of the medical staff in a central place. Through the hospital, in both its formal and informal processes, the physician learns of new developments in medical science. The hospital is also a center for education of other health personnel—not only nurses, but also technicians, physical therapists, social workers, record librarians, and aides of many types. It is also becoming more of a center for medical research and, to a limited degree, a channel for preventive service.

The expanded role of the hospital has induced reactions in the social structure of medicine, and we are witnessing in recent years a stress on strengthening so-called "out-of-hospital health services." This represents, in my view, not a swing in the social pendulum, but rather an effort to achieve in the other sectors of health care the same degree of organizational advancement that has been, with relative ease, attained in the hospital. There is certainly no sign of any reduction in importance of the hospital world, while a kind of reactive emphasis is being given to the extramural services. On the contrary, the hospital is being developed more fully as a center for service to ambulatory patients (while not reducing its bed-patient volume) through expanded clinic and "emergency room" services, connection with private medical offices, and so on.

The importance of the hospital, in my view, will continue to grow in the foreseeable future, not because it contains beds for the seriously sick, but because it is a practical locale for the increasing organization of health services in general. This movement is seen more clearly in countries like Chile, Soviet Russia, or India where the hospital is the official center for the ambulatory and preventive as well as the bed-care services in each district. It has become popular in our country to speak of the "public utility" character of hospitals, which is the American way of assigning an overall public responsibility to a service that may be legally under private ownership.

There is another reaction to the increasing place of hospitals in the health services which, in my view, has less significance than is often claimed. This is the alleged impersonality of patient care in the large institutional setting. All the firm statistical evidence suggests that patients are getting more and more personal attention than they have had in the past, precisely because of the automation of procedures like meal-serving or bed-pan washing and the release of more effective time of a greater ratio of personnel to serve the needs of patients. It is the demands and expectations of people in an increasingly educated society that are enlarging. One cannot object to this, but it should at the same time not distort perspective. This is a complex problem, meriting fuller discussion, but I believe it is safe to predict that the future holds still greater, rather than lesser, attention to the personal sensitivities of hospital patients.

The organizational enrichment within hospitals is matched also by an increasing network of connections between hospitals. The forms taken by regional or metropolitan associations of hospitals are varied, and time does not permit their elucidation, but they will doubtless expand in the years ahead. The requirement of "transfer agreements" between extended care facilities and general hospitals required in the new Medicare Law will promote a special aspect of these connections. The educational and patient-care provisions of the new federal legislation on "regional cooperative arrangements" for heart disease, cancer, and stroke will advance the movement along other lines. These specific legislative pushes, however, only represent the concrete expression of a movement brought about by the basic economic, biological, and social forces mentioned at the outset—a movement that may therefore be expected to mature further with or without legal inducement.

Medical Practice

The historical core of the medical system has been the individual healer, and his mode of work is obviously changing with the overall structure. The movement is likewise toward more organization, less isolation.

Within the private medical office, mechanization, record systems, auxiliary personnel, multiple examining rooms, all add to a framework for increasing productivity. Home calls have steadily declined (saving the doctor's time) and the patients seen by a doctor in the course of a day have doubled in the last 30 years. The telephone has widened patient contacts further. Medical history-taking is being automated and numerous procedures formerly requiring a physician are now delegated to others.

Specialization is, of course, a predominant feature of all the healing arts and in the physician's life it is central. The vast majority of new medical graduates are entering one of the 25 or 30 specialties. To put further order into their lives, specialists (as well as general practitioners) increasingly set up their practices in shared office facilities. About 45 percent of American physicians are now reported to have such shared quarters. The "medical arts building," containing a wide range of specialists and other paramedical personnel (optometrists, physical therapists, dentists) as well as laboratories and pharmacies, is becoming the model pattern in large cities.

A deeper response to the problems of specialization has been the group practice clinic. After a slow growth in the first half of this century, the rate of expansion of such teamwork in ambulatory medical service is now becoming rapid. About 15 percent of American doctors doing clinical work are now engaged in group clinics (by the usual definition of 3 or more doctors with shared income) and there is every reason to predict that this will increase further. The polyclinic or district health center of other countries finds its expression in the free enterprise American scene as the private medical clinic.

The typical American physician earns most of his income from fees paid for each service, whether the payment is from the patient directly, from an insurance plan, or from a governmental agency (e.g., a Welfare Department). But this pattern is also changing, and each year a higher proportion of doctors are paid through salaries. It is now about 35 percent on full-time salary and probably two-thirds if one considers part-time salaried appointments as well. The salary mechanism per se is less important, of course, than its meaning as a reflection of a social framework in which the doctor works. It means he is in a setting where some sort of continuing surveillance is exercised, as well as the other features of organizational dynamics. Even in fee-for-service private medical practice, moreover, the payment of fees by insurance or public programs usually means imposition of certain standards (sometimes quite weak, it is true) over the doctor's actions.

These organizing tendencies in ambulatory medical practice will doubtless continue. In the next 30 years, I would predict that purely isolated office practice will decline to very small proportions, except perhaps in very thinly settled rural areas. The attendant problem of the need for a personal or family doctor (non-specialized)—which most observers still recognize as valuable—would be met by a general physician attached to a group. Perhaps the specialist in internal medicine or pediatrics will play this role for the adult or child, with increasing frequency.

Public Health Services

There are scores of types of community health agencies in the structure of social medicine, but we may examine only one of these. The health department or public health agency is certainly the most ubiquitous, if not the strongest, of such organizations.

Initiated with a focus on the prevention of disease through environmental and other mass application measures, the local public health agency in the United States still retains this as its primary emphasis. But the changes are active. As early as 1910, attention began to shift from the communicable diseases to the promotion of health in children and pregnant women, although the approach remained preventive rather than therapeutic. In more recent decades, public health programs have widened to include dental health service, early detection of chronic disease (like cancer or diabetes), general health education, mental hygiene, and accident prevention. Various aspects of medical care and rehabilitation have also come under the health department bailiwick in certain local jurisdictions. At the state and national levels a wider range of responsibilities for the curative services have been assigned to public health agencies, including hospital construction planning and licensure, programs for treatment of crippled children, and treatment of specified populations like the indigent or merchant mariners.

The reduction of the communicable diseases, and the great strides in environmental sanitation, however, have occurred at a time when other agencies, in government and out, have widened their health service role. The welfare medical programs, Veterans Administration, workmen's compensation commissions, vocational rehabilitation agencies, and mental health departments have expanded enormously. In the voluntary sector, there are all the disease-specific societies, the visiting nurse associations, the hospital councils, the professional societies, and all the nongovernmental health insurance plans mentioned earlier. This atomization of social medicine has been a striking feature of the American scene, and it creates a special challenge for public health agencies.

My guess about the future in this sphere is that the public health agency will gradually change its role to that of a coordinating, planning, standard-setting, and perhaps supervising center in the arena of government. Rather than keeping its focus on the prevention of disease, and rendering direct services (like immunizations or restaurant inspections), it will oversee all aspects of organized health service, whether preventive or curative. The provision in the new Medicare Law that the state health agency should "certify" the providers of service, according to specified standards, is a bellwether of future patterns. If every small child becomes entitled to general health care under an insurance program, there will be little need for independent well-baby clinics. But the assurance of proper preventive procedures—whether by solo practitioners or medical teams—will require some continuing surveillance. The coordinating task among hospitals, ambulatory services, and mass preventive measures will be more difficult, but I believe it will evolve as the principal function of the health department we know today.

Health Personnel and Quality Surveillance

Just as hospitals are acquiring the status of public utilities, the whole range of health manpower is increasingly recognized as an essential corps for the public welfare. Physicians, dentists, nurses, pharmacists, technicians, therapists, and others are seen not merely as members of the healing arts selling their wares to the sick. They are viewed increasingly as essential servants required by society for its effective functioning—therefore, increasingly subject to both public support and public control.

The medical and related licensure laws, starting in nineteenth century America, were an early recognition of this concept. They were designed to protect the people against the ministrations of incompetent healers, although their implementation has often seemed more directed to limiting competition among professional tradesmen. The approach to health manpower today has become much more positive both in principle and in implementation.

The rigors of medical education in America have been steadily increased—more so, in fact, than in any other country. Following four years of baccalaureate education, the typical candidate attends medical school for four additional years, followed by two or three years of internship and residency in a hospital. If he wishes to attain certification by a "specialty board," his specialized hospital training must ordinarily summate to five years after medical school, followed by tough examinations. The specialty board procedures, interestingly enough, are not governmental, like the basic licensure, but voluntary innovations established by the medical profession itself.

Similar upgrading has been the general rule in dentistry, nursing, pharmacy, laboratory technology, and the allied professions. We still see cults outside this main medical stream, like chiropractic, but osteopathy is becoming so modified as to be approaching complete absorption into regular medicine (in the state of California, this has already occurred). After licensure or certification, the postgraduate educational process continues—at least among the more alert practitioners—for life.

As the primary practitioners in medicine and dentistry have increased their formal training, their relative numbers, as ratios to population, have not increased. The rising demand for health services, reviewed earlier, has been met in the main by the enormous expansion of nursing, technical, and other paramedical personnel. These have increased from a 1:1 ratio to physicians in 1900 to about a 9:1 ratio today. Each of the associated professions, moreover, gives rise to its own auxiliaries: the pharmacists to pharmacy clerks, the technicians to laboratory assistants, the nurses to a whole series of practical nurses, orderlies, and aides. New modalities in medicine breed new personnel, so that now we have the audiologist, the remedial gymnast, the inhalation therapist, and more. For each of the professions or health vocations (and a great deal of time is wasted, I fear, on exploring the distinctions between these two statuses) a set of prescribed criteria for training and official approval is developed.

As broadly based economic support for health service expands, the public expectations of a supply of personnel adequate to meet the demand also rise. Therefore, public subsidy of the training of health personnel is gradually enlarging. In medicine and dentistry, it takes the form of professional school establishment and operation by state government universities, as well as subsidy through federal research and also teaching grants. In nursing and other fields, it takes the form of loans, scholarships, and university grants, as well as direct operation of training centers. Basically, the social decision is to make sure that large enough numbers of health personnel are trained to meet the demands, if not the ultimate needs. The new National Advisory Commission on Health Manpower is only the latest of the signs of this social policy decision. One can safely predict that in the next generation or two, all types of health personnel will be trained mainly in publicly operated or supported schools, just as was done to assure the output of public school teachers in the past.

The public underwriting of professional education in this way may well affect the readiness with which government will feel free to influence the personal careers and locations of graduates. There are several states that now support the medical education of their native sons, with the proviso that they set up their future practices in rural locations of doctor shortage for a specified number of years. The concept in back of such laws may be expected to be applied more widely in the future.

Parallel with their quantitative output and distribution, public concern for the nation's health manpower will also probably be more and more applied to their quality of performance. In the past century, except for the basic licensure laws, the professions have mainly disciplined themselves. Hospitals, beyond state licensure, have developed the voluntary "accreditation" program, and we see this now being extended to nursing homes. Where self-policing of quality has not been effective—as in the drug production field—federal government intervention has become stronger. Specific federal or state laws on medical care for designated beneficiaries (like crippled children or industrially injured workers) may set standards for participating personnel higher than licensure. New York State has even recently passed a law authorizing the State Health Department to conduct "medical audits" in all general hospitals, as a measure for promoting quality of physician performance. The path seems clear toward a time when social controls—either governmental or voluntary—over both quantity and quality of medical service will permeate the entire framework of social medicine.

Categorical Health Care Programs

Finally, a few words may be said about the great medley of categorical programs for special population groups or special types of care or special diseases which have evolved in America. In a basically free enterprise medical economy, the decision to apply social measures to solve a problem is made only slowly and in small steps. When a human need becomes glaring, action is taken, but then only within the specific confines of the need. In the background of most social actions stands a large admonition: do not encroach on the free market more than is absolutely necessary.

Organized health services have been launched by government, therefore, for selected populations whose needs were compelling for the stability of society. Military personnel had to be protected for obvious national reasons, veterans for vast political reasons. As an aid in military recruitment in the peacetime 1950s, the dependents of military men were brought under a federal payment program. Merchant seamen had been enrolled in a compulsory health insurance program in the early years of the republic to help build up a fleet of trading ships. Indians came to be helped as a gesture of national guilt. These were all federal actions, while at the local and state levels, the poor have been the major recipients of public medical care. The story of their eligibility, under varying demographic status definitions, varying tests of poverty, and varying formulas of federal financial assistance is a saga of evolution of social responsibility for human welfare. Children and pregnant women are other groups for whom government has provided special services—although limited largely to prevention—and more recently migrant agricultural families. Organized health services have also been developed by numerous private resources, especially industry. In the interest of production, workers get special services—partially through the inducements of workmen's compensation laws. Fraternal lodges help their members and the Salvation Army helps the destitute.

Specific diseases have also summoned social actions from both governmental and private sources. For the care of serious mental illness, the state governments built a great network of mental hospitals, now becoming less custodial and more therapeutic and being complemented by a variety of clinics for ambulatory patients. Tuberculosis has been treated largely through public hospitals and clinics, as has much of venereal disease. Crippling conditions of many diagnoses in children and adults have come under governmental rehabilitation programs. Voluntary agencies have likewise tackled all these diseases, often long before government, as in the case of tuberculosis. In recent years they have concentrated on support of research and professional education, with some ancillary services for patients afflicted by cancer, heart disease, poliomyelitis, arthritis, cerebral palsy, and relatively rare diseases like hemophilia, cystic fibrosis, or leukemia. The general problems of chronic disease, especially in the aged, have summoned other social actions in both voluntary and governmental sectors, not the least result of which has been the new Medicare Law for health insurance of the aged.

Each of these categorical programs has meant some progress in meeting health needs. They have mobilized financial resources and often introduced certain new mechanisms for the organization of services, especially through clinics and hospitals. At the same time, they have led to an enormously complicated panorama of health care in the average community. The multiplication of facilities, personnel, and administrative services has often been wasteful and confusing. The relative attention accorded to certain problems corresponds more often to effective fund-raising than to objective appraisal of needs. As a result, a widespread demand has arisen for coordination of health agencies and services. One form of this demand has been a repeated call for integration of specialized programs into the "mainstream of American medicine."

The "mainstream" argument is quite complicated. It has been counterposed to categorical programs establishing separate facilities like public health clinics for babies, municipal hospitals for the needy, the Veterans Administration medical care system, or isolated rehabilitation centers for the disabled. By contrast, the "mainstream" is usually interpreted to mean the private doctor's office and the voluntary general hospital. The assumption is often made that the mainstream represents high quality of care, while separated arrangements mean mediocre or perfunctory care.

Unfortunately, the mainstream does not always represent the best application of medical science. Private offices and voluntary hospitals show a range of qualities, from very good to very bad. The organized, though separated, public clinic—if adequately financed and supervised—*can* represent superior quality service. Most important, these separate categorical programs would not have developed in the first place if the mainstream in a free enterprise medical economy had responded adequately to the total needs. One does not find this type of problem to any great extent in countries with "national health services" on the British or the Soviet model.

The dilemma will be solved in the years ahead, I believe, not by further medico-social fragmentation, but rather by a gradual yet major modification of the character of the mainsteam itself; then the categorical programs will be, in due course, absorbed within it. As suggested earlier, group medical practice clinics and regionalized systems of hospitals will probably eventually become the prevailing norm. When this happens, there will be no social justification for separate well-baby clinics operated by health departments, separate hospitals for veterans, separate schemes for vocational rehabilitation of disabled adults, or separate welfare medical programs for the poor. Instead, all these categories of persons and sickness will be served in the general network of health care facilities. Separate sources of financing may continue for a while, but the money will funnel into an integrated system. After a while, the source of financing will also probably be simplified, through levies on the whole population. The health department, as noted above, will provide the supervision to see that technical standards are met, whether they apply to preventive services for babies or job training for handicapped workers. In the long historical view, the current galaxy of categorical health care programs will be seen as having provided stepping stones toward a comprehensive health service for everyone. There will still be need for specialized skills within it, of course, but they will be offered as the tones in a symphony rather than the discordant noises of jammed-up city traffic.

The Principal General Trends

From this all too sketchy and oversimplified review of trends in the principal components of social medicine in America, a few generalizations emerge. While some of the detailed predictions offered above may be hazardous, on a more generic level the social directions may be predicted with greater assurance.

First, it seems quite clear that economic support for the health services will be increasingly collectivized. As we have seen, this may take many forms, but the principal ones are bound to be the insurance device and public taxation. There are endless varieties in these economic mechanisms, but the forces of our economy, at least in the health services, favor the path of taxation and its use at higher levels of government. Through national taxation, greater relative sums can be raised, and the process of redistribution of resources in relation to need can be more readily carried out.

The second general trend is clearly toward greater organization and systematization of technical services. Even if there were no movement toward collectivization of finances, this medico-social organization would continue, but the economic evolution accelerates it. For the public visibility of costs, which accompanies their collectivization, leads to wider public concern for economy and efficiency in the use of resources. This means increasingly rational organization (in the industrial sense of the phrase), so that a given action is performed by the person with the least training necessary to perform it properly, or by a machine. Thus, even more types and greater relative numbers of auxiliary or paramedical personnel will be trained and, to be used effectively, will be mobilized in structured organizations. Such organized patterns will doubtless characterize not only the personal health services (patient care and disease prevention) but also the process of professional education, construction of health facilities, and medical research.

Bound up with these two trends will doubtless be a third one, namely, the increasing application of social controls. To achieve both economy and quality of service, any system must be subject to continual monitoring. This may be built into the system in various ways. It may be put at the end of the "assembly line," so to speak, or all along the way. Because the flow chart for health services is long and complicated—indeed, it is several flow charts intermingled—the more pragmatic solution is to build in controls all along the way. The control of drugs, for example, must operate at the place of manufacture, the point of pharmaceutical distribution, the prescription by the doctor, and even at the point of consumption by the patient. For the diagnostic and therapeutic decisions of physicians, the process is far more complicated. The professional self-discipline now rapidly advancing in hospitals—with departmentalization, committee approvals, medical audits, utilization review procedures, and so on—will gradually extend and increase through all the sectors of health service.

There are corollaries of these three principal trends in the education of health personnel, the construction of health facilities, the conduct of research, the attack on specific problems like mental illness or cancer, and other features of social medicine. Since doctors, nurses, and other health workers are essential servants of society, their preparation will be more and more publicly financed, systematically organized, and subjected to quality controls. Likewise for hospital operation, research, and so on.

The character and ramifications of these basic trends need not be expounded further to clarify the issue that, we all know, disturbs many people. It is the issue of personal freedom. The problem concerning many is whether all the social organization—in health services as in other fields—deprives individuals of their freedom to enjoy life as they please.

The issue, of course, is very complicated and much confusion is caused even by the posing of it in such simple terms. Freedom is a many-splendored thing and our social order abounds with examples of trading one form for another—like the trade of a child's freedom to labor for an adult's freedom from ignorance through childhood attendance at public schools, or the trade of freedom to drive one's car at any speed for freedom from violent death on the highways. In the health services, it is evident that we are making vast trades of freedom to spend one's own money (foolishly perhaps), for freedom to have a hospital bed available in time of need (through mandatory insurance) or many other benefits that could be cited. We are continually restricting the individual doctor's freedom to do as he pleases in favor of a compulsion to meet certain scientific standards that are designed to save the lives of patients.

One can argue that the judgment of the collective authority may not always be sound; the individual may be right and the group wrong. Fortunately there are safety valves in any control system and my own view is that it is important to preserve them against the fallacies of the fathers. But in the long run, the judgment and actions of the group are more likely to promote the common welfare than the deviant decision of a random individual. While this may be endlessly argued in general politics, I think there is very little question about it in the sphere of science or the specific applications of science in medicine.

One corollary of personal freedom that concerns many is the problem of individualizing the care of the sick. With much higher utilization of health service than ever before, the pressure on a relatively constant ratio of doctors in the United States over the past half century has greatly increased. This pressure has been met mainly by a vast increase in the supply of paramedical personnel and greater recourse to the hospital, where these personnel are largely concentrated. Inevitably it is more difficult for a team of health workers to offer tender loving care than for a single bedside doctor, but the important fact is that a much greater proportion of persons are getting service today, and each person on the average is getting more service, than ever before.

As noted earlier, it is our expectations that have risen, and this is more a solid social force than a cliché. The whole social organization of medicine has come from the demands of humanism as well as science. The response to further enlargement of such demands will be not lesser but still greater organization of the health services. It is *through* organization that deficiencies are remedied and greater personal freedoms are achievable.

Social Medicine Research

This paper has hazarded a lot of predictions, based mainly on observation of past trends. But we might hope that the path to the future will be navigated with reason rather than fatalism. As in other phases of society, this demands research and planning.

In all sectors of health service we observe an adjustment to perceived needs through social organization. But there are diverse, and often intensely competitive, forms of organization applied. The most critical question for social medicine research, in my view, is to determine which form of organization gives the best results. The definition of "best" is, of course, very complex and depends on a variety of outcomes that may be defined. Once defined, however—whether in terms of end-results like mortality or morbidity rates, quantity of health service units, quality of service, economic costs, political by-products, personal satisfactions, or other parameters—they can be measured. Social policy-makers, as well as individual citizens, can then make rational decisions on which pattern of social organization should be promoted. One cannot escape from value-judgments in the mind of the decision-maker, and one person may count high personal satisfactions as worth more, for example, than low costs. But with a firm and quantified knowledge of the several outcomes of alternative systems of organization, decisions can be made rationally.

This basic research approach, of course, is the classical model for most clinical investigation in medicine. It is the design which compares the outcomes of alternative therapies applied to two or more matched series of patients. In this sense, social medicine research is also a type of "clinical investigation" except that its unit of study is not the individual patient, but rather the social group being subjected to an organizational therapy.

The applied questions to be answered in social medicine are numerous and pressing. Despite academic biases favoring non-applied or "basic" research, there is no reason why research on urgent medico-social problems should be considered less intellectually lofty or stimulating. Moreover, the history of science abounds with examples of great generalizations emerging from applied investigational efforts, ranging from Mendel's work with monastery garden peas or Pasteur's inquiries for the French wine-makers to the efforts of Fermi, Bethe, and others on the Manhattan Project.

Social medicine, because it inevitably concerns social change, is full of controversy. Through research, the student of social medicine can shed light on the probable outcome of different channels of change, so that decisions may be reached through the exercise, not of power, but of reason.

35

A National Health System: Analysis and Projection

In January, 1969, a quite conservative federal government administration took control in the United States, but the pressures propelling the health care system toward greater organization continued to grow. Three kinds of pressures could be identified: 1. pressures for universal accessibility to health care, 2. for protection of the quality of services, and 3. for control of escalating costs. The aggregate effect of these pressures, it is argued, was to move the nation toward a more orderly and effective national health system.

Subsequent national issues–especially the Vietnam War and the Watergate scandals–delayed the culmination of events anticipated in this paper. Elements of the "national health system," such as more systematic efforts at comprehensive health planning, evolved, but now a decade later, with a more liberal federal administration in office, the prospects of fundamental change in the health care system appear more likely. The chapter that follows was presented at the 1969 Annual Meeting of the Catholic Hospital Association.

SINCE 1965, the American health services system has been a boiling cauldron. The porridge, of course, was simmering for many years before that, but the enactment, in July 1965, of the Medicare amendments to the federal Social Security Act—30 years after Franklin Roosevelt signed the original law—brought a quantum leap in the turbulence of the mixture. To anyone who had studied health service developments over the previous years, the currents and cross-currents evident today were largely predictable—currents involving both the economic and the organizational dimensions of health care. In the same way, an examination of the current scene, or more especially the movements emerging since 1965, can provide important clues to the future shape of things.

Pluralistic Health Care System

It has been said that the United States does not have a health service system, but rather a "non-system." While the word gets across a certain message, it is not quite accurate. As does every nation of the world the U.S. has a health care system, but it is a very complicated one. Its complexity results from the many parallel and independent streams of social action that are part of the national heritage,

Chapter 35 originally appeared in *Hospital Progress* (the journal of the Catholic Hospital Association), September, 1969, pp. 71–77, and is reprinted by permission of that journal.

no less in the health field than in industry, agriculture, education, housing, and other basic endeavors. Especially prominent in American health service has been and is the robust private sector for both financing and delivery of health care. Voluntary forms of social organization have developed to meet the health needs of particular persons or the burden of particular diseases in a bewildering variety of ways. Even within the public or governmental sector, however, the social solutions to problems have been hardly any more systematized, because the decisions of lawmakers reflect the culture in which they function. The diversity of governmental health service programs for different persons, diseases, or technical services—functioning at local, state, national, and even other jurisdictional levels—is just as bewildering.[1]

In a very broad sense, the central meaning of the turbulence in the health services is a struggle or interplay of pressures to achieve order out of disorder. The pressures come from many sources and take diverse forms, but apparently are willy-nilly pushing in a certain direction. It is toward a much more orderly, economical, and effective national health system.

The ultimate social goal that inspires these pressures is simple enough to state: *good health care for everyone at acceptable cost*. The short-term inducements, however, are perceived much more specifically. They can be identified under three clusters of pressures implicit in the goal: 1. pressures for assurance of *good* health care—that is, promotion of quality; 2. pressures for assuring that the care reaches *everyone*—that is, achievement of economic, geographic, and psychological accessibility; and 3. pressures for assuring that the *costs* are acceptable—that is, control over the level of expenditures for health care, in reasonable relation to other competing demands in the economy.

There are endless ramifications to the expression of social pressures in each of these three channels. Some of the recent or current actions in each of the channels foretell the shape of a future national health system. With respect to several of these actions, a combination of pressures emanates from two or even all three of the channels, but for the sake of clarity each channel should be examined separately. Since the most fundamental feature of the health service goal is accessibility to everyone, the pressures toward this feature may be considered first.

Pressures for Universal Accessibility of Health Care

The primary purpose of the Medicare amendments was to assure accessibility to medical care of people needing it. Since the aged have the most illness, since they tend to have reduced incomes, and since 30 or 40 years of voluntary health insurance had managed to reach hardly half of them—with meagre insurance benefits at that—it was understandable that America's first national social insurance program for health care should concentrate on the aged.[2]

As elsewhere in the world, it was both the successes and failures of voluntary health insurance that led to social insurance—the successes in demonstrating the soundness of the idea and the failures in not accomplishing all that was needed. Also as elsewhere, the enactment of social insurance for a segment of the population is leading to further pressures for extension to cover more people. Within a year of Medicare's passage, proposals were made for extension of coverage to the totally disabled—that is, social security beneficiaries who are, in a sense, prematurely aged. In 1968 a leading Republican, New York Governor Nelson Rockefeller, testified before a Congressional committee to call for extension of the Medicare principle to the total national population. Texas Senator Ralph Yarborough, a leading Democrat, and chairman of the U.S. Senate Committee on Labor and Public Welfare—the committee that considers health legislation—recently advocated national health insurance. Thus, it is not only labor leader Walter Reuther's Committee for National Health Insurance that calls for universalization of the Medicare program, but leading spokesmen of the two national political parties.

Extensions of Medicare

While these are still only proposals for extension of coverage, actual enlargements of benefits under Medicare already have occurred. Additional general hospital days and all types of (instead of restricted) hospital outpatient services were included in 1967, along with certain podiatry services and additional physiotherapy services. Serious proposals have been made in Congress to add prescribed drugs to the regular benefits, as well as eyeglasses and optometric refractions. At the same time, removal of the heavy burden of the aged from the voluntary insurance plans has enabled them to further extend their benefits to the younger population.

Meanwhile, the federal-state Medicaid program has been extending accessibility of a broad range of medical services to the indigent and medically indigent in over 40 states. The "neighborhood health centers" of the Office of Economic Opportunity have increased geographic accessibility of teamwork medicine to the dwellers in urban ghettos. The special maternity and infant care program for high-risk mothers and babies has extended services beyond the conventional preventive focus of health department clinics in this field. Vocational rehabilitation and crippled children's programs have greatly extended their reach in recent years.

Yet all these programs that are dependent on general revenues to widen health care accessibility have run into serious cost problems. States such as New York, which attempted to apply a very liberal interpretation of medical indigency, have found the costs too high to support, and the federal government has now imposed a limitation on the definition of "medical indigency" to keep a ceiling on costs. It is significant that it is the Governor of New York State who advocates national health insurance, for this would permit coverage of low-income people with a lesser drain on general tax revenues. One is reminded of the pleas to manual workers by early 19th century British Poor Law authorities that they should join the "friendly societies" so that, on a rainy day, they could take care of themselves instead of becoming a burden on the state. Social insurance, it is sometimes overlooked, is actually a rather conservative form of taxation; under it, the low-income groups largely take care of themselves, instead of benefiting from the steeper tax levies on the rich.

All these pressures point to the high probability of nationwide extension of social insurance for general hospital and physician's care within the near future. This will happen regardless of the party in power nationally, although the administrative mechanisms would differ under one party or the other. Even under the Democrats, with the New Deal tradition of extending public authority, it may be noted that the 1965 Medicare program provided for the actual delivery of services almost entirely through the private medical establishment, and even the administration of the program is done in partnership with scores of private "fiscal intermediaries." The climbing costs of medical care and the rising expectations of people will, no doubt, lead to extension of financial access to care for everyone or almost everyone, whether Republicans or Democrats control the national administration.

Alternatives for Extensions

The precise route and staging of this extension process permit several alternatives. Some have proposed, as a next step, health insurance coverage of another age group—children—so that the dependent persons at both ends of the life span are governmentally protected, leaving the middle years of economic self-sufficiency for voluntary insurance (perhaps with public coverage also of the disabled of any age). Another approach would be through categories of service, as in Canada, where hospitalization insurance for everyone was provided in 1957, followed by physician's care in 1968. Still another approach might be the traditional social insurance sequence, starting with wage-earners and their dependents, followed by farmers, self-employed, and others. By any of these routes, there could be a variety of administrative mechanisms for coverage, ranging from direct national enrollment (like the old-age pension system), to mandatory enrollment in existing health insurance plans (like the old German system), and variants in between. Whatever path is chosen, it will gradually obliterate the line between the care of the affluent as against the indigent. The Medicaid program has not wiped out this line, despite its improvements over the past.

The various cost-sharing features of Medicare, the financial deductibles, and the maximums are, of course, carry-overs from the customs of commercial indemnity insurance. It has been said that while Medicare was passed through the massive effort of its supporters, the language of the law was written by its opponents. Most of the services for which the patient must partially pay, it may be noted, follow from the decision of the doctor rather than the patient, so that the cost-sharing requirements can hardly be expected to deter utilization. These payments, however, reduce the social insurance taxes that must be levied to support the program, and probably they will, therefore, be retained. It is likely, on the other hand, that the complicated distinctions in administration between the universal hospital insurance (Part A) and "voluntary" medical insurance (Part B) will eventually be eliminated, thereby extending the accessibility to physicians' services a little further, to reach everyone.

There are other important developments leading to wider accessibility to health care, beyond the various insurance and welfare medical programs. The increasing attention being given to expansion of the supply, and improvement of the efficiency, of health manpower is important among these. The President's National Advisory Commission on Health Manpower in its final report of November, 1967, recommended many actions which, in fact, had been under way for some years.[4] Most important was the call for a still greater output of physicians and dentists—through federal subsidy of professional schools—than had occurred since the similar recommendation of the Surgeon General's Bane Report of 1959.[5]

Greater numbers and new types of auxiliary health personnel were also recommended. In the last few years a number of important experimental training programs, like that for "physician's assistants" at Duke University or for "pediatric nurse practitioners" at the University of Colorado, have developed. The Commission also recommended a number of approaches to improving the efficiency of health care delivery, through so-called peer review of performance, increased automation and managerial skill in laboratories and hospitals, more judicious review of medical care utilization, and exploration of various innovations in the organization of health care. These recommendations obviously concern promotion of the quality, as well as accessibility.

A companion National Advisory Commission on Health Facilities gave its report to the President in December, 1968.[6] Its central thrust was a call for "comprehensive health care systems," which would assure good care to everyone. "The Nation must be prepared," said the Commission, "to finance comprehensive health services adequately to ensure the continued operation of efficient health care systems and the development of new components that will meet the full needs of the population." Funds might be derived from multiple public and private sources, but hospitals and related facilities should be expected to function in cooperation with "a community health planning council." To assure reasonable area-wide location and operation of health facilities, the Commission stated: "The power to approve governmental funding and to license health institutions and health agencies according to certain standards for quality care, safe construction, and evidence of needed services should be vested in a government body."

Of all the states, only New York has legislation with such mandatory hospital planning authority currently, but the ineffectiveness of voluntary planning agencies in several regions is leading other states to consider similar public policy. It is noteworthy that the American Hospital Association recently resolved that every member hospital should be obligated to cooperate affirmatively with area-wide community planning agencies.[7]

Social insurance, health manpower expansion, health facility planning, and innovative organizational forms are all designed to extend accessibility of people to needed health care. The pressures for these actions seem to continue in spite of the change in national political administrations, for the economic and technological forces in back of them persist. As already noted, the recommendations of various national commissions have been directed to qualitative improvements, as well as quantitative accessibility, but, in addition, several other important movements for quality promotion are in process.

Pressures for Quality Promotion

The social measures designed to protect people from the ministrations of poorly qualified health practitioners go back to the medical licensure laws of the 13th century.[8] The whole advancement of professional education in America, since the milestone Flexner Report of 1910, has been directed to improvement of the quality of health care. In recent years, a number of other national movements have evolved or accelerated, with the specific objective of strengthening the quality of medical services provided to anyone.

Only a few months after Medicare, the Congress enacted the "Heart Disease, Cancer, and Stroke Amendments of 1965."[9] While drawing public and Congressional support by focusing on the serious diseases constituting the three top causes of death in the nation, this legislation had the underlying objective of promoting a vitalized regionalization of all health services in order to improve their scientific quality. If there was any doubt of this basic intention, it has obviously been removed by the operation of the Regional Medical Program (RMP) during its first three years.

RMPs and Group Practice

The main thrust of the RMP movement is to bring to bear the influence of the larger medical centers, especially those associated with medical schools and teaching hospitals, on the practices of the average doctor in the average hospital. Much of this is done through the extension of formal programs of continuing education for physicians, nurses, and others. It is also done through organization of mobile consultation services from the larger centers, and assistance to the smaller peripheral facilities in establishing new types of effective service, like coronary care units or stroke rehabilitation programs. Screening programs for earlier detection of cancer or health educational programs designed to reduce the risk of heart disease or cancer are other approaches.

Quality promotion pressures are also seen in the deliberate actions of the U.S. Department of Health, Education and Welfare to foster the organization of group medical practices.[10] The group practice movement, of course, has been in process for many years, but since the end of World War II it has clearly accelerated. In 1949, about 3 percent of clinically active physicians were engaged in group practice (as defined by the U.S. Public Health Service, to include shared arrangements among three or more doctors) and by 1968 this had risen to 11 percent.[11] There are many consequences of medical teamwork in the sphere of productivity and costs and in doctor-patient relationships, but the main significance is doubtless its effect on the qualitative content of medical services. For in medical clinics—whether private, hospital-based, or prepaid—it is possible to achieve an integration of skilled personnel and equipment for sophisticated diagnosis, treatment, and also prevention, which is not feasible in the solo doctor's office.

There are other trends in the organization of ambulatory medical services with serious quality implications. The OEO neighborhood health centers have been mentioned; while some of them are having difficulties in reaching large enough numbers of poor patients, their impact is to permit an alternative for the ghetto-dweller which is qualitatively superior to the isolated general practitioner and humanistically better than the crowded clinic of the municipal hospital.[12] At the same time, hospitals are giving more and more attention to the structure and function of their outpatient departments. Under the increasing pressure of "emergency room" demands from people of all income groups, the OPD is no longer a resource restricted to the poor, and medical staffs are developing new patterns for providing these services in a qualitatively satisfactory manner.

Medical staff oganization in hospitals is in active ferment.[13] More hospitals are appointing directors of medical education whose duties usually go beyond the strictly educational sphere. Full-time chiefs of clinical services are increasingly being appointed in community general hospitals, emulating the university hospital pattern. Departmentalization is increasing, even in small hospitals, and various medical staff committees to review professional performance are taking their tasks more seriously. Utilization review committees are inducing greater group discipline for surveillance over admission, length-of-stay, and the content of patient care. The Professional Activity Study (PAS) is tabulating the elements of patient care in more hospitals, providing information by which medical staffs can review their work.[14] The Joint Commission on Accreditation of Hospitals is now engaged in a major upgrading of its standards, with particular reference to the rigor of medical staff policies. All of these actions are part of a swelling movement to fortify the quality of medical care in hospitals, in response to pressures from the general community.

Many of these quality-promotion trends were brought into sharp focus in 1968 by the report of the Secretary's Advisory Committee on Hospital Effectiveness.[15] It recommended many proposals on area-wide planning, similar to those made by the President's National Advisory Commission of Health Facilities, but with more specific details on franchising of institutions by a public body and on inter-hospital regional ties. There were also numerous recommendations on methods of improving internal hospital management in the interests of both quality and economy. The Commission sees the hospital as "the principal organizing focus of a new and more effective system for the delivery of health care" in each community. The recommendations of the report reflect, of course, the trends in widening hospital responsibilities for total health care in an area which has, in fact, been developing for many years.

Pressures to Stem the Tide of Rising Costs

Finally, among the pressures fostering a more orderly health care system in America are those directed to stemming the tide of rising costs. Throughout the world and for many years the costs of medical care have been rising, as the potentialities of medical science have increased and the technology to apply it has become more elaborate. A day of general hospital care in the United States today includes in its cost the wages of three persons or more, compared with one person 50 years ago; when other expenses are added to personnel, it is easy to see why hospitalization is approaching an average daily cost of $100. It is not difficult to understand why, in the 10-year period from 1958 to 1967, when the consumer price index for all items rose 16.3 percent, physician's fees rose 37.6 percent and hospital daily service charges rose 100.1 percent.

Other factors are also contributing to rising health care costs—factors relating to the classical vectors of supply-and-demand. The extension of health insurance and public financing of medical care has greatly increased the effective demand, while the supply of physicians, dentists, and hospital beds has not risen at a proportionate pace. These dynamics alone would cause a rise in prices, even if all the other technical changes were not occurring. Of course, the demand pressures have been met by training increased numbers and proportions of nurses, technicians, aides, and many other types of allied health personnel, or else the rise in prices and costs would have been even greater. These cost pressures reflecting supply-and-demand discrepancies, however, give the clue to their solution—namely, enlargement of the total supply of health personnel. Thus, the manpower developments mentioned earlier are, in large measure, a response to the problem of rising costs.

The pressure of rising medical costs is leading to serious explorations of many other approaches which would modify conventional patterns of medical care. In the last six months of the Johnson Administration, a series of regional conferences were held by the Secretary of HEW on the subject of "health care costs."[16] Hundreds of knowledgeable laymen and professional spokesmen came together to discuss the issues, and scores of suggestions were voiced. Again and again, there were proposals for increased use of auxiliary (and less expensive) health personnel, for automation of the diagnostic process, for administrative controls over medical and dental fees, for use of equivalent generic-name (in place of costly brand-name) drugs, for greater surveillance over hospital utilization, for reasonable control over the supply of hospital beds in each region, for organized home-care programs, for maximum promotion of preventive services, for merger of small hospitals into larger units, and other actions believed likely to reduce or at least hold the line on costs.

Also emerging from these regional conferences, as from many other sources, was repeated advocacy of the extension of prepaid group practice as a sounder pattern for provision of ambulatory health care. More than any other concrete measure, this pattern has actually demonstrated the feasibility of reducing the costs of medical care, compared with conventional arrangements, or of giving more services per dollar spent. The economies of prepaid group practice appear to be of two types: primary economies of scale and rationalization within the organized clinic, and secondary economies due to the more judicious use of hospitals, low-cost drugs, and other services outside the clinic.[17]

These secondary economies appear to be even greater when the group practice clinics are closely affiliated with hospitals, as in the Kaiser-Permanente Health Plan. This is the most significant approach to containment of rising medical costs being explored in the nation today, and it is bound to have a very large impact on the future. At the same time, the available evidence suggests that prepaid group practice yields a higher quality of medical care—in terms of lower mortality rates and other indices—than the conventional pattern of fee-for-service private medicine.[18]

To encourage cost reduction under Medicare and Medicaid, the Social Security Administration launched a plan in early 1968 for "Incentive Reimbursement Experiments."[19] These enable hospitals, physicians, and others to share in any savings that can be achieved, in relation to average experience, by innovative systems of medical care organization or payment mechanisms. Only a few of these local experiments have been authorized so far, but they may be expected to increase.

Constraints on Inflation

It is noteworthy that a change of federal administrations has not reduced the concern in high circles to halt the rise in medical and hospital costs. Former HEW Secretary Wilbur Cohen, in his final official act, declined to authorize an elevation of the Medicare voluntary medical insurance monthly premium from $4 to

$4.40 per month, calling on the nation's private physicians instead to exercise restraint in their charges to patients.[20] HEW Secretary Robert Finch has eliminated from the Medicare reimbursement formula to hospitals the 2 percent supplementation which had been designed to cushion the institutional budget with a contingency fund against unanticipated expenses. The actions of both Democratic and Republican secretaries have obviously been designed to impose constraints on inflationary tendencies in the national health care system.

In a recent interview, Secretary Finch said:

> I feel that in many cases, medicine is too hospital-oriented, in the sense that there's often no place to put a hospital patient during his recovery, so he remains there three or four days longer than he otherwise would. We've got to make better use of extended care facilities. And we've got to make better use of people other than doctors—even other than paramedical personnel. We need to beef up homemaker services and home health-aide services, so that people can be cared for in their own homes under medical supervision but at greatly reduced cost.[21]

The pressures exerted by rising costs lead to certain types of corrective action, almost regardless of political ideology. A conservative federal Congress and competitive demands from other national and international policy issues will, of course, affect the rate of legislative attention to health problems. Yet the solutions that are likely to be proposed are ones which will probably call for more attention to the total organization of medical services in a community, for an integrated and rationalized use of the various component elements in the health care system.

Indeed, the pressure of rising medical care costs, along with rising public expectations, may do more to stimulate an improved organization of national health care patterns than anything else. The pressures for achieving accessibility to care for everyone, along with quality maintenance, have been exerted for a long time, but it is the spiraling of costs that, in the minds of many legislators, lends an air of crisis to the situation and summons urgent responses.

The Striving for Order

A striving for order is the central meaning of all the turbulence in America's health services today. Three sets of pressures can be identified in this striving—pressures for accessibility, for quality, and for economy in health services. Beyond these, there are deliberate and conscious efforts to coordinate the hundreds of component parts of the complicated health care system in the combined interests of accessibility, quality, and economy.

The federal Comprehensive Health Planning Amendments of 1966 were landmark legislation in integrating several previous categorical health grants to the states into two streamlined types of "block grants."[22] One of these is based on an automatic formula, dependent on state population, economic need, and other factors; the other supports special projects for various innovative health service programs that any state or local community may propose. In addition, these amendments to the basic Public Health Service Act provide grants to the states and to regions within states (area-wide agencies) for the specific purpose of comprehensive health planning.

The law and regulations assign broad responsibilities to the state and area-wide agencies responsible for comprehensive health planning. Aside from control over the allocation of federal public health formula grant funds, the state agencies—usually the state health department—are expected to encourage coordination of all public and private health services in the state; the area-wide agencies are expected to do the same within their geographic jurisdictions, with special emphasis on the physical planning of hospitals. A majority of the members of the planning councils and boards, set up with these funds, must represent recipients rather than providers of health services. Their scope of concern is defined as including health manpower, health facilities, and health services.

Because the planning umbrella is intended to cover both public and private health activities, the 1967 version of the federal law came to be called the "Partnership for Health Act." The title underscores the pluralistic character of the American health system, with its contributions of money and activities from many different social sources. In practice, however, it is too early to tell how effectively this partnership planning will work out. Up to the present, there is little evidence from the states or regions of any major achievements in integration or coordination of previously discordant services.

Perhaps rapid progress in this type of formal planning should not be expected at the outset. For a few years, one may expect the board members of the planning agencies simply to be learning about their tasks. As self-education proceeds, it is likely that responsible board members will begin to see the need for attaining order in the health care system, regardless of the individual's politics or philosophy. The striving for order implicit in this nationwide program is, of course, not merely for the gratification that some people may get from a tidy organization chart; the chart may never be very tidy. It is to attain the accessibility, the quality, and the economy of health services that so many forces in society are pressing for.

Planning Agencies as Sounding Boards

The comprehensive health planning agencies will perform another important function. They will serve as a sounding board, a court for hearing the voices of social criticism from every segment of the community. There is hardly a major city in this nation, or a major university campus, that has not resounded with such cries for social change in the last five years. The angry words and the physical violence of the poor are directed against the many inequities in society, including the demeaning aspects of charity medicine.

The large urban public hospital, with its crowded wards and congested clinics for the poor, has become a national object of derision. Evidence of technical competence in these hospitals—many of them affiliated with fine medical schools—does not satisfy the grievances of assaulted personal dignity. This is just one of the issues which must be faced soon by the comprehensive health planning agencies. Organized labor will also call, as it already has done in several states, for greatly improved health insurance benefits, as it learns that many problems in health care cannot be solved within the bailiwick of the labor-management contract. Organized farm groups will call for a better deal in health services out in the villages and rural areas.

The net effect of all these demands, and all the other social pressures mentioned in this article, will be to propel the U.S. further toward an orderly and effective national health system.[23] It will be a system in which accessibility to care is assured financially and geographically for everyone in the nation—probably through combined use of social insurance and general revenue mechanisms. It will assure quality maintenance through a variety of organized patterns both for hospital care and for ambulatory services. Teamwork and use of auxiliary health personnel will be maximized. It will use the people's money with greater frugality than now demanded, through continuous surveillance and a rational ordering of the work of all health personnel and facilities.

There will be no decline in the freedom of doctors or hospitals, despite apprehensions that have been voiced over the years. Some personal autonomy may have to be traded for brotherly cooperation, but the freedom of the human spirit—through better health and greater opportunities for service—should be steadily enhanced.

References

1. Leslie J. DeGroot, editor, *Medical Care: Social and Organizational Aspects,* Springfield, Ill., Charles C. Thomas, 1966.
2. Herman M. Somers and Anne R. Somers, *Medicare and the Hospitals,* Washington, Brookings Institution, 1967.
3. Walter P. Reuther, *The Health Care Crisis: Where Do We Go from Here?* Washington, Committee for National Health Insurance, 1968.
4. *Report of the National Advisory Commission on Health Manpower,* Vol. I, Washington, Government Printing Office, November, 1967.
5. Surgeon General's Committee, *Physicians for a Growing America.* Washington, Public Health Service Publication No. 709, 1959.
6. National Advisory Commission on Health Facilities, *A Report to the President,* Washington, Government Printing Office, December, 1968.
7. "Hospitals Must Plan," *AMA News,* Feb. 24, 1969.

8. Henry E. Sigerist, "The History of Medical Licensure" in Milton I. Roemer, ed., *Sigerist on the Sociology of Medicine,* New York, M D Publications, 1960, pp. 308–318.
9. Robert Q. Marston, "A Nation Starts a Program: Regional Medical Programs, 1965–66," *Journal of Medical Education,* January, 1967, pp. 17–27.
10. U.S. Public Health Service, *Promoting the Group Practice of Medicine,* Report of the National Conference on Group Practice, Oct. 19–21, 1967, Washington, Government Printing Office, 1967.
11. Based on data in: B. E. Balfe and M. E. McNamara, *Survey of Medical Groups in the United States, 1965,* Chicago, American Medical Association, 1968.
12. David Kasanov, "Antipoverty Medicine: Atlanta to Watts," *Medical Economics,* July 8, 1968, pp. 123–143.
13. C. Wesley Eisele, ed., *The Medical Staff in the Modern Hospital,* New York, McGraw-Hill Book Co., 1967.
14. Vergil N. Slee, "The Physician as an Evaluator of Care," *Group Practice,* September, 1968, pp. 42–45.
15. Secretary's Advisory Committee on Hospital Effectiveness, *Report,* Washington, U.S. Department of Health, Education and Welfare, 1968.
16. For example, *The Secretary's Regional Conference on Health Care Costs,* San Francisco, Department of Health, Education and Welfare, Jan. 15–16, 1969.
17. Milton I. Roemer, and Donald M. DuBois, "Medical Costs in Relation to the Organization of Ambulatory Care," *New England Journal of Medicine,* May 1, 1969, pp. 988–994.
18. Sam Shapiro, "End Result Measurements of Quality of Medical Care," *Milbank Memorial Fund Quarterly,* April, 1967, pp. 7–40.
19. U.S. Social Security Administration, *Incentive Reimbursement Experiments,* Washington, October, 1968.
20. "Cohen's Farewell," *Modern Medicine,* Feb. 24, 1969, p. 41.
21. "Secretary Finch Sizes Up the Health Program," *Hospital Physician,* March, 1969, pp. 184–190.
22. Douglas Cater, William R. Willard, Ellis D. Sox, and Paul G. Rogers, "Comprehensive Health Planning," *American Journal of Public Health,* June, 1968, pp. 1,022–1,038.
23. Milton I. Roemer, "The Voluntary Hospital in an Organized Society—Fears and Prospects," *Hospital Progress,* September, 1966, pp. 81–86.

36

From Health Insurance to Health Care Systems—An International View

All over the world, one finds that the collectivization of health care costs through social insurance programs has often been a prelude to numerous modifications of health care delivery systems. Once major economic responsibility must be borne by the total or a substantial portion of the national population, political pressures mount for assuring that the health services are delivered in more efficient ways.

In Canada, nationwide hospitalization insurance was enacted in 1957 (after initiatives in several provinces), followed by national-provincial insurance for physician's care in 1966. By the late 1960s and early 1970s, the pressures for more systematic delivery patterns were keenly felt. This world review of corresponding developments in Europe, Latin America, Asia, and elsewhere was invited for presentation at the April, 1973, Annual Meeting of the Canadian Public Health Association. The text that follows has not been previously published.

Current Problems in Health Care

In spite of the vast improvements over the last century in levels of health throughout the world—improvements due as much or perhaps more to higher general standards of living than to personal health services—almost all countries are beset with problems in the field of health care. Scientific technology has made enormous strides, but access to it, in relation to needs, is by no means equitable. Even in the large proportion of countries, including Canada, where economic support mechanisms have minimized or eliminated financial barriers, there are obstacles of geographically uneven resource distribution, inadequate transportation, personal attitudes, or administrative complexity that still impede the receipt of appropriate services.

Second, the costs of medical care have been rising rapidly, usually at a rate which exceeds the general pace of price inflation for all goods and services. This rise is due both to increasing rates of utilization of personal health services and to higher costs per unit of service—the latter associated with richer technical content (for example, more diagnostic procedures within one day of hospital care) as well as higher salaries or incomes for health personnel. Whether or not we can demonstrate that these higher expenditures also yield higher benefits in health status and years of life (and I think we can), the escalation of costs has been a cause for social and political concern almost everywhere.[1]

A third general problem in health care is the complex and poorly coordinated organizational structure in many countries. There are numerous sovereignties in different sectors of the health arena which guard their independence, resulting in administrative waste for the system and confusing fragmentation of service for the patient.

These problems of inequitable access, escalating costs, and organizational complexities—and there are other problems involving quality of care permeating these—have stimulated increasing concern in most countries for improving the organization of health services. We are not the first generation, of course, to sense this need. It is, in fact, the very improvements of the past—the dialectics of previous progress—that have made so prominently visible today the need for further changes that would achieve an effective *system* of health service provision.

A Bit of History

If you will permit some oversimplification, the historical development of health services can be summarized along four paths, each starting at different periods but eventually running parallel with the others.

The first path was the whole development of science and its transmission to a body of trained manpower—initially the doctors and apothecaries, then gradually additional categories of health worker. Medical and other types of higher education became increasingly formalized, professional societies took shape, laws on licensure were enacted, and a whole field of "the healing arts" emerged. The relationships between healer and patient were traditionally individualistic, involving—as feudalism evolved into capitalism—a market transaction for buying and selling a skilled service.[2]

A second path, starting somewhat later, was motivated by religious concepts of charity, and offered protection for the seriously sick in hostels or hospitals. The line between custodial care of the destitute poor and medical service was originally not sharp, but gradually institutions for the sick came to be recognized as places where advanced scientific skills could be mobilized through special personnel and equipment. Hospitals became also centers of professional education and, because they were seen to fulfill technical as well as charitable functions, they came to be increasingly financed by governmental revenues.[3]

A third path took origin from recognition somewhat later that disease could be prevented by certain social actions to constrain the movements of people and control the environment. Long before micro-organisms were recognized as causes of disease, the city fathers of Europe learned that isolation, quarantine, and sanitation could reduce the occurrence of fevers. With the rise and extension of the public health movement in the nineteenth century, the scope of social action for prevention gradually extended to include concern for the general health of children, mothers, and industrial workers, and then for the control of diseases that were admittedly not infectious or communicable.[4]

A fourth path, important for understanding current health service problems, was not in the bailiwick of medicine—either healing or preventing—at all, but in the economic sphere. As cities grew, as industrialization developed, a large working class formed, dependent on wages for survival; sickness meant both loss of earnings and financial burdens to purchase the help of doctors (outside of hospitals) or drugs. The solution devised was periodic pooling of small sums when a worker was well, so that funds would be at hand to meet his needs or those of his family when sickness struck. And so health insurance, first private or voluntary, then mandated by government, evolved. After the 1880s, the same principle came to be applied to the liabilities of old age, unemployment, complete invalidity, and even the family obligations of child-rearing (family allowances). Social insurance or social security for working people eventually became statutory in every industrialized, and many developing, agricultural countries.[5] For non-working indigent people, public assistance—financed from general revenues—often became another source for supporting the costs of sickness and other social risks.

Some Early Health Insurance Developments

The first health insurance programs, as noted, were frankly intended as a form of economic protection. By the mid-nineteenth century, the patterns of health service delivery, as we now call it, had already taken shape along the first three paths: individual doctors or other healers for the self-supporting sick, hospitals for the poor with serious disorders, and public health action for community prevention of disease. The objective of health insurance, first made compulsory in Germany in 1883, was to ease the access of the working man or his dependents to a private doctor or pharmacist, to guard him from the indignities of a hospital ward or the social stigma of a hospital out-patient department, and to compensate for his wage losses during disabling sickness. Later, when hospitals came to be recognized as effective places for the scientific treatment of the non-indigent, health insurance was applied to payment for hospital rooms with more amenities than characterized the large medieval-style ward.

In spite of this frankly economic objective, it was not long before the health insurance societies of Europe came to realize that wise expenditure of the worker's and employer's insurance monies required something more than simply paying medical bills. By the early twentieth century, when preventive modalities on an individual, as distinguished from a mass or environmental, basis came to be appreciated, the German insurance societies began to set up special clinics for the early detection of tuberculosis, to launch periodic health examinations of workers at factories, to send health visitors to the home for assistance with communicable disease care, and even to subsidize local public health clinics for venereal disease treatment or maternal and child health promotion purposes.[6] The French social security system, offering medical benefits in 1928, likewise subsidized tuberculosis and MCH control services, and supported a whole corps of "assistantes sociales" to help working class families cope with health and social problems.

While these preventive and social services did not involve a major share of insurance expenditures, they demonstrate the fact that the health insurance idea was recognized as an instrumentality for organized disease prevention at least a half-century ago. Insurance monies were also used to change conventional patterns for treating the sick. In some of the large European cities, special centers for physical rehabilitation of workers were set up. Sections of medical school polyclinics, previously intended only for the poor, were opened to insured families under special contract with the insurance funds. Put in another way, the embryonic signs of evolution of health insurance into health care systems began to be evident well before the concept of "health planning" had diffused to the West from its earlier origins in the Soviet Union of the 1920s.

Outside of Europe, in fact, the health insurance movement from the beginning was associated with major modifications of the one-to-one pattern of doctor's care. In Japan, where social insurance was adapted through German influence in 1922, the initial model was factory-based clinics for treatment of workers. In Chile, where governmental health insurance was first launched in the Western Hemisphere in 1924, the pattern for ambulatory care was through special polyclinics constructed by the social security authority and employing teams of salaried doctors. A special "Preventive Medicine Law," furthermore, was enacted in Chile in 1938 to mandate annual screening tests of all insured workers for tuberculosis, syphilis, and heart disease.[7] Later in Peru, in 1940, an impressive "Hospital Obrero" was built for insured workers—starting a movement for special social security hospitals that are now found in the majority of Latin American countries. When European Jews went to Israel and organized the "Kupat Holim" in 1911, their insurance monies, while nongovernmental, were used to develop a network of health centers, polyclinics, and hospitals, rather than simply to finance care through the existing private sector.[8]

Moreover, national health insurance systems, both in Europe and elsewhere, served sometimes as the prelude to the inauguration of massive changes in health care organization, which are usually described as "national health services." The metamorphosis in the USSR, the world's first socialist country, was, of course, brought about by its 1917 social revolution, but the first stages of Soviet socialized medicine were built upon the limited health insurance schemes covering industrial workers in the Russian cities, with a separate organizational structure being developed for peasants in the rural areas.[9] Other such relatively abrupt changes in health care organization occurred in the Eastern European countries, where after World War II Fascist occupation was succeeded by Socialist governments, but in these countries, too—Czechoslovakia, Hungary, Poland, Bulgaria, and Roumania—the fully socialized programs evolved from earlier social insurance mechanisms, extending their coverage to rural and other previously non-protected populations.[10] In Cuba, also, after its 1959 Revolution, the universal program started with an extension of the prerevolutionary "mutualistas," a non-governmental network of health insurance societies.[11]

More relevant perhaps for Canada and other capitalist democracies has been the development from limited health insurance programs into "national health services" without social revolutions. The course of events in Great Britain after World War II is well known. The original structure of the National Health Service in 1948 was a clear outgrowth of the administrative lines and the power centers evolving over the previous 50 years or more: 1. the Executive Councils for general practitioner and other ambulatory services coming from the National Health Insurance framework initiated in 1911; 2. the Regional Hospital Boards from the wartime emergency services; 3. the independent teaching hospitals from the long tradition of autonomous universities and medical schools; and 4. the local health authorities from the structure of British local government with its public health legislation arising in the early nineteenth century. While the functions of all four of these components of the NHS were modified, it is obvious that the past was prologue.[12] The same sort of evolutionary process characterized the Chilean National Health Service of 1952, building upon the health insurance scheme started 28 years before.[13]

Thus, while the health insurance movement started everywhere as a social process to ease the economic pressures on working people, it soon became concerned with more efficient and effective patterns for providing care, and in several countries served as the prelude to massive changes in health care delivery systems. This process, of course, is still going on, and we may get a better appreciation of its meaning if we examine briefly some of the main new developments in health service organization around the world today.

Current Movements toward Health Care Systems

It has been fashionable in the United States, with its highly complicated and pluralistic arrangements for both financing and delivery of health services, to say that we have a "non-system." This rhetoric gets across a certain idea, but it is not accurate. Every country has a health care system, but this system may demonstrate varying degrees of efficiency and effectiveness—that is, varying degrees of achievement of goals in relation to the input of resources. C. West Churchman has said that "Systems are made up of sets of components that work together for the overall objective of the whole."[14] The thought in this simple statement which, in my view, is most salient for health care systems is: "components that work together"—in other words, the operation of relationships between and among different providers of health service, so as to attain the goal of healthy populations in the most efficient (or the least wasteful) way.

The relationships that have emerged as the important current issues in health care systems can be classified in many ways. A helpful approach, in the light of the brief glimpse we have taken of historical developments, is to identify four sets of relationships evident in all countries: 1. between preventive and curative service, 2. among different classes of health personnel, 3. among different facilities in geographic regions, and 4. between actual performance of health service and ideal standards. It is, in my view, the smooth and complementary operation of these four sets of relationships that can well define the movement toward more effective and efficient health care systems in any country.

As we noted above, the earliest application of preventive concepts involved impersonal control of the environment or police power to constrain the movement of persons, but with increasing knowledge we have learned the feasibility of affirmative personal services to promote health as well. Thus, the impending reorganization of the British National Health Service in 1974 has among its several objectives the integration of personal preventive services, now under local authorities, and the curative ambulatory services, now under Executive Councils, beneath the broader umbrella of Area Health Boards. The executive officer of these boards will not be the old-fashioned Medical Officer of Health but a new breed of "Community Medicine Specialist," whose skills will include the planning and administration of curative as well as preventive services.[15]

In countries at all points on the political spectrum, health services are being organized to assure to families conveniently accessible primary care, encompassing both prevention and treatment under the same roof and by the same team of health personnel. This is the policy in the health centers of India, where family planning advice also figures prominently in the preventive armamentarium. Integration of this sort is the keynote of the polyclinics of modern Cuba, serving populations of about 30,000 each, no less than in the Neighborhood Health Centers built in the slum areas of many American cities by the U.S. Office of Economic Opportunity (OEO). Malaysia illustrates a former British colony where the rural population is served by a network of health centers offering both preventive and curative services, given in different rooms but at the same hours every day.[16] Health education on hygiene, nutrition, and other preventive concepts is an official duty of the Soviet family doctor for a few hours every week.

Teamwork relationships among several types of health personnel, the second component in modern health care systems, are likewise growing at an increasing tempo around the world. In the United States, the proportion of clinical physicians engaged in group practice clinics has now reached about 20 percent. The worldwide character of the group practice movement, in the private professional sector, was vividly shown at the First International Congress of Group Medicine, held in Winnipeg, Manitoba, in April, 1970.[17] In Great Britain, after a slow start, health centers, bringing together general practitioners and several types of paramedical personnel supported by local authorities, have begun to mushroom since 1965. Similar developments have been occurring in France, with the combined support of the social security program and local governments.[18]

The rising costs of medical care have led most countries to put new emphasis on the training of ancillary health personnel, who can perform many functions previously regarded as requiring the expensive time of physicians or dentists. The former colonies of European powers in Africa long used minimally trained "dressers" or sanitary officers to treat the local populations, but with national independence, the thoroughness of these training programs is being increased and the health teams which offer the services are being expanded. Venezuela, which long resisted entrusting therapy to anyone but a physician, is now reaching its rural people better with a corps of auxiliaries trained in "medicina simplificada." And the People's Republic of China has impressed the Western world with the massive progress achieved through brief training (about three months) of "barefoot doctors," as well as the integration of the work of Chinese traditional healers with that of modern Western-style physicians.[19]

All these developments involving allied health manpower necessitate the organization of health care delivery by teams, in which each member does his part. Division of labor, specialization, teamwork—these constitute basic dimensions of an efficient system of health care, as distinguished from a conglomerate of small unrelated and independent units.

The third type of relationship in a system involves the coordination of components in geographic regions. Typically we think of regionalization as applying to hospitals of different levels of technical capability, but it also applies to relationships between hospitals and ambulatory care facilities. Evidence of a heightened appreciation of the need for this type of coordination is also coming from many countries.

Sweden has recently developed greater rationalization of its whole health care system by dividing its 25 counties among 7 regions. In each health region of about 1,000,000 people is a network consisting of four echelons of facility: a central hospital serving the whole region for super-specialty services; several county hospitals serving 250,000–300,000 people for the main medical and surgical specialties; numerous district hospitals serving 60,000–90,000 people for maternity, accidents, and common conditions; and fourth, a network of local health centers serving 10,000–20,000 people for ambulatory primary care, curative and preventive.[20] In the new British reorganization, the Regional Hospital Boards governing the 14 regions of England and Wales will be converted to Advisory Regional Health Councils with wide health care concerns; they will serve as a second echelon above the approximately 90 Area Health Boards which will, in turn, exercise certain controls over district hospitals within their borders.

In the United States, the regionalization idea has not really developed much beyond the planning of hospital construction, subsidized by federal funds (Hill-Burton Law of 1946), except in a few demonstration areas. The RMP legislation (Regional Medical Programs for Heart Disease, Cancer, and Stroke) of 1965 attempted to promote stronger professional ties between peripheral and central hospitals in health regions, but the sovereignty of each hospital was usually too proud. While many new services (like coronary care units or stroke rehabilitation centers) were started in smaller hospitals, little was changed in the way of inter-hospital relationships, and now under a conservative national government the entire RMP program is to be eliminated. On the other hand, about half the 50 states have now passed so-called certificate of need legislation, under which new hospital beds may be added—whether or not they are governmentally subsidized—only if they are demonstrably needed as part of a reasonable state plan for hospital development.[21]

In the socialist countries, regionalized networks of hospitals and health centers have been the standard strategy for years. The hospital of the USSR is usually regarded as not only the technical center for treatment of serious illness, but also as the administrative center for the surrounding ambulatory services in polyclinics or health centers, and also for the preventive services emanating from sanitary-epidemiological stations.[22] A goal espoused in these as well as free enterprise countries, but only sporadically achieved, is the establishment at the same site as the general hospital of facilities for the mentally ill and also for long-term care of the chronic sick.

The Latin American countries, since the 1940s, have been characterized by two major subsystems (sometimes three or four) of hospital care—the network of institutions under the Ministries of Health, including both hospitals and ambulatory service centers, and a parallel network under separate social security authorities. In the last decade, however, a strong movement has been mounting for coordination of these subsystems on a regional basis, in the interests of economy and efficiency. Aside from Chile, where such coordination was achieved through the "Servicio Nacional de Salud" in 1952, progress toward this end has been notable in Costa Rica, Venezuela, Brazil, and Ecuador.[23]

In New Zealand, where national health insurance has protected the entire population for most medical service needs since 1939, the hospital and specialist services have been administratively quite separate from the general practitioner services. An important sign of coordination, however, is reflected in the legislation of 1971 authorizing the statutory Hospital Boards to build and operate health centers for ambulatory care. Equally encouraging is the positive attitude of many New Zealand G.P.s toward transferring their practices to such centers, where the first steps would be taken in the way of strengthening their ties with hospitals.[24] The election of a new Labor Government in Australia in late 1972 may imply similar developments.

Finally, in the sphere of system relationships between the actual and the ideal, one sees the developments in all countries toward strengthening controls over the quality and costs of medical service. In the "direct systems" of health insurance or health care, found typically in most of the developing and all the socialist countries, such controls are built into the day-to-day hierarchical operations. The tasks of quality control are more difficult in the "indirect systems" of health insurance found in Western Europe and North America, as well as in Japan. The significant point, however, is the mounting movement toward more rigorous quality and cost controls in the latter type of country.[25]

In the administration of the health insurance programs in Germany or Belgium, statistical procedures have long been used to identify doctors or other providers whose patterns of service (as reflected by fee claims) deviate markedly from the norms. With greater computer capabilities, such controls have been getting more sophisticated at lower relative administrative costs. Such surveillance, even after the fact as it is, doubtless exercises a disciplinary influence on the future performance of doctors. In Japan, steeply rising costs in the two major statutory health insurance programs, and a staunchly laissez-faire attitude up to the present, have led to recent demands for much greater controls in that very rapidly industrializing nation of over 100,000,000 people.

The new slogan for this quality control movement in the United States has become promotion of "peer review." The escalating costs (compounded by the Medicare legislation for the aged and Medicaid for the poor), the mounting rate of malpractice suits, the rising voice of consumerism have all contributed to louder demands for social controls over the open market of medical care delivery. Fiscal intermediaries under both Medicare and Medicaid have applied various forms of automated monitoring on utilization and medical care prices, but with limited effectiveness. "Medical care foundations," organized by county medical societies, have expanded under a strategy of rigorous claims review. A major step toward increasing social controls was the inclusion in the 1972 Amendments (H.R.1) to Medicare and Medicaid of provision for PSROs (Professional Standard Review Organizations) to blanket every local area in the nation. These bodies would develop various techniques for overseeing the necessity and quality of all services for which government must pay fees on behalf of its beneficiaries; while initially limited to hospital-based services, the intent is clearly to extend the principle to all ambulatory services as well.[26]

These four sets of the relationships, discernable in so many countries, are all contributing to a worldwide movement toward more highly organized systems of health care. Increasing integration of preventive and curative service, greater personnel teamwork, more regionalized coordination of facilities, and heightened social controls over quality and costs—these trends are all pressing the many schemes of health care financing, especially through insurance, toward higher levels of concern about the content of services for which the people's money is being spent.

Some Significant U.S. Developments

In the United States, beyond the points already mentioned, there are certain other developments that might be of special interest. Most significant is the definite movement toward some type of national health insurance to cover all or nearly all of the population for most of the costs of medical care. Hardly five years after enactment of social insurance for hospital and medical services to the aged (persons past 65 years), the issue of extending the same concept to the rest of the population became so prominent that no less than 12 bills—from all points on the political spectrum—were introduced into the Congress in its 92nd session (1970–72). It is no surprise that liberal Democrats, led by Senator Edward Kennedy and backed up by the organized labor movement, should put forward such legislation. The notable fact, however, is that the American Medical Association and the commercial insurance industry—long foes of any governmental action in the health insurance field—should feel compelled to promote legislation of this sort. While modeled somewhat on the Australian concept of retaining a central role for existing voluntary insurance plans, these latter bills would subsidize membership of low income families in such plans, call for wider health benefits than are now typically offered, and require that the plans meet certain governmental standards.[27]

Even more notable is the introduction in Congress by a conservative federal administration of a bill which would mandate payment of the greater part (65 percent, then 75 percent) of insurance premiums by all employers for enrollment of their employees in governmentally approved health insurance plans, along with subsidy of the enrollment costs of low income persons not employed. There are numerous limitations in all these bills, by way of deductibles, cost-sharing, and so on, and the latest version of President Nixon's proposal has not yet been submitted to the 93rd Congress. Nevertheless, there seems little doubt that the United States is on the eve of some legislative action which will at least resemble Canada's statutory program for social underwriting of most medical care costs.

A second significant development on the United States medical scene is the support by both major political parties of a concept of medical care delivery previously considered avant garde, if not radical, but now dignified with White House backing and a snappy new phrase: the "health maintenance organization." HMOs are what we used to call cooperative health plans, or sometimes prepaid group practice plans, through which members would be assured a relatively comprehensive scope of medical and hospital services for one fixed annual premium. The doctors and others would usually be paid on a salary basis, but they could be paid by fees for each unit of service, as long as they assumed some risk which might entail fee reductions if the volume of services was very high. On the other hand, if there were savings due to the frugal use of expensive services, like hospitalization or certain diagnostic procedures, the doctors and others would enjoy greater earnings.[28]

Several bills have been introduced in the Congress to subsidize and promote the establishment of HMOs, beyond the small number that already exist, in the hope of using this strategy to gradually modify the traditional open-market, fee-for-service pattern of medical care delivery across the nation. The hope would be to create incentives for maximizing preventive and low-cost ambulatory services, rather than the curative and high-cost hospital services which have been so heavily fostered by previous U.S. health insurance patterns. Even before any of these bills has been enacted, however, the U.S. Department of Health, Education and Welfare in early 1971 established an administrative unit that began to subsidize the founding of new HMOs around the country—about 110 of them so far—under certain broadly defined legal authorities (Public Health Service Act, Section 314-e) that already existed.[29] Moreover, in the 1972 Medicare Amendments previously mentioned, authorization for enrollment of these aged beneficiaries in HMOs was, for the first time, specified. The future course of HMO development in the United States—even if legislation is soon enacted, which is likely—depends on many political and social forces, but one must conclude that the very promulgation of the idea is a sign that health insurance alone is recognized as an insufficient solution to the health care problem. Along with it, steps are needed to change the delivery patterns as well, everyone seems to agree.

A third current development of special significance in the United States is not so much in the legislative sphere as in the general social setting of health care delivery. I am thinking of the numerous eddies and currents through which the ambulatory services, both curative and preventive, are becoming increasingly organized. Some of this has, indeed, resulted from specific laws, like the approximately 100 "neighborhood health centers" for the poor built by the U.S. Office of Economic Opportunity, or the comprehensive M.I.C. (maternity and infant care) and the C. and Y. (children and youth) clinics launched by special funds from the Department of HEW. Most of the increasing provision of ambulatory services under organized mechanisms, however, has come through existing private resources. The rapid extension of group medical practice has already been mentioned. A great expansion of the services of hospital out-patient departments, both for scheduled clinic sessions and for emergency care, is another important trend. One study estimates that in 1970 some 18 percent of patient-doctor encounters in the United States occurred in hospital OPDs.[30] Still another trend is the broadening role of Health Department clinics in many localities, widening from their traditional focus on prevention to general ambulatory care. Health services in the schools and work-places are also continuing to develop, and a whole panoply of special clinic programs for mental problems (including drug abuse and alcoholism), for cancer detection, for crippling conditions, and for selected populations like migrant families or alienated youth are being established under both governmental and voluntary auspices.

All these organized patterns of ambulatory health care are, in aggregate, contributing to a general modification of the traditional model of private medical service in the United States. Even without the leverage of a national health insurance scheme, such as exists in Canada, a variety of social forces is pushing health care in the United States toward more sysematic arrangements.

From "Insurance" to "System"

In concluding this survey of developments in health insurance and other sectors of the health service field around the world, there would seem to be a few generalizations that are warranted.

1. Under all political ideologies, health care seems to be acquiring the status of a *civil right,* which governments feel impelled increasingly to guarantee through various mechanisms of social financial support.
2. With extension of nationwide health insurance as a major one of these mechanisms in the more industrialized countries, there is a natural tendency for *utilization of services and prices per unit to rise,* resulting in an enlarging proportion of GNP (gross national product) becoming devoted to health costs.
3. Rising costs, as well as the inherent human values of preventing serious illness, are leading most countries to seek methods of *maximizing prevention and ambulatory care* and of reducing the high expenditure for hospital care, which has had priority in the past and still absorbs the largest fraction of health expenditures.
4. This growing emphasis points increasingly to the organization of primary health services (curative and preventive) in various forms of *health center,* where teams of personnel work together, in contrast to the traditional model of the independent individual healer.
5. To cope with the problems of geography and large populations, nations are being divided into *health regions,* in which facilities are organized at various levels, in proportion to the technical capabilities required to cope with different types of disorder.
6. In recognition of democratic principles, a *balance* is evolving in each country—shaped by its particular political ideology—*between centralized and localized authority;* in general certain minimum standards of health resources and services are formulated at the central or national level, while their application and adjustment are delegated to local authorities with much input from consumers.
7. Because of the complexities of health service financing and delivery, and the inevitable competition between health attainment and other social goals, *national planning* is increasingly appreciated as necessary. The very process of planning creates pressures in government for progressive development of rational health care systems.

These seven conclusions would seem to apply to Canada and the United States as much as to other countries. While day-to-day problems can be discouraging, the long view would seem to give us cause for optimism that we are all moving toward health care systems that will more effectively serve human needs.

References

1. Joseph G. Simanis, "Medical Care Expenditures in Seven Countries," *Social Security Bulletin* (Washington), March 1973, pp. 39–42.
2. Milton I. Roemer, (Editor), *Henry E. Sigerist on the Sociology of Medicine,* New York: MD Publications, 1960, pp. 65–74.
3. Courtney Dainton, *The Story of England's Hospitals,* Springfield, Illinois: Charles C. Thomas, 1961.
4. George Rosen, *A History of Public Health,* New York: MD Publications, 1958.
5. Eveline M. Burns, *Social Security and Public Policy,* New York: McGraw-Hill Book Co., 1956.
6. Franz Goldmann and Alfred Grotjahn, *Benefits of the German Sickness Insurance System from the Point of View of Social Hygiene,* Geneva: International Labour Office, 1928.
7. Milton I. Roemer, *Medical Care in Latin America,* Washington: Pan American Union, 1963.
8. Th. Grushka (Editor), *Health Services in Israel,* Jerusalem: Ministry of Health, 1968, pp. 233–250.
9. H. E. Sigerist, *Medicine and Health in the Soviet Union,* New York: The Citadel Press, 1947.
10. E. R. Weinerman, *Social Medicine in Eastern Europe,* Cambridge, Mass.: Harvard University Press, 1969.
11. Vicente Navarro, "Health, Health Services, and Health Planning in Cuba," *International Journal of Health Services,* 2:397–432, August 1972.
12. Almont Lindsey, *Socialized Medicine in England and Wales: The National Health Service 1948–1961,* Chapel Hill, North Carolina: University of North Carolina Press, 1962.
13. Benjamin Viel, *La Medicina Socializada y Su Aplicacion en Gran Bretana, Union Sovietica, y Chile,* Santiago: Universidad de Chile, 1964.
14. C. West Churchman, *The Systems Approach,* New York: Dell Publishing Co., 1968, p. 11.
15. George A. Silver, "The Community-Medicine Specialist—Britain Mandates Health Service Reorganization," *New England Journal of Medicine,* 287:1299–1301, 21 December 1972.
16. Milton I. Roemer and Olive Manning, *Assignment Report on Strengthening of Health Services and Training of Health Personnel (Malaysia),* Manila: World Health Organization, February 1969.
17. *New Horizons in Health Care* (Proceedings, First International Congress of Group Medicine), Winnipeg: Wallingford Press, 1970.
18. Milton I. Roemer, *Evaluation of Community Health Centres,* Geneva: World Health Organization, 1972, pp. 17–19.
19. V. W. Sidel, "Some Observations on Health Services in the People's Republic of China," *International Journal of Health Services,* 2:385–395, August 1972.
20. Anne R. Somers, "The Rationalization of Health Services: A Universal Priority," *Inquiry,* 8:48–60, March 1971.
21. American Hospital Association, *Survey Report: Review of 1971 Certificate-of-Need Legislation,* Chicago, 1972.
22. World Health Organization, *Health Services in the USSR* (Report of a Study Tour Organized by WHO), Geneva: WHO, Public Health Paper No. 3, 1960.
23. Milton I. Roemer, "The Development of Medical Services under Social Security in Latin America," *International Labour Review* (Geneva), 1973.
24. J. S. Dodge (Editor), *The Organisation and Evaluation of Medical Care,* Dunedin, New Zealand: University of Otago, Dept. of Preventive & Social Medicine, 1970.
25. Milton I. Roemer, *The Organization of Medical Care under Social Security,* Geneva: International Labour Office, 1969.
26. Robert M. Ball, "Social Security Amendments of 1972: Summary and Legislative History," *Social Security Bulletin,* Vol. 36, No. 3, March 1973, pp. 3–25.
27. I.S. Falk, "National Health Insurance: A Review of Policies and Proposals," *Law & Contemporary Problems,* 35:669–696, Autumn 1970.
28. Paul M. Ellwood, "Health Maintenance Organizations: Concept and Strategy, *Hospitals,* Vol. 45, No. 6, 16 March 1971, pp. 53–56.

29. Gordon K. MacLeod and Jeffrey A. Prussin, "The Continuing Evolution of Health Maintenance Organizations," *New England Journal of Medicine,* 288: 439–443, 1 March 1973.
30. Nora Piore, Deborah Lewis, and Jeannie Seeliger, *A Statistical Profile of Hospital Outpatient Services in the United States: Present Scope and Potential Role,* New York: Assoc. for Aid of Crippled Children, 1971.

37

A National Health Service and Social Security

With the election of a more liberal federal administration in 1976, the prospects of enactment at last of a national health insurance program in the United States grew brighter. But some who had long advocated such legislation had become disillusioned with the idea because of the serious inadequacies exposed by enactment of Medicare for the Aged in 1965 within the framework of the existing system of private fee-for-service medicine. The spiraling costs and sometimes fraudulent practices led some to advocate abandonment of the social insurance idea entirely and immediate enactment of a "national health service," supported entirely by general revenue with all personnel and facilities controlled directly by government.

To expect such legislation in present-day America was not only politically unrealistic, but flew in the face of worldwide experience on the path to a national health service (NHS) in capitalist parliamentary democracies. In collaboration with S. J. Axelrod, I summarized the lessons of this global experience and the hazards of the "NHS now" position in the essay reproduced below.

WITH THE NEW federal administration, there is widespread belief that at long last some type of National Health Insurance legislation will be enacted in the near future. The scope of that legislation is bound to depend on the strength and unity of public demand. It is unfortunate, therefore, that at this critical hour voices should be raised rejecting National Health Insurance and calling for general revenue financing of a National Health Service. This is regrettable in the light of both worldwide and American experience on the issue.

Improved organization of health service delivery for everyone, through teams of salaried personnel in a regionalized network of public facilities, is clearly desirable. Worldwide trends are moving in that direction, and this pattern is a reasonable goal for the United States as well. To expect such a goal to be attained in current-day America, however, through "progressive taxes on personal wealth, taxes on corporate profits and general revenues"—in the words of the newly launched Committee for a National Health Service—is to flirt with a dangerous illusion.

To understand how a universal and effective system of comprehensive health service can be achieved in a free-market economy, such as characterizes the United States, requires analysis of the issue into its major components. One com-

Chapter 37 originally appeared in the *American Journal of Public Health,* 67:462–465, May, 1977, and is reprinted by permission of that journal.

ponent is the method of financing health services, and the other is the method of delivery of those services. Each of these components shows a clear evolutionary development in the capitalist world, and each has distinct political implications.

World-wide Experience

If we examine the relationships between the statutory patterns for 1. financing and 2. delivery of health care, that have developed around the world, we find at least four principal combinations. These may be schematized as follows:

Financing	Delivery	
	Individual	Organized
Insurance	(1)	(2)
Revenues	(3)	(4)

Only combination (4) corresponds to the National Health Service, as perceived by its advocates.

The realities are further complicated by the fact that in many nations—such as Sweden, Great Britain, or Chile—there are combinations of both forms of financing within one health care system. Moreover, there are often different patterns of delivery for hospital and ambulatory services in the same system. Thus in Great Britain's National Health Service, hospital care is delivered through organized arrangements, while ambulatory care is still predominantly on an individualistic basis. In Germany, most in-hospital medical care, though not all, is provided by organized staffs of salaried doctors, with ambulatory care by private doctors paid by fees, and this mixed pattern prevails in many European countries.

If we focus, for the sake of clarity, on general physician services for ambulatory care, we find that the above combinations may be illustrated in practice as follows:

Pattern	*Country*	*U.S. Program*
(1)	France	Medicare
(2)	Israel	Kaiser Health Plan
(3)	Great Britain	Medicaid
(4)	U.S.S.R.	Indian Health Service

The only countries in the world that have so far developed for their total population a predominantly organized pattern for delivery of ambulatory health services, combined with general revenue financing, are the socialist nations. In all countries, military personnel are served by such systems. Otherwise, the United States has applied this type of system only to certain economically depressed populations, such as American Indians or impoverished city dwellers served by "neighborhood health centers." Even veterans, who are entitled to certain inpatient services in highly organized hospitals, get much of the ambulatory care (to which they are statutorily entitled) through the "hometown program," using private doctors.

The above relationships are not accidental. In all the non-socialist or capitalist countries the use of general revenues, as the *initial* basis of financing a health care program, has only been applied to limited categorical populations, for whom the allocations may be reduced at any time. (We emphasize "initial" because the dynamics change after two or three decades of experience—see below.) In industrialized capitalist countries everywhere, the initial strategy for *broad* population coverage has been social insurance or social security financing. About 70 nations throughout the world, both industrialized and developing, have applied this strategy (although in developing countries, population coverage of social insurance is typically restricted to industrial workers).

The reasons for this worldwide strategy are clear. It has been largely because of the serious political hazards of the general revenue approach—its great vulnerability to major reductions in funding—that the social security approach has been so widely applied. This strategy has been supported not only by conservative parties, which launched it in 19th century Europe, but also by most left-wing political parties over the last 50 years. The rationale boils down to political realism and economic stability.

In free market parliamentary democracies, enactment of a new system of personal health service for all or even most of a national population, through general revenue financing, has simply not been politically feasible. Such financing has been acceptable for the poor (or for the mentally ill) not only because of their marginal status, but also *because* the funds could be frugally allotted and reduced at will—as, indeed, they usually are. The social insurance mechanism, on the other hand, has everywhere been contrasted to charity and "handouts"; everyone "pays his own way" and earns entitlement to benefits (medical or pensions or other) as a right. This concept has been politically acceptable to nearly all parties in capitalist nations. The United States in the 1970s is no exception.

Even more important is the second reason—stability. Because of the separate status of social security funds, outside the general national treasury, they have everywhere acquired an immunity from political or ministerial inroads. This has applied to the Trust Funds of the U.S. Social Security System, no less than to similar social insurance funds in nations throughout the world. As a result, the benefits payable from these funds have been remarkably assured over the years.

United States Experience

For those skeptical of the relevance of this reasoning to the United States, compare the experience of our Medicare and Medicaid programs over just their first 12 years. In both programs, of course, there has been waste and abuse associated with the private fee-for-service pattern of delivery and remuneration. Nevertheless, the Medicare program, based on social security, has had enlargement of its scope. The population covered has been expanded from the aged to include the permanently disabled and persons with severe kidney disease. As a result of both the 1967 and the 1972 amendments, benefits have also been somewhat expanded. When a conservative President (Gerald Ford) proposed a reduction in benefits to Medicare beneficiaries, the idea was ignored by Congress.

By contrast, the Medicaid program—financed from federal and state general revenues—has suffered repeated cutbacks. The provisions of the original Act, which required broadening the scope of care under the state plans and liberalizing eligibility, were first postponed and then eliminated. Entitlement to coverage for the medically indigent was restricted. Although the federal government has increased the list of mandated services, many states—under the pressures of financial stringency—have imposed various limits on mandated services and have reduced or eliminated optional ones.

The political likelihood of a universal health care system being enacted under general revenue support is extremely remote in America today. But even if, by some political twist, a program with modest coverage or benefits—e.g., a national service for children or for general hospital care—were legislated under general revenue support, one could soon expect the type of scuttling familiar under Medicaid. Regardless of the patterns of delivery, costs would inevitably rise and the voices of conservatism would call for "economies." By legislation or regulation, benefits and coverage would be reduced to save government funds. The introduction of a means test would soon follow. "Why should the taxpayer's money be used," we would hear "for those who can well afford to pay for their medical care?" If a salaried, organized system of delivery were embodied in the program, private practice would still remain. As in Chile, an increasing proportion of people, dissatisfied with a pinchpenny and congested public system, would resort to the private market. The more that demands increased in the private sector, the more the public sector would be deprived of resources. As the vicious cycle continued, the public system would become increasingly concentrated on the poor who could not afford private care.

Evolution of Social Security

This sequence has *not* occurred in countries that *initiated* their national programs of health service through the social security approach—even when they *later* shifted to general revenue support. Thus, in Great Britin, National Health Insurance for manual workers was started in 1911. Benefits were limited to general practitioner service and drugs, since most hospital and specialist care for this social class were available in public or charitable institutions at little or no charge. It took 37 years of experience with this program—and a World War against

Fascism—to pave the way in 1948 for the British National Health Service, supported predominantly by general revenues. Even so, 15–20 percent of NHS support is still derived from social insurance contributions, and general practitioners remain in private practice (paid about one-half by capitation and one-half by fees).

In New Zealand, National Health Insurance covering everyone for comprehensive benefits started in 1939. After 31 years, in 1970, financing was shifted to general revenues, but general practitioners, as in Great Britain, remain in private practice and are paid on a fee-for-service basis. Norway's voluntary health insurance, enacted in 1911, had reached coverage of about 70 percent of the population in 1956, when it was made mandatory to achieve universal coverage. After 16 years, in 1972, support was shifted to general revenues.

These and other national evolutions suggest strongly that, after many years of social insurance experience, the concept of health care as a right becomes so firmly established that no political party would think of eliminating or even reducing it. At this point, the support can be and often is shifted to general revenues without danger to the program.

It is worth recalling also that even in the Soviet Union, the world's first socialist nation, the concept of stability in the social security mechanism—protection of the funds from use for other purposes—was initially recognized. Although a system of organized health care delivery, through government-employed physicians working in public facilities, was established soon after the Revolution of 1917, the financing of services for city dwellers was through an earmarked social security fund. Not until 1937—20 years later—was the urban health care system combined with the rural and the financing shifted to the general government budget.

Within health care systems financed by social insurance, moreover, it is faulty to regard individualistic patterns of delivery and remuneration as inevitable. Combination (2) defined earlier is illustrated not only by Israel, but also by most Latin American countries and about 20 others. It is true that for out-of-hospital ambulatory care in Western European countries (also in Canada, Australia, New Zealand, and Japan), private delivery initially prevailed. In fact, health insurance has even fortified private practice in the early years. But in time, pressures for more organized and economical delivery patterns soon increase. Thus, even in individualistic France, hundreds of health centers with teams of personnel have been organized through stimulation of the social security system. In Great Britain, the majority of previously solo private general practitioners are now in small groups, and about 20 percent are in governmental health centers with teams of allied health workers. Canada, the Scandinavian countries, New Zealand, and Australia are all establishing health centers for ambulatory care within the framework of their health insurance systems.

In the developing countries, the introduction of social insurance for medical care has nearly always been through highly organized networks of health centers and hospitals, staffed entirely by salaried doctors and allied personnel. This is the pattern, as noted, in Israel, Latin America, and many other countries. In fact, taking a world view, about half the nations using social security financing have an organized delivery pattern, with salaried personnel working in public facilities owned and controlled by the health insurance system.

This combination of organized delivery with insurance financing in the less developed nations has resulted from the obvious need for economy in these countries. Yet, as noted above, the same pressures for economy and efficiency are also leading to increasingly organized service patterns in the more affluent industrialized countries.

Implications for U.S. Policy

In the light of this worldwide experience, as well as the lessons of public medical care programs in the United States, the wisdom of *initiating* a national health care system in America under the social security mechanism should be clear. When the system achieves political stability and is out of danger from financial cutbacks, it can and should be shifted to general revenue financing. Before that time, patterns of organized delivery can and should be promoted within the social security framework.

Considering the legislative measures actually before the U.S. Congress, the whole issue of posing general revenue financing versus social insurance financing is vastly oversimplified. The major proposal backed by organized labor and many other groups is the Kennedy-Corman Health Security Bill (H.R. 21 and S.3), which does, in fact, call for financing 50 percent from general revenues, the balance coming 35 percent from employers and 15 percent from employees. It is all-important, however, that the basic level of the health care funding is to be set by the social insurance contributions, since this amount is to be equally matched (hence 50 percent) by money from general revenues. European experience has shown this strategy to yield fiscal stability that simply does not occur with general revenue financing alone.

As for the so-called regressive nature of social insurance fund-raising, compared with general revenues (derived from progressive income taxes), this has been a price that labor and socialist parties throughout the world have been more than willing to pay for the substantial advantages reviewed above. Moreover, as social security leaders have long pointed out, the "regressive taxation" argument is, at best, a half-truth. For one thing, the contribution rates are the same regardless of family size; thus (unlike private insurance) large families—usually of lower income—pay less per member. Second, up to a ceiling (which in the U.S. will soon be $16,500 per year), contribution rates (shared by employers and workers) are proportional to earnings, and the regressive impact applies mainly to the minority of people earning more than this ceiling.

Third and most important, the "regressive" argument focuses only on the payment side and ignores the benefits of social security. The benefit structure in the United States (and most other countries) is slanted heavily in favor of low-income persons; thus contributors of low "premiums" receive relatively greater benefits than they have paid for, while higher contributors receive relatively lesser benefits. This is especially true of health care benefits, which are identical for all persons—under the Kennedy bill, as in the systems of other countries—regardless of the rate of contributions by each individual.

Thus, the attainment of a "National Health Service" in the United States requires far greater analysis of the political dynamics in a free market society than appears to have been made by the new advocates of this idea. Such analysis indicates that the path to a fully organized, comprehensive health service, covering everyone and financed by general revenues, is *through* the enactment first of a politically feasible National Health Insurance program. The Kennedy-Corman Health Security Bill needs all the support it can get. This bill, furthermore, offers many ways to improve health care delivery patterns. (To assume, as some do, that a more radical proposal helps the Kennedy-Corman Bill, by showing it to be "moderate," is dangerous; just as likely is the opposite boomerang effect, in which Health Security becomes cast as the insidious entry to fully "socialized medicine.")

It would be regrettable if the advocacy of an immediate National Health Service, aside from its naiveté, should lend strength to the many conservative forces opposing social security financing of health care for other reasons. History has too many stories of progress obstructed by divisiveness among the proponents of social change. One may hope that, with the prospect of National Health Insurance in America now brighter than in many years, all progressive groups will join in promoting it.

38

An Ideal Health Care System for America

In spite of the strategy argued in the previous chapter, based essentially on worldwide experience, it is helpful to envisage the outlines of an ideal health care system toward which America might move. With an understanding of a sound ultimate goal, better decisions can be made on intermediate steps that may be politically necessary and feasible along the way.

A crucial intermediate step in the present-day U.S. political and social climate is probably enactment of a program of universal insurance for health services, comprehensive in scope and preventive in emphasis. But this should be regarded as a step toward attaining a rational system in which all people are served by teams of salaried health workers employed in regionalized networks of ambulatory care and hospital facilities; quality should be protected by supervision built into the daily work, and representatives of the people should participate in policy formation and administration. The ultimate outlines of such an ideal health care system, published in a 1971 article, form the chapter that follows.

THE STRATEGY OF compromise and adjustment to political realities has so long influenced the design of American health legislation that seldom has anyone considered what an ideal health system might look like. Yet it has become fashionable to recognize that there is a "crisis" in our health services (the White House said so in July, 1969) and that the "system" is in need of basic overhauling.

The Private Medical Market

What is it that is basically wrong with the health service system in the United States? What would an ideal and really sound system look like? Aside from high and rising prices, inaccessibility of medical care for the poor and long waits for doctor and dentist appointments for everyone—all of which are symptoms rather than causes—there is little said in answer to the first of these questions. To the second question, one rarely sees any answer at all.

As to the first question, we can be brief. The basic fault in American health

Chapter 38 originally appeared as "Nationalized Medicine for America." Published by permission of Transaction, Inc. from *TRANSACTION,* vol. 8, no. 11, copyright © 1971 by Transaction, Inc. The chapter was republished under its present title in *Where Medicine Fails,* ed. A. L. Strauss (New Brunswick, N.J.: Trans-Action Books, 1973), pp. 77–93.

service is the discrepancy between our assertion of health care as a basic human right and our practice of treating it as a marketplace commodity. Even when we have taken steps to improve medical care for the poor, as under Medicaid, or for the self-supporting, as under voluntary health insurance plans, we have used a systematized flow of money simply to purchase the services of physicians or hospitals in the open market. We have not organized the provision or "delivery" of health services in the way that other services deemed essential to society have been organized, such as education or protection against fire.

So long as medical care remains a matter of private buying and selling—whether it be from a doctor, a dentist, a pharmacist, a podiatrist, a hospital, or a nursing home—it will be subject to all the profit-seeking vicissitudes of the commercial market. This will be true even if the hospital is "nonprofit," because, even without stockholders, it still must make the financial ends meet. And it will be true in spite of the noblest constraints of medical ethics, which may inhibit open fraud but hardly can influence subconscious monetary incentives.

Over the last 40 years or so there has been a steady increase in the demand for medical care in the United States. This has been due not only to the increasing potentialities of medical science but also to the rising knowledge and expectations of people, and the enhanced purchasing power furnished by expanded health insurance. This elevated demand for medical care has been met, of course, by increases in the supply of health care resources—personnel, facilities, and equipment—but, as in many commercial markets, at a rate slower than the rate of rising demand. The lag has been caused partly by 30 years of professional obstruction to increasing the output of doctors under the banner of "protecting quality," and partly by the especially high cost of producing medical resources—training doctors, building hospitals, and so forth. Because of these educational and capital costs, social funding (mostly state and federal tax revenues) has been called upon, but it has not been forthcoming at a rate commensurate with the needs.

And so we are faced with a mounting shortage of doctors and other health personnel. To cope with it, many ideas formerly rejected are now being implemented. Osteopaths, of decidedly meager educational background, are turned into M.D.s by law (California), and they are now counted in the national statistics as physicians. Graduates of foreign medical schools—partly foreign nationals and partly Americans denied admission to United States schools—are now welcomed here (about 25 percent of new medical licentiates each year!). Medical care is more and more shifted to the hospital, where large numbers of auxiliary personnel are regularly on hand, conserving the time of the doctor. And diverse new types of health personnel are being trained not merely to help the doctor but to replace him for certain tasks—the physician's assistant, the pediatric associate, the Medex, the nurse practitioner, and others.

At the same time, to cope with the medical "crisis," many limited and modest steps are being taken to "change the system." In a variety of forms, these involve the modification of individualistic medical practice toward more organized forms. Group practice of doctors—three or more banding together in a team—is steadily increasing, now engaging the time of about 15 percent of physicians. (While most of this remains private and entrepreneurial, it sets the stage for more socially oriented patterns.) More and more ambulatory care is being sought from hospital outpatient departments or emergency rooms, requiring hospital medical staffs to organize services to meet the demand. In these and other roles, physicians are entering full-time hospital employment in increasing numbers and rates. Neighborhood health centers, offering generalized ambulatory care rather than purely preventive service, are increasing, not only under the auspices of the United States Office of Economic Opportunity (OEO) but under a diversity of local agencies. Medical schools are organizing comprehensive prepaid health care plans based on medical teams, not only for teaching but for demonstration of sound patterns for the future. Even the Nixon administration is calling for the creation of "health maintenance organizations" like the Kaiser Health Plan.

These innovations—and many more (youth clinics, maternity and infant care centers, migrant family clinics, and the like)—are all straws in the wind. They depend, however, on private spending, voluntary health insurance, or special grants from government and sometimes on philanthropy. Significant as they are, their impact is spotty, and the vast majority of people are not reached. The 63 neighborhood health centers launched by the OEO, for example, altogether reach hardly 1.5 million people in the urban ghettos, while about 30 million Americans are estimated conservatively (15 percent of 200 million) to fall below the poverty line.

The "plight of the patient," as *Time* magazine put it, has many more facets than this. There are the grim and crowded conditions in large urban public hospitals serving the poor—beds in the corridors and packed benches in the clinics. There are the bleak realities in the office of the harassed practitioner in Appalachia. There is the squalor of most state mental hospitals. There is the multibillion dollar wastage each year on worthless (if not harmful) patent medicines, on naturopathic food faddism, on chiropractors and phony curative appliances. But most of all there are the daily inefficiencies of private medical and dental practice, with the design of what *Fortune* magazine calls a "pushcart industry." There are the inducements to unnecessary surgery, made all the more lucrative by much of the undisciplined voluntary health insurance coverage. There are the "shot doctors" who give every indigent patient an injection, because for this the welfare agency pays an extra fee.

What can be done about all this? At least five major bills have been introduced in the United States Congress to tackle the medical care cost problem, and some of them to go much further. The weakest of them— the "Medicredit" offering of the American Medical Association—would subsidize, from federal monies, voluntary membership of poor people in existing private health insurance plans. Other proposals call for mandatory enrollment in existing plans. The Nixon administration, following the nineteenth century German strategy of requiring employer and worker contributions to these plans, would cover about 90 percent of the population, but substantial deductibles and co-payments by the patient would obviously limit accessibility of low income people to needed care.

The strongest of the proposals—the "Health Security" bill proposed by the late Walter Reuther's Committee of One Hundred and introduced by Senator Edward Kennedy and others—would provide many incentives to modify the system. It would encourage group practice, health maintenance organizations, rural location of doctors, continuing professional education, systematic hospital planning, controls on drug prescribing, increased output of needed health resources and much more. It is clearly the best national health reform legislation ever introduced, using financial support as leverage to modify the health care system. It would certainly move us forward, and it deserves the strongest possible support. Yet the Kennedy bill would still depend on the effectiveness of various incentives, and we cannot be sure how well they would work. The mainstream of private, entrepreneurial medicine would probably remain predominant for many years. Moreover, much would depend on the ideology and spirit of the government in power, and its delegates at regional, state, and local levels

The Shape of an Ideal System

If an ideal and reasonable system of health care were to be achieved—to answer the second question posed at the outset—what, then, would it look like? Its design need not be so mysterious nor unknowable as some imply.

First of all, in every neighborhood, close to the homes of people, would be a health center staffed by a team of primary health personnel. The doctor would be a generalist—perhaps one of the new "specialists in family practice"—or else an internist, working in association with nurses, social workers, and clerks. On the team would also be "medical assistants" or "assistant physicians" who would be trained and authorized to handle simple cases on their own—the common cold, the minor injury, the mild gastroenteritis, or the follow-up visit after a previous medical service. These medical assistants would be supervised by the physician, and, of course, any case not recovering promptly would be referred to the doctor. They would not represent second-class medicine, because they would be properly trained for their duties and would have more time than the doctor to give sympathetic attention to each patient.

At this primary health center all the usual personal preventive services would also be provided. Babies and expectant mothers would get their checkups, immunizations would be given, dietary counseling and health education on various subjects would be offered. Screening tests would also be offered for detection of chronic disease, so that laboratory and X-ray technicians and appropriate equipment would have to be on hand. The basic health and medical record of each patient would be kept here, transferred to another health center if he should move, and temporarily lent to a hospital or other facility where he may be referred for care.

Depending on the distribution of the population, each such health center would be intended to serve about 10,000 people. In a sparsely settled rural area, it might be fewer, and in a very densely settled city it might be more. There would be one primary physician, along with the other allied health personnel, for about 2,000 persons; assuming this, a complement of five doctors per 10,000 might be divided between four generalists and a pediatrician. In addition, each health center should have a dental staff—dentists plus dental auxiliaries who, like the New Zealand "dental nurse," would do reparative work as well as prophylaxes on children. An optometrist would also be on the team for visual refractions. Drugs would be dispensed from the pharmacy within the health center.

Each person served by this health center would be attached to a particular doctor and his team of colleagues. Such attachment should ideally be on a geographic district basis, but this should not be rigid. If someone did not like the primary doctor covering his district, he should be free to change to another one in the same health center or, indeed, to a doctor in another center that was not too far away. Limits would have to be placed on the number of patients a popular doctor could attract, for the protection of quality; up to a certain level, however (perhaps 2,200 persons), the primary doctor should get additional rewards as an inducement to win the confidence of patients. Services of the neighborhood health center should be available 24 hours a day, but no individual doctor should ordinarily have to serve more than an eight-hour day, with the other hours covered on a rotation scheme.

For each four or five such health centers—that is, for population clusters of 40,000 to 50,000—there should be a district hospital. Assuming about three beds per 1,000 for the relatively common conditions handled at this hospital, it would have 120 to 150 beds. This facility would accommodate maternity cases, trauma, abdominal surgery of lesser complexity (appendicitis, hernial repair, gallbladder work), certain psychoneuroses, most cardiovascular cases, severe respiratory infections, and the like. It would be staffed by a team of specialists in surgery, internal medicine, orthopedics, obstetrics and gynecology, pediatrics, and psychiatry. Normal obstetrical deliveries would be done in the hospital by well-trained midwives—as they are now done in Great Britain with the results better than in America. Anesthesia would also, for the most part, be given by trained nurse-anesthetists working under the supervision of an anesthesiologist. The staff of hospital doctors would be essentially full-time, except for periodic visits they would make as consultants to the affiliated health centers. They would provide ambulatory specialist care through an active outpatient department, to which patients would be referred by doctors at the primary health centers. Except for obvious emergencies, all admissions to the hospital would be made through the outpatient department.

The 120 to 150 beds in the hospital would be organized into "progressively" staged sections for intensive, intermediate, and long-term care. The intensive care unit would have all the necessary emergency and monitoring equipment for the severe accident victim, for the postoperative patient, the acute coronary occlusion case, and so forth. The highest proportion of beds would be in the intermediate care unit—postoperative surgical patients and most medical patients being diagnosed and treated. The long-term unit would care for patients requiring skilled medical observation and nursing care, but in a chronic or convalescent stage of their illness. In this unit, plenty of provision should be made for diversion and self-help, and an active department of physical and occupational therapy should be attached to it. Patients should not remain here, however, for more than about 30 days, after which they would be transferred to another long-term care institution (extended care facility), if not to their own homes.

In the district hospital, probably near the long-term unit, there should also be provision for some mental patients. If they are not ready for discharge within about 30 days, they would be transferred to a mental hospital. Both the mental hospital and the long-term care institution referred to above would be affiliated with the district hospital administratively and professionally. Thus, the psychiatrist on the district hospital's medical staff would have an appointment on the mental hospital staff, as would the other physicians on the staff of the long-term care institution.

The next echelon of hospital care would be a regional hospital serving populations of about 500,000—in other words, the service areas of about ten district hospitals. Offering about 1.0 bed per 1,000 people, this larger hospital would have about 500 beds and would be devoted to the care of patients with more complex medical or surgical problems. Here is where the chest surgery (heart or lungs) would be done, the more complicated abdominal surgery, the kidney dialyses, the complex diagnostic workups. Here also would be an active program of medical research, along with training programs for nurses, technicians, and various other types of health personnel. Physicians and others from both the district hospitals and neighborhood health centers would come here also for periodic refresher courses on new developments in medical science.

At the highest echelon, serving the population under three to five regional hospitals (that is, from 1½ million to 2½ million people), should be a university medical center. Since this institution would provide the clinical experience for training medical students and certain other health professionals, it must not be limited to acceptance of only the most complex cases, like the regional hospitals. Assuming roughly 0.5 beds per 1,000 (that is, 750 to 1,500 beds), part of these beds would be devoted to simple cases (of the district hospital type), part to complex cases (of the regional hospital type), and part to special diagnostic categories on which the medical school staff was doing research. The latter type of patient might be referred from outside the territory served by each medical center, through intercenter agreements. For certain rare types of cancer, for example, on which critical research might be undertaken, the population required to yield enough patients for good clinical investigation might number 10 million to 20 million.

As described above, this "regionalization" network of health centers and hospitals is, of course, oversimplified; a perfectly accurate description would have to be much more elaborate. In the immediate surroundings of each medical center and regional hospital, for example—as well as in the service area of the district hospitals—there would have to be neighborhood health centers, so that each person would have convenient access to a primary doctor. Every hospital, from smallest to largest, would have to provide an outpatient department, not only to furnish specialist consultations but also to cope with emergencies at any hour of the day or night. Moreover, sections for long-term care and psychatric therapy—as well as the conventional medical, surgical, pediatric, and obstetrical departments—would be found in all levels of hospital.

As for care in the patient's home, this would be provided principally by the staff of the local health centers. Physicians would go when necessary—usually for acute emergencies—but most initial or follow-up home visits would be done by broadly trained nurses or medical assistants attached to the health center. If a patient discharged from the hospital must have continuing medically supervised care, this should be provided by the health center staff (aided by any special instructions or advice from the hospital staff) or occasionally by a "home care" staff dispatched directly from the hospital.

This entire network of services, it may be noted, is based on the locations of people's homes in cities, towns, or rural areas, but certain health services in an ideal system would have to be provided at places where people are occupied outside their homes. To be convenient for adults and children, therefore, health stations would also be provided at factories or other work places and at schools. These would be for first aid in emergencies, simple follow-up care, health education, immunizations, case-detection screening tests, and for other measures that can be more efficiently given where people are congregated. For any significant or continuing medical care, the child or adult would be referred to his local health center.

Economic Support and Administration

How would all this be paid for? Ideally health care should be a public service like schools or roads, paid for from general tax revenues. It is only because of our reluctance to accept this basic concept that we resort to all sorts of other collective devices which still signify individual responsibility, like voluntary health insurance or even social security. These are obviously reasonable methods to collectivize costs, up to a point, but their limitations in achieving comprehensive health care have been all too obvious. Conceivably, because of its political and psychological attractiveness, part of the costs of an ideal health service might be met by a social insurance tax (as is done for about 15 percent of the costs of the British National Health Service), but the great bulk should come from general revenues. These might be divided in some equitable way between federal and state governments. The tax burden should be adjusted according to individual or corporate ability to pay, and the health services offered should bear no relation to the origin of the funds.

For any services rendered within the social program described, there would be no charges made at time of sickness. It is often argued that the patient should bear at least a share of the cost of health services to deter him from unnecessary demands or "abuse." Without going into all the arguments and empirical data about "cost sharing" or "coinsurance" or "deterrent fees" or "deductibles"—whatever term is used—it should simply be realized that the vast majority of medical expenses are determined by the doctor, not the patient, and there is no evidence that cost sharing selectively discourages the unnecessary and not the needed services. This is quite aside from the unequal weight of cost sharing on persons of different wealth, and its administrative awkwardness. Basically, no financial barrier should inhibit the patient from seeking medical care; if he makes demands that are medically and psychosomatically unreasonable, it is up to the doctor to deny the service.

With monies raised from general revenues and no private cost sharing, the fee-for-service method of medical remuneration, with all its incentives to waste, would have no place. Just as nurses, technicians, pathologists, or professors are now paid by salaries, so would be all physicians, dentists, and everyone else in the health service system. Salaries, of course, should vary, according to qualifications, skills, and responsibilities, but each person would be paid for the proper value of his time.

Without the direct financial incentive to hard work of the fee system, how would the quality of medical care be assured, including sympathetic personal concern for the patient? The answer is: the way it is assured in any organization—by a framework of authority and responsibility, backed up by continuous education. Surveillance and reasonable professional controls would also be provided, with rewards and penalties as necessary. It must be realized that in any health care system there can be and should be incentives to excellence in the form of both honor and material rewards.

Another continuous safeguard of medical quality, especially along its personal dimension, should be advisory boards of citizens, made up of both consumers and providers of service, at all echelons of the system. These boards would exercise continuous influence on the appointments of personnel and the operations of the whole health care program. Minority groups should obviously be represented on these boards, but the militant slogan of "consumer control"—generated by today's inequities and professional chauvinism—would be replaced by a reasonable mix of consumer-professional collaboration in policy decisions within an ideal system.

Which brings us to the final topic of this account: the mode of administration of the entire system. Our spectrum of health services in America has conventionally been described as "pluralistic." More accurate would be to describe it as an irrational jungle in which countless vested interests compete for both the private and the public dollar, causing not only distorted allocations of health resources in relation to human needs but all sorts of waste and inefficiency along the way.

To administer the ideal program of health services there would be a single official health agency in each local area. This area is not so easy to define, but it would ideally be synonymous with the catchment area of a regional hospital—about 500,000 population. Subunits within this basic administrative area would operate at the level of a district hospital—that is, for about 50,000 population. Indeed, the health official serving as director for each of these hospitals might properly serve as the overall health director for the corresponding area. Thus, he would not be a "hospital administrator" in the conventional sense, but a "public health director" in the broadest social sense. Under this official would be administrative personnel for managing the hospital, but the functions of the health officer would be much wider. It would be his duty, backed up by the citizen boards mentioned above, to see that the whole health service operates effectively. He would be responsible for quality surveillance and for detection and correction of any deficiencies. He would be constantly alert to the opportunities for health prevention and health promotion, including the whole task of environmental health protection (which this article has not discussed). He would be responsible for coordination of the several parts of the system, through proper use of records, statistics and information exchange. He would observe trends and take steps to plan for the future.

Naturally, the "regional health director" should not be an absolute power but would be responsible to a health official above him. In the American political context, this would be a state health officer, whose responsibilities and duties would be, of course, much broader than they are now. State health officers, aided by a democratically constituted state board of health, would be responsible to a national official. With so large a responsibility, this person should be a member of the president's cabinet—the equivalent to the minister of health found in most countries.

Simplicity from Complexity

All this will strike some people as insufferably bureaucratic or naively utopian, depending on one's ideology. It also might seem hopelessly complicated. In fact, it would be a much simpler health care system than we have now, with its thousands (yes, thousands) of separate agencies for financing or providing different sectors or subsectors of health care. Bureaucratic? Yes. To meet health needs effectively in a complex society of 200 million people demands an organized framework. We take this for granted in much simpler matters, such as operating a post office or a school system. It is all the more necessary if the myriad tasks of assuring good health service are to be carried out. The trend, indeed, over the last 50 or 75 years has been toward increasing health care organization in order to apply the advancing science to increasingly perceived needs. The ideal system described here is essentially only an extension of the direction in which we have been moving.

As for the charge of "utopian," this is a question of timing. The system described could obviously not be achieved in the United States overnight. Even sweeping national legislation could not establish it. Quite aside from the tradition of private entrepreneurial medical practice, with all its inertia and resistance, there is manifestly a nationwide establishment of hospitals and health agencies that would require enormous readjustments to approach the ideal system. This would take great managerial skill and infinitely diplomatic human relationships. It would also require a great deal of money for new construction and new training. And it would take time.

Perhaps the health care system described could not be achieved short of a social revolution? One might be justified in holding this view if it were not for the historical lessons demonstrated in the achievement of a public school system, a sharply graduated income tax, and an extensive social security program in all the industrialized capitalistic countries of the world. Each of these vast social developments came in the face of substantial opposition. Each involved invasion of previously sacred rights of private property. Each was part of the program of revolutionary socialistic parties before accomplishment.

Regardless of how utopian or unrealistic the ideal health care program may appear, it has importance as a social goal. Only by having a clear goal ahead can one make sound decisions today—decisions along the scores of separate paths on which the health services are becoming organized. By formulating such an ideal system we can recognize that all the legislative measures now being considered in the national Congress—even the most advanced of them—are compromises, middle-of-the-road proposals adjusted to the political realities. The Kennedy "Health Security" Bill would undoubtedly be a great step forward, but we need not succumb to the charge that it is a radical proposal. At best, it would provide better economic support and long overdue incentives to move us a little more rapidly toward a reasonable health care system. It needs support precisely because it would help us to reach an ideal system. The challenge is to see the goal clearly, so that we can decide wisely what specific actions—at local, state, and national levels and in all health sectors—would retard and what ones would accelerate our attainment of a really sound health service for America.